ETHICS & ISSUES
IN CONTEMPORARY NURSING

Second Canadian Edition

Margaret A. Burkhardt

PhD, RN, CS, FNP

Alvita K. Nathaniel

MSN, RN, CS, FNP

Nancy Walton

RN, PhD (Collaborative Program in Bioethics);
Associate Professor, Daphne Cockwell School of Nursing,
Faculty of Community Services;
Chair, Research Ethics Board,
Ryerson University

NELSON / EDUCATION

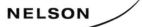

NELSON / EDUCATION

Ethics and Issues in Contemporary Nursing, Second Canadian Edition
by Margaret A. Burkhardt, Alvita K. Nathaniel, and Nancy Walton

Vice President, Editorial Higher Education:
Anne Williams

Publisher:
Paul Fam

Executive Editor:
Jackie Wood

Marketing Manager:
Alexis Hood

Developmental Editor:
Courtney Thorne

Photo Researcher:
Christine Elliott/2Birds Media

Permissions Coordinator:
Christine Elliott/2Birds Media

Production Service:
Cenveo Publisher Services

Copy Editor:
Susan James

Proofreader:
Lina Suresh

Indexer:
BIM Indexing Services

Manufacturing Manager:
Joanne McNeil

Design Director:
Ken Phipps

Managing Designer:
Franca Amore

Interior Design:
Carianne Sherriff

Cover Design:
Cathy Mayer

Cover Image:
James Osmond/Alamy

Compositor:
Cenveo Publisher Services

Printer:
RR Donnelley

Library and Archives Canada Cataloguing in Publication Data

Burkhardt, Margaret A.
Ethics and issues in contemporary nursing / Margaret A. Burkhardt, Alvita K. Nathaniel, Nancy A. Walton. -- 2nd Canadian ed.

Includes bibliographical references and index.
ISBN 978-0-17-650459-5

1. Nursing ethics--Textbooks.
I. Nathaniel, Alvita K. II. Walton, Nancy A., 1967- III. Title.

RT85.B872 2013   174.2
C2012-906922-1

ISBN-13: 978-0-17-650459-5
ISBN-10: 0-17-650459-1

Notice to the Reader

Publisher does not warrant or guarantee any of the products described herein or perform any independent analysis in connection with any of the product information contained herein. Publisher does not assume, and expressly disclaims, any obligation to obtain and include information other than that provided by the manufacturer.

The reader is expressly warned to consider and adopt all safety precautions that might be indicated by the activities herein and to avoid all potential hazards. By following the instructions contained herein, the reader willingly assumes all risks in connection with such instructions.

The publisher makes no representation or warranties of any kind, including but not limited to, the warranties of fitness for particular purpose of merchantability, nor are any such representations implied with respect to the material set forth herein, and the publisher takes no responsibility with respect to such material. The publisher shall not be liable for any special, consequential, or exemplary damages resulting, in whole or part, from the readers' use of, or reliance upon, this material.

CONTENTS

Preface   xii
Acknowledgments   xvii
Contributors   xviii

PART I   **Guides for Principled Behaviour   1**

Chapter 1   **Social, Philosophical, and Other Historical Forces**
                  Influencing the Development of Nursing   2
                  Objectives   2
                  Introduction   3
                  The Influence of Social Need   5
                  Gender and Spiritual Influences   6
                      Gender Influences   6
                      Spiritual/Religious Influences   7
                  Ancient Times   8
                  The Middle Ages   8
                  The Renaissance and the Reformation   11
                  The Modern Era   13
                  Summary   16
                  Chapter Highlights   17
                  Discussion Questions and Activities   17
                  References   18

Chapter 2   **Ethical Theory   20**
                  Objectives   20
                  Introduction   21
                      Ethics and Nursing   24
                  Philosophy   25
                  Morals/Ethics   26
                      Philosophical Basis for Ethical Theory   27
                  Theories of Ethics   28
                      Utilitarianism   30
                      Deontology   34
                      Virtue Ethics   37
                      Feminist and Relational Ethics   41
                  Summary   45
                  Chapter Highlights   45
                  Discussion Questions and Activities   46
                  References   46

Chapter 3   **Ethical Principles   48**
Objectives   48
Introduction   49
   Respect for Persons   49
Respect for Autonomy   49
Beneficence   59
Non-maleficence   62
Veracity   64
Confidentiality   69
   Limits of Confidentiality   73
Fidelity   75
Justice   76
Principles of the *Canada Health Act*   78
Summary   79
Chapter Highlights   79
Discussion Questions and Activities   80
References   82

PART II   **Developing Principled Behaviour   85**

Chapter 4   **Values Clarification   86**
Objectives   86
Introduction   87
What Are Values?   87
   Moral Values   88
Acquiring Values   88
Self-Awareness   90
Values in Professional Situations   94
   Impact of Institutional Values   96
   Clarifying Values with Patients   99
Summary   102
Chapter Highlights   102
Discussion Questions and Activities   103
References   104

Chapter 5   **Values Development   106**
Objectives   106
Introduction   107
Transcultural Considerations in Values Development   107
Theoretical Perspectives on Values Development   109
   Piaget's Stages of Cognitive Development   109
   Kohlberg's Theory of Moral Development   110

Gilligan's Study of the Psychological Development of
Women 111
Thomas's Levels of Moral Response 113
Some Nursing Considerations 115
Summary 118
Chapter Highlights 118
Discussion Questions and Activities 118
References 119

Chapter 6 **Ethical Decision Making 121**
Objectives 121
Introduction 122
Moral/Ethical Problems 122
Moral Uncertainty 122
Moral/Ethical Dilemmas 123
Moral Distress 124
Making Decisions 128
Nursing and Ethical Decision Making 128
Scientific Process and Ethical Decision Making 130
Ethical Decision Making 130
Emotions and Ethical Decisions 130
Process of Ethical Decision Making 132
Applying the Decision-Making Process 138
Summary 141
Chapter Highlights 141
Discussion Questions and Activities 141
References 142

PART III **Principled Behaviour in the Professional Domain 145**

Chapter 7 **Legal Issues 146**
Objectives 146
Introduction 147
Relationship Between Ethics and the Law 147
General Legal Concepts 149
Sources of Law 150
How Laws Are Made in Canada 151
Branches of Law 154
Negligence 156
Privacy and Confidentiality 160
Consent 164
Documentation 173

Technology and Documentation   174
Privacy and Confidentiality   175
Accountability in Practice   178
Summary   179
Chapter Highlights   179
Discussion Questions and Activities   180
References   180

Chapter 8   **Professional Issues   183**
Objectives   183
Introduction   184
Professional Status   184
   Nurses as Professionals   188
Expertise   189
Autonomy   189
Accountability   194
Authority   199
Unity   200
Summary   203
Chapter Highlights   204
Discussion Questions and Activities   204
References   205

Chapter 9   **Professional Relationship Issues   208**
Objectives   208
Introduction   209
Moral Integrity and Relationships   210
Problem Solving in Situations of Conflict   210
Nurses' Relationships with Institutions   216
Nurses' Relationships with Other Nurses   221
Challenges in Nurses' Relationships with Other Nurses: Workplace
   Incivility   222
   Workplace Harassment   224
Nurses' Relationships with Other Health Care Professionals   226
Working as Part of a Team   229
Moving Forward   230
Summary   231
Chapter Highlights   231
Discussion Questions and Activities   231
References   232

Chapter 10   **Practice Issues Related to End-of-Life Care   234**
Objectives   234
Introduction   235
The Use of Technology at the End of Life   235
Quality of Life   237
Medical Futility   245
Decision Making at the End of Life   255
Nursing Practice in the Midst of Technology   260
Summary   262
Chapter Highlights   262
Discussion Questions and Activities   263
References   264
Further Suggested Readings and Resources   267

Chapter 11   **Practice Issues Related to Patient Self-Determination   269**
Objectives   269
Introduction   270
Autonomy and Paternalism   270
    How Far Does Autonomy Go?   272
Informed Consent   273
    Ethical and Legal Elements of Informed Consent   274
    Nursing Role and Responsibilities: Informed Consent   277
Advance Directives   278
    Decision-Making Capacity   279
    Nursing Role and Responsibilities: Advance Care
    Planning   281
Choices Concerning Life and Health   285
Choices Regarding Recommended Treatment   286
    Complementary and Alternative Medicine (CAM)   290
    Controversial Choices   291
    Confidentiality   296
Summary   298
Chapter Highlights   299
Discussion Questions and Activities   300
References   301

Chapter 12   **Scholarship Issues   303**
Objectives   303
Introduction   304
Academic Honesty   304

Research Issues and Ethics   307
   Ethical Issues in Research   308
   Special Considerations: Vulnerable Populations   317
   More than Protection of Human Rights   317
Ethical Treatment of Data   319
Summary   321
Chapter Highlights   321
Discussion Questions and Activities   321
References   322

Chapter 13   **The Future of Canadian Health Care: Challenges and Priorities   324**
Objectives   324
Introduction   325
Federal and Provincial Responsibilities in Health Care Delivery   326
   Historical Influences on Our Modern Health Care System   328
Challenges in Our Current Health Care System: Perspectives   335
   Accessibility of Health Care   337
   Medically Necessary: Who Decides?   338
Health Care Systems and Sustainability: Global Concerns   338
Summary   341
Chapter Highlights   341
Discussion Questions and Activities   342
References   342

PART IV   **Nursing in Today's World: Challenges and Opportunities   345**

Chapter 14   **Health Policy Issues   346**
Objectives   346
Introduction   347
Politics   347
Health Policy   348
Nursing, Policy, and Politics   356
Lobbying   359
   Methods of Lobbying   360
   Preparing for Political Action of Any Kind   361
   Political Campaigns   363
Summary   364
Chapter Highlights   364
Discussion Questions and Activities   364
References   365
Websites   366

Chapter 15 **Economic Issues   367**
Objectives   367
Introduction   368
Overview of Today's Health Care Economics   368
Distributive Justice   371
    Entitlement   373
    Fair Distribution   377
    Distribution of Resources   378
    Theories of Justice   378
Recent Trends and Health Economic Issues   380
    The 1990s   381
    Today   381
Summary   387
Chapter Highlights   387
Discussion Questions and Activities   388
References   388

Chapter 16 **Social Issues   390**
Objectives   390
Introduction   391
Social Issues   391
    Poverty   392
    Homelessness   394
    Intimate-Partner Violence   397
    Increasing Elder Population   400
    Racism   402
Ethical Principles Applied to Social Issues   403
Personal Impediments to Intervening with Vulnerable Groups   405
    Victim Blaming   405
    Language of Violence   406
Social Issues and Scholarship   407
Summary   408
Chapter Highlights   408
Discussion Questions and Activities   408
References   409
Websites   412

Chapter 17 **Issues of Gender and Culture   414**
Objectives   414
Introduction   415
Historical Perspectives and Overview of Gender-Based Issues   415
    Societal Expectations   416
Gender Discrimination in Nursing   417

Expanding Numbers of Men in the Profession   418
Gender and Caring   418
Sexual Harassment in Nursing   420
Communication Issues Related to Gender   422
"The Doctor–Nurse Game"   422
Communicating with Patients   423
Modern Sexism   424
Sexual Orientation   425
Transcultural Issues   426
Summary   437
Chapter Highlights   438
Discussion Questions and Activities   439
References   440

Chapter 18   **Rural and Aboriginal Nursing in Canada   444**
Objectives   444
Introduction   445
Rural Nursing   445
Canada's Rural Environments   445
Rural Health   447
The Challenges of Rural Nursing   448
Professionalism in Rural Nursing   449
Boundaries, Obligations, and Confidentiality   450
Working with Constraints   452
Scope of Practice   453
Aboriginal Health in Canada   454
Factors Affecting the Health of Aboriginal Persons   456
Aboriginal Nursing   458
Recommendations for the Future of Rural and Aboriginal
Nursing   460
Summary   461
Chapter Highlights   462
Discussion Questions and Activities   464
References   464

Chapter 19   **Empowerment for Nurses   467**
Objectives   467
Introduction   468
Personal Empowerment   471
Professional Empowerment   474
Empowerment for Evolving Professional Nurses   477
Nurses and Patient Empowerment   478

Enhancing Patient Capacity for Decision Making   479
    Fostering Patient Empowerment   480
Barriers to Empowerment   482
Summary   483
Chapter Highlights   484
Discussion Questions and Activities   485
References   485

**APPENDIX A   The Canadian Nurses Association Code of Ethics
for Registered Nurses   488**

APPENDIX B   The ICN Code of Ethics for Nurses   506

Glossary   513
Index   525

PREFACE

Nurses and nursing students today face complex challenges in a wide array of modern practice settings. From the bedside to policy arenas, nurses work in environments where they face not only difficult clinical challenges but also thorny ethical questions. In grappling with these kinds of complex problems, we are cognizant of the fact that there is no single correct approach or solution that can be applied to each ethical problem in an attempt to find a one-size-fits-all solution. Instead, nurses must be sensitive to a myriad of possibilities and responses unique to each situation and person. We also must be aware of our own personal values and beliefs, and how these shape our responses to professional practice dilemmas. Our moral responses depend upon highly contextual factors, the relationships we have with others, and our own moral development and integrity, along with our past experiences. As professional nurses, we cannot simply set aside our own values and beliefs when we put on our uniform, enter a residence to provide home care, or step into our role as managers, administrators, or educators. Rather, we must be attuned to our own reactions, judgments, and priorities, and be aware of how these reactions are shaped by the ever-changing world around us.

In *Ethics and Issues in Contemporary Nursing*, Second Canadian Edition, it is our intention to acknowledge the role of the professional nurse as a moral agent and an advocate. As part of an ethically responsible profession, we also acknowledge that the role of the moral agent and advocate can be fraught with complications and worries, barriers and stumbling blocks. Developing skills as an effective and sensitive moral agent is an iterative process; one that requires patience, constant self-reflection, and an openness to new and diverse perspectives.

Dealing with ethical issues requires that we develop skills in reflecting upon and clarifying our values. As part of this process, we also develop skills in ethical decision making, the empowerment of self and others, cultural competence, and challenging social injustice. To help develop these skills, the text poses stimulating questions about contemporary issues and provides clear processes to resolve ethical problems with sensitivity and skill. Acknowledging and highlighting the fact that nurses work in a variety of settings and roles, the exercises and activities are designed to reflect real-life challenges, facilitate self-reflection, and encourage a stronger awareness of a number of different approaches to decision making. Our goal is for you to become engaged in active learning throughout the text through the use of *Case Presentations* based on everyday situations and *Ask Yourself* and *Think About It* exercises derived from the case presentations and other thought-provoking material.

With a strong groundwork of ethical theories and principles as presented in Part I, subsequent chapters deal with various issues relevant to ethics and ethical decision making. As you explore political, professional, legal, social, and gender issues, we encourage you to engage in the discussions by considering a problem in a variety of ways, moving back and forth between considering the more concrete actions and solutions to the more abstract exploration of principles, and from the perspective of a specific case to a more general, or even global perspective. Complex ethical problems can rarely be resolved by only considering one viewpoint, perspective, theory, or possibility. Rather, problems can begin to be resolved by recognizing the interrelatedness and importance of a diversity of factors, perspectives, rationales, and viewpoints. A key element of engaging in ethical problem solving is to recognize and acknowledge conflicting perspectives — especially those that are markedly different from your own. *Part I, Guides for Principled Behaviour,* presents ethical theories, models, and principles that can serve as guides for ethical action.

In *Part II, Developing Principled Behaviour,* we discuss in more depth the relationship between the personal and the professional, and explore values clarification, moral development, and ethical decision making. *Part III, Principled Behaviour in the Professional Domain*, presents an overview of professional and legal aspects of contemporary nursing. This section includes discussions about autonomy, accountability and integrity, scholarship issues, Codes of Ethics, and the use of technology. In *Part IV, Nursing in Today's World: Challenges and Opportunities*, we address health care challenges and changes that are imperative to consider in the contemporary health care system in which nurses practice. Considerations related to political, economic, social, gender, and transcultural issues are discussed in the context of nursing roles and professional practice. We address nursing in a variety of settings in this section and, in keeping with the goal of describing nursing and health care issues across many contexts, have added a new chapter to this edition on rural and Aboriginal nursing. To end the final section of the text, we focus on the nurse as an empowered advocate, and ethical leader, who can act with both sensitivity and courage to challenge social injustices across many different settings and contexts.

From a uniquely Canadian perspective, the text offers content and cases that reflect the diversity of nursing practice and patient populations from across our country, from both rural and urban settings, as well as a range of practice environments, from the bedside to the administrative office to the classroom. Landmark Canadian legal and ethical cases have been included, as well as important literature from Canadian ethicists and nurse scholars. As before, we continue to include even more real-life cases that reflect modern Canadian health care issues and challenges, as well as the realities of nursing across Canada.

For our second Canadian edition, we have revised the text in a number of truly exciting ways, in response to the changing landscape of nursing and thoughtful reviews from outstanding scholars, educators, and colleagues with expertise in the content areas. The entire text has been updated, reflecting the newest revisions of the *Canadian Nurses Association Code of Ethics for Registered Nurses*, which has been better integrated throughout the text and in discussions and cases. The newest revision of the *Tri-Council Policy Statement for the Ethical Conduct of Research* (2010) has been emphasized in the discussions of research ethics, accountability, and scholarship. We have added significant additional content on end-of-life care in Chapter 10, with emphasis on the nursing roles when providing care to dying patients and their families. In Chapter 6, we have added another decision-making model to provide a wider variety of perspectives on how to approach difficult ethical problems. More emphasis has been placed on interdisciplinary practice and relational ethics. Additionally, we have also tried to reflect the kinds of unique questions and challenges that today's nurse will face; e.g., what are some best practices related to the use of social media? What kinds of challenges do nursing students and new graduates face in today's health care settings? How can we face the challenges of increased use of technology as we provide nursing care?

In our discussions of nursing as a regulated profession in Canada, we have not only addressed the roles of the provincial regulatory bodies, but also have stressed the diversity of nursing practice across our country. This brings us to our most exciting and distinctive addition to the textbook: *Chapter 18, Rural and Aboriginal Nursing in Canada*. With increased attention to the importance of social determinants of health, the health of Canadians in rural and remote areas, and a recognition of the inequities in access to care between those living in rural and urban areas, nurses can be leaders in advocating for the fair allocation of appropriate health and social resources to communities in which they work. The needs of those living in busy urban centres such as Toronto, Montreal, or Vancouver are markedly different from people living in small towns, remote rural areas, or bedroom communities. You will find nurses providing needs-driven community and individual care in all of these areas — and nurses play a valuable role in addressing and rectifying health and social injustice across these diverse settings. When we look at the social determinants of health of Aboriginal groups and peoples of Canada, we see that there are historical, socioeconomic, and political legacies that have had an impact on the health and well-being of communities, and individual men, women, and children living in those communities, who are bearing an additional burden of health-related problems resulting from these legacies. In Chapter 18, we not only address the unique role of the rural nurse and the nurse working with Aboriginal communities, but we also hope to highlight inequities and vulnerabilities across contexts and communities.

Throughout the text, we hope to emphasize the nature of the iterative development of skills related to values clarification and ethical decision-making, on the journey to becoming an ethically responsible professional, an ethical leader, and an advocate for social justice and empowerment. We acknowledge that, as moral agents, we are each a *work-in-progress* and that the journey is often far more important than any perceived end point. As Florence Nightingale stated, "Were there none who were discontented with what they have, the world would never reach anything better."

INSTRUCTOR'S RESOURCES

About the Nelson Education Teaching Advantage (NETA)

The **Nelson Education Teaching Advantage (NETA)** program delivers research-based instructor resources that promote student engagement and higher-order thinking to enable the success of Canadian students and educators.

Instructors today face many challenges. Resources are limited, time is scarce, and a new kind of student has emerged: one who is juggling school with work, has gaps in his or her basic knowledge, and is immersed in technology in a way that has led to a completely new style of learning. In response, Nelson Education has gathered a group of dedicated instructors to advise us on the creation of richer and more flexible ancillaries and online learning platforms that respond to the needs of today's teaching environments. Whether your course is offered in-class, online, or both, Nelson is pleased to provide pedagogically-driven, research-based resources to support you.

In consultation with our editorial advisory board, Nelson Education has completely rethought the structure, approaches, and formats of our key textbook ancillaries and online learning platforms. We've also increased our investment in editorial support for our ancillary and digital authors. The result is the Nelson Education Teaching Advantage.

NETA Assessment is a key platform in the Nelson Education Teaching Advantage program. It relates to testing materials. Under *NETA Assessment*, Nelson's authors create multiple-choice questions that reflect research-based best practices for constructing effective questions and testing not just recall but also higher-order thinking. Our guidelines were developed by David DiBattista, a 3M National Teaching Fellow whose recent research as a professor of psychology at Brock University has focused on multiple-choice testing. All Test Bank authors receive training at workshops conducted by Prof. DiBattista, as do the copy editors assigned to each Test Bank. A copy of *Multiple Choice Tests: Getting Beyond Remembering,* Prof. DiBattista's guide to writing effective tests, is included with every Nelson Test Bank/Computerized Test Bank package. (Information about the NETA Test Bank prepared for *Ethics and Issues in Contemporary Nursing*, Second Canadian Edition, is included in the description of the Instructor Companion Website below.)

Resources on the Instructor Companion Website

Key instructor ancillaries are provided on the Instructor website at www.nelson.com/Burkhardt2CE. Our website gives instructors the ultimate tool for customizing lectures and presentations. Ancillaries include:

- **NETA Assessment (Test Bank).** The Test Bank was written by Monique Bacher of George Brown College. It includes over 250 multiple-choice questions written according to NETA guidelines for effective construction and development of higher-order questions. Test Bank files are provided in Word format for easy editing and in PDF format for convenient printing whatever your system.

  The Computerized Test Bank by ExamView® includes all the questions from the Test Bank. The easy-to-use ExamView software is compatible with Microsoft Windows and Mac OS. Create tests by selecting questions from the question bank, modifying these questions as desired, and adding new questions you write yourself. You can administer quizzes online and export tests to WebCT, Blackboard, and other formats.

- **Instructor's Manual.** The Instructor's Manual to accompany *Ethics and Issues in Contemporary Nursing*, Second Canadian Edition, has been prepared by Paula

Crawford-Dickinson of George Brown College. This manual contains an overview of the chapter, instructional strategies and suggested classroom activities, and a resource integration guide to give you the support you need to engage your students within the classroom.

- **Microsoft® PowerPoint®.** Key concepts from *Ethics and Issues in Contemporary Nursing,* Second Canadian Edition, are presented in PowerPoint format. The PowerPoint presentation was created by Carrie Mines of Mohawk College
- **DayOne.** Day One—Prof InClass is a PowerPoint presentation that you can customize to orient your students to the class and their text at the beginning of the course.

ACKNOWLEDGMENTS

The author and Nelson Education Ltd. would like to thank the following reviewers for their help in the development of the Second Canadian Edition of *Ethics and Issues in Contemporary Nursing*:

Judith Barnaby, Seneca College; Kathleen Carlin, Ryerson University; Denise English, Memorial University; Cathy Foster, Brandon University; Neghesti G. Gebru, Laurentian University; RaeAnn Hartman, North Island College; Shirlene Hudyma, Laurentian University; Katharine Hungerford, Lambton College; Dr. Wanda Pierson, Langara College

Part of writing this new edition has meant that I have also taken time to reflect upon just how many other people have helped this come to fruition. With her endless patience, fabulous sense of humour, and encouragement beyond what I ever expected, my developmental editor, Courtney Thorne, has made this process into a true pleasure. I could not have finished this without her perseverance, enduring support, and excellent advice. I would like to express my gratitude to Nelson Education, Jackie Wood in particular, and the entire team I have been fortunate to have alongside me in this effort. I would also like to acknowledge Susan Calvert and Devanand Srinivasan, production managers, my patient, good-natured, and incredibly thorough copy editor Susan James, and Franca Amore and Cathy Mayer for their work on the cover design. Anne Williams, Vice President, Editorial, deserves thanks for her role in getting this second Canadian edition published. I would like to acknowledge the original authors of the American edition for an already strong and thoughtful text with which to work. While I worked on this, many family members and friends provided support, childcare, patience, and understanding. I owe Dr. Chris MacDonald a debt of gratitude for continuing to support me in every way, having already provided valuable help in the preparation of the first edition. My lovely daughter Georgia also deserves a thank-you for her patience with a parent who works both days and nights. Finally I would like to thank my colleagues and my students, who, many without knowing it, have inspired, encouraged, and compelled me in this project. Writing a textbook that may be used in nursing classrooms across Canada is both a privilege and an honour. With each edition, I realize even more just how much we have to learn from each other and just how much there is out there to learn, and to bring alive both on the page and in the classroom. For the support and encouragement of each of these people and the inspiration every day from my students — past, present, and future — I am most grateful.

Nancy Walton

CONTRIBUTORS

Barbara C. Banonis, MSN, RN
Well-Being Consultant
LifeQuest International
Charleston, WV

Mary Jo Butler, EdD, RN
Former Associate Professor and
Director
West Virginia University
School of Nursing, Charleston Division
Charleston, WV

Sandra L. Cotton, MS, RN, C-ANP
Instructor
West Virginia University
School of Nursing
Morgantown, WV

Mary Gail Nagai-Jacobson, MSN, RN
Director, Healing Matters
San Marcos, TX

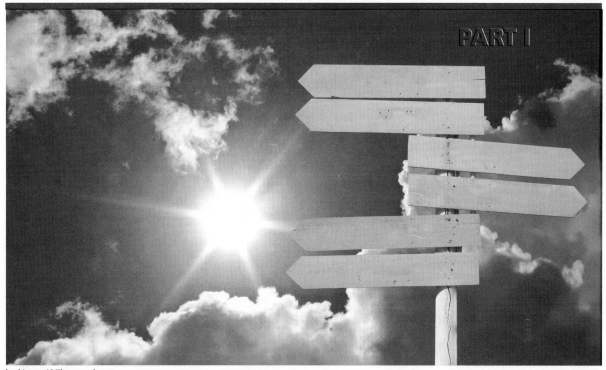
bochimsang12/Shutterstock.com

PART I

GUIDES FOR PRINCIPLED BEHAVIOUR

P art I lays a foundation for nurses to begin critically examining issues and systematically participating in ethical decision making. Examining the history and context of nursing in Western cultures, Chapter 1 gives nurses insight into the profession of nursing as part of an overall social system—focusing specifically on the influence of history, culture, and the status of women in society on the profession. Recognizing that knowledge of ethical theories and principles can help the nurse to develop a cohesive and logical system for making individual decisions, Chapters 2 and 3 describe philosophical perspectives, various classic ethical theories, and ethical principles.

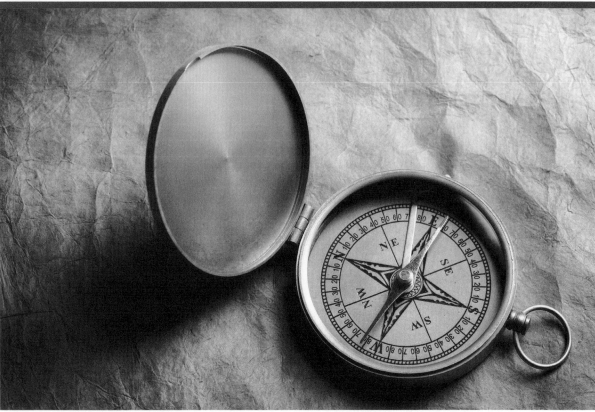

Alex Staroseltsev/Shutterstock.com

CHAPTER **1**

SOCIAL, PHILOSOPHICAL, AND OTHER HISTORICAL FORCES INFLUENCING THE DEVELOPMENT OF NURSING

OBJECTIVES

After completing this chapter, the reader should be able to:

1. Discuss the relationship between social need and the origin of the profession of nursing.

2. Briefly discuss the relationship between moral reasoning and the origin of nursing.

3. Describe the mutually beneficial relationship between the broader society and its professions.

4. Explain the effect of a culture's prevailing belief system on the practice of nursing.

5. Identify how issues such as gender, spiritual beliefs, and religious practices have influenced the evolution of nursing.

6. Discuss how the historical background of the status of women in various cultures is related to the practice of nursing.

7. Make plausible inferences relating the evolution of the practice of nursing to the current state of the profession.

INTRODUCTION

Although the development of the profession is difficult to trace, moral action is the historical basis for the creation, evolution, and practice of nursing. Nursing is considered to be "a moral endeavour" (Smith & Godfrey, 2002, p. 302). The spirit and substance of nursing are based on social and individual moral codes and often, in discussions of nursing and morality, social and Nursing has been called the "morally central health care profession" (Jameton, 1984, p. xvi). individual moral codes are highly intertwined. Florence Nightingale stated that the only way to become a good nurse was to first be a good woman (Baly, 1986). In this chapter, we look at three historical influences on nursing as a moral discipline—social need, spirituality/religion, and the role of women.

Morals and ethics affect nursing on more than one level. As nurses, our motivation to care for others is underpinned by moral reasoning. Collectively, moral beliefs of groups of people produce rules of action, or ethics. These culturally accepted rules are an integral part of both the experience and the profession of nursing. Expressions of ideals, discussions of moral issues, statements of moral principles, and codes of ethics are found throughout the history of nursing. In addition, Jameton (1984) says that nursing is morally worthy work since "caring for and treating the sick, and comforting and protecting the suffering, are basic benefits of human culture" (p. 1). As our modern health care technology extends the boundaries of what is possible, all of society is compelled to examine emerging ethical issues. We are faced with ethical tensions in a health care system that requires moral decision-making, yet sometimes restricts us from legitimate decision-making roles. We examine the history of nursing to help understand our position within the contemporary health care system and the evolution of nursing as a moral profession. The Canadian Nurses Association states the following, in a Position Statement addressing the value of nursing history,

> The practice of nursing takes place within larger cultural, economic, and political contexts that have helped shape the discipline. Nurses need to centre their research and development of professional practice within a knowledge and understanding of trends and patterns in the past. It is essential for nurse clinicians, educators, administrators, researchers, and policymakers to understand the challenges and

opportunities of the past in order to prepare direction for the future. Therefore, a historical perspective is important to the quality of care in all domains of nursing. (Canadian Nurses Association, 2007)*

One of our purposes in writing this text is to present nursing ethics in a manner that will encourage empowered decision-making. In an examination of nursing empowerment, Fulton (1997) proposes that nurses' perspectives can be constrained by historical forces that impart negative messages. According to Stevens, these distortions and constraints "impede free, equal and uncoerced participation in society" (1989, p. 58). Struggling to cope with impossible situations, nurses continue to believe negative messages about themselves and behave in ways that are neither constructive nor empowered (Roberts, 1983; Hedin, 1986). In other words, we can understand our present situation only in relation to our social and professional history (Harden, 1996). These ideas are related to critical social theory as proposed by Habermas (1971) and Freire (1993). The basic principle of critical social theory is that we can understand each aspect of a social phenomenon only in relation to the history and structure in which it is found. As humans existing within societal contexts, this theory assumes that we self-interpret based on the integrated ideas and positions of self, society, and history (Dickinson, 1999). The significance of ideas can be grasped only when we remove ourselves and objectively view them in the context of historical and social practices and entanglements of power and interest (McCarthy, 1990). Habermas (1971) proposes that as individuals we can assess the evidence and fully participate only when we are aware of, and free from, the hidden oppressions that are working on our lives. Insights gained from the study of nursing history enable us to see these conditions for what they are and find ways of interpreting and releasing them in order to move forward. To this end, we present some selected historical and social forces that have shaped the contours of our profession.

It is difficult to establish a clear and linear picture of the development of the profession of nursing through history. Medicine and nursing both emerged from a long history of healers. It is not possible for us to know the exact origin of either profession, since the earliest stages of each are so closely interwoven (Donahue, 2011). Even so, we know that the history of nursing is one in which people—usually women—have attempted to relieve suffering. Selanders writes, "Nursing's history is one of people, both ancient and modern. It has not evolved solely because of one individual or one event or with directed purpose. Rather, nursing's current status represents a collective picture of societal evolution in a health care framework" (Selanders, 1998a, p. 227). From the beginning, the motivation of nurses to care for others came from practical, moral, or spiritual influences. Our history is also the story of a profession inescapably linked to the status of women and changing notions of gender and power. The history of healers, and subsequently that of nurses, has gone through many phases and has been an important part of social movements. Ours is a narrative of a professional group whose status has always been affected by the prevailing standards of society (Donahue, 2011).

---

* Excerpt from Positioning Statement, *The Value of Nursing History Today* © 2007 Canadian Nurses Association. Reprinted with permission. Further reproduction prohibited.

THE INFLUENCE OF SOCIAL NEED

Helping professions find their origin, purpose, and meaning within the context of culturally accepted moral norms, individual values, and perceived social need. By serving others, and responding to their needs, we express moral belief. The term moral thought relates to the thoughtful examination of right and wrong, good and bad. **Moral reasoning** includes any level of this type of thinking. It may be complex and well developed, or it may be rudimentary. Why do we care about moral issues? Some moral philosophers propose that empathy is a motive for moral reasoning and action. For example, if we visualize the suffering of another person, we begin to imagine ourselves suffering. Some describe the desire to help others as a natural outcome of social consciousness and motivation similar to the golden rule, "Do unto others as you would have them do unto you." A universally popular precept, the "Golden Rule" is found in some form in most major moral traditions (Honderich, 1995). Some say that we follow the "Golden Rule" both to help someone in need and, to some degree, in the hope that someone will show us consideration if we are unfortunate enough to find ourselves in similar circumstances. Whatever our original motivation, ethical action is based on a desire to help others and the desired outcome of the action is the same: meeting the health needs of others. Even when not directly acting for others, nurses are almost always inherently concerned with the well-being of others within their care (Bishop & Scudder, 1996). As the morally central health care profession, nursing has historically responded to human suffering.

ASK YOURSELF

What Is the Motivation for Helping?

Imagine a utopian world in which all people are happy and healthy, and have satisfying relationships. There is neither illness nor death. Each person's needs are entirely met without the help of other people. Within this model society, because everyone is satisfied, healthy, and happy, there is no social disorder and no need for any helping profession: no police, doctors, nurses, lawyers, or social workers. Neither is there need for moral discernment. Now, imagine the social disorder that would follow the introduction of serious disease. Individuals who become ill are unable to care for themselves and to meet their own basic needs.

- How should the society deal with this problem?
- Are the ill entirely responsible for themselves?
- Should unaffected members of society continue to live the utopian existence, ignoring the suffering of others, or is the whole of society responsible for helping those in need?
- Should society allow the diseased members to suffer, or do healthy members act to help those afflicted, thus altering their own "perfect" lives—and in turn the prevailing social order?

It is likely that at least some members of the hypothetical community described in the *Ask Yourself* exercise below will recognize the importance of helping those in need. These people will begin to exercise moral thinking as they examine their beliefs. Ethics will emerge in the form of rules of action that are specifically related to solving the moral problem. Those committed to helping the sick will devise methods to utilize individual abilities to the best advantage, and fairly distribute the burden of providing services and resources. As this example implies, nursing can be described as a profession that exists to meet certain needs of individuals and groups, and thus is a product of the moral reasoning of people in society.

As we will see in later chapters, the needs of society at a given time, combined with the technological capabilities and knowledge base, determine the existence and parameters of a profession. Societies establish dynamic boundaries of a profession that move and change as needs change. Our profession is a part of society and, to continue to exist, our professional interest must continue to aim to serve the interests of individuals, families, groups, and communities (International Council of Nurses, 2006).

THINK ABOUT IT

What Makes People Service Oriented?

- Why do you think people are motivated to help those who are in need?
- The actions of those who choose to help others in specific situations might be described as based on self-interest, altruism, or a combination of other motives. How would you describe the motivation to care for others within the healing professions today?
- Think about your own reasons for entering nursing. What were they? Are they the same today? If not, why do you think they have changed?

The nursing profession was created by society for the purpose of meeting specific health needs. In response, the profession has made an implicit promise to ensure, by various means, that its members are competent to provide that service, and further, that these are the *only* members of society who can qualify to provide the service. The relationship between social need and our motivation to care for others is complementary. It is fortunate that human nature is such that some of us, for whatever reason, are interested in serving others.

GENDER AND SPIRITUAL INFLUENCES
Gender Influences

One of the factors that most influences nursing practice is the role of women in society. In every culture women have traditionally been healers. Because nursing has generally been a profession of women (from the beginning, the majority of nurses have been women), women's status in society is central to determining the extent of freedom and respect granted to nurses. Contours of the profession have been shaped, in large part, by social forces that determine gender roles in society. As a result of the perception that women are more humane and more caring by nature, they have been viewed as naturally endowed with nursing talents. Even Florence Nightingale wrote, "Every woman . . . has, at one time or another of her life, charge of the personal health of somebody, whether child or invalid—in other words, every woman is a nurse" (Nightingale, 1859, preface). Gender stereotyping has been both a blessing and a curse to nursing.

It has also created discouragement and, at times, barriers for men wishing to enter the nursing profession. Because nursing is labelled by some as a calling that is inherently female, instead of a legitimate and highly skilled profession, male nurses often find themselves ridiculed or challenged. As well, even in today's world, society may allow or fail to allow women to assume roles of knowledge and authority, roles that allow independent decision making or even limited participation in decision-making processes. One would hope that today, in a world with both an increased awareness of the unique skills and knowledge of nursing alongside more progressive notions of gender, these would no longer be issues. Unfortunately, they are.

Spiritual/Religious Influences

The spiritual and religious foundations of past and present cultures are intertwined with many aspects of health care. Spiritual belief and religious practice have made major contributions to the moral foundation of nursing and other healing professions; they have also influenced both the gender and, to some degree, much of the activity of healers. Spirituality and religious doctrine have also influenced beliefs about the value of individuals, and about life, death, and health. Historically, many of the dominant religious institutions have made judgments about the origin and essence of healing, endorsed (and sometimes certified) those who would hold positions as legitimate healers, and put barriers up to prevent others from becoming leaders or taking part in healing practices. The path that nursing has taken since ancient times has not been smooth. There have been advances and setbacks; libraries have been destroyed; widely diverse groups have held the title of nurse; and those who were the nurses in some early cultures left few records. Nevertheless, nursing in some form has existed in every culture, and has been influenced by spiritual beliefs, religious practices, and related cultural values.

There are documented periods in history in which women were the honoured sole practitioners of the healing arts, and other periods when women were forced into submissive and subservient healing roles. It remains that the status of women and the role of nurses in society have always been intertwined. This is sometimes referred to as the feminization of nursing. Although there are more males in nursing now, and the recognition of nursing as a profession is not necessarily tied to gender in the modern world, some of these more archaic beliefs still persist.

ANCIENT TIMES

To examine nursing from a historical perspective, we must keep in mind that, throughout history, the sociological view of gender and the historical connection between spirituality and healing have both influenced the evolution of health care and nursing. While we can and must separate Church and State in the modern view of health care and health care ethics, throughout history, religion and spirituality have played greater roles than secular legal frameworks in how nursing care is considered and delivered and how moral dilemmas in health care have been approached and solved.

We will begin by looking at nursing and health in the Middle Ages, a significantly large expanse of time from the fall of the Roman Empire in the fifth century until approximately the sixteenth century, the dawn of the early Modern Age. While there is much to document about ancient times and the early Middle Ages in terms of healing and views of illness, we see more evidence of direct influence on nursing in Canada from the later Middle Ages onward.

THE MIDDLE AGES

The period called the Middle Ages was a time of great change and growth for the scientific and political landscape of Western Europe. During this time, the urbanization of much of Northern and Western Europe occurred, and many political geographical boundaries were established that persist today. But most of all, this millennium was a period of significant scientific change, as much of the Islamic world was making advances in science and technology, including astronomy, medicine, and research, as well as establishing degree-granting universities — advances that ultimately reached Europe as well.

As the early Middle Ages began, many people believed that the world was falling into ruin. During this time, disease, large-scale food shortages, and war interacted to produce a predictable sequence: war drove farmers from their fields and destroyed their crops; destruction of the crops led to famine; and the starved and weakened people were easy victims to the onslaught of disease (Cartwright, 2004). During this time, monasticism and other religious groups offered the only opportunities for men and women to pursue careers in nursing. Much of hospital nursing was carried out by repentant women and widows called sisters, and by male nurses called brothers.

Women who entered nursing orders donated their property and wealth to the Christian Church and devoted their lives to service. Although in many cases "nursing" care was given by slaves or servants, religious orders offered the only route through which respectable women and men could serve as nurses.

The overall belief system of a culture influences the extent to which members accept various healing methods and health care practices. An example of this can be seen in historical accounts of the healing arts in the Middle Ages. The term **empirical** relates to knowledge gained through the processes of observation and experience. Many people, especially those involved with the Christian Church, had deeply anti-empirical beliefs. Consequently, people were more likely to seek healing through religious intervention, touching of religious relics, visiting of sacred places, chanting, and other methods approved by the Church. Because of religious fervour at the time in Christian Europe, empirical treatment (particularly if provided by anyone not explicitly sanctioned by the Church), even if it was successful, was thought to be produced by the devil, since the position of the Church was that only God and the devil had the power to either cause illness or promote healing.

Beginning in 1096, the Crusades were military campaigns driven by mostly Christian Western Europe against opponents, such as the Muslims, Jews, those identified as pagans, the Greek Orthodox church, and anyone else viewed as a political or ideological enemy of the papal legacy. These holy wars led to deplorable sanitary conditions, fatigue, poor nutrition, diarrhea, and the spread of communicable diseases. These health problems in turn led to a need for more hospitals and greater numbers of health care providers. For most of the Middle Ages, the Roman Catholic Church held tremendous influence over the people and governments of European countries. Powerful leaders within the Church determined the appropriateness of various healing practices. Official credentialing of physicians, nurses, and midwives was left in the hands of the Church. Even after civic legislation became common, the Church continued to enforce the law and monitor practitioners (Achterberg, 1990).

Accounts of the actual treatment of patients in early times vary. In some hospitals operated by religious orders, patients were treated as welcome guests. People sometimes pretended to be ill to be admitted. In contrast, there are reports that some groups of patients were treated inhumanely, even by members of nursing orders. The treatment of persons with mental illnesses was based on the idea that they were possessed by devils or that they were being punished for their sins (Dolan, 1973). They were often put in chains, starved, and kept under filthy conditions. There was even a time when it was thought that torture was useful in driving out what was labelled at that time as "madness." Because the public perception of mental illness was based on religious beliefs related to demon possession and punishment for sin, the mentally ill were treated inhumanely.

During the Middle Ages, the status of women also declined in much of Europe. In many ways this was directly related to Christian doctrine. St. Thomas Aquinas, ironically known within the Church as the "angelic doctor" (Donahue, 2011), wrote that one should "only make use of a necessary object, woman, who is needed to preserve the species or to provide food and drink . . . . Woman was created to be man's [helper], but her unique role is in conception . . . since for all other purposes men would be better assisted by other men" (Thomas Aquinas as cited by Achterberg, 1990, p. 68). Religious leaders like Aquinas were helping to set the stage for the persecution of women, which would last for hundreds of years and leave a persistent legacy of misogyny.

During the Middle Ages, religious and Church–sanctioned secular nursing orders afforded the only legitimate avenue for women wishing to be nurses. The Church popularized the ideals of virginity or chastity, poverty, and a life of service. By the end of the thirteenth century, an estimated 200 000 women served as nurses within these orders (Achterberg, 1990). It was often the case that these orders were subordinate to the men's communities (Donahue, 2011). Nevertheless, some speculate that within the structure of the Church, these women exercised a degree of independence and autonomy and contributed to the health care of the time.

During the Middle Ages, the Church and the newly formed medical profession in Europe were actively engaged in the elimination of lay female healers. Women were excluded from the newly formed degree-granting universities. Except for those devoting their lives to serving in religious nursing orders, women were not allowed by the Church to practise the healing arts. Nevertheless, some women continued to secretly practise the healing arts, both inside and outside the home, using knowledge handed down for generations, intuitive knowledge, and empirical knowledge.

Although the medical profession was officially sanctioned by the Church, and male physicians were beginning to be trained in the university setting, there was scant scientific knowledge. Physicians relied solely on superstition (Ehrenreich & English, 1973). University-trained physicians used bloodletting, astrology, alchemy, and incantations. Their patients were almost exclusively wealthy. Physicians' treatments were usually ineffective, often dangerous, and inaccessible to the majority of the poor.

Much of the time, during and after the Crusades, people formed small communities around lords or "masters," who were often bishops or barons, usually with power related to land ownership or religion. Under this feudal system, peasants or serfs had serious problems related to poor sanitation and hygiene because of their poor living conditions. Without antibiotics, the discovery of which would not occur until centuries later, most people died of infections, exposure, and diseases.

At this time, concepts such as the four humours were popular notions of how the body worked. Directly related to the environment, the four humours existing in the human body were considered to be related to fire (yellow bile), earth (black bile), water (phlegm), and air (blood). Illness and death were thought to be related to an imbalance of humours or to "sins of the soul," and most treatments for ailments were related to creating balance in the humours through methods such as bloodletting, pilgrimages, and praying.

Peasant women were often the only healers for people who had no doctors and suffered bitterly from poverty and disease (Ehrenreich & English, 1973). These folk healers had extensive knowledge about cures that had been handed down for generations via oral tradition. They constantly improved their practice through empirical methods of observation, trial, and evaluation. While physicians continued to rely on superstition, these women developed an extensive understanding of bones and muscles, herbs, drugs, and midwifery (Barstow, 1994; Ehrenreich & English, 1973). Some authorities believed these peasant folk healers were actually practising some form of magic or witchcraft (Barstow, 1994). This atmosphere set the stage for Church–sanctioned crimes against women in the form of the witch hunts. In a sweep across Europe, the witch hunts lasted from the fourteenth to the seventeenth century. The atmosphere that led to the witch hunts was a critical mixture of war, disease, and poverty, combined with religious fervour, superstition, and political unrest. Women, particularly women healers, represented a political, religious, and sexual threat to both Church and State, which were, during the Middle Ages, tightly bound together. An atmosphere of superstition and a widespread belief in magic set the stage that would allow terrible crimes to be perpetrated against women (Achterberg, 1990; Barstow, 1994; Ehrenreich & English, 1973) as a result of these witch hunts and trials.

What crimes were the women accused of? Any woman who treated an illness, even if she applied a soothing salve to the diseased skin of her child, was likely to be accused of witchcraft. If the treatment failed, she was thought to have cursed the patient. If the treatment succeeded, she was believed to be in consort with the devil. Although women were permitted to practise midwifery (no one else wanted to do it), these women were in danger of being accused of witchcraft if anything went wrong with either mother or baby.

No one knows how many women were killed during the witch trials. When records were kept, they were abysmal. The most authoritative estimate of the number of executions is 200 000, although some estimates are as high as ten million. Women comprised 85 percent to 95 percent of those killed (Barstow, 1994). It is difficult to comprehend the effect of the witch hunts on European society. Women silently watched the public humiliation, torture, disfigurement, and death of other women. Barstow believes that this public acknowledgment of the evil nature of the female sex left all women humiliated and frightened. Because both the accused and those viewing the proceedings were powerless to prevent the torture and executions, the witch craze served to undermine women's belief in the ability and power of women. Indeed, this was likely the inference made by all of society. Achterberg writes, "women were never again given full citizenship in any country, nor was their role in the healing professions reinstated" (1990, p. 98). Even after the end of this terrible time, women were prohibited from independent healing professions by law in every country in Europe. This created a climate in which, under the protection and patronage of the ruling classes, men became the authoritative medical professionals (Ehrenreich & English, 1973). Although accounts of the witch hunts are absent in most popular nursing history texts, these events had a significant influence upon the profession.

THE RENAISSANCE AND THE REFORMATION

The sixteenth century heralded the beginning of two great movements: the Renaissance and the Reformation. Resulting from a revolutionary spirit and quest for knowledge, the Renaissance produced an intellectual rebirth that began the scientific era. The Reformation was a religious movement precipitated both by the widespread abuses that had become a part of the Roman Catholic Church, and by doctrinal disagreement among religious leaders (Donahue, 2011).

The Renaissance gave birth to the scientific revolution and a new era in the healing arts. Beginning its gradual escape from the control of the Church, the scientific community made advances in mathematics and the sciences. René Descartes is credited with proposing a theory that quickly altered philosophic beliefs about the separation of mind and body. He proposed that the universe is a physical thing, and that everything in the universe is like a machine, which can be analyzed and understood. Descartes further theorized that the mind and body are separate entities (Durant, 1926), and that people are set against a world of objects that they must seek to master (McCarthy, 1990). Based on Descartes' work, **Cartesian philosophy** began to replace religious beliefs related to the physical and spiritual realms of humankind. As a direct result, a separation was created between the acts of caring and curing in the healing arts. The arrival of this philosophy, while elevating the sciences and making scientific inquiry possible, did not improve the status of nursing. Achterberg identifies this time as an important turning point. Regarding Cartesian philosophy, she says, "When spirit no longer is seen to abide in matter, the reverence for what is physical departs. Hence medicine no longer regarded itself as working in the sacred spaces where fellow humans find themselves in pain and peril, and where transcendence is most highly desired" (1990, p. 103). As Cartesian philosophy became popular, nurses' place in the health care system became limited to the "caring" realm. Caring was given lower priority than curing within the hierarchy of the healing arts. Some would argue that this legacy remains with nursing yet today.

In Canada, the earliest records of nursing begin in the seventeenth century, just after Jacques Cartier and Samuel de Champlain's historic voyages to establish the settlements along the St. Lawrence River that would later become Canada, then known as New France.

At the time of the establishing settlements, there were a number of prevailing systems of health care. Aboriginal persons living in the region had traditional healing methods, with remedies and treatments specific to their culture and beliefs. Other health care was provided by male priests who immigrated to New France and, while promoting Christianity, found themselves also caring for the ill and dying. While their main goal was promoting Christianity, they found that they needed help caring for the sick and sent pleas back to France for nurses to join the new settlements and help provide care, thus freeing the time and energies of the priests to carry out their missions.

The nursing traditions in Canada were by and large established with influence from France, not Britain. At that time, there were significant differences between the state of nursing as a profession or activity of women in Britain and France. In Britain, tensions between the Catholic Church and the monarchy had resulted in the closing of the monasteries and subsequent release of nursing care from the nuns into the hands of incompetent lay staff. As conditions in Britain became deplorable, it was known as the "Dark Period of Nursing" (Donahue, 2011).

From France, laywomen such as Marie Rollet Hébert came to Canada to assume nursing roles and be trained in providing care for the sick and dying. Her attitude towards Aboriginal persons and their practices established her as compassionate and open-minded. She demonstrated respect for their beliefs and practices, and collaborated with them in providing health care, which was novel at the time. Instead of trying to change their beliefs or convince them to adopt different practices, she embraced the differences in beliefs and practices, and shared resources.

Jeanne Mance was another noteworthy woman in early nursing in Canada. One of the first female settlers, she was responsible for the first hospital established in the

New World, what we now know as Hôtel-Dieu de Montréal, in 1645. Although, like Marie Hébert, she was a laywoman, her hospital was staffed by nurses who belonged to the religious order of Sisters of St. Joseph. Mance is seen as not only the founder of a hospital, but also one of the founders of the city of Montréal.

Later, into the modern era, women such as Marguerite D'Youville (founder of the Grey Nuns), Ethel Bedford Benwich, and Florence Nightingale all had important roles in the development of Canadian nursing.

THE MODERN ERA

Nursing as we know it today in North America began to emerge in the modern era. Known as the founder of modern nursing, Florence Nightingale (1820–1910) in her life and writing reflects the influence of the Renaissance and Reformation. As a person, Nightingale remains an enigma. As a nurse, she remains a pioneer: researcher, leader, and scholar. She saw nursing as a profession separate from the Church, yet she began her career as the result of a mystic experience (Simkin, 2001). Nightingale's religious beliefs were evident in her practice and beliefs about nursing care. She claimed that God spoke to her four times, calling her into his service when she was sixteen years old (Selanders, 1998b). Nightingale's description of nursing as "caring for the mind and the body" was one of the first references to holistic nursing in the modern era.

Florence Nightingale became a model for all nurses. She was a nurse, statistician, sanitarian, social reformer, and scholar. She was politically astute, intelligent, and single-minded. Contrary to accepted Victorian social conventions, Florence Nightingale addressed moral issues with courage and conviction. She also rebelled against the traditional expectations for women of that era: to become good wives and mothers. Her work was foundational in many ways. During the Crimean War, the rates of soldiers dying from poor living conditions and ailments related to sanitation and hygiene was incredibly high. Nightingale, on the front lines, recognized the importance of clean conditions in which to eat and provide nursing care, with separation between the clean and dirty areas of the soldiers' camps. What is basic knowledge to us today, when introduced and operationalized by Nightingale (her nurses went to work rearranging the camps and cleaning), remarkably decreased the mortality rate of soldiers on the front lines. Nightingale provided clear support and evidence of what eventually became known as the germ theory of disease. Having strong opinions on women's rights, she did not hesitate to challenge the established male hierarchy. Nightingale argued for the removal of restrictions that prevented women from having careers (Simkin, 2001). Her writings instructed nurses to "do the thing that is good, whether it is 'suitable for a woman' or not" (Nightingale, 1859, p. 76). Nightingale has been criticized, however, for situating the moral agency of nursing within a gender-specific context. Her belief that a good nurse is both qualified and signified by being female has been described by some as furthering the "gender essentialism" (LeVasseur, 1998, p. 286) that is apparent in many discussions of morality and nursing (Walker and Holmes, 2008). Some go on to argue that Nightingale was not a feminist, though her writings indicate that she felt women should have a more important place in the social structure. She wrote, "Passion, intellect, moral activity—these three have never been satisfied in woman. In this cold and oppressive conventional atmosphere, they cannot be satisfied" (Nightingale, 1852/1979, p. 29). It is certain that she did not subscribe to the then-current Cartesian notion that women had neither minds nor souls, but were put on the earth solely for man's purpose and pleasure (Roberts & Group, 1995).

Another of nursing's great modern leaders is Lavinia Lloyd Dock (1858–1956). Considered a radical feminist, Dock actively engaged in social protest, picketing, and parading for women's rights in the United States (Roberts & Group, 1995). She was concerned with the many problems plaguing nursing, warning that male dominance in the health field was the major problem confronting the nursing profession. Lavinia Dock's contemporaries ignored her concerns, and twentieth- and twenty-first-century nurses have found themselves fighting the same battles.

From the 1840s onward, the force of nursing was moving through the country as settlement into the West increased. With the leadership of the Grey Nuns, missions were established throughout the West and nursing became a part of quality health care available to new settlers.

Ethel Fenwick (1857–1947), a British nurse, made a strong case that nurses should have their own professional organizations and that work needed to be done to raise standards for the educational preparation of nurses and to increase respect and legitimacy for the profession of nursing. Her work was fundamental in establishing what we now know as the International Council of Nurses in 1899. Furthermore, she influenced the formation of nursing professional associations in both Canada and the United States.

In Canada, Mary Agnes Snively established the first national organization for nurses in 1907, known as the Canadian Society for Superintendents of Training Schools for Nurses. Snively was the first Ontario nurse to be trained in the Nightingale method of nursing. The following year, the Canadian National Association of Trained Nurses (CNATN) was established, again with Snively as president. Some years later, this organization, by then with memberships from nursing schools situated in hospitals across the country, would become a formal part of the International Council of Nurses, further legitimizing the profession of nursing in Canada. The CNATN later became the Canadian Nurses Association (CNA). Snively was also superintendent of the Toronto General Hospital's School of Nursing and had significant influence on the standing of the profession in Canada, the improvement in hospital-based training of nurses, and the formation of leading nursing groups such as the CNA and the professional organizations of nurses in Ontario.

Nursing further evolved as more identified needs and roles emerged. Public health nursing and military nursing were both important new avenues in the first half of the twentieth century, and significant leadership in both areas was seen in Canadian nursing. Nurses played important roles in both World Wars. Nurses held ranks of officers, lost their lives, and tended to the wounded and dying in precarious and gravely dangerous situations. At this time, the image of nursing was described using words such as bravery, courage, loyalty, and dedication (Kalisch and Kalisch, 1987). The evolving image of nurse from unskilled helper of the physician to independent and brave professional was an important step in improving the image of nursing in the public eye.

The mid-1900s heralded great advances for nurses. During these decades nurses moved into spheres of professional, social, and political responsibility. Through this political activism, the profession gained acceptance as a legitimate health care force.

After the World wars, the Canadian Red Cross Society provided grants and certification for nurses to become experts in public health nursing through university programs. Both the Society and nurses alike recognized that the entrenchment of health care in the hospital system isolated many in communities and focused care on episodic, acute problems. Many persons, it was noted, suffered from chronic, manageable ailments and diseases, which could be better managed outside the hospital system by qualified caregivers such as public health nurses. In addition, there was recognition at that time of the need for strong well-established public health programs, health education, immunization, hygiene, and care for those living in poverty or without basic social determinants of health. This trend is seen as one of the most important in health care today, articulated in documents such as the Romanow Commission Report (2002), the Kirby report (2003) and the more recent Drummond report in Ontario (2012). The most vocal and consistent supporters for strong and well-supported public health programs, as well as the most prominent providers of public health today, are still nurses. The establishment of the goal of "Health for All by the Year 2000" by the World Health Organization out of the Alma-Ata Declaration in 1978 is being embraced and acted upon by organizations such as the Canadian Nurses Association (2008). The CNA's vision for the future of nursing embraces the varied roles that nurses must play in order to provide holistic care to a diverse and changing Canadian population, ever mindful of the role of public health and the importance of the determinants of health for all Canadians (CNA, 2006). In *CNA's Preferred Future: Health For All,* the CNA states that,

> The need for equitable access has not changed, nor has it been met. And we are also facing new challenges on many fronts: shifting demographics, growing and unmet health needs, human resources shortages, as well as the globalization of economies and diseases. Other trends have created new opportunities through partnerships, research, innovation and evolving technology. The Canadian Nurses Association (CNA) accepts the challenge to re-frame and reinvigorate our approach to health care and human resources issues, from how nurses are educated and licensed to how their competencies are used to best advantage. Nursing education, job design and responsibilities must change as the country moves from the traditional model of treating illness to one that focuses on keeping people well, with both care and support for maintaining health delivered in the community. Making this model of health care a reality will require breaking down divisions within nursing as well as barriers between nursing and other professions. (CNA, 2008)

Many nurses have now claimed legitimate authority to provide independent skilled health care and assume institutional and political leadership positions. Perceiving a health care crisis of growing proportions, and recognizing a need for comprehensive, accessible, and sustainable health care, society has challenged established institutions to foster greater use of nurses in expanded roles. Encouraged by a society in which health care has become a scarce resource, nurse practitioners, nurse midwives, and other advanced nurses have begun to assert themselves as independent professionals.

Entering the twenty-first century, nursing in Western culture has been shaped by spirituality and religion, ideas about gender roles, and cultural influences of the past. As a tapestry woven over time, nursing owns the heritage of those early times. Although many nurses have overcome social and institutional barriers to practise as full members of the profession, others continue to struggle within a patriarchal, institutional hierarchy. Recognizing the legitimate need for both the caring and curing aspects of healing, nurses, committed to holistic practice, are charged with working together to improve their status and to ensure that the problems of the past are not repeated. Today's health care system is experiencing rapid change. Health care reform and proposed new models of health care delivery offer nurses opportunities and challenges. The position of the professional nurse within these systems is far from assured. Recalling lessons from the past, nurses remain acutely aware of threats to newly won professional recognition.

SUMMARY

Nursing is a profession that was created for the purpose of meeting specific perceived health needs. The profession is bound by the duty to competently meet the needs for which it was created. Individual nurses, therefore, have a duty to uphold the fiduciary commitment involved in being professionals.

In all cultures, the profession has been profoundly influenced by various aspects of gender roles, spirituality, and the dominant values and beliefs. Ideas and notions about health, illness, death, and the provision of care have always been influenced by prevailing ideas arising out of religion, scientific enquiry, philosophy, art, and literature. Sociological and anthropological approaches to examining the role of nursing in societies have uncovered ideas around the status of women and the valuing of feminized work that have had lasting effects on the legitimacy of nursing care and the status of nurses as autonomous professionals. In many cultures, women have been healers. Women's status in societies has directly determined the freedom they are given to become educated, to think and act independently, and to participate fully in the provision of skilled and unique health care. There were periods in history when women had freedom and responsibility, and there were periods when women lived in subjugation. Even in the modern world, the notion of nursing as women's work persists, not only from a historical perspective but also in the kinds of challenges and unfortunate barriers that many males who seek to enter nursing still encounter. Nursing today is at a crossroads, free of many of the restrictions and oppressions of the past, yet not fully franchised as a profession with power and authority.

Many religions have strong value-based statements about moral issues at the boundaries of life and death and, by virtue of this, have often had a profound influence on how many people, in the past and today, think about issues in health care. Throughout history, the strong relationship between religion and power has meant that the values of societies often were those espoused by the most powerful. Power gained through religion, historically, has often not been gained legitimately and has often come at the expense of others' well-being or values. Today, nursing and health care tend to be influenced by the State rather than the Church. In countries like Canada, where there are many religions and belief systems, it is important to realize the historical influence of religion on nursing but to remember that in the modern world, there is not one set of overarching values and beliefs; instead, there is a legitimate and highly valued diversity of ideologies.

CHAPTER HIGHLIGHTS

- Throughout history, spiritual beliefs, religious practice, cultural norms, and political factors have influenced evolutionary changes in nursing. These factors continue to influence the practice of nursing today.
- Social need is the criterion for the existence of all professions.
- The practice of nursing is focused on meeting the health care needs of others; therefore, the practice of nursing originates in moral thinking.
- Many social forces have had an impact on the evolution of the profession of nursing.
- Because nursing is primarily a profession of women, the social status of women affects the status of the profession.
- The status of the nursing profession determines its members' ability to practise with freedom and responsibility.

DISCUSSION QUESTIONS AND ACTIVITIES

1. Talk with nurses and physicians in your clinical practice setting. Ask about why they have chosen a profession with a main goal to help others in need. In class, analyze and compare the responses.
2. Discuss the historical developments that caused the separation of the professions of medicine and nursing. How were the distinctions drawn that led to the boundaries of the professions? If you could, how would you change the boundaries today?
3. Search the Internet for information on Florence Nightingale. Critically discuss how she is presented and discussed. Pictures and a short history can be found at http://www.spartacus.schoolnet.co.uk/REnightingale.htm
4. What is the relationship between the historical roles of women and the current status of nurses?

5. What is the relationship between the role of women ***today*** and the status of nurses?

6. Do you think that the role of women in today's society still has a significant effect on the image of nursing, now that more men are involved in nursing? Why or why not?

7. Discuss the relationship between the role of nurses in the health care system today and their role in ethical decision-making in the clinical setting.

8. Discuss the challenges that the profession of nursing has faced and continues to face related to attaining or maintaining an authoritative role in the health care system of the present and the future.

REFERENCES

Achterberg, J. (1990). *Woman as healer*. Boston: Shambhala Publications.

American Nurses Association (1980). *Nursing: A social policy statement*. Kansas City, MO: Author.

American Nurses Association (1996). *Nursing's social policy statement*. Washington, DC: Author.

Baly, M. E. (1986). *Florence Nightingale and the nursing legacy*. London: Croom Helm.

Barstow, A. L. (1994). *Witchcraze: A new history of the European witch hunts*. San Francisco: HarperCollins.

Bishop, A. H., & J. R. Scudder (1996). *Nursing ethics: therapeutic caring presence*. Sudbury, MA: Jones and Bartlett.

Canadian Nurses Association (2006). *Towards 2020: Visions for nursing*. Ottawa: Canadian Nurses Association.

Canadian Nurses Association (2007). *Position Statement: The value of nursing history today*. Ottawa: Canadian Nurses Association.

Canadian Nurses Association (2008). *CNA's preferred future: Health for all*. Ottawa: Canadian Nurses Association. Retrieved/from December 8, 2008 http://www.cna-aiic.ca/CNA/resources/webcastOct8/preferred_future/default_e.aspx.

Cartwright, F. F., & M. D. Bidiss (2004). *Disease and history*. Sutton: Stroud, UK.

Dickinson, J. (1999). A critical social theory approach to nursing care of adolescents with diabetes. *Issues in Comprehensive Pediatric Nursing, 22*(4), 143–152.

Dolan, J. A. (1973). *Nursing in society: A historical perspective* (13th ed.). Philadelphia: Saunders.

Dolan, J. A., M. L. Fitzpatrick, & E. K. Herrmann (1983). *Nursing in society: A historical perspective* (15th ed.). Philadelphia: Saunders.

Donahue, M. P. (2011). *Nursing: The finest art*. St. Louis, MO: Mosby.

Drummond, D. (2012). *Commission on the Reform of Ontario's Public Services*. Queen's Printer for Ontario: Toronto.

Durant, W. (1926). *The story of philosophy*. New York: Washington Square Press.

Ehrenreich, B., & D. English (1973). *Witches, midwives, and nurses: A history of women healers*. New York: The Feminist Press.

Freire, P. (1993). *Pedagogy of the oppressed* (New rev. 20th Anniversary ed.). New York: Continuum.

Fulton, Y. (1997). Nurses' views on empowerment: A critical social theory perspective. *Journal of Advanced Nursing, 26,* 529–536.

Habermas, J. (1971). *Communication and the evolution of society.* Boston: Beacon Press.

Harden, J. (1996). Enlightenment, empowerment and emancipation: The case for critical pedagogy in nurse education. *Nurse Education Today, 16*(1), 32–37.

Hedin, B. A. (1986). A case study of oppressed group behavior in nurses. *Image: Journal of Nursing Scholarship, 18*(2), 53–57.

Honderich, T., ed. (1995). *The Oxford companion to philosophy.* Oxford, U.K.: Oxford University Press.

International Council of Nurses (2006). *The ICN code of ethics for nursing.* Geneva: ICN.

Jameton, A. (1984). *Nursing practice: The ethical issues.* Englewood Cliffs, NJ: Prentice-Hall.

Kalisch, P., & B. Kalisch (1987). *The changing image of the nurse.* Toronto: Addison-Wesley.

Kirby, M. J. L. (2003). *Reforming Health Protection and Promotion in Canada: Time to Act.* The Standing Senate Committee on Social Affairs, Science and Technology. Health Canada: Ottawa.

LeVasseur, J. (1998). Plato, Nightingale, and contemporary nursing. *Image – The Journal of Nursing Scholarship 30*(3), 281–285.

McCarthy, T. (1990). The critique of impure reason. *Political Theory, 18*(3), 437–469.

Nightingale, F. (1859). *Notes on nursing: What it is, and what it is not.* London: Harrison & Sons.

Nightingale, F. (1979). *Cassandra.* Old Westbury, NY: Feminist Press. (Original work published in 1852).

Roberts, J. I., & T. M. Group (1995). *Feminism and nursing: An historical perspective on power, status, and political activism in the nursing profession.* Westport, CT: Praeger.

Roberts, S. J. (1983). Oppressed group behavior: Implications for nursing. *Advances in Nursing Science, 5*(4), 21–30.

Selanders, L. C. (1998a). Florence Nightingale: The evolution and social impact of feminist values in nursing. *Journal of Holistic Nursing, 16*(2), 227–243.

Selanders, L. C. (1998b). The power of environmental adaptation: Florence Nightingale's original theory for nursing practice. *Journal of Holistic Nursing, 16*(2), 247–263.

Simkin, J. (2001). *Florence Nightingale.* Retrieved January 14, 2001, from http://www.sparticus .schoolnet .co.uk/REnightingale.htm.

Smith, K. V., & N. S. Godfrey (2002). Being a good nurse and doing the right thing: A qualitative study. *Nursing Ethics, 9*(3), 302–312.

Stevens, P. E. (1989). A critical social reconceptualization environment in nursing: implications for methodology. *Advances in Nursing Science, 11*(4), 56–68.

Walker, K. & C. A. Holmes (2008). The 'order of things' – tracing a history of the present through a re-reading of the past in nursing education. *Contemporary Nurse, 30,* 106–118.

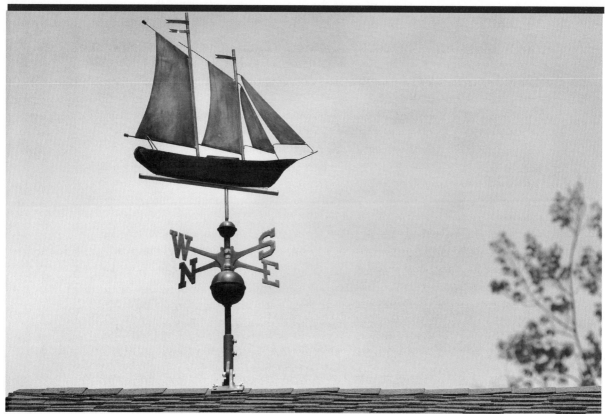

Mark Herreid/Shutterstock.com

CHAPTER 2
ETHICAL THEORY

OBJECTIVES

After completing this chapter, the reader should be able to:

1. Discuss the purpose of philosophy.
2. Define the terms "moral philosophy" and "ethics."
3. Discuss the importance of a systematic study of ethics to nursing.
4. Discuss the importance of ethical theory.
5. Describe utilitarianism.
6. Describe deontological ethics, defining the terms "categorical imperative" and "practical imperative."
7. Define the terms "virtue" and "virtue ethics."

INTRODUCTION

At its core, nursing deals with issues and situations that have elements of ethical or moral uncertainty. A growing dependence on technology and the resultant longer lifespans and higher health care costs, coupled with increasing professional autonomy, creates an atmosphere in which we are faced with problems of ever-increasing complexity. We need to be able to recognize situations that have ethical and moral implications, and to make coherent and logical ethical decisions based upon recognized ethical principles and theory. This text will prepare you to examine the issues and, in doing so, help you to come to logical, consistent, and thoughtful ethical decisions.

In order to be ethically aware professionals, nurses need to be able to recognize ethical issues and components of practice. This involves four key elements: having an awareness of our own beliefs and values; appreciating the diversity of views on ethical issues; recognizing that an issue is, in fact, an ethical dilemma or that the issue has ethical significance; and, finally, having some sound basic knowledge of ethical theories and decision-making models.

While being an ethically aware nurse entails being prepared to engage in ethical decision-making processes as part of a collaborative and interprofessional team, it also means that you must be prepared to examine your own values and beliefs. This can be a challenging, and at times enlightening, process. It may mean acknowledging that your values or beliefs differ from those of the institutions or agencies in which you work. It may also mean discovering that your values and beliefs are markedly different from your patients' or your co-workers' beliefs or cultural norms. This is a necessary and important part of evolving as an ethical professional—taking responsibility for your own beliefs while acknowledging and appreciating diversity. It requires moral courage and a willingness to be open not only to your own views, but also to the views of others and the to ways that you might be viewed by others for holding particular opinions or beliefs. It also requires active avoidance of quick judgments of or assumptions about others. Finally, patience, sensitivity to the concerns and priorities of others, and insight are all key attributes of an ethically aware professional nurse, who makes dealing directly with ethical issues a priority in practice.

Ethical dilemmas or problems or, more broadly, ethical challenges rarely have easy answers and often require time, effort, and attention to try to sort out. Situations that involve ethical implications or challenges can often be resolved in a number of realistic ways, each of which might be pleasing to some stakeholders but problematic for others. In order to deal effectively with such situations, one must first learn to recognize when something is, in fact, an ethical problem or situation and not, for example, a purely professional or policy issue. Sometimes ethical problems may involve professional demeanour, practice, or policy, but that doesn't mean that you will necessarily find a clear answer in professional codes of ethics, institutional policies, or agency handbooks. When we refer here to ethical problems or ethical dilemmas, we also acknowledge that this does not imply that every situation with ethical dimensions will present as a "problem" or "dilemma." Often these sorts of situations will not present as isolated "problems" which, once resolved, will be over and done with.

Instead, situations with ethical dimensions come in many sizes and shapes, from those involving individual patients and nurses to those that have broader implications for entire institutions or groups of persons.

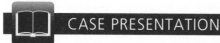

CASE PRESENTATION

Facing a Difficult Problem

Ahmed is a new nursing graduate on a busy surgical floor. His preceptor, Marta, and he have a collegial and friendly working relationship and Ahmed is grateful to Marta for her help and patience as he orients to the floor. He is concerned, however, with the apparent level of stress Marta seems to be under, and he knows from their conversations over meals and coffee, that she has a difficult home life, as she is going through a divorce and custody hearings for her children. Today, when Ahmed enters the medication room, he sees Marta closing the controlled medication cupboard, and then taking two pills at the sink, with a glass of water. For the rest of the day, Marta seems calmer and more focused. At the end of the busy shift, the narcotics count is short two tablets of lorazepam, an anti-anxiety medication. Ahmed is concerned and approaches Marta privately about his suspicion, in a caring and concerned way. Marta admits to Ahmed that she took two lorazepam tablets, as she has been very anxious and feeling unable to cope with the level of stress, over the last few days. She tells Ahmed she regrets doing this, has never done this before and won't do it again, and asks him for his continued support and confidence, while apologizing for putting him in this situation. Ahmed knows that Marta's actions are wrong, from a legal, professional and institutional policy perspective and that his professional obligation is to report Marta the manager or encourage her to talk to the manager herself, in order to support both her and the patients she provides care for, and fulfil his professional obligations. He knows that, if he referred to the hospital's policy on medications, the policies and practice standards from the professional College, and documents outlining the legal obligations of Registered Nurses, they would all be in agreement that Marta's actions are professionally irresponsible, illegal, and could potentially put patients at risk. However, that doesn't help him decide what is the right thing to do at this moment, even though he clearly knows what he **should** do. The problem is not a simple one—although Ahmed's professional obligations are clear, he also wants to support Marta, a nurse he respects and feels he "owes," in the best possible way, and continue to be her friend and colleague.

In this example, we see that there are clear and available answers to Ahmed's dilemma in professional codes of ethics, institutional policies, and nursing practice standards. However, while these answers clearly prescribe what Ahmed's next steps should be, it is understandable that doing what is professionally required would not be easy for Ahmed. Even if a code of ethics or a policy is clear about **what to do**, it often doesn't tell you **how to do it**. Furthermore, referring to a code of ethics or a policy guideline does not mean that a nurse's own moral judgement becomes irrelevant. While Ahmed knows that he needs to report Marta's actions, he also finds himself thinking about Marta's home life, her unconditional support of him through difficult times, and her genuine remorse at her actions, as well as her promise never to do this again. The kinds of guidelines provided in professional or policy documents don't always provide all the kinds of answers that nurses need when they find themselves involved in these types of complex situations.

Having knowledge of ethical theories and ethical decision-making models, both of which are provided in this textbook, does not mean that you will find it easier to solve ethical dilemmas that may arise in your practice. However, this kind of knowledge can equip you to approach an ethical problem in a way that everyone can understand and a way that all stakeholders can participate in. Such knowledge may also help you to identify the most logical, fair, or rational decisions. Ethical theories can help you to understand a markedly different worldview than your own on a specific issue. Decision-making models may help you by taking you step-by-step through a difficult and complex issue. They may even help you to identify useful resources, or discover alternative points of view that you may not have initially considered.

CASE PRESENTATION

Nursing Students Face an Ethical Dilemma

Santos and Lydia are two senior nursing students assigned to work in the intensive care unit with a critically ill patient. The patient, Mr. Dunn, is an eighty-seven-year-old retired ironworker. He lives alone in an old two-storey frame house. Mr. Dunn is diabetic. He is nearly blind and has moderately advanced prostate cancer and Alzheimer's disease. Mr. Dunn was admitted to the intensive care unit after he was discovered unconscious in his home by a neighbour. At that time he was ketoacidotic and had a very severe necrotic wound on his left leg. The surgeon attending Mr. Dunn is planning amputation of his left leg but has been unable to get consent from either Mr. Dunn or his next of kin, a niece who lives out of town.

Santos is proud of his efficiency as a nursing student. He makes rapid decisions. He insists that Mr. Dunn must have the amputation. He suggests to the physician that he have a substitute decision maker appointed for Mr. Dunn so that the surgery can proceed. The course appears clear to him. Lydia, on the other hand, is not certain of the correct course of action. She talks to Mr. Dunn and his niece about his condition. She wonders if the amputation is the best solution to his problem. She thinks about his quality of life after the surgery. She worries about his ability to care for himself and about his state of mind should he be forced to live in a nursing home. She thinks about what she would want for her father if he were in the same situation. Lydia falls asleep at night pondering these thoughts.

(Continued)

She does not know how to go about solving the problem. Santos is impatient with Lydia. He sees no benefit to the time and energy spent worrying about this problem when the solution is obvious to him.

In this example, we see nurses at two extremes. Santos makes quick decisions. In all likelihood he fails to recognize the ethical nature of the problem, the bearing the outcome may have on the people involved, or the conflicting possible solutions. He has great pride in his ability to make decisions, and has confidence in the correctness of those decisions. Lydia, being more insightful and sensitive, recognizes intuitively that the problem presents no clear solution. She is troubled by the situation, but has no tools she can use to deal with the predicament. One of the most important first steps to approaching an ethical dilemma is realizing that one exists. While Santos feels that there is a clear solution, he fails to recognize that there is more than one perspective in this situation, resulting in an ethical dilemma. By identifying that, in fact, there is no straightforward solution, Lydia has initiated the process of ethical decision making and deliberation. Both of these nurses will benefit from a study of nursing ethics.

THINK ABOUT IT

Facing Ethical Dilemmas

- What alerts you to the presence of an ethical dilemma?
- How do you feel when confronted with difficult ethical decisions?
- What resources do you use to help you deal with ethical dilemmas?

Ethics and Nursing

Nursing is a profession that deals with the most personal and private aspects of people's lives. From the beginning of time, and by definition, nurses, whether called healers, caretakers, nurturers, or nurses, have cared for those in need in a very personal and intimate way. Nurses are often attentive to patients' needs over long periods of time. They may have made home visits and may know patients' families. They may have ongoing relationships with clients at clinics and community centres. They may care for patients at their bedsides for hours and days on end. It is through the intimacy and trust inherent in the nurse–patient relationship that nurses become critical participants in the process of ethical decision making.

As participants in a dynamic profession, we are faced with ethical choices that affect the profession itself. For example, as the needs and demands of society change, the boundaries of the domain of nursing contract and expand. This forces us to make decisions about such issues as the delegation of traditional nursing functions to non-nurse caregivers and the expanding boundaries of nursing. Because nursing is a regulated profession, we are obligated to review and discipline peers. This holds many ethical implications as we attempt to balance desires to protect the public, advance the profession, and maintain professional cohesiveness.

Nurses may also be called upon to take part in decision making on a broader scale. More than ever before, we now participate as members of policy-making bodies. Community, provincial, and national task forces; committees; and boards of advisors are just some of the health care decision-making groups in which nurses have become integral and respected members. It is imperative for nurses who participate in decision making at this level to be aware of the ethical implications of the decisions, particularly decisions dealing with the fair allocation of resources. These decisions affect both individuals and populations and, as such, compel those involved to cautiously deliberate every decision. A working knowledge of ethical theory enhances our ability to deal with difficult ethical dilemmas by helping us to appreciate diverse perspectives, to explore rationales and interests that may be markedly different from our own, and to understand our own approach to these kinds of complex issues. While knowledge of ethical theory does not guarantee that ethical decision making will necessarily be easier, it helps to ensure that an ethical dilemma does not become an ethical impasse.

PHILOSOPHY

Philosophy is the intense and critical examination of beliefs and assumptions. It is both natural and necessary to humanity. Philosophy gives coherence to the whole realm of thought and experience. It offers principles for deciding what actions and qualities are most worthwhile. Philosophy may also make apparent inconsistency in meaning and context (Kneller, 1971). There are many philosophical schools of thought. Because of the nature of philosophy, it is impossible to verify philosophic beliefs or theories; nevertheless, the study of philosophy helps give order and coherence to beliefs and assumptions. It gives shape to what would otherwise be a random chaos of thoughts, beliefs, assumptions, values, and superstitions.

Philosophers examine questions dealing with life's most important aspects. Typical questions include the following: What is the meaning of life? Is there a God? What is reality? What is the essence of knowledge? How can something be known? What is happiness? What is the ideal or virtuous human character? How can one understand human beliefs, values, and morals? Questions such as these have been asked by the most widely studied philosophers. Buddha asked, "How can one find the path that leads to the end of suffering?" Confucius asked, "What is the remedy for social disorder?" Socrates asked, "How should one live?" Through the centuries, philosophy has been concerned with topics that define the essence of human life. Martin Buber said, "With soaring power [man] reaches out beyond what is given him, flies beyond the horizon and the familiar stars, and grasps a totality" (1965, p. 61).

Ayn Rand, author and social philosopher, expressed her thoughts eloquently when she wrote the following:

> A philosophic system is an integrated view of existence. As a human
> being, you have no choice about the fact that you need a philosophy.

Your only choice is whether you define your philosophy by a conscious, rational, disciplined process of thought and scrupulously logical deliberation—or let your subconscious accumulate a junk heap of unwarranted conclusions, false generalizations, . . . undefined wishes, doubts and fears, thrown together by chance, but integrated by your subconscious into a kind of mongrel philosophy and fused into a single weight: self doubt, like a ball and chain in the place where your mind's wings should have grown. (1982, p. 5)

Raphael (1994) describes philosophy as essentially divided into two branches: the philosophy of knowledge and the philosophy of practice. The philosophy of knowledge is attentive to the critical examination of assumptions about matters of fact and argument. Included in this branch are epistemology (the study of knowledge), metaphysics (the study of ultimate reality), philosophy of science, philosophy of the mind, and philosophical logic. Philosophy of practice, on the other hand, focuses on the critical examination of assumptions about norms or values and includes ethics, social and political philosophy, and philosophy of law. It is philosophy of practice, particularly moral philosophy, that provides the groundwork for discussion of many of the troubling issues that nurses must face.

Ethical theory provides a framework to guide cohesive and consistent ethical reasoning and decision making. This chapter is devoted to an examination of the two ethical theories that have had the greatest influence on contemporary bioethics: utilitarianism and deontology. A description of virtue or character ethics is also included. There are many ethical theories, some more sound than others, and some consisting of combinations of other theories. Theories related specifically to resource allocation, such as libertarianism, are described in Chapter 15. Nurses who are interested in a more detailed examination of specific theories should read works by the original theorists as well as analysis by contemporary writers.

MORALS/ETHICS

Ethics is concerned with the study of social morality and with philosophical reflection on its norms and practices. Moral issues are those that are essential, basic, or important, and deal with important social values or norms, such as respect for life, freedom, and love; issues that provoke the conscience or such feelings as guilt, shame, self-esteem, courage, or hope; issues we respond to with words like *ought, should, right, wrong, good, bad;* and issues that are uncommonly complicated, frustrating, unresolvable, or difficult in some indefinable way (Jameton, 1984). Morality refers to traditions or beliefs about right and wrong conduct (Beauchamp & Walters, 1999). Morality is a social and cultural institution with a history and a code of learnable rules. Morality exists before we are taught its rules—we learn about them as we grow up (Beauchamp, 2001). **Moral philosophy** is the philosophical discussion of what is considered good or bad, right or wrong, in terms of moral issues.

Ethics addresses the question, "What should I do in this situation?" Ethics offers a formal process for applying moral philosophy. The study of ethics gives us a basis for making thoughtful and consistent decisions. These decisions may be based upon morality or formal moral theory. In the end, though, ethics does not tell us what we ought to do. We must decide that for ourselves.

Philosophical Basis for Ethical Theory

Unlike mathematics or other empirical sciences, there are no clear and absolute rules governing ethics. Mathematicians can say for certain that two plus two always equals four, regardless of the time factors, circumstances, feelings, or beliefs of those involved in the calculations. Ethical rules are less clear, and are difficult or impossible to prove. For example, while some people believe that killing for any reason is always wrong, others might argue that euthanasia can be beneficial either for the individual or the society, that abortion to save the life of the mother is permissible, or that killing during war or for purposes of self-defence is justified. There are reasonable arguments, based upon opposing viewpoints, to support any of these beliefs. How can rational people reach such different conclusions? The answer to this question may lie in the particular perspectives of the people involved.

Ethical theories are derived from either of two basic schools of thought: **naturalism** or **rationalism**. An examination of these perspectives will help clarify the various theories.

ASK YOURSELF

What Is Your Personal Code of Ethics?

- Do you believe that there are some actions that are absolutely wrong in all circumstances? Why?
- Do you believe that you have an innate knowledge of right and wrong?
- How did you learn right and wrong? What was the influence of your parents? Society? Other forces

Naturalism. **Naturalism** is a view of moral judgment that regards ethics as being dependent upon human nature and psychology. Naturalism attributes differences in moral codes to social conditions, while suggesting that there is a basic congruence related to the possession, by nearly all people, of similar underlying psychological tendencies (Raphael, 1994). These similarities suggest that there is universality (or near-universality) in moral judgment. This viewpoint allows each group or person to make judgments based upon feelings about particular actions in particular situations. It further suggests that most people's judgments in similar circumstances will be much alike. Naturalism does not explain what others may consider to be aberrant, selfish, or cruel choices that are made by apparently rational people.

Naturalism holds that, collectively, all people have a tendency to make similar ethical decisions. Though there are many value differences among cultures, the variations are not as great as they may seem. Most people desire to be happy, to experience pleasure, and to avoid pain. There seems to be a natural tendency to sympathize with the wishes and feelings of others and, as a consequence, to approve of helping people in need. Raphael outlines similarities among cultures:

> All societies think that it is wrong to hurt members of their own group at least (or to kill them unless there are morally compelling reasons); that it is right to keep faith; that the needy should be helped; that people who deliberately flout the accepted rules should be punished. (1994, p. 16)

Raphael points to **sympathy** as a motivating factor in moral decision making. Sympathy is the sharing, in imagination, of other people's feelings. This entails imagining ourselves in the shoes of the other and consequently sharing their feelings. Sympathy involves such feelings as pleasure, the tendency have positive feelings about one who has pleased another, pain, and the tendency to feel hostile toward one who has caused pain to another. Sympathy, according to some, is a natural tendency and is the basis for moral reasoning.

Rationalism. The opposing school of thought is **rationalism**. Rationalists argue that feelings or perceptions, though they may seem similar in many people, may not actually be similar. Rationalists believe there are absolute truths that are not dependent upon human nature. They argue that ethical values have an independent origin in the nature of the universe, and can become known to humans through the process of reasoning. Rationalists believe there are truths about the world that are necessary and universal, and that these truths are superior to the information that we receive from our senses (Raphael, 1994).

To rationalists, moral rules are necessarily true. Rationalists see the knowledge gained through the senses as only contingently true (Raphael, 1994). For example, the grass is *perceived* as green, but the actual colour may be different—or may be seen as different by some. One who feels bad when hearing of the misfortune of another may not feel the same way about all others. On the other hand, moral or ethical rules, originating from a higher source and being free of the variances in human nature, are always true. For example, rationalists argue that it is good to help those in need, and the truth of this maxim will not change based upon different circumstances or perceptions.

The differences between the two schools of thought revolve around the question of the origin of ethics. Is ethics a matter of feeling, or of reason? Are individuals free to make ethical choices based upon predictable human nature, or is the foundation of ethics based upon universal or theological truth? The comparison between naturalism and rationalism is seen clearly in the study of ethical theories. We are challenged to consider these two viewpoints when learning about ethical theory.

THEORIES OF ETHICS

Moral philosophy is the branch of philosophy that examines beliefs and assumptions about the nature of certain human values. Ethics is the practical application of moral philosophy; that is, given the moral context of good or bad, right or wrong, *"What ought one to do in a given situation?"* The philosopher reveals an integrated global vision in which elements, like pieces of a puzzle, have a logical fit. By developing theories of ethics, the philosopher hopes to explain values and behaviours related to cultural and moral norms. Each theory is based upon the particular viewpoint of the individual philosopher, and maintains, within itself, philosophical consistency. The discussion related to naturalism and rationalism explains, in part, one basic difference among moral philosophers. We chose utilitarianism and deontology for inclusion in this chapter because they are two of the major theories central to medicine, nursing, and bioethics.

CASE PRESENTATION

Conflicting Duties

Hannah is the director of a visiting hospice outreach service for a large rural area. This week, she received notice that funding to the hospice service from the provincial governments was being drastically decreased. Without this funding, cuts must be made in the services provided to clients. When Hannah meets with the advisory board, they agree that one of two programs must be eliminated in order to cope with the decreased funding. One program is a common outreach program that provides assistance with activities of daily living for clients. This program helps a large number of clients, has been in place for many years and is consistently inexpensive to run. The other program is more innovative and costly, providing an opportunity for clients with highly complex and specific needs to get their nursing care at home, instead of visiting the local hospital on a regular basis, for specialized services. This program benefits a very few clients but does so in a significant way. While Hannah and the board recognize the importance of helping with complex, specific needs of the few, they are hesitant to advise eliminating a program that has been proven to help large numbers of clients.

THINK ABOUT IT

- What kinds of factors should Hannah and the board consider when making their decision? Why?

- What is the responsibility of the board to the large number of clients who would be denied assistance with daily living activities if the first program was eliminated?

- How would you decide what to do in this situation? What would you use to guide your decision making?

- As you continue to learn about the following ethical theories, return to thinking about this case and comment on what a utilitarian or a deontologist might do, and why?

Utilitarianism

Utilitarianism, sometimes called **consequentialism**, is a form of teleological theory. "Telos" comes from the Greek and literally means "end." Utilitarianism is the moral theory that holds that an action is judged as good or bad in relation to the consequence, outcome, or end result derived from it. Utilitarianism is an important ethical philosophy that has its basis in naturalism. According to the utilitarian school of thought, the right action is that which has greatest **utility** or usefulness. No action is, in itself, good or bad. Utilitarians hold that the only factors that make actions good or bad are the outcomes, or end results, that are derived from them. Utilitarianism is, essentially, forward looking. In other words, a utilitarian is always looking into the future, assessing the potential outcomes and consequences of various courses of action, and considering factors such as motivation, intention, or reasons behind actions to be irrelevant in assessing the ethical soundness of a proposed action.

"Utilitarianism" is a broad term that relates to a number of important theories. One of the first utilitarians was the Roman philosopher Epicurus, whose teachings date to about 300–200 B.C.E. Epicurus believed that both good and evil lie in sensation, pleasure being good and pain being evil. He taught that pleasure could be gained by living a life of moderation, courage, and justice, and by cultivating friendship. Epicurus also believed that deities dwelt apart from humans, and were not concerned with the state of human existence; that therefore, humans control their own destinies (Honderich, 1995).

There was a rebirth of interest in utilitarian philosophy in the late eighteenth and early nineteenth centuries. Jeremy Bentham (1748–1832), a leading political philosopher of that time, is considered to be the father of modern utilitarianism. According to Bentham's theory, actions can be considered to be right when they increase happiness and diminish misery, and can be considered to be wrong when they have the opposite effect. Following is Bentham's definition of the "principle of utility":

> By utility is meant that property in any object, whereby it tends to produce benefit, advantage, pleasure, good, or happiness … or … to prevent the happening of mischief, pain, evil, or unhappiness to the party whose interest is considered: if that party be the community in general, then the happiness of the community: if a particular individual, then the happiness of that individual. (Bentham, 1948, p. 2)

Bentham attempted to create a science derived from the principle of utility. He proposed that we should measure the product of an act in terms of the value of a proposed pleasure. Six criteria used to measure the pleasure included intensity, duration, certainty, propinquity (nearness in place or time), fecundity (the chance of it being followed by more sensations of the same kind), and purity (the chance of it not being followed by sensations of the opposite kind). Bentham proposed that each criterion be given a value, and that the sum of the values related to the pleasure be weighed against a similar sum of values related to the pain that might result from any given act. The person should act in accordance with the result of this mathematical formula, resolving ethical decisions based upon the sum total of the value of a given act.

Many critics describe Bentham as having a purely hedonistic tendency, as his theory is often referred to as hedonistic utilitarianism. **Hedonism** can be defined as the pursuit of pleasure as the highest achievable ***good***. We see, though, that Bentham is interested in more than simply physical pleasure. He wrote that *pleasure* is synonymous with many other terms such as *good, profit, advantage, benefit,* and so forth. In fact, his interest in the common good of the community refutes those who charge that his theory is hedonistic. He describes a type of justice in which action should have a tendency to augment the happiness of the community as a whole, rather than diminish it.

John Stuart Mill (1806–1873) was a leading nineteenth-century British moral philosopher. Like Bentham, Mill was a utilitarian. He described utilitarianism in terms of judging acts according to the end result. He wrote, "All action is for the sake of some end; and rules of action, it seems natural to suppose, must take their whole character and colour from the end to which they are subservient" (Mill, 1910, p. 2). The phrase *"the end justifies the means"* relates to Mill's theory. According to Mill, the only right actions are those that produce the greatest happiness. His "greatest happiness principle" holds that the right action in conduct is not the agent's own happiness, but the happiness of all concerned. He further believed that sacrifice is good only when it increases the total sum of happiness. For Mill, the object of virtue is the multiplication of happiness. He cautioned, however, that we must carefully attempt to avoid violating the rights of some people in the process of maximizing the happiness of others.

Mill defined his concepts in ways that make the meaning of this theory clearer. He described happiness as a state of pleasure that is not restricted to physical pleasure alone. In fact, Mill made a strong argument in favour of prioritizing pleasures, with intellectual pleasure having greater priority than physical or hedonistic pleasure. Further, Mill condemned those who chose sensual indulgences to the detriment of health. He described the greatest sources of physical and mental suffering as "indigence, disease, and the unkindness, worthlessness, or premature loss, of objects of affection" (Mill, 1910, p. 14).

There are two basic types of utilitarianism. **Act utilitarianism** suggests that people choose actions that will, in any given circumstance, increase the overall good. **Rule utilitarianism**, on the other hand, suggests that people choose rules that, when followed consistently, will maximize the overall good.

Act utilitarianism. Act utilitarianism states that, when faced with a choice, the action should be chosen that, in that specific situation, will increase the overall good. The act utilitarian measures, or calculates, the overall good produced in a single act only, rather than considering what would happen if the single act was carried out over and over again, that is, treated as a rule. Therefore, act utilitarianism can allow for different, and sometimes opposing, actions in different situations. For example, while act utilitarians probably believe that it is best to tell the truth (or keep promises, or avoid killing, and so on), they recognize that there are times when the overall consequences will be better for everyone concerned if this guideline is not followed, even if the rights of some individuals are violated (Beauchamp & Childress, 2008; Smart, 1997). Act utilitarians recognize that tenets such as "lying is wrong" should be treated as guidelines rather than strict rules.

Rule utilitarianism. Rule utilitarianism, on the other hand, suggests that people should act according to rules that tend to maximize happiness and diminish unhappiness in terms of outcomes. Rule utilitarianism requires that people tell the truth (keep promises, avoid killing, and so on) in all circumstances, because the overall good is maximized by consistently following such rules. An example of rule utilitarian thinking regarding truth telling comes from the writing of Dr. Worthington Hooker, a prominent nineteenth century figure in medical ethics:

> The good, which may be done by deception in a few cases, is almost as nothing, compared with the evil which it does in many, when the prospect of its doing good was just as promising as it was in those in which it succeeded. And when we add to this the evil which would result from a general adoption of a system of deception, the importance of a strict adherence to the truth in our intercourse with the sick, even on the ground of expediency, becomes incalculably great.
>
> (Hooker, W. as cited in Beauchamp & Childress, 2008, p. 340)

The argument of this rule utilitarian was that even though the patient's health is sometimes maximized through the use of deception, a widespread use of deception will eventually cause more harm than good. Thus, though rule utilitarians recognize that in some instances good might result from a particular act, in the end, the overall good is maximized by the strict following of rules in all situations.

In other words, in some cases, the rule utilitarian will act in a way that, for example, the act utilitarian would not approve, as the good consequences of a particular act are not maximized. This is because the rule utilitarian seeks to follow the rule that will, overall, maximize good even though, in some specific cases, it might not lead to a decision that maximizes good.

Though utilitarianism is a widely accepted ethical theory, there are a few problems inherent in its use. Utilitarianism does not give sufficient thought to respect of persons. In fact, it is possible that harm can be done to minority groups or individuals in the name of overall good. It gives little recognition to the principle of autonomy, particularly when we consider utilitarian decision making relative to distributive justice. Critics argue that utilitarianism sacrifices the rights of individuals in favour of the overall good.

Other limitations that are cited when referring to utilitarianism include the difficulty with defining what constitutes happiness or a "good" outcome. In a diverse world, there are many subjective and variable ideas about what defines a "good" consequence. When we consider the practical application of a utilitarian ethical theory, we also realize that our ability to accurately predict the future consequences of actions is limited and that many times, there are unpredictable or unforeseeable factors that influence outcomes.

Many people criticize utilitarian approaches for aiming solely to optimize pleasure or happiness without considering that there may be other values that we should seek to optimize; there may be other values that are just as or more important than our own satisfaction or happiness.

Finally, utilitarianism provides no room for special relationships or interests. In evaluating what constitutes a "good" outcome, the interests of one person are considered as equal to those of any other person. This notion was revolutionary at its inception: a time of strong hierarchy, stringent notions of class and socioeconomic status, and feudal law. However, today, it is recognized that in some contexts and relationships, persons have and should be given special consideration or priority. Utilitarianism simply does not provide for this.

Even though there are problems inherent in utilitarianism, this ethical theory captures the imagination as an attractive moral philosophy. Its appeal lies in the simple precept of promoting happiness for as many people as possible. It is particularly useful as a method of deciding issues of distributive justice.

ASK YOURSELF

Is Utilitarianism Useful?

- What useful guidelines does utilitarianism provide in terms of distributing resources?

- To what degree is it permissible to sacrifice the rights of one to provide for the welfare of many?

- To what degree is it permissible to sacrifice the rights of many to provide for the welfare of one?

- Think about the strengths and weaknesses of utilitarianism in today's health care environments.

CASE PRESENTATION

Martin is a public health nurse in a large urban centre. This week there has been an outbreak of viral coughs, fever, and flu in the downtown community. Fearing a potential pandemic, public health has taken the extreme precaution of asking all health care professionals who work in acute care centres, or in public health involved in direct client care, to be quarantined when not at work. Martin is allowed to drive to work and home again but is prohibited to leave the house or have visitors at his home at all other times until the outbreak is controlled or the quarantine is deemed no longer necessary. While it is an extreme precaution, Martin knows that these kinds of measures are necessary to prevent further spread of an unknown viral illness and adheres strictly to the guidelines for quarantine.

(Continued)

Leila is also a nurse in public health who is on home–work quarantine. While she also recognizes the importance of the quarantine, she is anxious to visit her mother, who lives a few kilometres from her house. She thinks to herself, "Well, no one will know and besides, who could it hurt? I'm only going to visit my mother for an hour and then I'll go straight home."

THINK ABOUT IT

- What kinds of factors should Hannah and the board consider when making their decision? Why?
- How is quarantine justified, from a utilitarian perspective?
- From a utilitarian perspective, is Leila's rationale for not following quarantine guidelines acceptable? Why or why not?
- How would you decide what to do in this situation? What ethical theories or principles would guide your actions?

Deontology

Deontological theories of ethics are based upon the rationalist view that the rightness or wrongness of an act depends upon the nature of the act, rather than its consequences. The term **deontology** is taken from the Greek word for "duty." Occasionally, deontology is called **formalism**; some writers refer to this type of ethical theory as **Kantianism**. Kantianism is based upon the writings of the German philosopher Immanuel Kant, who shaped many deontological formulations. For the purpose of this chapter, the terms *deontology* and *Kantian ethics* are used interchangeably.

Kant was born at Königsberg, Prussia, in 1724. After an uninspiring academic career, he surprised the world with his groundbreaking ethical theory. Late in his life, Kant published volumes of philosophical writings that shook the religious and political systems of his day, and continue to have strong influence on contemporary ethical philosophy. Kant contended that ethical rules are universal, and that humans can derive certain consistent principles to guide action. The awareness of these moral rules is the product of pure reason, rather than experience, as naturalists would maintain. Kant asserted that moral rules are absolute and apply to all people, for all times, in all situations. He believed that ethical rules could be known by rational humans. Knowledge of the right course of action in any given situation could be obtained by following a maxim that he called the **Categorical Imperative**. *Categorical* refers to moral rules that do not admit exceptions; *imperative* denotes a command that is derived from principle. Kant said there is only one Categorical Imperative:

> Act only according to that maxim by which you can at the same time will that it should become a universal law. (1959, p. 39)

In other words, when making a decision, one should imagine that, in all similar cases, the same decision should be made. As an example, Kant related a moral problem in which a man needs money to feed his family. He knows that he will not be able to repay it, but knows that nothing will be lent to him if he does not promise to repay it at a certain time. In order to satisfy himself that the act of breaking the promise to repay the money is morally correct, the man asks himself the question, "Should every person always make promises which they know will not be fulfilled?" Through reasoning, the man can see that this could not become a universal law, because no one would ever believe what has been promised. As a consequence, promise-making would hold no meaning. Kant gave similar examples of situations related to suicide, squandering of talent, and helping others. Rather than compile a list of specific ethical rules, Kant proposed that each rational person should use the test of the Categorical Imperative to guide his or her actions.

Following after the first formulation of the Categorical Imperative, Kant also described the a second formulation, which directs persons to do the following:

> Act so that you treat humanity, whether in your own person or that of another, always as an end and never as a means only. (1959, p. 47)

To treat another person as a means according to Kant, is to use another person to fulfil your own needs or meet your own agenda. However, to treat a person as an end is to make their needs, agenda, or desires ends in themselves, and work toward them as you might work toward fulfilling your own needs or desires. Raphael (1994) makes the point that Kant's second formulation of the Categorical Imperative automatically shows that domination of one person over another is morally wrong. Domination makes no allowance for the dominated person's power of decision-making. He also notes that acting toward another as you would toward yourself mandates that, whenever possible, you must help people who need help. The second formulation of the Categorical Imperative requires that we must fulfil certain duties owed to others, while keeping their needs foremost.

Following the first and second formulations of the Categorical Imperative, the third formulation implies that each person is a member of a *realm* or *kingdom of ends*. Kant calls this "a systematic union of rational beings through common objective laws" (1959, p. 51). This requires that we act as members of a community of equal and autonomous individuals, and that each member treats all others as moral beings, as both ends and means in themselves. Each person should have regard for the desires of others, and allow them freedom of decision; in other words, respect their autonomous decisions. In Kantian theory, there is an inherent recognition that all rational people are equal, and equally competent to make autonomous, universal decisions. According to Raphael (1994), "Kantian ethics is in fact an ethics of democracy. It requires liberty, equality, and fraternity" (p. 57).

Deontology also implies that ethics are derived from fulfilling duties. When judging the ethical soundness of a proposed action, we are always backward looking. In other words, one must always pay particular attention to the duties that lie behind our proposed actions, which motivate or drive us. An ethical person must act for the sake of duty or obligation. Kant believed that all *imperatives of duty* could be deduced from the first formulation of the categorical imperative (one should act as if one's actions could become universal law for all people) and must also comply with the second formulation (treat all people as ends, none as means to an end). Deontology does not require that we never look forward to the possible consequences or results of possible actions, merely that we attend to the duties that underpin our actions, thereby making our actions ethically sound. Kant also believed that an action done from duty has its moral worth based upon reverence for the law and carrying out one's duty, rather than the results or outcomes of the act (Paton, 1961). Most professional codes of ethics are based upon Kantian principles. Nurses' codes of ethics stress the importance of fulfilling duties that are inherently owed to patients, and the importance of preserving the dignity and autonomy of each individual patient.

There are some acknowledged weaknesses with the practical application of deontological ethics. It has been noted to be exceptionless and rigid, with no acknowledgment of special relationships and subsequent duties that result. Deontologists do not tell us how to decide between conflicting duties. Often, nurses find that they have clear, ethical duties that seem to present conflicts. How do we decide which duty has priority? Deontologists, such as Kant, offer little advice, noting only that a rational person will simply know his or her duties.

Finally, it does seem reasonable to assume that by failing to consider the possible consequences of given actions, we might create difficult, if not tragic or disastrous, situations.

Like utilitarianism, deontology is an attractive ethical theory. It is, in fact, a most popular foundation for many contemporary beliefs. It provides clear guidelines for judging the rightness or wrongness of action. It recognizes the dignity and autonomy of individuals, and allows all people equal consideration. It serves as a basis for much of the contemporary ethical thinking that guides health care delivery.

CASE PRESENTATION

Weighing Rights and Duties in Questions of Justice

Sumiko is the home health nurse for Mrs. Bingham, an eighty-nine-year-old widow who lives in the home that she and her husband shared until his death five years earlier. Mrs. Bingham suffers from severe rheumatoid arthritis and has a new colostomy. The colostomy was performed as a last resort for severe ulcerative colitis. Mrs. Bingham is unable to care for herself because of the advanced state of her arthritis. Her daughter, son-in-law, and two teenage grandchildren moved into her home to take care of her daily needs. After many months, the family feels that caring for the elderly woman has become an unbearable burden. They ask Sumiko to help arrange long-term care in a local nursing home. Mrs. Bingham wants to continue to live in her home.

THINK ABOUT IT

Whose Rights Are More Important?

- Does Mrs. Bingham have the right to stay in her home, even if the entire family is made unhappy by her presence?
- According to deontology, what factors must the family consider in deciding?
- To whom does Sumiko owe a duty?
- To what degree should the rights of the other family members bear on the decision that Sumiko makes?
- Apply the categorical imperative to Sumiko's options.
- What would you do if you were Sumiko? On what basis would you make your decision?

Virtue Ethics

Virtue ethics, sometimes called **character ethics**, represents the idea that the actions of individuals are based upon a certain degree of innate moral virtue. First noted in the writings of Homer, and subsequently in the works of Plato, Aristotle, and Socrates, the idea of cardinal virtues emerged: wisdom, courage, temperance, justice, generosity, faith, hope, and charity (Kitwood, 1990). Modern and contemporary writers also include such virtues as honesty, compassion, caring, conscientiousness, responsibility, integrity, discernment, trustworthiness, and prudence. Virtue ethics is re-emerging as an important framework for examining ethical decision making and behaviour.

The concept of virtue ethics presents a challenge to deontological and utilitarian theories. These theories conceive of the demands of morality similarly; ethics provides guidelines to action that begins with the question, *"What ought we to do?"* (Beauchamp, 2001). In contrast, virtue ethics does not ask this question; instead, it posits that the basic function of morality is the moral character of persons and it shifts the focus from the action to the character of the actor. In doing so, it also moves away from the external to a greater involvement of self, persons, and relationships (Gardiner, 2003). Beauchamp (2001) suggests that virtues should not be thought of as moral require-ments, because this confuses them with principles or rules. Rather, we could say that virtues are character traits that are socially valued. A *moral* virtue is a character trait that is morally valued, such as truthfulness, kindness, or honesty. A person with moral virtue has both consistent moral action and a morally appropriate desire.

The term "ethics" was derived from Aristotle's word *ethika,* which refers to matters having to do with character. Aristotle (384–332 B.C.E.) considered goodness of character to be produced by the practice of virtuous behaviour, rather than virtuous acts being the end result of a good character. According to Aristotle, virtues are tendencies to act, feel, and judge that are developed from a natural capacity by proper training and exercise. He believed that practice creates a habit of acting in a virtuous way, and that virtue can be learned and improved. Virtue, according to Aristotle, depends on "clear judgment, self-control, symmetry of desire, and artistry of means" (Durant, 1926, p. 75). He considered virtue to be the fruit of intelligent pursuit. "It is not the possession of the simple [person], nor the gift of innocent intent, but the achievement of experience in the fully developed [person]" (Durant, p. 75). He considered excellence to be won by training and habituation, and believed that virtuous character is created by repeatedly acting in a virtuous manner. Aristotle provided three criteria for traits of a virtuous character:

First, virtuous acts must be chosen for their own sake. Second, choice must proceed from a firm and unchangeable character. Finally, virtue is a disposition to choose the mean.

Aristotle did not make a list, *per se,* of actual traits but did discuss moral habits or behaviours such as courage, temperance, and justice. For him, the basic moral question was not "what should one *do*" but rather "what should one *be*" (Mayo, 1958).

The third criterion refers to a mean. The *golden mean* of virtuous behaviour, for Aristotle, meant practising moderation: avoiding both excess and deficiency. To put it simply, virtuous habits should be exercised in a *moderate* way. Consider the following examples. Honesty is considered by many to be a virtue. However, to be not truthful enough (deficient) means that one would be deceptive. On the other hand, to be too truthful would imply that someone might be too forthright. Neither deception nor absolute forthrightness is considered virtuous. Think about this from a perspective of nursing: a deficit of honesty might result in a nurse deceiving or misinforming a patient. Alternatively, an excess of honesty might result in a breach of confidentiality. Compassion is another example of a virtuous principle. Too little compassion implies disinterest, while an excess of compassion may result in entanglement. Again, neither disinterest nor entanglement is considered to be virtuous in and of itself and both are extremes of the more moderate virtuous behaviour.

Phillipa Foot adds another perspective to Aristotle's concept of a virtuous person. Foot proposes that virtue lies not only in engaging in virtuous acts, but also in will. She defines will as "that which is wished for as well as what is sought." According to Foot, a positive or moral will is sometimes the necessary ingredient in success. She says,

> sometimes one man succeeds where another fails not because there is some specific difference in their previous conduct but rather because his heart lies in a different place; and the disposition of the heart is part of virtue. What this suggests is that a man's virtue may be judged by his innermost desires as well as by his intentions and this fits with our idea that a virtue such as generosity lies as much in someone's attitudes as in his actions. (1997, p. 330)

According to Foot, virtue is not like a skill or an art. It cannot merely be a practised and perfected act: it must actually engage the will. In other words, an act, though apparently kind or generous, for example, cannot be considered to be virtuous if the intention is not good. Although Aristotle's idea of virtue is one of hope (everyone has the capacity to learn virtuous action through exercising one's "moral muscles"), Foot makes the road to virtuous character less easily travelled.

Focal Virtues. In the discussion of virtue as related to biomedical ethics, Beauchamp and Childress note that "What often counts most in the moral life is not adherence to moral rules, but reliable character, good moral sense, and emotional responsiveness." (2008, p. 30). Like Aristotle, these authors suggest that although people have different character traits, all have the capacity to learn or cultivate those traits that are important to morality. Beauchamp and Childress propose that there are five **focal virtues** that are more pivotal than others in characterizing a virtuous person: compassion, discernment, trustworthiness, integrity, and conscientiousness. Focal virtues can be described as core virtues, or those that are central to the character of the virtuous health care professional (Beauchamp & Childress, 2008). They present these five focal virtues as underpinnings for an overarching or fundamental virtue: caring. Together, these six virtues, according to Beauchamp and Childress, "provide a moral compass of character for health professionals." (2008, p. 38).

Caring. The virtue of **caring** is a fundamental and central virtue. It influences what we do and how we do it, what motives underlie our actions, and whether we are able to promote positive relationships. Caring involves "emotional commitment to, and deep willingness to act on behalf of, persons with whom one has a significant relationship." (Beauchamp & Childress, 2008, p. 36). The following five focal virtues help in the development and orientation of caring within the context of health care.

Compassion. **Compassion** is the ability to imagine oneself in the situation of another. Beauchamp and Childress define the term in the following manner: "The virtue of compassion combines an attitude of active regard for another's welfare with an imaginative awareness and emotional response of sympathy, tenderness, and discomfort at another's misfortune or suffering" (2008, p. 38). Compassion is so important that many times the patient's need for a compassionate and caring presence outweighs the need for technical care. We must be careful, however, that compassion does not impede our ability to make objective or impartial decisions.

Discernment. The virtue of **discernment** is related to the classical concept of wisdom. "The virtue of discernment brings sensitive insight, astute judgment, and understanding to action. Discernment involves the ability to make fitting judgments and reach decisions without being unduly influenced by extraneous considerations, fears, personal attachments and the like." (Beauchamp & Childress, 2008, p. 40). Discernment gives an insight into appropriate actions in given situations. It requires sensitivity and attention attuned to the demands of a particular context. For example, a discerning nurse will recognize when a patient needs comfort and reassurance rather than privacy. Discernment requires that we continually strive to recognize and understand important nuances in human behaviour.

Trustworthiness. **Trustworthiness** is another focal virtue for nurses. "Trust itself is a confident belief in and reliance upon the moral character and competence of another person, often but not always a person with whom one has an intimate or established relationship. Trust entails a confidence that another will act with the right motives and in accordance with appropriate moral norms." (Beauchamp & Childress, 2008, p. 41). Trustworthiness is measured by others' recognition of the nurse's consistency and predictability in following moral norms. In practical terms, trustworthiness is accounted for in the reputation we have among co-workers. This virtue is important for us in relationships with patients, physicians, and other nurses.

Integrity. **Integrity** is perhaps the cardinal virtue. **Moral integrity**, according to Beauchamp and Childress , means "soundness, reliability, wholeness and integration of moral character." (2008, p. 42). Integrity refers to two parts of a person. First, it refers to the integration of all parts of a person, which can include aspects such as values and beliefs, along with emotions, wishes, and actions. Second, it encompasses the moral trait of holding steadfastly to one's values and beliefs and standing up for them, even when facing adversity. It also refers to our continuing to follow moral norms over time. A person with integrity has a consistency of convictions, actions, and emotions and is trustworthy. Integrity is compromised when the nurse acts inconsistently, or in a way that is not supported by professed moral beliefs. Deficiencies in moral integrity may include hypocrisy, insincerity, and bad faith.

Conscientiousness. A person acts in a conscientious way, according to Beauchamp and Childress (2008), if he or she consistently, with explicitly good intentions, tries to do what is right, after putting an effort into determining what constitutes the "right" choice of action. **Conscientiousness** involves significant effort and strong intentions to do what is right.

While there are many different writings on virtues, there is no set list of virtues. Ancient writings tended to consider virtues as existing on a spectrum, from excess to deficiency. For example, when considering truthfulness as a virtue, the deficient extreme is deception, while the excessive extreme is forthrightness. Similarly, in considering the virtue of compassion, the deficient extreme is disinterest, while the excessive extreme is entanglement. If we examine conscientiousness, the deficient extreme might be carelessness, contrasted with the excessive extreme of obsession. Finally, when thinking about the virtue of integrity, we can identify that the deficient extreme would be corruption, while the excessive extreme would be self-righteousness (Gardiner, 2003). Considering the virtues as existing along a spectrum demonstrates that one can have "too much" of what might be considered a good virtue, and that in turn, this excess might be just as problematic as a deficiency.

Virtue Ethics Today. How does the concept of virtue or character ethics fit with nursing today as a principled profession? It is likely that principled behaviour, while not the sole domain of a good moral character, is more likely to occur in the presence of one. Certainly Florence Nightingale thought virtue was an important trait of the good nurse and she cites this many times in her writings. Although the Nightingale Pledge was not composed by Florence Nightingale herself, the Pledge emphasizes virtues of character as outlined by Nightingale, as nurses promise purity, faith, loyalty, devotion, trustworthiness, and temperance (Miracle, 2009). Although the Pledge uses language that is considered quite dated today, the principles of maintaining confidentiality and always keeping the welfare of patients in mind still resonate with nurses today. It is reasonable to say, according to the Pledge, that good character is the cornerstone of good nursing, and that the nurse with virtue will act according to principle. If Aristotle was correct in his belief that virtue can be practised and learned, then we can learn, through practice, those acts which, by their doing, create a virtuous person.

Virtue theory is not without its limitations. One assumption is that there are shared virtues, or a kind of meta-narrative about what constitutes virtue. While many people may agree that compassion or truthfulness is a virtue, this view may be neither universal nor shared. Additionally, virtue theory assumes that all agents share a goal of becoming more virtuous as they grow and evolve. This, in turn, leads to the assumption that all people share this goal and aim of becoming as virtuous as possible. Moreover, if virtuousness does in fact, then, exist in degrees, how do we approach those with "evolving" virtuousness?

One critically important feature of virtue theory is that it shifts the locus of ethical decision making from outside the person, driven by ethical principles or theories, to the actual person, and her views, attributes, and inner motivations. This may be a more realistic view of how people make difficult ethical decisions, on the one hand. On the other hand, expecting everyone to be virtuous decision makers fails to acknowledge the fact that when motivations and emotions play a part in judgment, we may not succeed at setting those emotions aside and acting in the most virtuous way. However, it is a strength of virtue ethics theory that it recognizes that good decision making may in fact be strengthened by habit, and that virtue and virtuous character traits may be developed over time.

Feminist and Relational Ethics

Typically, traditional ethical theories have focused on abstract approaches (couched in philosophical theories) to complex ethical issues. In the past decades, feminist perspectives on ethics and bioethical issues have challenged these traditional approaches to solving moral dilemmas, which often aim to uncover the rational, just, and fair course of action or solution. Relational ethics approaches emphasize, like feminist ethics, the importance of the relationships between the "players" in ethical dilemmas.

Many of the potential problem-solving methods and plausible outcomes to moral dilemmas from traditional perspectives, such as utilitarianism or deontology, tend to focus on justice and the rights of persons, and not attend to issues of power or the nature of relationships. Relational ethics requires that we focus on *the relationship* as the significant and central aspect of healthcare ethics. Rather than being considered as oppositional to other ethical theories or models of ethical decision-making, relational ethics claims to, instead, build upon the strengths of other ethical theories, principles, and decision-making models to create a more modern, inclusive approach with an emphasis on relationships (Bergum & Dossetor, 2005). Bergum and Dossetor state that the defining nature of health care professions lies in the relationships that health care professionals engage in and demonstrate commitments to. However, these fundamental relationships are often overshadowed by the more demanding and more obvious kinds of issues in modern health care that tend to be more individualistic in nature: consumer and rights-based movements in health care, new technologies, legal and bureaucratic processes, and the protection of the autonomous choices of individuals. Without attention to the kinds of relationships health professionals engage in, the **ethical space** or the place where ethical practice can occur, is virtually ignored. While more traditional ethical theories such as deontology or utilitarianism focus on principles, these principles take actual shape and animation and are, essentially, brought to life through an emphasis on relationships (Bergum & Dossetor, 2005). Relational ethics, as outlined by Bergum and Dossetor, emphasizes four major themes: *mutual respect, engagement, embodiment and environment* (Read Paul, n.d.). Mutual respect is characterized by an interactive respect for, and attention to, difference. Engagement refers to a quality of a relationship in which there is striving for authenticity and connection. Embodiment refers to the relationship in which not only is the person treated in a holistic manner but there is consideration of emotion, and of subjective experiences, alongside more empirical or scientific knowledge. Finally, the theme of environment refers to the inevitable relationships that individuals engage in, which connect them to larger social groups, systems, and communities (Bergum & Dossetor, 2005). Relational ethics is an important ethical theory for nurses, since the relationships we have with our patients are ones that, by their very nature and intentionality, are always morally relevant (Austin, Lemermeyer, Goldberg, Bergum & Johnson, 2005).

Feminist ethics theorists posit that ethical dilemmas, especially in social constructs such as health care, are often laden with issues of power and an imbalance of power. Along with those using relational ethics, they say that when considering an ethical situation, one must attend to the relationships between the persons involved, and to the consequent power differentials, perceptions of hierarchy, marginalization, or oppression of persons involved (Keatings & Smith, 2000; Sherwin, 1992).

 THINK ABOUT IT

Consider the case of an illiterate woman, Grace, without legal status, who is new to Canada, faced with a complex health system that is difficult to access and navigate, who has a sick child. Her visa as a visitor has expired and she cannot return to her country of origin. She knows that there is a local medical clinic near the shelter where she is currently living, but has no idea if they will see her, since she has no identification and no money. She has a small network of people who help her out, and they have identified that her child is very ill and should see a doctor immediately. They cannot reach the physician who comes to the shelter once a week in time for her child to be seen today.

Consider that she is a refugee from a country where she has endured civil unrest and, along with other women in her family, has been physically beaten and oppressed with a threat of rape or further violence if she remained in her country of origin. This is not an unrealistic or unusual case. When faced with barriers to accessing care for her child—barriers that may include her own gender; her poor comprehension of English and inability to read or understand in a predominantly English-speaking system; her illegal status; her fear of being uncovered as a person without legal status; and her feeling that she would take significant personal risks to access care for her child—all these things make her vulnerable.

Add to that the oppression and violence she endured in her home country, and her resulting fear of males in authority positions. The relationships she has experienced and those that she might experience as part of her health care experience are clearly all important to sort through when considering her case from a perspective of feminist ethics.

- What kinds of issues make Grace *most* vulnerable, in your opinion?

- Grace does not have provincial coverage for health care, as she is not a citizen, landed immigrant, or permanent resident. Her lack of legal status is not her fault, as she has emigrated here to escape torture and possibly death for herself and her children. Do you think it is fair that she, technically, cannot access adequate health care? What would a feminist ethicist say?

- If you were a nurse who first encountered Grace in a local medical clinic, how would you go about making her comfortable and addressing her needs? What are the priorities?

That ethical approaches such as utilitarianism or deontology do not allow for considerations of important contextual issues, like past experiences, relationships, or vulnerability, as is clear in the case above. The traditional theories fail to acknowledge or address issues of vulnerability, the nature of special relationships (e.g., mother and child, adult child and elderly parent), and caring roles and duties, often traditionally taken on by women in society and unrecognized as unique and important in history. Often classified as systematic and based on primarily male-biased perspectives, these traditional ethical theories are seen to be limited in their usefulness for approaching the kinds of complex, contextual, relational, and sometimes gendered health care dilemmas that arise in the modern world.

CASE PRESENTATION

Mr. Wey is an eighty-three-year-old retired bus driver who is being seen in the respirology clinic today, as he has had some unusual shortness of breath over the past few weeks, accompanied by transient pain and discomfort. He is

(Continued)

accompanied by his wife and by his son, Francis, who is a physician in the radiology department of the same hospital.

When the tests are completed and Mr. Wey is getting changed down the hall, Mr. Wey's son Francis asks the respirologist what, if anything, was found in his father's tests. The respirologist and Francis are close colleagues, and the respirologist looks concerned. He quietly discloses to Francis that they have found a significantly large growth in his father's lungs and it is likely cancerous. He wants to schedule more tests, a biopsy, and likely surgery, as soon as possible. He asks Francis if he agrees with the proposed course of treatment and the two physicians engage in a discussion of the course of treatment. Francis explains the details of the discussion, briefly, to his mother.

After a few minutes of discussion, Mr. Wey's wife and son ask that the doctor not tell Mr. Wey his diagnosis now. They inform him that they have a family trip planned, on a cruise ship and then at a resort in the southern United States. The trip will take about a month and a half. Mrs. Wey tells the doctor that they have been saving for this trip for two years. They will finally be able to see their eldest daughter again, who has been overseas and estranged from them for over ten years, and meet their only grandchildren for the first time.

Francis also adds that Mr. Wey has a history of depression and alcohol abuse, which has been very hard on the family and especially their eldest daughter, who left home because of the strained relationship with her father. Francis feels that it is a good idea to withhold the information from his father at this time, to let him enjoy his family trip and then, upon his return, inform him and begin treatment.

Before Mr. Wey returns, the family and his physician quickly agree not to tell him until after his trip. They feel that by allowing him to enjoy his trip and reconnect with his daughter, they are acting in his best interest.

THINK ABOUT IT

- What would a deontologist do, and why?
- What would a utilitarian recommend, and why?
- What virtues should the family and physician exercise in making a decision?
- What ethical principles are most important to consider in this situation?
- Should the physician have shared the patient's information with his son without first telling the patient? Why or why not?
- Mr. Wey's son and the respirologist are close colleagues. Is this a justifiable reason for disclosing information about Mr. Wey without his consent?

- If you were the physician, would you tell Mr. Wey of his diagnosis? How would you justify your decision?

- Think about Mr. Wey's perspective. How might he feel, in either case, if he is told right now or after his trip?

SUMMARY

Ethical theory helps us understand the origin and process of ethical and moral thinking and behaviour. Two theories are particularly important to nursing ethics. The ethical theory of utilitarianism was developed in part by Jeremy Bentham, and later refined by John Stuart Mill. Utilitarianism suggests that ethical decisions should be made in regard to the outcome or end result. Accordingly, no action in itself is inherently right or wrong. This theory also provides for the greatest good for the greatest number. Utilitarianism is particularly useful in situations of distributive justice but tends to ignore the rights of the minority or the individual.

Deontology, or Kantian ethics, was initially developed by Immanuel Kant. This theory, through the use of the categorical imperative, assists one in making ethical decisions. The categorical imperative demands that the agent ask the question, *Can this action be a law for all people in all circumstances?* Additionally, the theory presents the practical imperative, which requires that we treat all individuals as if they were ends only, rather than means. Kantian ethics provides clear guidelines for making ethical decisions, but does not provide for making decisions when there are conflicting duties or obligations.

Virtue, or character, ethics, as described by Aristotle, describes each person as capable of practising and learning virtue through repetition of virtuous acts. Thus, the virtuous person is one in whom virtue is habituated. Virtue ethics complements other ethical theories, and can be used to nurture or predict character in individuals.

Relational ethics offers a more modern and nursing-relevant ethical theory, with emphasis on the relationships that are fundamental. Ethical theories can help us understand ethical decision-making models, and assist in developing a cohesive and logical system for making individual decisions.

CHAPTER HIGHLIGHTS

- Philosophy is the intense and critical examination of beliefs and assumptions.

- Moral philosophy is the philosophical discussion of what is considered to be good or bad, right or wrong.

- Ethics is a formal process for making logical and consistent decisions, based upon moral philosophy.

- As the morally central health care profession, nursing requires astuteness regarding moral and ethical issues.

- Ethical theories explain values and behaviour related to cultural and moral norms.

- Utilitarianism holds that right action is that which has the greatest utility or usefulness, and no action is in itself either good or bad.

- Deontology is based upon the rationalist view that the rightness or wrongness of an act depends upon the nature of the act, rather than the consequences that occur as a result of it.

- Kantianism is a particular deontological theory developed by Immanuel Kant.

- The categorical imperative is the Kantian maxim requiring that no action can be judged as right which cannot reasonably become a law by which every person should always abide.

- The practical imperative is the Kantian maxim requiring that one treat others always as ends and never as means to an end.

- Virtue ethics, usually attributed to Aristotle, represents the idea that individuals' actions are based upon innate moral virtue.

DISCUSSION QUESTIONS AND ACTIVITIES

1. Describe the differences in beliefs about the origin of ethical rules.

2. Describe a hypothetical situation in which an ethical dilemma exists, and discuss solutions to the dilemma in terms of act utilitarianism and rule utilitarianism.

3. Identify specific health care funding policies, and discuss them in terms of utilitarian theory.

4. Identify different ethical codes, including professional codes, that are based upon Kantian or deontological ethics.

5. Describe a real or hypothetical situation in which there is an ethical dilemma. Relate a solution to the dilemma, using the rule of the categorical imperative.

6. List and describe the virtues that you feel are important for nurses.

7. Consider the following situation: Two nursing students are discovered to have cheated on several assignments. After being questioned by the instructor, both students deny having cheated, even though the evidence is irrefutable. Discuss these students in terms of virtue ethics and Kantian ethics. Do these students have integrity? Do these students have the character to become good nurses? How would you apply the categorical imperative?

REFERENCES

Austin, W., G. Lemermeyer, L. Goldberg, V. Bergum, & M. S. Johnson (2005). Moral distress in healthcare practice: The situation of nurses. HEC Forum, *11*(3), 33–48.

Beauchamp, T. L. (2001). *Philosophical ethics* (3rd ed.). Boston: McGraw Hill.

Beauchamp, T. L., & J. Childress (2008). *Principles of biomedical ethics* (6th ed.). New York: Oxford University Press.

Beauchamp, T. L., & L. Walters (1999). *Contemporary issues in bioethics.* Belmont, CA: Wadsworth.

Bentham, J. (1948). *An introduction to the principles of moral legislation.* New York: Hafner Press.

Bergum, V., & J. Dossetor (2005). *Relational ethics: The full meaning of respect.* Maryland: University Publishing Group.

Buber, M. (1965). *The knowledge of man: A philosophy of the interhuman.* New York: Harper & Row.

Durant, W. (1926). *The story of philosophy.* New York: Washington Square Press.

Foot, P. (1997). Virtues and vices. In C. Sommers & F. Sommers, eds., *Vice and virtue in everyday life: Introductory readings in ethics* (4th ed., pp. 328–343). Fort Worth, TX: Harcourt Brace College. (Reprinted from P. Foot, *Virtues and vices,* Berkeley, CA: University of California Press)

Gardiner, P. (2003). A virtue ethics approach to moral dilemmas in medicine. *Journal of Medical Ethics, 29,* 297–302.

Honderich, T., ed. (1995). *The Oxford companion to philosophy.* New York: Oxford University Press.

Jameton, A. (1984). *Nursing practice: The ethical issues.* Englewood Cliffs, NJ: Prentice-Hall.

Kant, I. (1959). *Foundations of the metaphysics of morals* (L. W. Beck, trans.). Indianapolis: Bobbs-Merrill.

Keatings, M., & O. B. Smith (2000). *Ethical and legal issues in Canadian Nursing.* (2nd ed.) Toronto: Saunders.

Kitwood, T. (1990). *Concern for others. A new psychology of conscience and morality.* New York: Routledge.

Kneller, G. F. (1971). *Introduction to the philosophy of education.* (2nd ed.). New York: John Wiley & Sons.

Mayo, B. (1958). *Ethics and the moral life.* London: MacMillan.

Mill, J. S. (1910). *Utilitarianism.* London: Dent & Sons.

Miracle, V. A. (2009). National Nurses Week and the Nightingale Pledge. *Dimensions of Critical Care Nursing, 28*(3), 145–146.

Paton, H. J., trans. & ed. (1961). *The moral law.* London: Hutchinson & Co.

Rand, A. (1982). *Philosophy: Who needs it?* New York: Bobbs-Merrill.

Raphael, D. D. (1994). *Moral philosophy* (2nd ed.). New York: Oxford University Press.

Read Paul, L. (n.d.) Relational ethics: the full meaning of respect. Book review, *Provincial Health Ethics Network,* Alberta, Canada. Retrieved on December 15, 2011 at http://www.phen.ab.ca/library_books/docs/Relational_Ethics.pdf

Sherwin, S. (1992). *No longer patient.* Philadelphia: Temple University Press.

Smart, J. J. C. (1997). Utilitarianism. In C. Sommers & F. Sommers, eds., *Vice and virtue in everyday life: Introductory readings in ethics* (4th ed., pp. 110–123). Fort Worth, TX: Harcourt Brace College. (Reprinted from J. J. C. Smart & B. Williams, eds., *Utilitarianism: For and against,* New York: Oxford University Press)

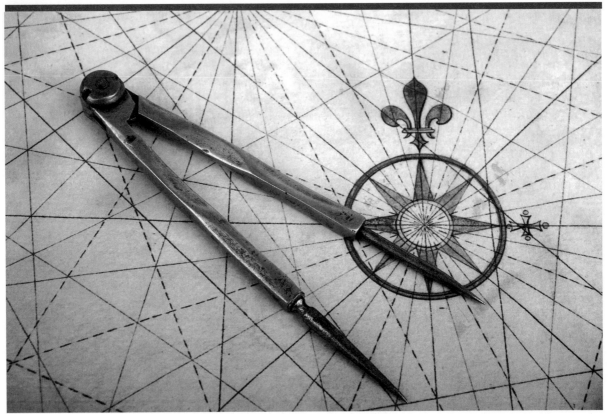

Lagui/Shutterstock.com

CHAPTER **3**
ETHICAL PRINCIPLES

OBJECTIVES

After completing this chapter, the reader should be able to:

1. Discuss the principle of respect for autonomy in terms of patients' rights, informed consent, parentalism, and noncompliance.
2. Discuss the principle of beneficence as it relates to nursing practice.
3. Define the principle of non-maleficence, and weigh actions in terms of harm and benefit.
4. Relate the principle of veracity to nursing practice.
5. Examine the principle of confidentiality in nursing practice, recognizing legal implications and reasonable limits to confidentiality.
6. Discuss the principle of justice as it relates to the delivery of health care goods and services.

7. Relate the principle of fidelity to nursing's promise to society.

8. Discuss situations in which there is a conflict between two or more ethical principles.

INTRODUCTION

Ethical issues are commonly examined in terms of a number of **ethical principles**. Ethical principles are basic and obvious moral truths that guide deliberation and action. Major ethical theories utilize many of the same principles, though either the emphasis or meaning may be somewhat different in different theories. For example, autonomy is a dominant principle in deontological theory but is less important in utilitarian theory. It is vital for nurses to understand ethical principles and be adept at applying them in a meaningful and consistent manner. (See Figure 3–1.) It is the authors' contention that consistent adherence to principle is an important basis for ethical practice in nursing. This chapter examines the following ethical principles: autonomy, beneficence, non-maleficence, veracity, confidentiality, justice, and fidelity.

FIGURE 3–1 **PRINCIPLES OF ETHICS**

Respect for Autonomy
Beneficence
Non-maleficence
Veracity
Confidentiality
Justice
Fidelity

Respect for Persons

All of the principles discussed in this chapter presuppose that nurses have respect for the value and uniqueness of persons. Occasionally viewed as an ethical principle in its own right, **respect for persons** implies that one considers other people to be worthy of high regard. Certainly, genuine regard and respect for others serves as the cornerstone of any caring profession. Discussion of the ethical principles in this chapter is based upon the belief that we value the principle of respect for persons. In other words, the principles that follow here are principles to guide our behaviour with regard to those who are, first of all, respected as persons.

RESPECT FOR AUTONOMY

The word **autonomy** literally means self-governing. Autonomy is a word that is frequently used, yet poorly understood. We are told to respect the autonomy of patients, but are given little guidance in understanding the meaning of this abstract concept. The term is more frequently used as a contrast to undesirable states such as dependency, coercion, paternalism, thoughtlessness, and habit (Jameton, 1984). We are expected to understand the concept and be advocates to ensure that autonomy is maintained for all patients.

Aveyard (2000) suggests that the ambiguous use of the term *autonomy* should be replaced by a concept with a specific meaning and working definition. The term *autonomy* denotes having the freedom to make choices about issues that affect one's own life. Autonomy is closely linked to the notion of respect for persons, and is an especially important principle in cultures where all individuals are considered to be unique and valuable members of society. In cultures that do not regard all members as being of equal worth or that respect social structure above individual rights, autonomy is less important. Autonomy implies that each person has the freedom to make decisions about personal goals. It is a state in which each of us is free to do as we wish, and not be forced or coerced to do something against our will (Yeo, Moorhouse, Khan & Rodney, 2010). In societies where slavery exists, where women are expected to be subservient to men, where there is a lack of respect for cultures, races or religious identities, or where children are exploited, the notion of autonomy is less meaningful and may be applied only to those who are privileged in that society. Autonomy cannot thrive in a climate that does not allow either the independent planning of personal goals or the privilege of examining and choosing options to meet goals.

Implied in the concept of autonomy are five basic elements. (See Figure 3-2).

FIGURE 3-2 **THE FIVE BASIC ELEMENTS OF AUTONOMY**

> ### The autonomous person must:
> 1. be respected.
> 2. be able to set goals.
> 3. be able to formulate a plan of action in order to meet goals.
> 4. be able to reflect upon values and beliefs involved in goals and choices.
> 5. have the freedom to act upon choices in order to meet goals.

First, the autonomous person is respected. It is logical that those choosing the nursing profession would inherently value and respect the unique humanness of others. This element is essential to assuring autonomy. Second, the autonomous person must be able to choose personal goals. These goals may be short-term or long-term and may be explicit or less well defined. Goals are as diverse as people are. For example, one patient with advanced cancer may have a goal of going into remission and returning to some active roles, while another may have a goal of peaceful palliative care in a chosen setting. In each case the patient develops personally chosen goals that are consistent with a set of values and beliefs and a particular lifestyle. In keeping with the notion of choice as an expression of one's lifestyle, values, and beliefs is the notion of autonomy as authentic articulation. When considering the choices made by persons who are ill, in pain, or frightened, one must try to ensure that their choice reflects who they are, in a broader sense, and that the choice they might make today would be the same as or at least similar to the choice they might make on any other day, when pain-free, well, and less scared or burdened (Yeo, Moorhouse, Khan & Rodney, 2010, p. 148). The challenge for the nurse is to try, with the help of the patient, to determine what constitutes a transient reaction to illness or prolonged pain and what is truly consistent with the character and authentic choices of the patient. Third, the autonomous person should have the capacity to decide on a plan of action. The person must be able to understand the options and the meaning of the choice to be made and to deliberate on the various options, while understanding the implications of possible outcomes. Imagine, for example, ordering from a restaurant menu written in a language you do not understand. You have the freedom and responsibility to make a choice, but cannot make a meaningful choice without an understanding of the various foods offered. Understanding, reasoning, and deliberating through a choice is, according to some, the most important aspect of exercising autonomy (Yeo, Moorhouse, Khan & Rodney, 2010, p. 148).

Fourth, a person must be able to demonstrate a kind of moral reflection, not just the ability to understand the differences between the choices from a practical perspective. In other words, autonomous persons must be able to reflect upon the values and beliefs that they hold when weighing options and making decisions. This also implies that the individual has adopted these values and beliefs in a meaningful and iterative way and not simply through a process lacking in critical contemplation or conscious choice (Yeo, Moorhouse, Khan & Rodney, 2010). When we believe that a patient is not able to comprehend the meaning of choices, goals, or outcomes, we may say that the person is incompetent to make decisions, or lacks decision-making capacity. There are certain groups of patients that are generally thought of as unable to make fully informed choices. Children, fetuses, and those with some types of developmental or intellectual disabilities may be among these groups.

Fifth and finally, the autonomous person has the freedom to act upon choices. In situations where persons are capable of formulating goals, understanding various options, and making decisions, yet are not free to actually implement their plans, autonomy is either limited or absent. Autonomy may be limited in situations where the means to accomplish autonomously devised plans do not exist. An example is seen in the case of a person living in a remote region of Ontario, who does not have the same access to timely, inclusive care as the person living in downtown Ottawa or Toronto. In order to assure autonomy, each of the five elements must be present to a reasonable degree.

A number of intrinsic factors may threaten patient autonomy. In health care settings, the patient's role is often a highly dependent one. The patient seeks health care assistance because of a real or perceived need and, as a result, can be thought of as being dependent upon the health care provider. The role of the health care professional, on the other hand, is one of power. Health care providers are often perceived as gatekeepers to care and because of this, patients are dependent on them for access to health care services and care. This role inherently involves power that is based upon special knowledge, access, and authority. The complementary relationship between a patient seeking care and a health care provider who can give access to care, while a necessary one, can potentially lead to violations of patient autonomy.

ASK YOURSELF

Is the Patient Role a Dependent One?

- Describe a time when you or a family member experienced the role of hospitalized patient.
- How did you or your family member feel when interacting with members of the health care team who were dressed in the uniforms of professionals, while you or your family member were in pajamas or a hospital gown or, worse yet, naked?
- Describe the degree to which you or your family member was able to maintain dignity and autonomy.

Certain aspects of the health care system may contribute to the erosion of patient autonomy, and health care professionals may not always be aware of this. Patients are often forced to comply with rules that require them to be and act dependent, often without consideration of individual, religious, or cultural differences, beliefs, and practices. Immediately upon admission to a hospital, patients are disrobed, asked questions about personal and private matters, forced to relinquish money and belongings, and expected to remain in a bed, emphasizing the dependency inherent in the patient role. Patients are placed in rooms with doors that are seldom closed and asked to wear pajamas. Workers, who are strangers to the patients, freely enter and leave the patients' rooms, making privacy impossible. Regardless of patients' personal habits or knowledge of their own health care, they are forced to bathe at specified times, eat at specified times, take medications at specified times, and are often prohibited from practising self-care measures that may have been their habits for many years. Patients are expected to follow each plan that is made. Otherwise, they may be labelled difficult or *noncompliant*. While there is strong emphasis on the importance of autonomy, health care professionals are often guilty of creating a climate of dependency for patients—of coercing otherwise autonomous, intelligent, and independent adults essentially into a very dependent role. Moreover, often patients lose their sense of self as they are acclimatized to a standard routine and care plan. While individualized and holistic care should always be the goal of nursing care, constraints on time and resources often prohibit the extra effort and time it takes to consistently deliver individualized care.

Recognizing Violations of Patient Autonomy

Often, nurses and other health care workers fail to recognize subtle violations of patient autonomy. This especially occurs when nurses believe the best choices to be self-evident. At least four factors are related to this failure (See Figure 3-3).

FIGURE 3–3 **FOUR WAYS PATIENTS' AUTONOMY IS VIOLATED**

1. Assuming that patients and nurses share the same values and goals.
2. Failing to recognize that people process information in unique ways.
3. Assuming that patients have more or less knowledge than is reasonable for us to presume them to have.
4. Focusing solely on the task-driven "work" of nursing—doing procedures, giving medications, documenting care—and in doing so, neglecting to provide individualized and responsive care.

First, nurses may falsely assume that patients have the same values and goals as they themselves have. This state of mind compels some nurses to believe that the only reasonable course of action is the one that is consistent with their own values. This leads to faulty conclusions. For example, if an elderly person chooses to stay in her own home, even though to others she seems to be incapable of caring for herself, the choice might be viewed as unreasonable and might become grounds to believe the patient incompetent to make decisions. In other words, "If you don't make the choices that seem correct to me, you must be incompetent to make decisions." In truth, the elderly person may recognize that life is drawing to a close and may want to remain in familiar surroundings, maintain dignity, remain independent, and prevent needless depletion of her life savings. The decision is based upon her thoughtful consideration of the consequences of staying home versus the consequences of living in a long-term care facility. There are some who would insist that she should be allowed to stay at home, even if she places herself at considerable danger, as long as she does not jeopardize the autonomy of others.

CASE PRESENTATION

Noncompliance Versus Autonomy

Cora is a forty-five-year-old woman who looks years older than her stated age. She has very limited monthly income. Cora smokes two and a half packs of cigarettes per day. She has severe COPD with constant dyspnoea and frequent exacerbations. The nurse who sees her at a local clinic is interested in at least preventing further problems, and speaks to Cora often about the importance of quitting smoking. The situation becomes very frustrating for all involved when

(Continued)

Cora returns repeatedly for increasingly severe problems, having failed to quit smoking. Cora, becomes labelled by the health care team as noncompliant. During a particularly severe exacerbation, the nurse says to Cora, "You know you are committing suicide by continuing to smoke." Cora's reply is, "You don't understand. I live alone. I have no money, no friends, no family, and will never be able to work. I know the damage I'm doing, but smoking is the only pleasure I have in life." (Nathaniel, 2000)

? THINK ABOUT IT

Do Nurses Coerce Patients?

- In attempting to persuade Cora to stop smoking, to what degree is the nurse infringing upon Cora's right to autonomy?
- Does Cora have the right to choose to continue smoking?
- If rights and responsibilities are two sides of the same coin, how should the clinic respond to Cora's continuing to smoke? Would you suggest that the clinic continue to serve Cora, even though she is not following the plan of care? How might Cora be better included in creating a collaborative care plan?
- To what degree is coercion employed in situations such as Cora's? Is coercion ever an appropriate strategy?
- What would you do?

The second cause of failure to recognize subtle violations of patient autonomy lies in our failure to recognize that individuals' thought processes are different. Discounting a particular decision as incorrect may not take into consideration the fact that people process information in different ways. For example, there are those whose thought processes are very logical and methodical; others think in ways that are more creative and free-flowing. It is particularly important to recognize these types of differences when several people are working together to come to a common decision. What is obvious to one will not be obvious to all—not necessarily because of a difference in values, knowledge base, or intellect, but because of different backgrounds and styles of thinking (Harrison & Bramson, 1982). This is an important consideration when collaborating with patients, families, and other professionals.

The third cause of failure to recognize subtle violations of patient autonomy lies in our assumptions about patients' knowledge base. It is easy for us to forget that we have gained a specialized body of knowledge through our programs of basic nursing education and clinical experience. Knowledge about such things as basic anatomy and physiology, disease processes, the mechanism of action of drugs, and so forth is so ingrained in our minds that it is easy to presume everyone has at least some of the same type of knowledge. In the modern age, we may assume that patients have done extensive research on the Internet (which varies significantly in quality and accuracy) and may be more knowledgeable than they actually are. Assuming a level of knowledge, without assessing and evaluating just how much the patient knows and wishes to know, may result in an inadvertent violation of a patient's autonomy. Recall that an understanding of the choices, outcomes, and implications is inherently necessary for autonomous decision making. The nurse must accurately assess the patient's level of understanding in order to assure autonomy.

The fourth cause of our failure to recognize subtle violations of patient autonomy lies in the unfortunate fact that in some instances the "work" of nursing becomes the major focus. This produces a climate of industrious habit. As we go about our work—doing procedures, giving medications, writing care plans, and trying to keep up a frantic pace—attentiveness to assuring patient autonomy is sometimes neglected. In today's climate of advanced technology, fiscal uncertainty, staffing reductions, and bottom-line management, we should guard against focusing solely on work to the exclusion of caring.

Autonomy for patients is more frequently discussed in terms of larger issues, such as informed consent, paternalism, compliance, and self-determination. Let us review this principle as related to these and other recurrent themes.

Barriers to Autonomy

Autonomy exists within the confines and constructs of the world around us. We exercise our autonomy within the contexts of relationships with others. As we have noted, it is often difficult for patients to express autonomous choices in various kinds of health care settings. However, there are also social, political, and relational contexts that may affect the ability to express an autonomous choice. Many of us have had our autonomy restricted at one time or another. Think about how that felt. Many people who are poor, institutionalized, or marginalized feel this way on an ongoing basis, as their autonomy is constrained by their position in the world. Their social status, position, relationships, perceptions, and visible or invisible attributes may severely limit their choices and make them unable to exercise their autonomy to its fullest extent. As nurses, we must always be keenly aware of broader social, political, or relational constraints on persons that might affect them and their ability to be free and autonomous decision makers for themselves.

Informed Consent

The term **informed consent** refers to a process by which patients are informed of the possible outcomes, alternatives, and risks of treatments, and are offered the opportunity to exercise their autonomy. The same barriers and facilitating factors relevant to autonomy also apply to the informed consent process. The process of informed consent assures the legal protection of a patient's right to personal autonomy in regard to specific treatments and procedures. The concept of informed consent is one that has come to mean that patients are given the opportunity to autonomously choose a course of action in regard to plans for medical care. Obtaining consent formally, through the use of a consent form, is usually discussed in relation to surgery and complex medical procedures, but there are also situations in which consent should be sought on a less formal basis. Each time a nurse approaches a patient to take vital signs or help with bathing, the nurse must take care to check with the patient that this activity is acceptable to them, at that particular time. While this may be a less formal consent process, it is no less important and should be a routine part of ethical nursing care and respect for autonomy. Informed consent will be discussed in more depth in Chapter 11.

Paternalism/Parentalism

Paternalism is a gender-biased term that literally means acting in a *fatherly* manner. The traditional view of paternal actions includes such role behaviours as leadership, benevolent decision making, protection, and discipline. As commonly used in nursing, the term *paternalism* carries negative connotations, particularly related to implied dominant male versus submissive female roles.

The term **parentalism** is a more modern, gender-neutral alternative to the term **paternalism**. In the health care arena, the concept of parentalism applies to professionals who restrict others' autonomy, usually to protect that person from perceived or anticipated harm or with a goal of acting in that person's best interests. Parentalism may be appropriate when a patient is judged to be incompetent or to have diminished decision-making capacity. As advocates, we choose to do for the patient that which it is reasonable to believe the patient would choose for him- or herself, if that were possible. We can consider parentalism a form of advocacy when we combine genuine concern for the patient with a well-founded belief that the patient is unable to make autonomous decisions. However, this combined concern can be misguided if it is used to coerce, control, or exert influence over persons, or if the person's best interests are not carefully considered and thoroughly articulated.

The risk of harm is not enough by itself to judge a person incompetent. Virginia Henderson, the well-known nursing leader and author, recounts her experience as a hospitalized patient:

> I was in the room with another patient, and I couldn't stand being in bed any longer, and I would sit in a chair. This nurse came in and saw me sitting in the chair, and she said, "Ms. Henderson if you keep doing that, we are going to have to tie you down" . . . I thought, You just try it . . . . (Goldsmith, 1992, p. 4)

Even though Ms. Henderson was ninety-four years old at the time of her hospitalization, she was certainly competent to make decisions for herself. Patients who are competent must be allowed to act autonomously—even if the choices can be predicted to cause them harm or render them incompetent (Quinn & Smith, 1987). One exception that can be made is that even competent persons cannot be allowed to act in a way that would cause harm to others.

The term *paternalism* generally evokes negative sentiments among nurses and other health care professionals. This is due in part to a recognition that in the past patients' autonomy was frequently violated in the name of beneficence. Professionals sometimes make the dangerous assumption that they are uniquely qualified to make health care decisions by virtue of their professional knowledge and, further, that professional knowledge is the only knowledge needed to make decisions for patients. "Health care professionals often [believe they] understand better than patients do the full clinical implications of health risks, for they have seen the clinical results of its total actual results" (Quinn & Smith, 1987, p. 37). This kind of thinking allows us to ignore multiple contextual factors that might be unrelated to physical outcomes, but that nonetheless affect the whole person. These factors include, among others, past experiences, economic considerations, lifestyle, values, role, culture, and spiritual beliefs. In making decisions, all possible factors must be taken into consideration. This dictates that the patient must be autonomously engaged in the decision-making process and considered as an individual with unique beliefs, values, and lifestyle choices. In today's health care environments, it is widely accepted that patients are "experts" with regards to themselves and only they can provide the important contextual information that is necessary for autonomous decision-making processes.

It is interesting to compare discussions of the concept of paternalism in the nursing and medical literature. Nursing literature generally describes paternalism in a negative way. Nurses often think of paternalism as behaviour that precludes autonomy. Medical literature, on the other hand, traditionally discusses paternalism as a benevolent quality. Consider the following excerpt from a medical ethics text that illustrates this point:

> In its strong version, the principle of paternalism justifies restricting someone's autonomy if by doing so we can benefit her. In such a case, our concern is not only with preventing the person from harming herself, but also with promoting her good in a positive way. The principle might be appealed to even in cases in which our actions go against the other's known wishes. (Munson, 1992, p. 43)

The differences between the nursing and medical communities in relation to beliefs about paternalism probably relate to historical, cultural, and gender factors. However, in medicine, just as in nursing, the beliefs and practices concerning the patient as autonomous have evolved markedly and paternalistic approaches to medical care are becoming a thing of the past. Interdisciplinary discussion and teamwork is needed in order to continue to evolve towards a health care environment in which respect for autonomy is encouraged and paternalistic approaches are discouraged.

ASK YOURSELF

Who Should Make Decisions?

- How do you feel when someone else makes a decision about you without your input?
- Since nurses and doctors may know more about the science of health care, is it ever appropriate for them to make decisions about the health care regimen without participation of the patient?

Noncompliance

The term **noncompliance** is generally thought of as denoting an unwillingness on the part of the patient to participate appropriately in health care activities. This commonly entails lack of participation in a regimen that has been planned by the health care team but that must be carried out by the patient. Examples of such activities include taking medication as scheduled, maintaining a therapeutic or weight loss diet, exercising regularly, and quitting smoking. Use of the term *noncompliance* is just as likely to represent the failure of the nurse as that of the patient. Discussion of noncompliance and of care of the noncompliant patient centres around two basic factors. First, the autonomous participation of the patient in the health care plan is essential to success. When patients are fully aware of their options and alternatives in health care therapies and the consequences of nontreatment and are encouraged to make health care decisions, they are more likely to assume ownership of them and, as a result, to participate in care. In nursing, this is sometimes discussed as the empowerment of patients (Chas. Skinner & Cradock, 2000). Often nurses formulate plans of care that have a firm scientific basis but that seem unreasonable to the patient, or that fail to recognize the diverse or unique needs or qualities of individuals. The nurse is amiss if she does not do her best to ensure that the patient is an autonomous participant in the formulation of the plan. Second, nurses and other health care professionals must assess patients' abilities to follow plans of care. Patients may be unable to adhere to plans of care for a variety of reasons, including lack of resources, lack of knowledge, lack of support from family members, psychological factors, and cultural beliefs that are not consistent with the proposed plan of care. Many times, patients are unable to participate in plans of care because they have not been included in the crucial planning processes and, because, as a result, their needs are not reflected in the proposed plans. An example of patients' inability to comply with a plan of care is seen every day in physicians' offices and emergency departments. Often patients are given prescriptions for medications that are prohibitively expensive. Many patients do not have private insurance or workplace plans to cover the costs of medication. These costs are not covered by the *Canada Health Act*, and so are generally not paid for by provincial health insurance plans. When they return with the same symptoms, not having taken the prescribed medication, they are invariably labelled as noncompliant. The problem is not one of compliance, but rather health care professionals' negligence in assessing patients' ability to follow a plan of care. Another example might involve a South Asian patient failing to adhere to a specific diet regimen tailored for a cardiac patient, as outlined by a dietician in hospital, after surgery. Often therapeutic diets and food guides reflect a very standardized Western diet and fail to accommodate the unique diet and traditional foods of other cultures. With a few simple questions and assessments, a healthy-heart diet could easily be adapted to the patient's dietary habits, traditional foods, and preferences.

What are we to do, however, when patients are well informed and apparently able to follow plans of care, yet do not do so? One hears stories of physicians who refuse to continue to care for patients who do not comply with instructions—smoking cessation, for example. In a climate of limited resources, this is a question worthy of contemplation. Codes of ethics for nurses universally support respect for individuals and individual choice, and such respect should not be restricted by considerations of social or economic status (Canadian Nurses Association, 2008; ANA, 2001; ICN, 2006). Further, the nurse must not be influenced by patients' individual differences in background, customs, attitudes, and beliefs. Because health care practices are an integral part of patients' backgrounds, customs, and beliefs, refusal to participate in a plan of care, regardless of the outcome, is the prerogative of the patient, and must not affect the care given by the nurse. Ultimately, choices about health care practices belong to patients. If allowed to choose, patients should not be labelled in a negative way for choices that nurses do not agree with. Furthermore, patients should not be chastised or labelled for making choices in a particular way. While some people prefer to make decisions in an independent way, others may depend much more on their family or their community to assist them with decisions. Requiring a patient always to make decisions in an individualistic way may not be in keeping with the way that they make decisions in other aspects of their life, and care must be taken to ensure that patients' methods for seeking advice and input into decisions is respected. The *Code of Ethics for Registered Nurses* states, "Nurses recognize that patients may place a different weight on individualism and may choose to defer to family or community values when decision-making" (CNA, 2008; p. 11). It is not appropriate for professionals who express the belief that all competent patients have the right to autonomous choice to then make value judgments about the choices made or the decision-making processes used, and subsequently to label patients as noncompliant (Nathaniel, 2000).

BENEFICENCE

The principle of **beneficence** is one that requires nurses to act in ways that benefit patients. There is no controversy as to whether nurses are obligated to act beneficently—beneficent acts are morally and legally demanded by our professional role (Beauchamp & Walters, 2001). The objective of beneficence provides nursing's context and justification. It lays the groundwork for the trust that society places in the nursing profession, and the trust that individuals place in particular nurses or health care agencies. Perhaps this principle seems straightforward, but it is actually very complex. As we think about beneficence, certain questions arise: *How do we define beneficence—what is **good***? *Who should decide what is good? Should we determine what is good by subjective, or by objective, standards? Furthermore, is it even possible to have an objective definition of the notion of good? When people disagree about what is good, whose opinion counts? Is beneficence an absolute obligation and, if so, how far does our obligation extend? Does the trend toward patient autonomy outweigh obligations of beneficence?* As Veatch (2000) asks, "Is the goal really to promote the total well-being of the patient? Or is the goal to promote only the *medical* well-being of the patient?" (p. 41) We must keep these questions in mind as we reflect upon our own practice.

The ethical principle of beneficence has two major components: doing or promoting good, and preventing harm. As noted above, it maintains, first, that we ought to do or promote good (Beauchamp & Childress, 2001). Even with the recognition that *good* might be defined in a number of ways, it seems safe to assume that the intention of nurses in general is to do good. Questions arise when, in particular situations, those involved cannot decide what is *good*. For example, consider the case of a patient who is in the process of a lingering, painful, terminal illness. There are those who believe that life is sacred and should be preserved at all costs. Others believe that death is preferable to a life of pain and dependence. The definition of *good* in any particular case will determine, at least in part, the action that is to be taken.

FIGURE 3–4 **BENEFICENCE**

Do or Promote Good
Prevent Harm
Remove Evil or Harm

CASE PRESENTATION

Making a Difficult Decision

Anthony is 23 years old and has been in a vegetative state for over three years. At the age of 19, he and his friends were diving off a rugged cliff face on a graduation trip to Costa Rica. When Anthony dove, he struck a rock. Hours passed before he received medical attention and he has never regained consciousness since that day.

Anthony is now in a long-term rehabilitation centre and has had numerous severe complications, including infections, respiratory illnesses, and serious pressure sores, despite excellent nursing care. In the past few months, he has had more serious respiratory infections and may require ventilation if these episodes continue. The nurses have mentioned to the physician that they recommend that a "Do not resuscitate" order be placed on Anthony's chart, in case of a respiratory or cardiac arrest.

His mother and father visit daily, and the strain is beginning to show. They also note that Anthony appears to be deteriorating. They have been told, from the beginning, that there is no chance of recovery and that the remainder of his life would be spent in a vegetative and unresponsive state.

His parents feel that, with the increased respiratory infections, he may be suffering. They call for a health care team meeting. His mother agrees with the nurses; she does not wish him to be placed on a ventilator and wishes that he not be resuscitated in the case of a respiratory or cardiac arrest. She tells the health care team that would be more "merciful" to her son and that he would have wanted this. On the other hand, Anthony's father disagrees and insists that his son have all measures taken in case of any serious adverse event. He tells the team that he is a "good Catholic" and believes that by not doing all that could be done, he would be allowing his son to be "murdered." He also believes that it is in his son's best interests to be kept alive, "in case something new comes along and he can be helped. After all," his father continues, "he is still so young and has so much promise. He loved life and would want me to fight for him."

? THINK ABOUT IT

- In this case, what does each person or group of persons (his mother, his father, the nurses) consider to be in Anthony's best interest, and why?
- How could Anthony's best interest be determined, if at all?

Second, the principle of beneficence also maintains that we ought to prevent evil or harm (Beauchamp & Childress, 2001). In fact, some believe that doing no harm, and preventing or removing harm, is more imperative than doing good. All codes of nursing ethics require us to prevent or remove harm. For example, the International Council of Nurses (ICN) *Code of Ethics for Nurses* (2006) says, "The nurse takes appropriate action to safeguard individuals, families and communities when their health is endangered by a co-worker or any other person" (p. 3). Similarly, the Canadian Nurses Association *Code of Ethics for Registered Nurses* (2008), states:

> Nurses question and intervene to address unsafe, non-compassionate, unethical or incompetent practice or conditions that interfere with their ability to provide safe, compassionate, competent and ethical care to those to whom they are providing care, and they support those who do the same. Nurses are attentive to signs that a colleague is unable, for whatever reason, to perform his or her duties. In such a case, nurses will take the necessary steps to protect the safety of persons receiving care. (CNA, 2008, p. 41)

Appendix D of the 2008 revision of the Canadian Nurses Association *Code of Ethics* outlines practical suggestions for the application of the *Code of Ethics* in minimizing the possibilities of potential harm to others in various, specific circumstances (See Appendix B). Some examples of specific ethical circumstances include when job action (such as a strike) is involved, when involved in working relationships with nursing students, or when providing nursing care during a pandemic. As a result of the SARS outbreak in 2003 in Toronto, there was acknowledgement that explicit guidelines were needed to assist individual practitioners, groups, and health care institutions to manoeuvre through critical situations such as a natural disasters, disease outbreaks, or pandemics. In addition to practical guidelines, there was also a need for guidelines that would address the ethical challenges of providing care in these kinds of contexts (Benatar *et al.*, 2003). In their 2008 revision of the *Code of Ethics*, the CNA has acknowledged that situations such as pandemics or disease outbreaks can create unique ethical challenges, such as the restriction of individual rights through quarantine or restricted movement, providing safe and competent care when there is a potential for risk to self, and prioritizing duties to the profession, family, and self in a crisis situation. The *Code of Ethics* provides basic ethical guidelines for nurses to consider in advance of a pandemic and while working during a pandemic, such as engaging in fair processes, helping to determine when other nurses may need to withdraw from direct care, and being familiar with guidelines and policies at a number of levels. Overall safe, competent, and compassionate care is emphasized in this unique situation, just as it is throughout the document.

While each specific circumstance outlined in this appendix to the *Code of Ethics* is unique in terms of context, the principles and values are consistent. For example, confidentiality is emphasized in more than one specific contextual circumstance, as is ensuring safe and competent care. The purpose of outlining these specific circumstances is to acknowledge that while it is important to be always aware of our overarching ethical obligations, context clearly does matter when nurses are involved in complex, dynamic, and ethically charged situations.

NON-MALEFICENCE

The principle of **non-maleficence** is related to beneficence. This principle requires us to act in such a manner as to avoid causing harm to patients. Included in this principle are requirements to avoid deliberate harm, risk of harm, and inadvertent harm that occurs during the performance of beneficial acts. Most ethicists today tend toward the Hippocratic tradition that requires that health professionals first do no harm (the principle of non-maleficence), placing this principle above all others (Beauchamp & Childress, 2001). It is obvious that we must not commit acts that cause deliberate harm. This principle prohibits, for example, experimental research that assumes negative outcomes for the participants, and the performance of unnecessary procedures for economic gain or solely as a learning experience. Non-maleficence also means avoiding, where possible, doing harm as a consequence of doing good. In such cases, the harm must be weighed against the expected benefit. For example, sticking a child with a needle for the purpose of causing pain is always bad—there is no benefit. Giving an immunization, on the other hand, while causing similar pain, results in the benefit of protecting the child from serious disease. The harm caused by the pain of the injection is easily outweighed by the benefit of the vaccine. In day-to-day practice, we encounter many situations in which the distinction is less clear, either because the harm caused may appear to be equal to the benefit gained, because the outcome of a particular therapy cannot be assured or accurately predicted, or as a result of conflicting beliefs and values. For example, consider analgesia for patients with painful terminal illness. Narcotic analgesia may be the only type of medication that will relieve very severe pain. Such medication, however, may hasten death when given in the amounts required to relieve pain (Boyle, 2004). Cammon & Hackshaw (2000) offer another common example. Orders for patients to receive nothing by mouth before procedures and tests are common practice, unquestioned by most nurses. The authors cite examples in which elderly patients were denied food for up to six days as tests and procedures were completed. The consequences of starvation in the elderly are unquestionable, yet the practice of following NPO orders for long periods of time is seldom questioned. As nurses, we must be alert to situations such as these in which harm may outweigh benefit, taking into account our own values and those of patients.

CASE PRESENTATION

Beneficence Versus Non-maleficence

A middle-aged nurse recounts an incident that she believes relates to the principle of non-maleficence. As a senior nursing student she was responsible for the care of a man who had a shotgun wound to his abdomen. Surgery had been performed, and the surgeon was unable to adequately repair the damage. The man was not expected to survive the day. He was, however, awake and strong, though somewhat confused. He had a fever of 107° Fahrenheit. He was receiving intravenous fluids and had continuous nasogastric suction. The man begged for cold water to drink. The physician ordered nothing by mouth in the belief that electrolytes would be lost through the nasogastric suction if water were introduced into the stomach. The student had been taught to follow the physician's orders. She repeatedly denied the man water to drink. She worked diligently—giving iced alcohol baths, taking vital signs, monitoring the intravenous fluids, and being industrious. He begged for water. She followed orders perfectly. After six terrible hours she turned to find the man quickly drinking the water from one of his ice bags. She left the room, stood in the hallway, and cried. She felt she had failed to do her job. As a result of the gunshot wound, the man died the next morning. Today her view of the situation is different and she notes that if faced with a similar situation in her practice now, she would approach the physician and discuss her concerns regarding the goals of care for such a patient.

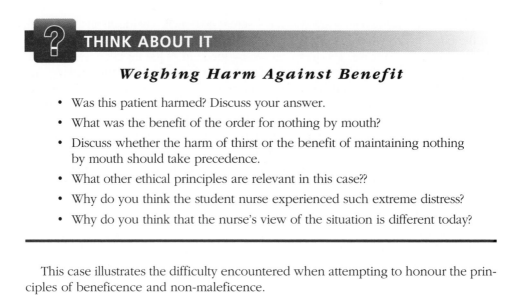

THINK ABOUT IT

Weighing Harm Against Benefit

- Was this patient harmed? Discuss your answer.
- What was the benefit of the order for nothing by mouth?
- Discuss whether the harm of thirst or the benefit of maintaining nothing by mouth should take precedence.
- What other ethical principles are relevant in this case??
- Why do you think the student nurse experienced such extreme distress?
- Why do you think that the nurse's view of the situation is different today?

This case illustrates the difficulty encountered when attempting to honour the principles of beneficence and non-maleficence.

VERACITY

The term **veracity** refers to the moral value of truth-telling. It is linked to the principles of respect for autonomy and dignity of persons. While truth-telling is valued in and of itself, veracity encompasses a broader principle. It emphasizes our moral obligation, as health care providers, to provide individuals with truthful, objective, and complete information in all interactions. (Collier & Haliburton, 2011). Truthfulness is widely accepted as a universal virtue. Most of us were taught as children to always tell the truth. The philosophers most frequently cited in nursing literature, Immanuel Kant and John Stuart Mill, agree in *favour* of telling the truth. Nursing literature promotes honesty as a virtue and truth telling as an important function of nurses. However, there are some differences in perspective among health care professionals. Bioethicists disagree about the absolute necessity of telling the truth in all instances, but in most cases, it is agreed that truth telling is better than deception (Hébert, Hoffmaster & Glass, 2008).

ASK YOURSELF

Is Telling the Truth Always Beneficent?

- A patient's family member asks you to lie to the patient about the seriousness of their diagnosis or prognosis, in order to "protect the patient." How would you feel? What would you do?

- A fellow nurse discloses to you, over lunch, that she mistakenly gave an incorrect dosage of medication to a patient earlier that day. She adds that the patient hasn't experienced any adverse effects due to the lower dose and that he is unaware of the mistake. She asks you to keep it a secret. What would you do? Is the patient owed the truth, despite the lack of serious adverse effects? Why or why not?

- One of your patients is being seen by a new clinical clerk from another medical service, who is very busy and overwhelmed with referrals. The patient asks the clerk about the results of the tests that were done two days ago, stating that she is very anxious and worried about the possible results. The clerk tells the patient "not to worry" and that the results aren't in yet, but they'll probably be just fine. When you read the chart, you see that in fact the results are there, and they indicate a serious condition and need for further surgery and treatment. When you confront the clerk about what he told the patient, he tells you, "She isn't my primary patient. I need to leave it up to her attending physician to give her that news. I just don't have the time or the knowledge of her case to tell her all that." What could the clerk have done instead? What would you do now?

- You are a registered nurse in a public health clinic in an underserved area of the city. You see many patients with a variety of social and economic challenges every day. One of your regular patients, a young single mother with three children, comes in to see you today, in obvious distress. She has run out of her medication because she has sold some of it on the street in order to make some extra money to buy food, as the food banks are tightening up their allowances for families. She begs you to provide her with more medication, as she now requires it. You know that you can dispense more medication to her, but you need to have the approval of the nurse practitioner to do so. You also know that the nurse practitioner will not approve dispensing medication if she knows that the patient sold it on the street. You decide that you will tell her that the patient simply lost the medication and now requires extra. Are health care professionals owed the same right to truth telling and veracity as patients? Who might be harmed as a result of not telling the truth in this case?

We can support nurses' practice of telling the truth in many ways. Truth telling engenders respect, open communication, trust, and shared responsibility. It is promoted in all professional codes of nursing ethics. Truth telling advances and ensures the genuineness and trust between patient and the health care professional, and establishes an environment of authenticity and openness.

A very general interpretation of the ideas of the contemporary philosopher Martin Buber (1965) suggests that true communication between people can take place only when there are no barriers between them. Lying or deception creates a barrier between people and prohibits both meaningful communication and the building of relationships. Recognizing that communication is the cornerstone of the nurse–patient relationship, an argument can be made that nurses must be truthful in order to communicate effectively with patients. While not addressed at length in the *Code of Ethics for Registered Nurses*, the Canadian Nurses Association considers honesty to be an inherent part of accountability in practice (CNA, 2008, p. 18).

Violating the principle of veracity shows lack of respect. Telling lies, or avoiding disclosure, implies that the specific priorities of the nurse or other person involved are more important than the patient or, at the very least, the autonomy of the patient. Jameton (1984) suggests that manipulating information for the purpose of controlling others is like using coercion to control them. In essence, this keeps them from participating in decisions on an equal basis. Used to benefit the patient, deception amounts to paternalism; used against the patient, it may amount to fraud (Myers, 2000).

Jameton (1984) also suggests that deceiving others may constitute an unnecessary assumption of responsibility. When unfortunate consequences occur as a result of deception, the one responsible for the deception can also be assumed to be responsible for consequences. It is often impossible to foresee all potential future negative consequences of deception, and the use of deception often begets further deception. When bad consequences occur after we have reported the truth, we can more easily attribute responsibility to unfortunate circumstances. Furthermore, it is much easier to deal realistically with unfortunate circumstances or outcomes if lies or deception are not involved at the outset.

Telling the truth, on the other hand, builds trust. We can make the argument that truth telling is imperative in assuring that patients continue to trust nurses and other health care professionals. It is by virtue of the trust in these relationships that patients are willing to suspend some measure of autonomy and seek help in meeting their health care needs. Without this trust, the nurse–patient relationship would be destroyed.

Veracity is described as a key element in professional–patient relationships more generally (Beauchamp & Childress, 2001; Hébert, Hoffmaster & Glass, 2008). The American Medical Association notes that physicians must be honest in all dealings with patients (AMA, 2001). While many documents mention truth telling or honesty as an ethical attribute and a professional obligation, veracity as an overarching notion is rarely addressed and is not explicitly mentioned in the *Code of Ethics* of either the Canadian Nurses Association or the Canadian Medical Association. Veracity compels health care professionals to provide "comprehensive, accurate, and objective transmission of information, as well as [referring to] to the way the professional fosters the patient's or subject's understanding" (Beauchamp & Childress, 2001, p. 284). Veracity refers to an overarching approach to practice that continually reflects the values of truth, accuracy, and comprehensiveness in all that we communicate to patients and other health care professionals.

As with other principles, there is some discrepancy between nursing and medical literature in regard to veracity. Recognizing that health care is an interdisciplinary effort, and that disclosure of information to patients involves both nurses and physicians, along with other members of the health care team, it is important for us to understand differing perspectives on the notion of veracity. It is also imperative to note two important considerations in this discussion. First, this discussion does not suggest that "all physicians" believe that the truth should be withheld in specific circumstances nor does it advance a mistaken belief that all nurses believe in veracity in all circumstances. This would be an error, based on an inaccurate assumption and a furthering of stereotypes about groups of health care professionals and the differences between these groups. Second, the perspectives and views on veracity in the medical, nursing, and bioethics literature and in practice are always changing, responsive to other trends in medical care, and legal and ethical obligations, as well as specific contexts or situations. A review of the literature suggests that, generally, patients tend to prefer to know the truth and have physicians and nurses treat them in an honest and straightforward way, even when communicating bad news (Tuckett, 2004).

Some medical literature makes the claim that patients do not want bad news, and that truthful information has the potential to harm them. Lipkin (1991) argues that physicians should sometimes deceive their patients or withhold information from them. It is his view that patients do not have sufficient information about how their bodies function to interpret medical information accurately, and sometimes do not want to know the truth about their illness. Nyberg (1993) agrees, noting that sometimes deceiving patients may avoid potential harm and that, therefore, a physician's duty includes not telling the patient the complete truth regarding a situation. Joseph Ellin (1991) discusses special considerations that have been posed by the medical profession in relation to truth telling. He suggests that it does not seem beneficent to adopt an ethic of absolute veracity in which it is an obligation to cause avoidable anguish to someone who is already ill, especially when hope and positive outlook may promote healing and help prolong life. He writes, "One could hope to avoid this dilemma by holding that the duty of veracity, though not absolute, is to be given very great weight, and may be overridden only in the gravest cases . . . " (p. 82). Ellin draws a distinction between lying and deception: lying is the deliberate telling of untruths, whereas deception is usually accomplished through nondisclosure. He argues that there is an absolute duty not to lie to patients but that there is no duty not to deceive. Examples he gives include withholding information about a poor prognosis or giving placebo medication. Consider the following situation: a mother of four is admitted to the emergency department after an automobile accident in which two of her children are killed. Recognizing that she is in very serious condition, according to Ellin, it would be appropriate to avoid telling her of the death of her children at this point in time. If, however, she asks about their condition, she must be told the truth.

This theme is reiterated in more recent literature, in which the notion of avoiding harm through deception or attempting to benefit the patient through withholding information may be promoted, e.g. not providing a patient with an early diagnosis of cancer in order to avoid a patient living "in the shadow of cancer" (Laurance, 2010, p. 2138). Other studies have demonstrated that providing increased amounts and depth of information to cancer patients resulted in higher levels of anxiety (Jenkins, Fallowfield & Saul, 2001). What the literature demonstrates is that there are variations in how much truthful or frank information some patients want to be told and how patients wish to be informed. To further complicate this, there is most certainly some degree of disagreement among health care professionals over how truth-telling should be handled in difficult or complex situations (Hébert, Hoffmaster & Glass, 2008). Each situation will vary according to the context, the patient, and the health care professionals involved in care. Clearly care must be taken to both explore and appreciate the perspective of the patient in approaching a difficult or tragic situation and our obligation to treat patients with dignity and with respect for autonomy underlies our obligation to tell the truth.

ASK YOURSELF

Is the Truth Sometimes Harmful?

- Do you think it is acceptable to deceive a patient in order to prevent unnecessary suffering?
- How would you feel if you were a patient and the health care team and your family conspired to deceive you—if, for example, you were ill and you had a bleak prognosis?

Bok (1991) examines the practice of physicians deceiving patients in the name of beneficence. She writes that lying to patients has historically been seen as an excusable act. "Some would argue that doctors, and only doctors, should be granted the right to manipulate the truth in ways so undesirable for politicians, lawyers, and others" (p. 75). In fact, truth telling has never been a principle that was given consideration in the medical literature. Veracity is absent from virtually all medical oaths, codes, and prayers. Even the Hippocratic Oath makes no mention of truthfulness. The 1847 version of the American Medical Association *Code of Ethics* endorses some forms of deception by stating that the physician has a sacred duty to avoid "all things which have a tendency to discourage the patient and to depress his spirits" (Bok, 1994, p. 1683).

Nursing and medicine view veracity from two different perspectives. It is clear that physicians have traditionally seen disclosure or nondisclosure to be a facet of care within their control that can have implications for patient welfare, and have exercised veracity in ways that were felt to be in the best interest of their patients. To withhold bad news is often considered a beneficent act if disclosure of the information is expected to harm the patient. However, what we see now in the medical literature reflects an increased tendency towards truthfulness to facilitate informed decision-making, enable trust, avoid harm, and respect persons. In other words, truth and truth-telling are more likely to be seen as inherent values in medicine today (Hébert, 1997). Nursing upholds veracity as supporting individual rights, respect for persons, and the principle of autonomy. However, there is significant discussion in the nursing literature, particularly in areas like critical care and cancer care, of the ethical challenges involved in disclosure and truth-telling, and the subsequent link to increased moral distress for many nurses working in these complex areas. It is fair to say that truth-telling is not a "black-and-white" issue in either nursing or medicine, and that it can be viewed quite differently even by members of the same profession. Recognition of the viewpoint of other members of the health care team is imperative for professionals who must collaborate. Chapter 4 discusses methods of making decisions about ethical problems when there are differences of perspective among those involved.

CONFIDENTIALITY

Confidentiality is the ethical principle that requires nondisclosure of private or secret information with which one is entrusted. Support for this principle is found in codes and oaths of nursing and medicine dating back many centuries. Nursing codes of ethics require that we maintain confidentiality of patient information. According to the ICN *Code of Ethics for Nurses* (2006), "The nurse holds in confidence personal information and uses judgement in sharing this information." Similarly, the Canadian Nurses Association *Code of Ethics for Registered Nurses* (2008) directs nurses to maintain confidentiality. Confidentiality is the only facet of patient care mentioned in the Nightingale Pledge, recited for decades by graduating nurses: "I will do all in my power to elevate the standard of my profession and will hold in confidence all personal matters committed to my keeping and all family affairs coming to my knowledge in the practice of my profession." The Hippocratic Oath is also very clear: "Whatever, in connection with my professional practice, or not in connection with it, I see or hear, in the life of men, which ought not to be spoken of abroad, I will not divulge, as reckoning that all such should be kept secret." Though there are compelling arguments in favour of maintaining confidentiality, there is disagreement about the absolute requirement of confidentiality in all situations. Furthermore, there are situations in which it may be permitted, or even required, to breach confidentiality.

Privacy is a term widely used in academic and legal discussions as well as in everyday life. While it is difficult to find one definition that will capture all the many facets of what we consider to be privacy, one definition might be "the condition of not having undocumented personal information about oneself known by others" (Parent, 1983). The ability to maintain privacy in one's life is an expression of autonomy. The capacity to choose what others know about us, particularly intimate personal details, is important, because it enables us to maintain dignity and preserve a measure of control over our own lives. Markus and Lockwood discuss the importance of privacy:

> Privacy is thus a value closely related to, and perhaps ultimately grounded on, the value of personal autonomy. To take this value of privacy seriously is to subscribe to a number of familiar precepts. It means that we should be reluctant to pry, that we should respect personal confidences, and that when we enter into relationships with others that render us privy to sensitive or intimate personal information, we should be [careful] about passing this information on, even in the absence of any specific request not to do so. (1991, p. 349)

Thus, maintaining the confidentiality of information about patients is an expression of respect of persons and, in many ways, is essential to the nurse–patient relationship. Consider the following case presentation.

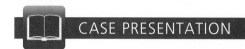

CASE PRESENTATION

Making the Best Choice

Lora is a seventeen-year-old high school student. She comes to the local family planning clinic requesting birth control pills. In the process of completing the initial physical examination, the nurse practitioner finds evidence of physical abuse, including a recent traumatic perforated ear drum. Lora hesitantly and tearfully admits that her biological father slapped her across her left ear prior to her coming to the clinic. She reports that she recently moved into his home after living most of her life with her mother and stepfather. She tells the nurse practitioner that her stepfather was sexually abusive to her and that she wishes to remain with her biological father. She says that she can tolerate her father hitting her occasionally, and she does not want to get him in trouble or be forced to move back to her stepfather's home. The law requires that the nurse report any suspicion of child abuse to adhere to mandatory reporting laws. However, the CNA *Code of Ethics* requires the nurse to maintain confidentiality.

THINK ABOUT IT

To Tell or Not to Tell

- What are the principles involved?
- Does the nurse's obligation to report the incident of child abuse supersede the obligation to maintain confidentiality—particularly considering that the patient requested confidentiality? What if Lora was fourteen years old?
- What are the options for the nurse?
- What are the possible outcomes of the different options?
- Does Lora's autonomy outweigh the nurse's responsibility to report the abusive situations?
- Review the legal obligation in Canada to report cases of suspected child abuse. What other kinds of situations require mandatory reporting?

There are at least two basic ethical arguments in favour of maintaining confidentiality. The first of these is the individual's right to control personal information and protect privacy. The second argument is one of utility, one we were introduced to in Chapter 2.

The *right* to privacy flows from autonomy and respect for persons. Patients have the right to expect that personal and private information will not be shared unnecessarily among health care providers. Patient information is not an appropriate topic for elevator or dinner conversation. It is most likely that violations of this nature were what authors had in mind when writing early creeds and oaths that promise confidentiality. Nurses and other professionals often casually discuss private patient matters but doing so may be in appropriate. Nurses have a professional responsibility to keep in mind the number of people who have legitimate access to patient records. In a hospital setting, patient charts are accessible to many personnel. Nurses, physicians, dieticians, respiratory therapists, students, clerks, physical therapists, and many others have legitimate reason to view patient records. Information of a sensitive and private nature that the patient intends for the nurse or physician alone can become widely known in a large health care facility. Care must be taken in choosing information to be recorded in patients' charts. Special care must be taken to avoid inadvertent breaches of confidentiality (Erlen, 1998), including those involved with electronic records (Muldoon, 1996). It is important for nurses to be aware of the many threats to patient confidentiality.

Confidentiality is particularly important when revealing intimate and sensitive information has the potential to harm the patient. Harm can take various forms, such as embarrassment, ridicule, discrimination, deprivation of rights, physical or emotional harm, marginalization, and loss of roles or relationships. Consider the plight of many HIV-positive people whose diagnoses have become public knowledge without their consent. Confidentiality is particularly important when dealing with vulnerable populations (Derlega *et al.*, 2010; Winston, 1988).

The second argument is one rooted in utility. If patients suspect that health care providers reveal sensitive and personal information indiscriminately, they may be reluctant to seek care. Government policy makers recognize this problem. In Canada, significant privacy legislation exists at both the federal and provincial levels to protect the confidentiality of personal information for Canadians. At the federal level, Canada has two privacy laws. The *Privacy Act*, first enacted in 1983 (and most recently amended in April of 2011), outlines the obligations of federal government agencies and institutions to respect the privacy rights of citizens by treating the collection and disclosure of personal information with great care. It also clearly states that individuals have the right to access their own information—information about themselves—without interference or constraints (Office of the Privacy Commissioner of Canada, 2004). Second, the *Personal Information Protection and Electronics Document Act*, also known by the acronym PIPEDA (2000) sets out rules for how personal information should be sought and managed by private-sector organizations and in commercial activities (Kardash & Penta, 2005). Each province, in turn, has individual legislation governing the management of personal and health information. For example, Alberta has the following legislation and acts pertaining to personal and health information: the *Freedom of Information and Protection of Privacy Act*; the *Health Information Act*, which took effect in 2001; and the *Personal Information Protection Act* (PIPA) which came into force January 1, 2004. Ontario has the *Freedom of Information and Protection of Privacy Act* and the *Personal Health Information Protection Act*, which came into effect in 2004.

Each province has its own privacy commissioner to oversee relevant legislation and the challenges that arise with complex legislation and rules governing the collection, use, storage, and dissemination of personal identifiable information, which includes health information, across a variety of contexts, including education and health care. The Privacy Commissioner of Canada has a Web site that describes the kinds of oversight the federal government and each province exercise in regard to private information about Canadian citizens (http://www.priv.gc.ca/index_e.cfm). Because of the intimate and private nature of reproductive health issues, the confidentiality of those seeking family planning services, for example, is mandated. Those caring for patients with HIV-positive status and AIDS also recognize the need to maintain confidentiality, or selective, thoughtful disclosure, creating safe, supportive communities for patients with HIV-positive status and avoiding potential discrimination (Derlega *et al.*, 2010). According to Derlega and colleagues, many people who work with HIV-positive patients find such arguments particularly compelling, believing that disclosure of a patient's antibody status or diagnosis of AIDS may result in the patient being unfairly stigmatized, subject to experiences of "rejection, prejudice and discrimination" (p. 259). There are other diagnoses, such as mental illness, alcoholism, and drug addiction, that, if revealed without the permission of the person involved, could lead to disruptions in patients' relationships and family support, or to public scorn, and subsequently discourage individuals from seeking care. One clear example of an issue in which disclosure may result in individuals not seeking medical care is the mandatory reporting of gunshot wounds in much of Canada. Today, most provinces have mandatory reporting laws that require health care professionals to report gunshot and stab wounds. British Columbia was the most recent province to enact such a law. This kind of legislation, while seeking to be protective and to encourage reporting of illegal activities, provides us with an example of the kind of situations in which it is acknowledged that victims of gunshot wounds may well avoid seeking medical treatment for fear of criminal charges or police involvement.

 CASE PRESENTATION

Angelo is a new graduate nurse, working in a busy downtown hospital. Today, he has a quick lunch by himself. He hasn't had time yet to make good friends and finds himself very busy, as a fresh graduate on a new unit. A group of more senior nurses from the unit are having lunch at an adjoining table, close by. Angelo hears them discussing a particularly challenging patient quite loudly, disclosing details about the patient and his wife and joking about them. He recognizes that it was a very difficult morning and that his fellow nurses are "letting off steam." He also notes that at nearby tables, there are patients, families, and staff from other units, who can also easily hear the conversation.

One of the nurses catches Angelo's eye and motions, in a friendly way, for him to come over and join the group. This is the first time that they have extended this kind of friendly invitation to him and he is eager to join them. However, he is very uncomfortable with discussing patients in a crowded cafeteria. He also thinks that he should mention something to them about not talking about patients in public places, but he is afraid that they will then not allow him to be part of the group.

 THINK ABOUT IT

- What should Angelo do, and why?
- Have you ever been in a similar situation? How did you feel? What did you do?
- What ethical principles are important to consider, in this case?
- What might a utilitarian or a deontologist advise Angelo to do, and why?

Limits of Confidentiality

Should the principle of confidentiality be honoured in all instances? There are arguments that favour questioning the absolute obligation of confidentiality in certain situations. These arguments include those rooted in the principles of harm and vulnerability (Winston, 1988). An example of a reasonable limit to confidentiality might be seen in a case where the nurse or other professional recognizes that maintaining confidentiality will result in preventable wrongful harm to innocent others. The harm principle states that the actions or autonomy of others can be limited in order to avoid harm to others. Originally stated by John Stuart Mill (1859) in his essay "On Liberty," this principle supports exercising power over another person to limit their autonomy, often against their will, in order to prevent harm. Mandatory testing of pregnant women for HIV and syphilis, for example, is intended to prevent the spread of a serious communicable disease to the fetus. In this instance, society chooses to override the privacy of the individual to protect the health of the innocent. While directing nurses to maintain confidentiality and to advocate for continuous policy development and safeguards for protection of privacy, the CNA *Code of Ethics* (2008) notes that in some situations the obligation of confidentiality is not absolute. The *Code of Ethics* states that if disclosure of information without a person's authorization is practically necessary or legally required, it must be carried out with great care, by disclosing the minimum amount of information to the fewest number of persons in order to satisfy the needs of the situation. Additionally, the persons in a nurse's care must always be told that their information is being disclosed to others, and be informed about the rationale for doing so. Finally, the *Code of Ethics* compels nurses, when disclosing health information without a person's consent, to do so in ways that do not further marginalize or stigmatize that person, their family, or their community, as a result of having that information known by others.

In rare instances, case law supports the violation of confidentiality in order to protect third parties. In July of 1976, the California Supreme Court ruled that a psychologist, Dr. Lawrence Moore, and his superior, Dr. Harvey Powelson, and the agency they worked for, were liable in the wrongful death of Tatiana Tarasoff. Prosenjit Poddar killed Tatiana Tarasoff in October of 1969. According to Tatiana's parents, Poddar had confided his intention to kill Tatiana to his psychologist, Dr. Moore, two months before the event. Though Dr. Moore initially tried to have his patient involuntarily committed, Dr. Powelson intervened and allowed Poddar to return home. Neither Tatiana nor her parents were informed of the patient's threats. The court found that the defendants were responsible for the wrongful death of Tatiana because they knew in advance of the patient's intentions. The obligation to protect the innocent third party superseded the obligation to maintain confidentiality. According to the majority opinion in this case, the duty to warn arises from a special relationship between the patient and the psychologist that imposes a duty to control the patient's conduct (Tobriner, 1991).

Foreseeability is an important consideration in situations where confidentiality conflicts with the duty to warn. The nurse or other health care professional should be able to reasonably foresee harm or injury to an innocent other in order to justify violating the principle of confidentiality in favour of a duty to warn. This consideration precludes blanket disclosure of private information that might predict harm to others. The Tarasoff case exemplifies reasonable application of the duty to prevent harm. Subsequent court cases support the decision in the Tarasoff case. Courts have found that privacy is not absolute and is subordinate to the state's fundamental right to enact laws that promote public health and safety.

The principle that says that confidentiality may be violated in order to prevent harm is strengthened when one considers the vulnerability of the innocent (Haggarty, 2000). The duty to protect others from harm is stronger when the third party is dependent on others or is in some way especially vulnerable. This duty, known as the *vulnerability principle,* states that moral agents have special duties to protect those who are vulnerable or highly dependent upon the choices or actions of others (Goodin, 1985). Goodin states that we must pay particular attention to the fact that the source of our special responsibility to protect the vulnerable and avoid harm to them is their degree of dependence on us to make choices and to carry out actions that are in their best interests. Vulnerability implies risk or susceptibility to harm when vulnerable individuals have a relative inability to protect themselves (Winston, 1988). The state of vulnerability may mean that individuals are also unable to protect their own best interests, and so others must be committed to doing so (Goodin, 1985). For example, nurses have a legal and absolute duty to report child abuse or suspicion of child abuse or neglect. Because children are dependent and vulnerable, they are at greater risk of harm. Coupling the harm-prevention principle with the vulnerability principle produces a strong argument for abandoning the principle of confidentiality in certain instances.

THINK ABOUT IT

Can Nurses Violate Confidentiality?

- How do you think confidentiality and the harm-prevention and vulnerability principles can be reconciled?
- How would you feel if a relative of yours contracted a sexually transmitted infection from a source who public health officials knew was infected, and had reason to believe would infect your relative, but neglected to warn your relative?
- How would you feel if your health care provider violated your right to confidentiality?

Actions that are considered ethical are not always found to be legal. Though there is an ethical basis for overriding the principle of confidentiality in special circumstances, and there is some legal precedent for doing so, there is a legal risk to disclosing sensitive information. There is dynamic tension between the patient's right to confidentiality and the duty to warn others. Nurses need to recognize that careful consideration of the ethical implications of actions will not always be supported by bureaucratic and legal systems.

FIDELITY

The ethical principle of **fidelity** is often related to the concept of faithfulness and the practice of keeping promises. Society has granted nurses the right to practise nursing through the processes of licensure and registration (*Regulated Health Professions Act*, 1991). The process of licensure ensures that no other group can practise within the domain of nursing as defined by society and by the profession or practise using the label of "registered nurse." Thus, to accept licensure and become legitimate members of the profession mandates that nurses uphold the responsibilities inherent in the contract with society and inherent in being a member of a regulated profession. Members are called to be faithful to the society that grants them the right to practice— to keep the promise of upholding the profession's code of ethics, to practise within the established scope of practice and definition of nursing, to remain competent in practice, to abide by the policies of employing institutions, and to keep promises to individual patients. To *be* a nurse is to *make these promises*. In fulfilling this contract with society, nurses are responsible to faithfully and consistently adhere to these basic principles.

On another level, the principle of fidelity relates to loyalty and faithfulness within the nurse–patient relationship. It gives rise to an independent duty to keep promises or contracts (Veatch, 2000) and is a basic premise of the nurse–patient relationship. Problems sometimes arise when there is a conflict between promises that have been made and the potential consequences of those promises in cases where keeping the promises will cause harm in other ways. Though fidelity is the cornerstone of a trusting nurse–patient relationship, many would agree that there are no absolute, unconditional duties to keep promises—that, while there is a very strong presumption in favour of promise-keeping, any harmful consequences of the promised action should, in every case, be weighed against the benefits of keeping the promise. Consider the example of suspected elder abuse. Recall that, in some situations, there are strong arguments against keeping the promise of confidentiality in the nurse–patient relationship. Situations such as disclosure of the suspicion of elder abuse implies an ethical obligation to disclose information and thus break the promise of maintaining confidentiality. While there are mandatory reporting laws for child abuse, corresponding laws do not exist specifically for abuse of elderly persons in most provinces, unless they are living in a long-term care setting or health care institution. For elderly persons living in the community, there are no specific laws requiring others to legally report suspicions of elder abuse. However, there remains an arguably strong ethical obligation to act or assist in such a situation and this may entail breaking the promise of confidentiality. Many would agree that this disclosure is justified, based on the comparison of potential harm against the potential benefit of keeping such information secret. Again, it is difficult to assert that we have an absolute responsibility to always keep every promise we make within a therapeutic relationship, without also considering the context of each promise made and the possible harmful consequences.

JUSTICE

Justice is the ethical principle that relates to fair, equitable, and appropriate treatment in light of what is due or owed to persons, recognizing that giving to some will deny receipt to others who might otherwise have received these things. Within the context of health care ethics, the relevant application of the principle focuses on distribution of goods and services. This application is called **distributive justice**. Unfortunately, there is a finite supply of goods and services, and it is impossible for all people to have everything they might want or need. One of the primary purposes of governance systems is to formulate and enforce policies that deal with fair and equitable distribution of scarce resources.

Decisions about distributive justice are made at a variety of levels in Canada. The federal and provincial governments are responsible for deciding policy about broad public health access issues, such as establishment of new programs or hospitals. These decisions are made at a "macro" level. Hospitals and other organizations formulate policy at an institutional or "meso" level, and deal with issues such as how decisions will be made concerning who will occupy intensive care beds and how patients will be triaged in emergency rooms. Nurses and other health care providers frequently make decisions of distributive justice on an individual basis or, literally, at the bedside. For example, having assessed the needs of patients, nurses decide how best to allocate their own time (a scarce resource) between their assignments of patients, all with varied needs and levels of required care. These kinds of issues occur at a "micro" level.

There are three basic areas of health care that are relevant to questions of distributive justice. First, what percentage of our resources is it reasonable to spend on health care? Second, recognizing that health care resources are limited, which aspects of health care should receive the most resources? Third, which patients should have access to the limited resources of health care: highly qualified staff, equipment, and so forth? (Jameton, 1984).

When making decisions involving distributive justice, one must ask the question, *"Who is entitled to these goods or services?"* Philosophers have suggested a number of different ways to choose among people. Figure 3–5 lists examples of some of the ways that people have historically made these types of decisions.

FIGURE 3–5 **DISTRIBUTIVE JUSTICE**

To each equally
To each according to need
To each according to merit
To each according to social worth
To each according to the person's rights
To each according to preference
To each according to individual effort
To each as you would be done by
To each according to the greatest good to the greatest number

There are those who believe that all should receive equally regardless of need. On the surface, nationalized health care systems would seem to meet this criterion, since all citizens are eligible for the same services. However, because some citizens would necessarily require more health care services than others, nationalized systems also are required to meet the criterion of need. Countries with different health care systems do this in different ways. In Canada, the allocation of health care resources, through what is known as universal health care, is based upon an egalitarian model—one in which everyone receives an equal share of available resources. The values underlying this approach include equal access to health care and the preservation of basic human rights through health care, social democracy, and social justice and humanitarianism. These values are closely related to our identity as Canadians and many persons feel that they should be upheld and protected closely (Romanow, 2002). Since the development of the first steps toward universal social health care programs, the health care system has continued toward addressing the varied health needs of the constituents and supporting the poor, elderly, and disabled through complex social systems. Dramatic cuts in health care funding and changes in the method by which the federal government provided health care funding to the provinces in the 1980s had dramatic effects on social programs, such as health care, education, and social support; however, the values underlying the system, even one constrained by financial limitations and sustainability concerns, have remained constant. Whether or not these values can be sustained in our current system is the most important question for the future of health care in Canada.

As health needs differ between persons, some citizens necessarily "use" more resources while others "use" less. However, the notion that a universal system is there, if we require it, is a fundamental value inherent in the Canadian system.

The principles of the *Canada Health Act* outline the values and their practical application and administration within the Canadian health care system. These principles are discussed in much more detail in Chapter 13, but are important to consider here as we reflect upon the principles underlying our health care system that influence how we allocate direct funding, resources, and efforts.

PRINCIPLES OF THE *CANADA HEALTH ACT*

The following are principles of the *Canada Health Act*. These principles are conditions provinces and territories must abide by in order to continue to receive federal funding for health. The five principles are: public administration, comprehensiveness, universality, portability, and accessibility (Canadian Nurses Association, 2000; Oberle and Bouchal, 2009).

1. Public Administration: This principle states that provinces and territories must deliver health care through plans and programs that are operated on a not-for-profit basis. This further implies that the provinces are fully accountable to the public for how health care funds are spent and used.

2. Comprehensiveness: This principle states that the provinces, in their health care programs, must ensure that all "medically necessary" (Canadian Nurses Association, 2000) services are provided to Canadians. These include services such as in-hospital care, physician services, and dental surgery, as well as, in some cases, services by other health care professionals. The degree of coverage of other professional services is decided upon by each province or territory differently.

3. Universality: This principle states that all Canadians are entitled to the health services that are insured by the provincial plans. It also refers to the fact that no Canadians should be paying health care insurance premiums in order to be able to receive services.

4. Portability: The principle of portability means that Canadians who move from one province or territory to another will still be able to access insured health care services in their new province, after a minimum amount of waiting time. After the waiting period, the new province or territory of residence assumes health care coverage for the new resident.

Canadians who are temporarily absent from their home provinces or territories, or from the country, must also continue to be covered for insured health care services. This allows Canadians to travel for business, go on vacation, or be absent, within explicitly stated limits of time, from their home in Canada but still retain their health insurance coverage when they return.

The principle of portability, however, does not entitle a person to seek preferred services in another province, territory, or country, but rather simply to ensure that Canadians who travel or vacation can be assured that their health care coverage will continue.

5. Accessibility: Accessibility refers to the fact that Canadians must have access to the services covered by provincial and territorial health care plans without paying user fees, extra charges, or bills. (Canadian Nurses Association, 2000; Oberle and Bouchal, 2009).

The perspective embodied in the *Canada Health Act* is not the only possible perspective, of course. The German philosopher Friedrich Nietzsche had a perspective that differed from the egalitarian model outlined above. He believed that there are superior individuals, and that society's goal should be to enhance these "supermen." For Nietzsche, the choice of distribution was a clear one—to each according to his present or future social contribution (Durant, 1926). Other perspectives: the slogan "To each according to that person's rights" indicates a libertarian viewpoint; "To each as you would be done by" by is a reflection of the golden rule. The idea that each should receive according to effort is a common belief in our culture, and indicates the traditional "work ethic." Entitlement programs in the United States generally award benefits based upon a combination of need and the greatest good that can be accomplished for the greatest number of people. In other words, the American system is often viewed as a libertarian system. Chapter 15 discusses the application of the principle of distributive justice in greater detail.

SUMMARY

As we participate in meeting the health care needs of society, we must be constantly aware of ethical implications inherent in many situations. Each nurse must develop a philosophically consistent framework on which to base contemplation, decision, and action. It is this framework that gives shape to our understanding of various ethical principles. Those ethical principles, again, discussed in this chapter presuppose nurses' innate respect for persons. Ethical principles include autonomy, beneficence, non-maleficence, veracity, confidentiality, justice, and fidelity.

CHAPTER HIGHLIGHTS

- All ethical principles presuppose a fundamental a respect for persons.
- Autonomy denotes having the freedom to make choices about issues that affect one's own life.

- Various intrinsic and extrinsic factors may threaten patient autonomy.
- The principle of beneficence maintains that one ought to do or promote good, prevent evil or harm, and remove evil or harm.
- The principle of non-maleficence requires one to avoid causing harm, including deliberate harm, risk of harm, and harm that occurs during the performance of beneficial acts.
- The principle of veracity relates to the universal virtue of telling the truth.
- Confidentiality is the ethical principle that requires nondisclosure of private or secret information with which one is entrusted.
- Justice is the ethical principle that relates to fair, equitable, and appropriate treatment in light of what is due or owed to persons, recognizing that what is given to some will be denied to others who might otherwise have received these things.
- Fidelity is the ethical principle that relates to faithfulness and keeping promises.

DISCUSSION QUESTIONS AND ACTIVITIES

1. Find the CNA *Code of Ethics for Nurses* on the CNA Web site. Read the *Code* and discuss how the various statements relate to the principles discussed in this chapter.

2. Read the following hypothetical situation and answer the questions that follow:

An elderly gentleman presents himself to the emergency department of a small community hospital. The patient has contractures and paralysis of his left hand; he apparently has complete expressive and at least partial receptive aphasia. Upon questioning, the man takes off his right shoe and points to his right great toe and grimaces, apparently indicating a problem in that area. The nurse is unable to gather any further information from him because of his difficulty in communicating. In attempting to help him, she asks if he has a neighbour or friend accompanying him. He shakes his head, indicating that he is alone. Curious, the nurse asks him how he came to the hospital. The patient smiles and proudly produces a driver's licence from his shirt pocket. Subsequently, the nurse leaves the room and returns a few minutes later to find that the patient has left the hospital, having received no care. The nurse suspects that because of his current physical condition the man is unsafe to drive a motor vehicle.

- What are the ethical implications in this situation?
- What ethical principles are involved?

- Should the nurse pursue avenues to locate the patient and ensure that he is not endangering himself or others by driving? Would this be a breach of confidentiality? Autonomy?
- How does the nurse express fidelity in this situation?
- What is the beneficent action?

3. Describe situations you have witnessed in which decisions were made for patients in a paternalistic manner. Discuss your perception of the appropriateness of paternalism in given situations.

4. Read the following hypothetical case and answer the questions that follow:

> Martha is a seventy-five-year-old woman who has terminal cancer of the bladder. During the course of her therapy, she sustains third-degree radiation burns to her lower abdomen and pelvic area. Her wounds are extensive and deep, involving her abdominal wall, bladder, and vagina. The physician orders frequent medicinal douches and wound irrigations. These treatments are very painful, and the patient wants the treatments discontinued but is too timid to actually refuse them. She tells the nurse that she "can't take any more" and asks for her help.

- Discuss the situation in terms of beneficence and non-maleficence.
- What is the nurse's responsibility in assisting the patient to maintain autonomy?

5. Do you think health care professionals should disclose information to patients that is related, for example, to a poor prognosis, even though the information may cause distress? Discuss your views in depth.

6. Jameton (1984) says that for nurses to be less than competent is unethical. Discuss this statement in terms of fidelity.

7. Read the following hypothetical case and answer the questions that follow:

> Micah Johnson is a forty-year-old disabled former truck driver. He was injured several years ago in a trucking accident. He subsequently has had back surgery but continues to have severe pain. He has been seen by every local neurosurgeon and, for one reason or another, is not pleased with the care he has gotten. Because of the seriousness of his initial injuries, there is little doubt that Mr. Johnson has chronic back pain. Even though the local emergency room policy of not prescribing narcotic analgesics for chronic pain is clearly stated on signs in the waiting area, Mr. Johnson comes there frequently complaining of severe back pain. He reports a history of gastric ulcers and allergy to nonsteroidal anti-inflammatory drugs (NSAIDs). The nurse practitioner who sees Mr. Johnson is faced with a man who is in obvious pain. She wishes to help him relieve the pain he is experiencing. At the same time she realizes that narcotic analgesia is not appropriate for this type of problem, and is unable to prescribe NSAIDs because

of his reports of gastric ulcers and allergy. He says he has tried exercises and a local pain clinic, neither of which was effective. He is aware of the emergency room policy regarding narcotic analgesics for chronic pain, but he comes there in desperation. He insists that his pain is relieved only by narcotic analgesia.

- What ethical principles are involved in this case?
- Does the benefit of pain relief outweigh the harm potentially caused by long-term narcotic analgesic use for this patient?
- Should Mr. Johnson's perceived need for narcotic pain medications be honoured even though the nurse practitioner feels he has a problem with drug dependence?
- How does the nurse do what she thinks is right and yet respect Mr. Johnson's autonomy?
- Is it important whether or not the nurse's actions please the patient?

REFERENCES

American Medical Association (2001). *Principles of Medical Ethics.* Chicago: American Medical Association. Retrieved August 15, 2012 from http://www.ama-assn.org/ama/pub/physician-resources/medical-ethics/code-medical-ethics/principles-medical-ethics.page

American Nurses Association (2001). *Code of Ethics For Nurses with Interpretive Statements.* Maryland: American Nurses Association. Retrieved August 15, 2012 from http://nursingworld.org/MainMenuCategories/EthicsStandards/CodeofEthicsforNurses/Code-of-Ethics.pdf

Aveyard, H. (2000). Is there a concept of autonomy that can usefully inform nursing practice? *Journal of Advanced Nursing, 32*(2), 352–358.

Beauchamp, T. L., & J. Childress (2001). *Principles of biomedical ethics* (5th ed.). New York: Oxford University Press.

Beauchamp, T. L., & L. Walters (2001). *Contemporary issues in bioethics.* Belmont, CA: Wadsworth.

Benatar, S., M. Bernstein, A. Daar, B. Dickens, S. McCrae, & R. Zlotnik Shaul (2003). Ethics and SARS: Lessons from Toronto. *British Medical Journal, 327*(7427), 1342–1345.

Bok, S. (1991). Lies to the sick and dying. In T. A. Mappes & J. S. Zembaty, eds. *Biomedical ethics* (pp. 74–81). New York: McGraw-Hill.

Bok, S. (1994). Truth telling. In W. Reich, ed., *Encyclopedia of bioethics* (pp. 1682–1686). New York: Macmillan.

Boyle, J. M. (2004). Medical ethics and double effect: The case of terminal sedation. *Theoretical Medicine and Bioethics: Philosophy of Medical Research and Practice,* 25(1), 51–60. Reprinted in J. Fisher, ed., (2009) *Biomedical ethics: A Canadian Focus.* Toronto: Oxford University Press.

Buber, M. (1965). *The knowledge of man: A philosophy of the interhuman.* New York: Harper & Row.

Cammon, S. A., & H. S. Hackshaw (2000). Are we starving our patients? *American Journal of Nursing, 100*(5), 43–46.

Canadian Nurses Association (2000). *The Canada Health Act*. Ottawa: Canadian Nurses Association.

Canadian Nurses Association. (2008). *Code of ethics for registered nurses*. Ottawa: Canadian Nurses Association.

Chas. Skinner, T. & S. Cradock (2000). Empowerment: What about the evidence? *Pract Diab Int., 17*(3), 91–95.

Collier, C. & R. Haliburton (2011). *Bioethics in Canada: A Philosophical Introduction*. Toronto: Canadian Scholars Press.

Derlega, V. J., B. A. Winstead, K. A. Gamble, K. Kelkar & P. Khu Anghlawn (2010). Inmates with HIV, stigma and disclosure decision making. *Journal of Health Psychology, 15*(2), 258–268.

Durant, W. (1926). *The story of philosophy*. New York: Washington Square Press.

Ellin, J. S. (1991). Lying and deception: The solution to a dilemma in medical ethics. In T. A. Mappes & J. S. Zembaty, eds., *Biomedical ethics* (pp. 81–87). New York: McGraw-Hill.

Erlen, J. A. (1998). The inadvertent breach of confidentiality. *Orthopedic Nursing, 17*(2), 47–50.

Goldsmith, J., ed. (1992). Virginia Henderson, RN: Humanitarian and scholar. *Reflections, 18*(1), 4–5.

Goodin, R. (1985). *Protecting the vulnerable. A Reanalysis of Our Social Responsibilities*. Chicago: University of Chicago Press.

Haggarty, L. A. (2000). Informed consent and the limit of confidentiality. *Western Journal of Nursing Research, 22*(4), 508–514.

Harrison, A. F., & R. M. Bramson (1982). *Styles of thinking*. New York: Doubleday.

Hébert, P. C., (1997). Bioethics for clinicians: Truthtelling. *Canadian Medical Association Journal, 156*(2), 225–228.

Hébert, P. C., B. Hoffmaster & K. C. Glass (2008). Truth telling. In P. Singer & A. M. Viens, eds., *The Cambridge textbook of bioethics*. Cambridge, England: Cambridge University Press.

International Council of Nurses (2006). *The ICN code of ethics for nurses*. International Council of Nurses, Geneva Switzerland. Retrieved January 23, 2001, from the World Wide Web: http://icn.ch/indes.html/

Jameton, A. (1984). *Nursing practice: The ethical issues*. Englewood Cliffs, NJ: Prentice-Hall.

Jenkins, V., L. Fallowfield & J. Saul (2001). Information needs of patients with cancer: Results from a large study in UK cancer centres. *British Journal of Cancer, 84*(1), 48–51.

Kardash, A., & A. Penta, eds. (2005). *A compendium of Canadian legislation respecting the protection of personal information in health research*. Ottawa: Canadian Institutes of Health Research.

Laurance, J. (2010). Ignorance can be preferable? *The Lancet, 375*(9732), 2138.

Lipkin, M. (1991). On lying to patients. In T. A. Mappes & J. S. Zembaty, eds., *Biomedical ethics* (pp. 72–73). New York: McGraw-Hill.

Markus, A., & M. Lockwood (1991). Is it permissible to edit medical records? *British Medical Journal*, 303, 349–351.

Mill, J. S. (1859). *On Liberty*. Oxford: Oxford University Press.

Muldoon, J. D. (1996). Confidentiality, privacy and restriction for computer-based patient records. *Hospital Topics, 74*(3), 32–37.

Munson, R. (1992). Major moral principles. In *Intervention and reflection: Basic issues in medical ethics* (4th ed., pp. 31–45). Belmont, CA: Wadsworth.

Myers, M. T., Jr. (2000). Lying for patients may be a violation of federal law. *Archives of Internal Medicine, 160*(4), 2223–2224.

Nathaniel, A. (2000). *An examination of ethical principles as they relate to noncompliance. Continuing education case study.* Sigma Theta Tau International Honor Society of Nursing. Retrieved January 13, 2001, from the World Wide Web: http://www.nursingsociety.org/

Nyberg, D. (1993). *The Varnished Truth*. Chicago: University of Chicago Press.

Oberle, K., & S. R. Bouchal (2009). *Ethics in Canadian Nursing Practice: Navigating the Journey.* Pearson: Toronto.

Office of the Privacy Commissioner of Canada (1985) *Privacy Act*. Retrieved July 6, 2011, from the World Wide Web: http://laws-lois.justice.gc.ca/eng/acts/P-21/index.html

Parent, W. A. (1983). A new definition of privacy for the law. *Law and Philosophy, 2*, 305–338.

Quinn, C. A., & M. D. Smith (1987). *The professional commitment: Issues and ethics in nursing.* Philadelphia: Saunders.

Romanow, R. (2002). *Building on values: The future of health care in Canada.* Commission on the future of health care in Canada. Final report. Canada.

Tobriner, M. O. (1991). Majority opinion in *Tarasoff v. Regents of the University of California*. In T. A. Mappes & J. S. Zembaty, eds., *Biomedical ethics* (pp. 165–169). New York: McGraw-Hill.

Tuckett, A. (2004). Truth-telling in clinical practice and the arguments for and against: A review of the literature. *Nursing Ethics, 11*(5), 500–513.

Veatch, R. (2000). *The basics of bioethics*. Upper Saddle River, NJ: Prentice Hall.

Winston, M. E. (1988). AIDS, confidentiality, and the right to know. *Public Affairs Quarterly, 2*, 91–104.

Yeo, M., A. Moorhouse, P. Khan & P. Rodney (2010). *Concepts and cases in nursing ethics* (3rd ed.). Peterborough, ON: Broadview Press.

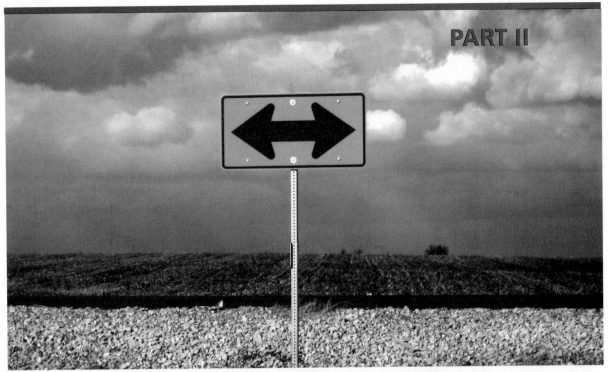

PART II

DEVELOPING PRINCIPLED BEHAVIOUR

Recognizing that values and beliefs are culturally relative, Part II describes theories related to moral development and clarification of values. This section examines the process of ethical decision making and its application to clinical situations. Because personal values and moral development influence perceptions and decisions, readers are encouraged to become aware of their own values and to examine personal levels of moral development in light of the different theories presented in Part I. Benefiting from this knowledge, readers can begin to be more sensitive to the perspectives, decision-making abilities, and tendencies of other people and to acknowledge the influence of their own values and moral development on decision-making processes.

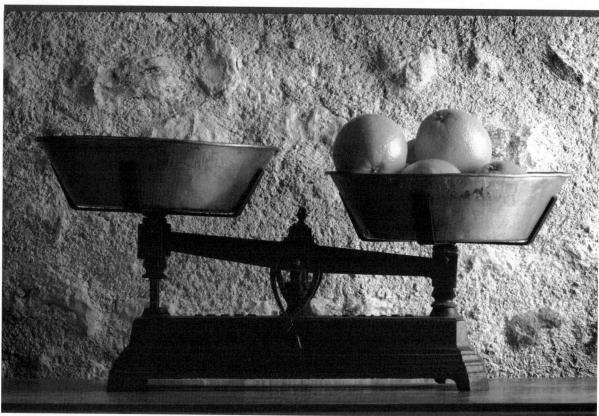

CHAPTER **4**
VALUES CLARIFICATION

OBJECTIVES

After completing this chapter, the reader should be able to:

1. Define and differentiate personal values, societal values, professional values, and organizational values.
2. Discuss how values are acquired.
3. Discuss self-awareness as a tool for ethical practice.
4. Explain the place of values clarification in nursing.
5. Describe values conflict and its implications for nursing care.
6. Consider the interaction between personal and institutional values.
7. Discuss the importance of attending to both personal values and patient values.

INTRODUCTION

Principled behaviour flows from personal values that guide and inform our responses, behaviours, and decisions in all areas of our life. Ethical decision making requires self-awareness and knowledge of ethical theories and principles. Such awareness of self includes knowing what we value or consider important. The branch of philosophy that studies the nature and types of values is called **axiology**, a word that comes from the Greek for *worth* or *worthy*. Axiology includes the study of aesthetics, such as the study of "beauty" in art or "tunefulness" in music, as well as ethics, the study of what is "right" or "wrong" in human relations and conduct.

If we listen to composer Arnold Schoenberg's *Six Little Pieces* (Opus 19, 1911), a work known for its atonal quality, many of us might find it difficult to listen to and not as harmonious as a piece such as *Claire de Lune*, a piano movement by Claude Debussy (part of the Suite Bergamasque, 1905), which is felt by many to be one of the most beautiful and melodious pieces of classical music ever written. Other people, however, may well feel that Schoenberg's atonal work is much more interesting, more vivacious, and far less predictable than Debussy's work and would claim that it is, therefore, better. There are as many diverse views and values as there are people. Just as tastes in music vary, so do our views on what may be "right" or "wrong" in terms of social or personal behaviours. Most of us are keenly aware of what music we find most harmonious and prefer to listen to. In turn, we also need to be aware of other kinds of values and preferences we hold, as these underpin our words, choices, and actions. This chapter discusses the importance of being aware of our own personal values and of how these values influence the way we relate to ourselves and others within both the personal and the professional arenas.

WHAT ARE VALUES?

Values are ideals, beliefs, customs, modes of conduct, qualities, or goals that are highly prized or preferred by individuals, groups, or society. Omery (1989) notes that the fundamental nature of values includes a pattern of a "subjective, strongly motivational preference or disposition toward a person, object, or idea that is more likely to be manifest in an affective situation ... and [is] more likely to be mobilized by the individual in a hierarchical order" (p. 500). Values, which are learned in both conscious and unconscious ways, become part of a person's makeup and provide guidance as we set priorities. When we are faced with choices, our preferences and their hierarchy become evident. For example, if we value truth telling in all types of situations without exception, others may see us as overly forthright or direct. What we value becomes apparent in how we conduct ourselves on a daily basis. When a friend asks how her new haircut looks, if we indeed value truth telling, we may well choose to tell her that the cut does not suit her. These kinds of decisions, and how we enact our values on a daily basis, shape who we are as moral persons and how those in our world perceive us. Our values influence our choices and behaviour, whether or not we are conscious that the values are guiding those choices. Values provide direction and meaning to life and a frame of reference for integrating, explaining, and evaluating new experiences, thoughts, and relationships. Values may be expressed overtly, as espoused behaviours or verbalized standards, or may manifest in an indirect way through other kinds of verbal and nonverbal behaviour.

Moral Values

As discussed in Chapter 2, individual cognitive evaluations of right and wrong, good and bad, reflects **moral thought.** Flowing from this, preferences or dispositions that reflect right or wrong in human behaviour are considered **moral values** (Omery, 1989). Moral values constitute a special type of values, because the particular circumstances that call them forth deal with ethical issues or dilemmas. These kinds of values are what we refer to, implicitly, when we are deciding, *"What is the right thing to do?"* We are often faced with moral or ethical dilemmas that challenge our beliefs or force us to articulate our values in an explicit way, through our actions or decisions. These kinds of ethical dilemmas may be encountered in a professional context or in our personal lives, as we interact and form relationships with others. Moral values help us to decide what we ought to do, or should do, according to our deeply held beliefs and priorities. These kinds of values are acquired over a lifetime, may be dynamic and iterative, and are influenced by any number of contexts or factors, such as our family, culture, spirituality, education, friendships, philosophical orientation, workplace, or profession, to name a few. These values may be acquired within contexts and social constructs such as the family, through our religious, educational, or philosophical orientation, or through our profession.

ACQUIRING VALUES

Personal ethical behaviour flows from values held by an individual that develop over time. Cultural, ethnic, familial, environmental, educational, and other experiences of living help to shape our values. We begin to learn and incorporate values into our beings at an early age and continue the process throughout our lives. As noted previously, values are acquired in both conscious and unconscious ways. Values may be learned in a conscious way through instruction by parents, teachers, mentors, religious leaders and educators, and professional or social group leaders. Many values are formally adopted by groups and are written in professional codes of ethics, religious doctrines, societal laws, and statements of an organization's philosophy. Socialization and role-modelling, other ways values are acquired, lead to more subconscious learning. Some values stay with us for much of our lives, and others may change or be altered in response to our own development and experiences. "The most important step in values formation is one's freedom to choose those values that are most cherished and to relinquish those that have little meaning" (Seroka, 1994, p. 11). The process of value formation, as Seroka calls it, and the choosing or rejecting of values, might also be referred to as the development of one's **moral autonomy**.

As children, we often adopt the values and beliefs of our parents. We are told what school we will attend, what religion we are affiliated with, and, in our interactions with those all around us, we encounter our culture, environment, and socioeconomic status relative to others. In one sense, we simply assume the values and beliefs of those with the most influence over us. Adolescents often identify more strongly with friends and peer groups, social networks, and both school and extracurricular activities. Through exploration of the world around them in a more independent way, adolescents may find that they are questioning the values of their parents, religion, culture, or the environment that surrounds them as they are growing up. This is often referred to as "teenage rebellion," and it is an important step in the development of our moral autonomy. By moral autonomy, we are referring to taking responsibility for our values and beliefs and embracing them as our own. As we develop increased moral autonomy, we move away from simply adopting the values of others, such as our parents or peers, and instead embracing our own values that we demonstrate to others through our words, our actions, and our choices. In essence, we become more independent in terms of our moral life and commit to "owning" our convictions, as opposed to being simply guided by others (Yeo, Moorhouse, Khan & Rodney, 2010).

Later in youth, as we take on new roles away from home, as college or university students, as workers, new professionals or careerists, we are compelled to again explore new sets of values, beliefs, and priorities, and find a way to incorporate or overlap these new values into our existing set of values and beliefs.

As we develop new relationships with people outside our immediate families, who may come from diverse cultures, environments, or religions than our own, we also may reflect upon our own values, and, as Seroka notes, discover which of our held values are especially important, while renouncing those without meaning. In addition to these processes, we may also adopt or assume new values, or change our values based on our experiences, relationships, and environments.

While many of us have "core" values that we find are relatively unchanging over time, even these values may be adaptable as we learn new perspectives or worldviews. Additionally, we may find a new perspective that helps us to better articulate our long-held values in a novel way. For example, consider Beatrice, a young nursing student who was raised by parents who identified themselves as agnostic and who instead focused their moral teaching toward Beatrice on doing good for others in all aspects of one's life and rejecting money or possessions as motivation for action or success. After travelling to do missionary work in Nepal, Beatrice found herself drawn to Buddhism. She identified strongly with the messages and philosophical stance of Buddhists and decided to embrace Buddhism in her own life. While she did not change her own values, she found that her identification with Buddhism provided with her a means to articulate the values that were instilled by her parents in a new and meaningful way.

Because values become a part of who we are, they often enter into decision making in less-than-conscious ways. We constantly make judgments that reflect our values, not always realizing that we have a given set of values or that these values are affecting our decisions (Davis, Aroskar, Liaschenko, & Drought, 1997; Engebretson &

Headley, 2000; Simon, Howe, & Kirschenbaum, 1995). Becoming more aware of one's own values is an important preliminary and ongoing step in being able to make clear and thoughtful decisions. Reflecting upon one's own values in a conscious way, and being able to help others to articulate their values clearly, are particularly important in the area of ethical decision making.

ASK YOURSELF

How Have Your Values Developed?

Think of three ideals or beliefs that you prize in your personal life. For example, you may value a clean house and an orderly life, or you may place a lower value on keeping your house clean and tidy and instead focus on valuing quality time with your children each day. As another example, you may find that you place a high value on being married, while others may feel that it is not necessary to be married to have a long-term, meaningful relationship. Or you may set priorities in your working life to work fewer hours and spend more time relaxing and with your family, but have less disposable income, while others may value working harder and longer hours in order to provide their family with more disposable income and time away on luxurious vacations.

When you think of what you value, your ideals or beliefs, try to think back to how those beliefs or values came into your awareness. Reflect upon how each belief or ideal evolved to become something that you identify as important or a priority. Try to trace each belief or ideal back to the earliest time in your life when you were aware of its importance or presence.

- When and how did you learn to view each belief or ideal as important?
- How have they changed or evolved over time?
- Where do you find your support for them?
- How prevalent do you think these beliefs or ideals are among other people?
- What do you think of people who hold different beliefs or ideals?
- Think of a time in your life when one of these beliefs or ideals has been challenged. How did you feel? How did you react?

SELF-AWARENESS

Ethical relationships with others begin with self-knowledge and the willingness to express that awareness to others honestly and appropriately. Self-knowledge is an ongoing, evolving process that requires us to make a commitment to know the truth about ourselves. This is not an easy commitment to make. We must remember that what we believe to be the truth is always coloured by our perceptions and surrounding contextual factors, and can change over a time (Covey, 1990). Keep in mind that most situations are not black-and-white, that is, with just two opposite sides. Many sides are present in each situation. Like looking through a camera, what we see in any situation depends upon where we are standing and the angle we are looking from. From this perspective, there can be many views of a situation, depending upon how many people are picturing it. Understanding the truth of a situation is usually more accurate if people appreciate that there can be different views, and openly share these perspectives (Banonis, 1997). While sharing diverse perspectives is key to any kind of exercise in which we identify or explore values, we must keep in mind the importance of remaining open to multiple perspectives. While we can never "walk in the shoes" of another person, truly; we can, however, remain open to how others' realities, experiences, cultures, spirituality, and environments have shaped their perspective. We also need to attend to and actively understand the reasons and rationales that others have for the decisions they make and the priorities they set, especially if they differ from what our own decisions or actions might have been in a similar situation. The ability to be open to multiple perspectives, to try to understand the reasons others have for their decisions or actions, is an important part of becoming an ethically aware person. In a professional context, developing this ability is essential to interacting with and providing holistic and client-centred care to a diverse population.

The term **values clarification** refers to the process of becoming more conscious of and articulating what we value or consider worthy. It is an ongoing process that is grounded in our capacity for reflective, intelligent, self-directed behaviour (Gaydos, 2000; Keegan, 2000). By devoting time, energy, and attention to reflecting on our values, we shed light on our personal perspective and discover our own answers to many concerns and questions. Developing insight into our values improves our ability to make value decisions. No one set of values is appropriate for everyone; we must appreciate that values clarification may lead to different insights for different people (Engebretson & Headley, 2000; Gaydos, 2000). Engaging in values clarification promotes a closer fit between our words and actions, enabling us to more clearly "walk our talk," thus enhancing personal integrity. As noted in Chapter 2, **integrity** refers to adherence to moral norms that is sustained over time. **Moral integrity** could also be called **authenticity**. Authenticity, in terms of moral development, refers to the attribute of maintaining and articulating consistent fundamental values and beliefs over time. As we noted above, sometimes our values and beliefs may change or iterate as we age, question, and learn new perspectives. However, for many of us, our very fundamental "core" beliefs persist over time, despite being exposed to many different influences. These might include fundamental beliefs such as believing that hurting others is wrong, that telling the truth is preferable to deception, or that those who are vulnerable or who depend on our care must be protected from harm. Being authentic, or maintaining moral integrity, signifies that we hold such beliefs or values in a way that is consistent and unwavering. Note, however, that this does not imply that, as persons with strong moral integrity, we automatically reject others who hold markedly different beliefs. Instead, we must be as steadfast in exploring, understanding, and appreciating the values of others as we are in holding onto our own. Trustworthiness and a consistency of convictions, actions, and emotions is implicit in integrity. It is only to the extent that we appreciate our own values that we can begin to understand the values of another.

Since values include dimensions of knowing and of feeling, the process of becoming more clear about what we consider to be overarching values needs to address both the cognitive and the affective domains. Through analyzing our own behaviour and becoming more in touch with our feelings, we learn to discern which choices are rational, thoughtful, and dynamic, and which are the result of preconditioning (Seroka, 1994). Assessment of personal values requires a readiness and willingness to take an honest look at our ideals and behaviours; at our words, actions, and motivation; and at the congruencies and incongruencies among them. Moving toward the point of choosing our own values, rather than merely acting out prior programming, is a goal of the process and part of our ongoing development of our moral autonomy.

Enhancing Self-Awareness

Self-awareness is the ultimate tool for living a personally ethical life. Values clarification and **self-awareness** go hand in hand. The first and most important step in awareness of the self is the conscious intention to be aware. Being conscious of our thoughts, feelings, physical and emotional responses, and insights in various situations can promote appreciation of our values. Conversely, by identifying and analyzing personal values, we become more self-aware (Burkhardt & Nagai-Jacobson, 2002; Rew, 1996; Rew, 2000). We can enhance insight by developing the ability to step back and see what is going on in any situation, and by being aware of ourselves and our reactions in the present moment. Self-awareness can begin with as simple an act as tuning in to our breathing, noting its rate, rhythm, depth, and other characteristics without any effort to change it. Self-awareness is a way of becoming conscious of an act that usually occurs quite unconsciously. Another way to become more aware is to pay attention to how we are feeling physically and emotionally in any given situation— to name the feelings without judging them. We might ask, "What do I think I am reacting to here, and can I identify where that reaction comes from?" or "Why am I uncomfortable with this person's choice or decision?" For example, when you see a beautiful sunset, you might note a feeling of peace, exhilaration, or relaxation, and realize you are responding to beauty, with an ensuing memory that your mother was always one to be observant of natural beauty in her world. You thus recognize that you learned this value, at least in part, from your mother. Introspection, observation, reflection, meditation, journaling, art, writing, therapy, reading, discussion groups, and feedback all assist us in expanding self-awareness.

Individual reflection and discussion with another person or in small groups help us to become more aware of and to analyze our values. Group discussion enables us to react and to hear the reactions of others. Such processes may lead us to see more clearly those values we have accepted because of programming, and to articulate better those values we have chosen. These processes may also lead us to modify our perspective based on the insights of others. Active listening and reflection upon the diverse views and beliefs of others is an important part of these processes. Alongside listening and reflecting, self-awareness requires that we maintain on openness to the views of others, as we reflect upon our own. Other tools that open our perspective include taking the other side of a debate, interviewing people with differing opinions, walking in another's shoes and defending his or her position, and asking for feedback on our positions. Another way to look at values is to ask general questions like, "If I knew I would die in six weeks, what would I be doing today?" or "If I had to leave my house and could take only three things with me, what would they be?" or "Where would I like to be five/ten/twenty years from now?"

Simon and colleagues (1995) suggest that the valuing process includes three areas:

Prizing and cherishing one's own beliefs and behaviours, which includes knowing what one does and does not support and communicating this to others;

Choosing one's own beliefs and behaviours by evaluating values received from others, which includes examining alternatives and their consequences, then deciding what is one's own;

Acting on these beliefs with a consistent pattern that reinforces actions supportive of the values.

The intent of values clarification is to help us become more aware of our own values and the valuing process in our lives; it does not aim to impose or instil particular values in our lives.

Journaling

Kolkmeier (1995) describes **journals** as "records that are kept on a periodic or regular basis and contain factual material and subjective interpretations of events, thoughts, feelings, and plans" (p. 336). For many people, keeping a diary or journal of experiences and personal reactions to situations is a useful tool in developing awareness. For evolving professionals, reflecting upon and keeping a record of how we sort out our values, deal with difficult situations or interpret events around us, can help us as we grow into our professional roles. Part of being a responsible and accountable professional is monitoring our own practice and reactions to difficult or challenging situations (Billings & Kowalski, 2006). Being aware of one's values is a key first step in clarifying them, yet we spend little time actively thinking about our values and beliefs. Journaling provides us with time that is purposely set aside for precisely that—thinking about and reflecting upon our reactions, beliefs, and values. The process of journaling may help us as we deal with difficult patient situations that challenge us and force us to reflect upon, or even re-evaluate, our values and beliefs. A number of books and scholarly articles such as those by Progoff (1992), Kahn (1996), and Boud (2002) are available to guide someone new to journaling. Figure 4–1 offers guidelines that may help students utilize the journaling process to gain insight into personal values. The following are a few general considerations that may enhance the ability to gain insight through journaling. When writing in a journal, let your thoughts flow as freely as possible without censoring or judging what you are writing. Allow yourself time and privacy when you are journaling, and keep the journal in a place where you feel comfortable that you control who has access to it. Commit to journaling on a regular basis. Recognize that journaling is a personal process, so go with your style. If a format such as that suggested in Figure 4–1 helps you, go for it! If not, write as the thoughts flow from you.

FIGURE 4–1 **JOURNALING FOR VALUES AWARENESS**

- Describe a situation in your personal or professional experience when you felt uncomfortable or felt that your beliefs or values were being challenged, or when you felt your values were different from those of others involved.
- As you record the situation, include how you felt physically and emotionally at the time you experienced the situation.
- Write down your feelings as you remember the situation. Are your reactions now any different from when you were actually in this situation?
- What personal values do you identify in the situation? Try to remember where and from whom you learned these values. Do you completely agree with the values, or is there anything about them that you question?
- What values do you think were being expressed by others involved? How are they similar to or different from your values?
- What do you think you reacted to in the situation?
- Can you remember having similar reactions in other situations? If yes, how were the situations similar or different?
- How do you feel about your response to the situation? Is there anything you would change if you could repeat the scene? Rewrite the scene with the changes or alternative endings.
- What do you need to do to reinforce behaviours, ideals, beliefs, or qualities that you have identified as personal values in this situation? When and how can you do this?

VALUES IN PROFESSIONAL SITUATIONS

Values clarification is important to nurses in several ways. To know and appreciate our own value system provides a basis for understanding how and why we react and respond in decision-making situations. Knowing our own values enables us to acknowledge similarities and differences in values when interacting with others, which ultimately promotes more effective communication and care. Commitment to developing more awareness of personal values enables us to be more effective in facilitating the process with others. In the professional realm, these others may be colleagues, patients, families, or institutions.

Values Conflict

When personal values are at odds with those of patients, colleagues, or the institution, internal or interpersonal conflict may result. This can subsequently affect patient care and can have serious personal and professional implications for the nurse. Dealing in an effective way with **values conflict** requires conscious awareness of our own values, as well as awareness of the perceived values of the others involved. Such awareness enables the nurse to be more alert to situations where the behaviours of others are judged according to his or her own values, or where personal values are being imposed upon another. When differences in values are identified, the nurse can choose to respond to the other's viewpoint in a way that seeks understanding and common ground, rather than reacting in a "knee-jerk" fashion. In this way the integrity of the caring relationship can be maintained.

The following case presentation provides an example of values conflict. As you read the case, think about the values that are evident in the situation. Put yourself in the position of each of the participants and ask yourself what you might do if you were in their shoes.

CASE PRESENTATION

A Conflict of Values

Nine-year-old Ryder is a patient on the pediatric unit with a diagnosis of terminal stage Ewing's sarcoma. He has three sisters, aged seven, six, and three, who are currently being cared for by a grandmother. His father is self-employed and works long hours. His mother has never worked outside the home. Both parents have high school educations, and their primary activities outside the family are church-related. They belong to a small nondenominational rural church and state that they hold fast to what is taught in the Bible and put their faith in the word of God.

Prior to his illness, Ryder, a healthy child, had been brought to the clinic only for acute health concerns. Shortly after entering second grade two years ago, he began limping. The family attributed the limp to a playground injury. When he continued to complain of pain and the limp persisted after three months, his mother took him to a local health clinic. Above-the-knee amputation followed diagnosis, but metastasis was evident in nine months. Chemotherapy has been only palliative.

The physician has discussed Ryder's poor prognosis with the parents, recommending comfort care. The parents say they want everything possible to be done for him, and the father conducts nightly prayer sessions at Ryder's bedside, affirming that God is healing Ryder. Although Ryder has asked whether he is going to die, his father refuses to allow staff to speak with him regarding fears or concerns about his condition. When asked what Ryder has been told, the father responds, "He knows God is trying us and we must have faith." The mother, who

(Continued)

appears less confident of a healing, is there twenty-four hours a day. She supervises Ryder's care relentlessly, at times irritating staff with questions and demands. She keeps a notebook record of her son's care, including medication, times of care, intake and output, and personal assessments. Although Ryder used to talk to staff, he now appears frightened and remains quiet, sleeping off and on.

THINK ABOUT IT

Dealing with Values Conflict

Respond to these questions from the vantage point of the nurse in the situation:

- What is your first personal reaction to this situation? Identify your values relative to the situation.
- What do you perceive to be the values of the others involved?
- Identify value incongruity that might lead to conflict. Give specific examples of how such a conflict can potentially affect patient care.
- Describe specific nursing interventions aimed at managing the conflict in a professional manner, and give examples of how nursing practice standards or Codes of Ethics might help to guide such actions.
- Describe your own strengths and limitations as you consider how you might deal with this situation.

Impact of Institutional Values

Nurses need to be conscious of both the spoken and unspoken values in their work settings. Values of individual institutions and organized health care systems that are explicitly communicated through philosophy and policy documents, such as mission or vision statements, are called **overt values**. Overt values are also found in Codes of Ethics, such as the Canadian Nurses Association *Code of Ethics for Nurses*, which lists eight core values of nursing (2008). These include "providing safe, compassionate, competent and ethical care; promoting health and well-being, promoting and respecting informed decision making, preserving dignity, maintaining privacy and confidentiality, promoting justice, and being accountable" (CNA, 2008, p. 3). While these are broad and, to some degree, highly interpretable values, they provide a reference for the public to understand the explicit values that nurses must embody in their everyday practice. We may have many different ways of, for example, preserving dignity or promoting justice, depending on the situation, but these two values should clearly be the motivating factor behind the actions of nurses as they provide care in a variety of contexts.

Values may also be implicit in expectations that are not in writing. Implicit or **covert values** are often identified only through participation in or controversies within the setting (Omery, 1989). When seeking employment, nurses should identify congruencies or incongruencies between their personal values and those of the institution, because accepting employment implies committing to the value system of the organization. Consider, for example, Maya, who has worked for many years at a small but busy downtown hospital that provides care for HIV and AIDS patients and is especially sensitive to the community of gay and transgendered individuals who live locally. Many of the staff there are members of that community and identify with the unique needs and concerns of their clients. Clients, in turn, feel supported and treated in a holistic and meaningful way. A decision by the provincial government has resulted in an amalgamation between Maya's small hospital and a larger hospital, located on the other side of town. Traditionally, the larger hospital has been affiliated with the Catholic Church but now, as the merger approaches, it has publicly acknowledged that the amalgamated hospital structure will be one that embraces diversity and provides holistic, client-centred care for all persons. While Maya appreciates this public acknowledgement, she is worried that there may well be difficulties in merging the collective but diverse values of the two groups of staff members. She has heard from some friends who work there that some of the staff members at the larger hospital are not in favour of the merger and do not wish to provide care to HIV-positive or AIDS patients who are gay or transgendered. She worries that her clients may not be treated in a way that is respectful or inclusive, and that they may feel further marginalized, despite what the public announcements have portrayed. Maya's worries about the institution are well-founded. Having markedly divergent personal values from the institutions we work in can easily lead to disagreements, control issues, and job dissatisfaction. In health care settings, this can have serious implications for patient care. Maya will be faced with a difficult decision as she decides whether or not she can work, or help to enact change, in the culture of the new amalgamated hospital setting.

If there is a conflict between our values regarding patient care and the values of the institution, physician, or family, we may experience moral distress. **Moral distress** is the reaction to a situation in which there are moral problems that seem to have clear solutions, yet we are unable to follow our moral beliefs because of external restraints. Jameton notes that moral distress is "knowing the morally right course of action to take" (Jameton, 1984, p. 542), but being prevented from taking it, due to institutional conflicts, structures, or constraints. This distress is often evidenced by anger, dissatisfaction, frustration, and poor performance in the work setting. We will be discussing moral distress in greater detail in Chapter 6, where we examine models of ethical decision making.

ASK YOURSELF

How Should Values Influence Job Selection?

Maria, a recently divorced mother of two, desperately needs to return to work, but nursing jobs in her area are scarce. There is one opening at a women's health clinic that provides advice on contraception and sexuality, and provides non-judgmental counselling and referrals for women who are seeking therapeutic abortions. The clinic is located close to a day care centre that can accommodate Maria's children. The job, which offers excellent salary and benefits, looks great to Maria, except that abortions are contrary to her personal and religious beliefs. A friend who works at the clinic said that, unless they are short staffed, Maria would not have to counsel women who are seeking abortions if she had objections.

- What dilemmas are evident in this situation?
- What are the clear differences in values between those that the clinic is founded upon, and Maria's?
- What are your values related to this situation?
- What factors should Maria consider in deciding whether to take the job?
- Although Maria's friend offers a possible solution, can you foresee any problems related to this proposed solution?

Gingerich and Ondeck (1993) describe one process for defining and making organizational values more explicit. This process includes determining what is valued by staff, board members, management, and health care professionals regarding the elements of the organization's philosophy, and identifying specific expectations for each group. Exercises focused on self-awareness, clinical priorities, and opinions about value-laden issues are conducted within each of the groups to develop awareness of and consensus around the values. This allows all involved to have an investment in the value system.

The Hartman Value Profile is another approach to looking at values within an organization (Edwards & Davis, 1991; Hartman, 1967). The process involves having the institution select a number of employees representing two groups within the organization: those considered to be the "shining stars," and those considered least satisfactory. The selected employees complete the profile, which is a forced ranking, from best to worst or most despicable, of eighteen items relating to how persons perceive the world around them and eighteen items related to how they perceive their inner selves. Patterns are identified by analyzing the participants' responses, utilizing a computerized mathematical system that identifies how each item compares with the others that are ranked. The resulting information provides a profile of the underlying values within the organization. Decision makers can use this information to examine how prevailing belief systems are influencing performance, and to seek potential employees whose values are most consistent with those of the organization.

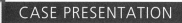

CASE PRESENTATION

Differences in Personal and Organizational Values

Joan has been the nurse manager of her unit for the past ten years and is highly regarded by the hospital's administration. For the past several months, however, she has been feeling more frustrated and less satisfied with her work because of staffing cuts and other institutional decisions. Attending to patient needs has always been the most rewarding part of her job. However, many of the institutional decisions, in Joan's opinion, have negatively affected patient care. Recently she feels that she has been forced to overlook these needs and attend more to the needs of the organization. She considers leaving, but she has seniority, good benefits, and two children to support. She is also aware that her distress at work is affecting her family, because she carries a lot of the frustration home with her.

THINK ABOUT IT

How Values Affect Choices

- Identify values evident in this situation. Which of these reflect your personal values?
- What conflicts might arise from these values?
- What do you think Joan should do?
- If you were in Joan's position, what beliefs, ideals, or goals would guide you in making a decision to stay or leave? Identify potential consequences of each choice.

Clarifying Values with Patients

Values of both nurses and patients influence patient care situations. Since patients are the recipients and consumers of health care, it is good to know what they expect or value. Patient and provider perceptions of what constitutes quality care can be quite different. Great discrepancies in these perceptions may lead to patient dissatisfaction. This can have a variety of consequences, including affecting a patient's attitude and decisions regarding following recommendations for care and treatment (which may affect recovery), marring the reputation of the health care agency or institution or potentiating poor relationships between patients and providers. Allanach and Golden (1988) describe the process of a service audit aimed at identifying patient expectations and clarifying their opinions about the level of service. Nursing care behaviours identified as valued by patients in this study relate to the amount of care and time spent with patients and to the technical quality of nursing care. Consider the potential conflict of values when patients expect nurses to spend time with them and the institution puts more emphasis on getting the tasks done.

ASK YOURSELF

What Would You Do?

- You are busy and two call lights go on at the same time. What factors enter into deciding which one you respond to first?
- Consider that in the above situation one patient is in serious condition and has been verbally abusive to staff, while the other is not quite as serious and is someone you really enjoy being with. Whom would you respond to first and why?
- Your patients let you know how much they appreciate the extra care and time you give them compared to the other nurses. At the same time, your evaluation is coming up and your supervisor has indicated that you need to be more efficient with your time. What would you do in this situation and why?

When working with patients regarding health care decisions, nurses need to be aware of personal values and patients' values pertaining to health. When the health values of the nurse and those of the patient are different, the patient may become labelled as "difficult," unco-operative, self-destructive, noncompliant, ignorant, or unwilling to take responsibility for her or his own health. Part of being an ethical practitioner involves the ability to see the world from others' perspectives and to realize that they are just as valid as our own, although they may be markedly different. Cultural differences in values, beliefs, and choices should be viewed as opportunities for learning and expanding our understanding of the world around us, without assuming that our perspective is the "right one." Instead, these differences are often seen as variances from a cultural "norm" and efforts are put less into understanding the divergent views of others, and more into trying to change these views to more closely resemble our own. This is a dangerous stance to take and one that is ethically problematic, at the very least. In today's world, **globalization** and the multicultural nature of most societies compel us to attend to, engage with, and be respectful of the varied views, values, and choices of others. We'll discuss respect for diverse views, values, and norms in much more detail in Chapter 18.

Pender (1996) discusses the role of values in health promotion. She notes that knowing personal values is important, as is the need to avoid imposing our values on patients. Consider, for example, this client at a youth outreach centre: an impoverished young woman living on the street, with few supports and almost no financial arrangements. She admits to drug use, cigarette smoking, and alcohol abuse. She also discloses to you that she has had sex with men for money, drugs, and alcohol. While she admits it is dangerous, she uses condoms and ensures that she always works with another friend, in order to be safe. She tells you that she likes "partying," doing drugs and drinking, and while living on the street would not be a choice for many, for her it represents an escape from a home life that was, according to her, highly abusive and much more oppressive and dangerous. If priorities on her care plan include improved nutrition, stopping sexual activity for money, smoking cessation, drug rehabilitation and cessation, and alcohol abstinence, while well-intentioned, these goals may simply demonstrate nursing values being imposed on the client. Instead, exploring the client's wishes, reasons for seeking care, and ways to advocate, support her, and help ensure her safety in her chosen lifestyle, at this time, would be a more meaningful and worthwhile health promotion activity.

With self-awareness, the nurse can be more effective in helping patients to identify their own values. Assisting patients to clearly articulate their values is important, because a lack of clarity about values may result in inconsistency, confusion, misunderstanding, and inadequate decision making. It can also lead to feelings of being influenced or coerced among patients who do not have an opportunity to clearly articulate their values, choices, and rationales. The ability to make informed choices, including the process of informed consent, is enhanced by having clarity about our values. "Assisting clients to clarify values; understand the personal and social consequences of acting on current values; achieve greater consistency among values, attitudes, and behaviours; and plan health-related experiences that may result in self-initiated changes in value hierarchies" are key nursing actions (Pender, 1987, p. 161). Many instruments, surveys and processes are available to facilitate exploring values in general and health values in particular. Here are a few examples of such instruments. From the simplest exercises to the most complicated psychological tools, exploring one's values can be done in many ways.

? THINK ABOUT IT

Here are some basic exercises for clarifying general values and those related to our health and well-being. Try them on your own or work through them with others, and compare your answers:

- Write a personal "mission statement." Include your thoughts on questions such as "If I could do the last ten years over, what would I change?", "What are the five things I feel most passionate about?", "If I only had one month left to live, how would I spend my time?", "Where would I like to be in five years, in terms of my personal life, career and financial status?", or "If I died tomorrow, what would people say about me?"

(Continued)

- Construct a list of your goals, as well as your strengths and weaknesses. Examine the list and ask yourself how your strengths may be better used to achieve goals that are aligned with your values. Then ask yourself how your weaknesses may make it more difficult to achieve your goals.

- Rank a list of ten health values from most important to least important. The list includes a comfortable life, an exciting life, a sense of accomplishment, freedom, happiness, health, inner harmony, pleasure, self-respect, and social recognition (Pender, 1987, p. 165). For this exercise, Pender notes that if health appears within the top four on the list, you tend to place a high value on health. Remember, however, that definitions of health will vary, since each person defines health according to personal beliefs and values.

- Identify a list of ten health-related behaviours you engage in, and then provide an answer for why you do each one. Behaviours might include activities such as exercising three times per week, eating healthy food, limiting the amount of alcohol you drink, taking medications carefully, talking to a close friend or relative about worries, or having sex with or without using a condom. Doyle (1994) notes that the response to *why* a behaviour is practised provides insight into values surrounding the behaviour, such as choosing not to exercise in order to have more free time, or choosing to exercise because it helps in weight control.

SUMMARY

This chapter has discussed the importance of self-awareness regarding values and the valuing process. Values are learned, and change in response to life situations as a person develops. The process of values clarification enables persons to begin to identify and choose their own values rather than merely act out of prior programming. The interaction between personal values and those of patients and organizations can affect job satisfaction and patient care. The reader is encouraged to explore various processes that facilitate values clarification, both those presented in this chapter and those found in other resources.

CHAPTER HIGHLIGHTS

- Values are highly prized ideals, behaviours, beliefs, or qualities that are shaped by culture, ethnicity, family, environment, and education, and are acquired in both conscious and unconscious ways.

- The process of incorporating values begins at an early age and continues throughout life. Some values remain constant, while others change in response to growth and life experiences.

- Awareness of personal values undergirds the ability to make clear and thoughtful decisions, and enables us to acknowledge similarities and differences in values when interacting with others, thus promoting more effective communication, care, and facilitation of values clarification with others.

- Values clarification is not intended to instil values; rather, the aim is to facilitate awareness of personal values and the valuing process in order to move toward the point of choosing our own values rather than merely reacting from prior programming.

- The valuing process includes prizing and cherishing, choosing, and acting on beliefs and behaviours.

- Dealing effectively with values conflict requires attention to personal values, the perceived values of others, and the ability to recognize both overt and covert expressions of values in a situation.

- Congruence between personal values and those of an institution is an important consideration for a nurse seeking employment.

- Assisting patients to articulate their values and beliefs, an important part of nursing care, may help prevent deleterious consequences related to not addressing differences in values between patients and providers.

DISCUSSION QUESTIONS AND ACTIVITIES

1. A non-nursing classmate asks you what studying personal values and beliefs has to do with nursing. How would you respond? Incorporate your understanding of the nature of values and how they become part of us into your response.

2. What values guide your personal life? How did you learn these values? Select something that you consider important in professional nursing practice and trace how you learned this value.

3. Identify a societal value. Then explore whether or not you also value this personally, and how you express this value as an individual. Some examples of societal values might include: wealth, technology, fairness, equity.

4. Identify the overt and covert values of your health care agency or school. Then identify both overt and covert values of nurses, educators, and others within the agency or school setting. Explain the importance of knowing about both.

5. Describe a situation in which you experienced someone (it could be you) reacting from values that were not conscious at the time. How did this affect the interaction?

6. Determine the health values of three patients or people you do not know well and discuss why nurses need to be attentive to what patients value.

7. Describe a situation in which you experienced values conflict and how you dealt with the conflict.

8. Find current examples of public or professional figures whose personal values seem at odds with their professional or public trust. Discuss your reaction to the discrepancy in values that you identify and the interplay between personal values and professional integrity.

REFERENCES

Allanach, E. J., & B. M. Golden (1988). Patients' expectations and values clarification: A service audit. *Nursing Administration Quarterly, 12,* 17–22.

Banonis, B. C. (1997). *Principled behavior applied to everyday life.* Charleston, WV: Unpublished manuscript.

Billings, D., & K. Kowalski (2006). Journaling: A strategy for developing reflective practitioners. *Journal of Continuing Education in Nursing, 37*(3), 104–105.

Boud, D. (2002). Using journal writing to enhance reflective practice. *New Directions for Adult and Continuing Education.* DOI: 10.1002/ace.16

Burkhardt, M. A., & M. G. Nagai-Jacobson (2002). *Spirituality and healing.* Albany, NY: Delmar Publishers.

Canadian Nurses Association (2008). *Codes of ethics for Registered Nurses.* Canadian Nurses Association: Ottawa.

Chinn, P. L. (1995). *Peace and power: Building communities for the future* (4th ed.). New York: National League of Nursing Press.

Covey, S. R. (1990). *The seven habits of highly effective people.* New York: Simon & Schuster.

Davis, A. J., M. A. Aroskar, J. Liaschenko, & T.S. Drought (1997). *Ethical dilemmas and nursing practice* (4th ed.). Norwalk, CT: Appleton & Lange.

Doyle, E. I. (1994). Recognizing the value-health behavior connection: "What I do and why I do it." *Journal of Health Education, 25,* 116–118.

Edwards, R. B., & J. W. Davis (1991). *Forms of value and valuation.* Lanham, MD: University Press of America.

Engebretson, J. C., & J. A. Headley (2000). Cultural diversity and care. In B. M. Dossey, L. Keegan, & C. E. Guzzetta, eds., *Holistic nursing: A handbook for practice* (3rd ed., pp. 283–310). Gaithersburg, MD: Aspen Publishers.

Gaydos, H. L. B. (2000). The art of holistic nursing and the human health experience. In B. M. Dossey, L. Keegan, & C. E. Guzzetta, eds., *Holistic nursing: A handbook for practice* (3rd ed., pp. 51–66). Gaithersburg, MD: Aspen Publishers.

Gingerich, B. S., & Ondeck, D. A. (1993). Values incorporation throughout the organization. *Caring Magazine, 12,* 18–23.

Hartman, R. S. (1967). *The structure of value.* Carbondale, IL: Southern Illinois University Press.

Jameton, A. (1984). *Nursing practice: The ethical issues.* New Jersey: Prentice-Hall.

Kahn, S. (1996). *The nurse's meditative journal.* Albany, NY: Delmar Publishers.

Keegan, L. (2000). Holistic ethics. In B. M. Dossey, L. Keegan, & C. E. Guzzetta, eds., *Holistic nursing: A handbook for practice* (3rd ed., pp. 159–170). Gaithersburg, MD: Aspen Publishers.

Kolkmeier, L. G. (1995). Self-reflection: Consulting the truth within. In B. M. Dossey, L. Keegan, C. E. Guzzetta, & L. G. Kolkmeier, eds., *Holistic nursing: A handbook for practice* (2nd ed.). Gaithersburg, MD: Aspen.

Omery, A. (1989). Values, moral reasoning, and ethics. *Nursing Clinics of North America, 24,* 499–507.

Pender, N. J. (1996). *Health promotion in nursing practice* (3rd ed.). Norwalk, CT: Appleton & Lange.

Progoff, I. (1992). *At a journal workshop.* New York: Tarcher.

Rew, L. (1996). *Awareness in healing.* Albany, NY: Delmar Publishers.

Rew, L. (2000). Self-reflection: Consulting the truth within. In B. M. Dossey, L. Keegan, & C. E. Guzzetta, eds., *Holistic nursing: A handbook for practice* (3rd ed., pp. 407–424). Gaithersburg, MD: Aspen Publishers.

Seroka, A. M. (1994). Values clarification and ethical decision making. *Seminars for Nurse Managers, 2,* 8–15.

Simon, S. B., L. W. Howe, & H. Kirschenbaum (1995). *Values clarification: A handbook of practical strategies for teachers and students.* New York: Hart.

Yeo, M., A. Moorhouse, P. Khan, & P. Rodney (2010). *Concepts and cases in nursing ethics* (2nd 3rd ed.). Peterborough, ON: Broadview Press.

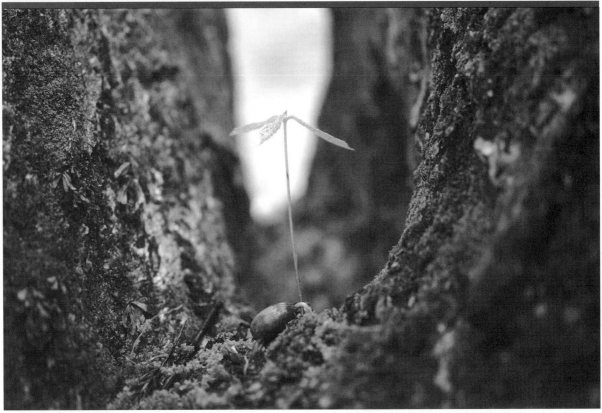

MC_PP/Shutterstock.com

CHAPTER **5**
VALUES DEVELOPMENT

OBJECTIVES

After completing this chapter, the reader should be able to:

1. Discuss influences of culture on values development.
2. Contrast theoretical approaches to moral development.
3. Describe and differentiate between an ethic of care and an ethic of justice.
4. Evaluate the personal phase of moral development.
5. Discuss gender bias and cultural bias in relation to theories of moral development.

INTRODUCTION

In Chapter 4, we learned about how to clarify and identify our individual values. Value clarification exercises can help us to realize just what it is we most appreciate, or hold in high esteem. Why is it important to know this? Why is there so much emphasis on clarifying our own values in nursing? Nurses frequently encounter situations that involve differing values or beliefs. In providing care to diverse patients and families, we will inevitably encounter persons who hold far different values than we do. We may well find ourselves in situations that force us to question our own values, or challenge us to be more accepting of other values that are divergent from ours. When forced to question our own values in a difficult situation, we may feel that it is that much harder to know what is clearly the "right" thing to do. In some situations the "right" choice seems quite evident, while in other circumstances a considerable lack of clarity about what is "right" may exist. How do we come to know what is right or how to respond in a principled way in a given situation? This chapter reviews factors that influence values formation, theoretical perspectives related to stages of values development, and considerations for nursing regarding moral development.

TRANSCULTURAL CONSIDERATIONS IN VALUES DEVELOPMENT

Human values development, often referred to as **moral development**, is a product of the sociocultural environment in which we live and develop. We learn what is considered right and wrong within the culture in formal ways, such as by precept and admonition, through informal processes such as role modelling, and by technical learning, as in a teacher-to-student process (Hall, 1973). Norms for etiquette and ethical behaviour that are "known" within the culture may be acquired by an outsider through technical learning; however, they are often appreciated by a neophyte only when a transgression has occurred and corrections to, or sanctions for, the behaviour have been imposed. There is an innate human capacity for developing an ethical stance to life that emerges through this process.

Leininger (1978; 1984) and Tripp-Reimer (1987) speak of culture in terms of values, beliefs, customs, and behaviours that are learned within and shared by a group of interacting persons. Because values are *learned* within the context of a particular culture, moral values are culturally relative (Gostin, 1995). This suggests that a value such as individual autonomy may be regarded highly in a culture that prizes independence and individualism. However, the same value may be considered contrary to the norm in a society where persons are defined by their relationships to others or in a community. Fowler (1981) notes that "we are formed in social communities and that our ways of seeing the world are profoundly shaped by the shared images and constructions of our group or class" (p. 105). Understandings of principles such as justice and care may vary in different cultures. In the ensuing discussion regarding stages of values development, it is important to be aware that the norms described have been derived primarily from Anglo-American and Anglo-European populations and, for the most part, are values that exist within a more Western-centric tradition. Although significant work has been done, there is a need for continued validation of these theories within a transcultural context.

ASK YOURSELF

How Did I Learn My Values?

Think about a ***personal*** situation in which you felt your values were challenged or you experienced a value conflict. Here are some examples:

- Erica values truthfulness over all other values. She discovers that Andrew, her friend's husband, is having an extra-marital relationship. Andrew asks her not to tell her friend about the relationship in order to protect her from being hurt, and promises Erica that it will end. Erica feels strongly that she should tell her friend the truth, but Andrew begs her not to tell.

- Sebastian values accountability and thoroughness in his work as an architect. He has been asked to rush through a very important client project, as his colleagues were careless and fell behind in the introductory part of the project. His colleagues told him to just "skip a few steps" to get the project done more quickly.

- Connor is a part-time teacher in an inner city school who values the strong personal connections he makes with some of his most troubled students. He started an "after school support program" for students who are having personal challenges to talk about their problems, get support, and share possible solutions. The students and their parents speak highly of this group, and it has become very important to the students who are involved, and to Connor. The Principal approached Connor to say that while he thinks this is a great initiative, many of the other teachers felt that it is inappropriate for a teacher to be leading a group that addresses students' personal problems, and not academic concerns. Additionally, some had said that they felt unduly pressured to do the same kind of thing and felt that wasn't fair to them.

Each of these examples above illustrates situations in which individuals were asked to do something that, for each person, went against their deeply held values. Everyone has very likely experienced a situation just like these ones above, at one time or another. Take a minute and think about a time when your values have been challenged.

- What made it a difficult situation for you?
- How did you decide the best course of action to take?
- What factors did you consider in making your decision?
- What values or principles guided you in this process?
- When and how did you learn these values or principles?
- Consider how you might have approached this same problem five or ten years ago. What, for you, has changed? Why?

THEORETICAL PERSPECTIVES ON VALUES DEVELOPMENT

Discussions of moral development found in current literature flow primarily from frameworks developed by Kohlberg (1981) and Gilligan (1982). An overview of the theoretical work of each of these scholars is presented in this section, followed by a discussion of how they contribute to understanding moral reasoning within nursing. Kohlberg's theory, which suggests that cognitive development is necessary though not sufficient for moral development, draws upon Piaget's (1963) original work on cognitive development in children. Thus, a brief review of Piaget's theory is included here. As you review the theories highlighted here, remember that **theory** is a proposed explanation for a class of phenomena. A given theory is not necessarily truth or reality, but it may shed light on truth. Engage critical thinking and intuitive knowing as you read, being attentive to what rings true in your own experience. At the same time, use your critical thinking skills to consider other perspectives on moral development.

Why is it important to discuss and understand these kinds of theories? Well, when we are talking about how we embrace values for ourselves as individuals, personally and professionally, we must also be aware that, as social beings, we evolve through stages of values development. Understanding that everyone is "on a journey" of values development, and not at end points, can help us to be flexible and realistic about how we work through values conflicts. Furthermore, it is very important to understand that there are social and psychological forces that have an influence on shaping what we value and how we grow as moral beings. Knowledge of these foundational theories on human moral development is key to understanding the development of self and others as moral beings in social contexts.

Piaget's Stages of Cognitive Development

Piaget's (1963) description of stages of cognitive development addresses how the mind works, that is, how we develop our intellectual capacities through childhood, from birth to about fifteen years of age. Piaget notes that cognitive development progresses through four stages, provided there is an intact neurological system and appropriate environmental interaction and stimuli. Although Piaget suggests specific ages for each stage, there may be variation due to environmental factors or innate intellectual capacities. Piaget's stages include the following. First, the sensorimotor stage (from birth to 24 months) includes learning about the world through reflexive behaviours, such as grasping, observing, and mouthing objects of interest. Second, as a baby develops into a toddler, this very physical way of interacting with the world develops into habits, which are driven by curiosity and goal orientation. Third, the Preoperational stage (age 2–7), is more focused on the development of mental operations, such as being able to represent objects through images, magical thinking, and some reasoning. As language use develops, so does the development of memory and imagination. While the child can now play and pretend in a social context, much of the world is still viewed through an ego-centric perspective. Fourth, in the

Concrete operations stage (age 7–11), children develop the ability to use logic and develop specific skills for working through many kinds of concrete problems. Piaget's fifth and final stage, the Formal operations stage (from age 11 into adulthood), brings development of the ability to deal with abstract problems, apply logical reason, and form ideas and conclusions that are relevant not only to concrete and abstract situations but also to hypothetical situations. The ability to utilize both inductive and deductive reasoning develops, as well as the ability to approach a problem in a more step-wise, methodical, and systematic way. This final stage continues into adulthood (Santrock, 2008).

Kohlberg's Theory of Moral Development

Kohlberg's (1981) theory of moral development was derived initially from interviews conducted with boys distributed in age from early childhood to late adolescence. In these interviews he asked participants to respond to hypothetical ethical dilemmas, such as a man considering stealing a drug to save his dying wife because he cannot afford the drug and has exhausted other possibilities of paying for it. The pattern of the responses that he observed, coupled with inferences about the reasoning behind the responses, suggested a progression in moral reasoning spanning three levels, each of which includes two stages. These levels and stages are summarized as follows:

Level I

The *Preconventional Level* has an egocentric focus and includes two stages. In Stage 1, *The Stage of Punishment and Obedience*, rules are obeyed in order to avoid punishment. In Stage 2, *The Stage of Individual instrumental purpose and exchange*, conformity to rules is viewed to be in our own interest because it provides rewards. Fear of punishment is a major motivator at this level.

Level II

The *Conventional Level* is focused more on social conformity and includes two stages. In Stage 3, *The Stage of Mutual Interpersonal Expectations, Relationships, and Conformity*, concern about the reactions of others is a basis for decisions and behaviour, and being good in order to maintain relations is important. In Stage 4, *The Stage of Social System and Conscience Maintenance*, we conform to laws and to those in authority because of duty, both out of respect for them and in order to avoid censure. For persons in this level, fulfilling our role in society and living up to expectations of others is important, and guilt is more of a motivator than the fear of punishment, as noted in Level I.

There is a transitional phase between Stages 4 and 5 in which emotions begin to be recognized as a component of moral reasoning. This transition includes an awareness of personal subjectivity in moral decision making and a recognition that social rules can be arbitrary and relative.

Level III

The *Post-Conventional and Principled Level* has universal moral principles as its focus. It includes two stages. In Stage 5, *The Stage of Prior Rights and Social Contract or Utility*, the relativity of some societal values is recognized, and moral decisions derive from principles that support individual rights and transcend particular societal rules such as equality, liberty, and justice. In Stage 6, *The Stage of Universal Ethical Principles*, internalized rules and conscience reflecting abstract principles of human dignity, mutual respect, and trust guide decisions and behaviours. Persons at this level make judgments based on impartial universal moral principles, even when these conflict with societal standards.

This theory proposes a linear movement through hierarchical stages, whereby each stage presupposes having completed the prior stage and is the basis for the subsequent stage. It is the pattern of a person's utilization of a particular level of reasoning that determines the stage, noting that each successive stage requires more advanced levels of moral reasoning. Research utilizing this framework indicates that not everyone moves through all the stages, and that few people actually progress to the postconventional level (Colby & Kohlberg, 1987). Within this theory, women tend to focus on relational stages, such as Stage 3. Men tend to focus on adherence to duty and the rules of authority, as highlighted in Stage 4. Kohlberg's model is generally considered to be an **ethic of justice**, because it is an approach to ethical decision making based on objective rules in which choices are made from a stance of separateness or individuality. This is in contrast to Gilligan's work, which describes what we call an **ethic of care**.

Gilligan's Study of the Psychological Development of Women

Gilligan, a former student of Kohlberg, studied the psychological development of women, arguing that women approach moral decision-making from a different perspective than men (Gilligan, 1982; 1987 and Gilligan *et al.*, 1988). In contrast to the ethic of justice described by Kohlberg, in which personal liberty and rights are primary, Gilligan noted that women utilize an **ethic of care**, in which the moral imperative is grounded in relationships with and responsibility for one another. "Women's construction of the moral problem as a problem of care and responsibility in relationship rather than of rights and rules ties the development of their moral thinking to changes in their understanding of responsibility and relationship, just as the conception of morality as justice ties development to the logic of equality and reciprocity" (Gilligan, 1982, p. 73). Gilligan's research did not say that most women think in the care perspective, while most men think in the justice perspective. Rather, as Little (2000) points out, she identified the default perspective that women use, the perspective they feel most comfortable with, and that they would turn to first. She noted that many women do, in fact, think in the justice perspective, about one-third of the population are mixed between them, and, when pressed, all people can shift to the other perspective. However, women tend to start off from the care perspective, so if you leave women out of the study, you leave out the care perspective.

Gilligan's research suggests a progression of moral thinking through three phases, each of which reflects greater depth in understanding the relationships between self and others, and two transitions that involve critical re-evaluation of the conflict between responsibility and selfishness. The sequence described proceeds from an initial concern with survival, to focusing on goodness, to reflectively understanding care as the most adequate guide for resolving moral dilemmas.

Phase 1

In this phase, *the concern for survival*, the focus is on what is best for the self, and includes selfishness and dependence on others. The *transition* to Phase 2 involves an appreciation of connectedness, and that responsible decision making takes into account the effects of decisions upon others.

Phase 2

The phase of *focusing on goodness* includes a sense of goodness as self-sacrifice, in which the needs of others are often put ahead of self, and there is a sense of being responsible for others, so that one is regarded positively. This focus on goodness reflects an awareness of relationship with others and may be used to manipulate others through a "see how good I've been to you" attitude. In the *transition* to Phase 3 there is a shifting from concern about the reactions of others to greater honesty about personal motivation and consequences of choices and actions. Responsibility to self is taken into account, along with responding to needs of others.

Phase 3

The phase of *the imperative of care* reflects a deep appreciation of connectedness, including responsibility to self and others as moral equals, and a clear imperative to harm no one. We take responsibility for choices, in which projected consequences and personal intention are the motivation for actions, rather than concern for the reactions of others. Although Gilligan does not clearly associate particular ages with each phase of development, she suggests a linear process moving from one phase to the next through the transitions.

ASK YOURSELF

Where Are You in Your Values Development?

- Where do you think you fit, in terms of your values development, in each of the above theoretical perspectives?

- Where would you place your parents? Classmates? Friends? Professors? Government leaders?

- Where would you place the following noteworthy spiritual leaders: Gandhi, Mother Teresa, or the Dalai Lama?
- Based on your critical thinking and intuitive knowing, which perspective makes the most sense for you, as an individual?

Kohlberg and Gilligan suggest that values development moves from a focus on self and survival, through responding to external forces such as perceived authority or the opinions of others, toward being motivated and guided by universal considerations. They also note that it is more common to find adults functioning in the middle phases of relying on external authority as guideposts for moral decisions than to find adults who base their actions and decisions on internalized universal guides that transcend codified rules. Within this pattern it is conceivable that, in response to life-changing experiences, persons may spiral back to an earlier stage and move through the stages again from a renewed perspective.

Thomas's Levels of Moral Response

When we consider difficult moral or ethical situations in which we are required to respond or act, our moral development and our subsequent level of moral autonomy informs our decisions, reactions, and actions. Thomas outlines three levels of moral response: the expressive level, the pre-reflective level, and the reflective level (Thomas, 1990). Consider asking someone why they oppose the legalization of abortion or euthanasia.

At an expressive level, while the person does express an opinion, the response is usually embedded in personal preferences, feelings, or emotional expressions. In and of themselves, these preferences and opinions are not reasons that are based on active reflection, research, and consideration of multiple perspectives. An example might be "I am against euthanasia because I don't like to think of anyone or anything being killed."

At a pre-reflective level, the rationale for the voiced opinion is usually provided in terms of unanalyzed values that have not been critically examined. Often the reasons for one's choice might be a reference to a widely held religious or cultural belief or a professional code of ethics. While this is considered, by some, to be more reflective than an expressive level of moral reasoning, others see this as representing a less-developed sense of moral reflection, as it is viewed as the "blind following of standards set by somebody else." (Thomas, 1990, p. 5). These kinds of sets of conventional rules and codes are helpful to establish norms and guidelines for behaviours within particular contexts; however, it is also important for there to be personal and critical reflection on how these norms, rules, and codes are integrated with our own personal moral convictions. In other words, there needs to be some internalization of these kinds of rules, along with an evaluation of their relevance, importance, and moral justification. At a pre-reflective level, according to Thomas, this has not yet occurred. At example of a pre-reflective moral response might be,

"I oppose euthanasia because my professional duty precludes the taking of a life in any way."

Finally, at a reflective level, reasons or justifications of moral views are provided based on rules, values, or principles that have been internalized, critically examined, and reflected upon. They may be rules or values espoused in a code of ethics or a widely held belief; however, instead of a blind acceptance of these rules, without critical analytical consideration of their relevance, there is some consideration of whether or not these are the kinds of rules and values that individuals should be expected to live by. An example of a statement at a reflective level might be, "I oppose euthanasia because the sanctity of all life and the principle of non-maleficence takes precedence over the autonomy of the individual person to choose." Note the complexity of the reasoning and articulation of that process of reasoning through a difficult and often emotionally driven moral dilemma.

CASE PRESENTATION

Three Nursing Students

Tanya, Randa, and Kuan are discussing experiences they had in clinical today in their post-clinical conference. Tanya describes feeling distressed because a decision was made, at a meeting involving the medical team and the patient's family, to withdraw food and fluids from her patient who has dementia and end-stage cancer. Her patient was not included in the meeting, as he has advanced dementia and has been deemed incapable of providing consent, but Tanya notices that he is able to communicate simple wishes and objections related to food and activity preferences. This morning he refused a bed bath, as he said he was in pain. She also notices that he appears to take some pleasure from food. Tanya understands that he may not be able to fully participate in decision making, but feels that he should have been included, in some way, in the decision-making process as he does demonstrate wishes and preferences. Randa responds to Tanya's situation, saying, "It's probably okay, he's not really 'with it' most of the time, Tanya. He couldn't really take part in a meeting and understand it. Besides, his family really seems nice. They seem to care about him, from what I've seen. That's what I would want if I was him – my family to take care of the hard decisions." Kuan also responds, reminding Tanya and Randa that the policy of the unit clearly notes that decisions about end-of-life care are made using a family meeting and that if a patient has been found incapable of providing consent, their substitute decision-makers will provide consent in lieu of the patient.

? THINK ABOUT IT

Indicators of Values Development

- What insights into the values of each of these students can you glean from this discussion?

- Which level of moral response (expressive, pre-reflective, reflective) does each student demonstrate in her approach to this situation?

- How do you think you would have responded in the situation described by the students? What values would guide your response?

SOME NURSING CONSIDERATIONS

Gilligan (1982; 1987) and others (Gilligan, Ward, Taylor & Bardige, 1988; Kittay & Meyers, 1987; Larrabee, 1993; Little, 2000; Noddings, 1984) have suggested that there are gender differences in approaching moral decision making: women tend to utilize a care or relational perspective, whereas men more frequently use the justice perspective. These authors note that Kohlberg's perspective on moral development tends to portray women's choices as deficient in terms of moral capacity. Many authors claim that research related to differences in ethical decision making based on gender is inconclusive and that the justice perspective is, and can be, used by both women and men (Colby & Kohlberg, 1987; Duckett, Rowan-Boyer, Ryden, Crisham, Savik, & Rest, 1992; Walker, 1993). When considering developmental norms for moral development, nurses must be alert for gender and cultural factors, norms, and bias in order to avoid simply classifying particular groups as lacking in moral capabilities.

Kohlberg's and Gilligan's work highlights and informs the debate on an **ethic of care** versus an **ethic of justice**, in which the former is viewed as an approach that encompasses notions of relationships and responsibilities to others. The latter, an ethic of justice, is focused on notions that are more concerned with social conformity, principles, rules, and clear hierarchies (Gremmen, 1999). The ethic of care, as iden-tified by Gilligan, has been subject to significant criticism, as it differs so markedly from the principle-based approach to moral decision making emphasized in most health care ethics education and textbooks (Woods, 2011). The literature offers an ongoing deliberation about the ethic of care versus the ethic of justice. An ethic of care approach has been embraced by nursing, despite claims that an ethic of justice is more impartial, rational, and universally understood. Many nursing theorists claim that, in fact, an ethic of care is a key theoretical foundation of nursing and nursing practice. Notwithstanding the assertions of many nursing theorists that a nursing ethic of care is absolutely foundational, there are many others, even from within nursing, who feel that caring is neither a sufficiently rigorous or well-understood foundation upon which to construct a theory of nursing moral reasoning. It is clear that nurses are moral agents and that they approach many moral problems from a perspective that acknowledges the meaningfulness of the needs of others, the significance of relationships, and the overriding importance of caring and avoiding harm to others (Bowden, 2000; Gremmen, 1999; Woods, 2011).

A comparison of the two perspectives reveals that the justice framework requires choices to be made from a stance of separateness, based on much more objective or universal rules and principles, to ensure the fair treatment of all persons (Botes, 2000). The care perspective emphasizes relationships with particular others in which the choice is contextually bound and requires responding to others on their own terms, developing strategies that maintain connections whenever possible, and striving to hurt no one. Moral concern within the ethic of justice is with rights and responsibilities; in the ethic of care the concern is with competing needs and responsibilities in relationships. Although much of the discussion in the literature focuses on the dichotomy between the two, we recognize that, rather than negating each other, the perspectives of justice and care offer different, and at times complementary, perspectives from which to examine problems. Offering balance to each other, these perspectives broaden the view from which to see the situation as a whole, and collectively constitute a more comprehensive moral perspective (Cooper, 1989; Little, 2000). Hekman (1995) suggests that a paradigm shift is occurring that requires a reconceptualization of morality and moral language away from the notion of universal morality toward a recognition of a plurality of moral voices. Furthermore, there are some who argue that viewing each of these perspectives as "mutually exclusive opposites" (Gremmen, 1999, p. 516) is an exercise that holds little value and functions to only try to resolve any discussion or debate by deciding "which is best." Instead of an attempt to decide which approach is "best," an exercise that is of little value, some theorists have instead proposed that by viewing the two perspectives as complementary, integrated, or comprehensive when considered together, a more relevant and fruitful discussion may ensue instead of a debate on the comparative value of each approach (Botes, 2000; Davis, 1992; Gremmen, 1999). It has also been suggested that nursing move beyond current models of biomedical ethics to a model that encompasses at least the concepts of care and justice (Cooper, 1990).

Because of nursing's concern for relational caring, an ethic of care may more thoughtfully reflect nursing's experience than a primary focus on justice (Cooper, 1989). Little (2000) notes that one of the lessons the ethic of care offers to health care professionals is the directive to meet the needs of *particular* others, recognizing that these needs are not always clear. This means caring about persons as individuals, and developing processes to help them figure out what they need. Part of this process, she suggests, is developing, through caring, a recognition that emotions are a constitutive part of the moral life. Considering the politics of caring, she speaks to the need for restructuring our health care systems to value caring through supporting and justly compensating those who do the sometimes emotional and taxing caring work.

We need to understand that there are different perspectives from which moral decisions are made, so that we can better appreciate our own and our patients' approaches to ethical dilemmas. We need to identify honestly our own phases of values development and ethical perspective in order to better understand personal responses to situations and to recognize more effectively how our approaches may differ from those of colleagues or patients. Acknowledging differences and similarities may prevent making inappropriate judgments about another's moral capabilities, and make possible better communication and collaboration in care.

CASE PRESENTATION

A Difficult Decision

Reba's eighty-two-year-old father has been hospitalized with a stroke that has left him severely incapacitated, requiring total care. She has been informed that her father is ready for discharge, and the physician is suggesting that he go to a nursing home. Reba feels that she should take him home with her because her faith says she should provide care for her parents, but her house is small and would need a bathroom added to the ground floor. She also has concerns about being able to care for her father because she works full time and has three small children. She has considered quitting her job, but the family needs her income because her husband's work is seasonal. When visiting her father, she tells the nurse, Moira, that she does not know what is best for him, noting that her sister in another province told her it is her duty to care for their father, but her husband says it is too much to take on with all her other family responsibilities. She asks Moira what she should do.

THINK ABOUT IT

Justice or Care—Is One Way Better?

- What values has Reba clearly articulated?
- What factors and forces do you think weigh most heavily in this situation?
- How would you respond if you were Moira?
- How would you approach this situation from the perspective of justice? From the perspective of care? Do you think one approach is better than the other? Explain.
- How would you describe Reba's phase of moral development? Her husband's? Her sister's?

SUMMARY

This chapter has presented an overview of theoretical perspectives related to values development, the importance of recognizing that values and beliefs are culturally relative, and that nursing considerations are related to moral development. Students are encouraged to explore and critique each model of values development in order to formulate a personal knowledge base to guide their own processes of development. Each perspective provides insight into what is true.

CHAPTER HIGHLIGHTS

- Human values development, which is a product of our sociocultural environment, reflects the content and process of learning what is right and wrong within the culture.
- Values development moves from a focus on self, through responding to external forces, toward being guided by universal considerations.
- Moral values are culturally relative.
- Current models of values development need further transcultural and transgender validation.
- Kohlberg's model, often referred to as an ethic of justice, suggests that choices are based on objective rules and principles and are made from a stance of separateness.
- In Gilligan's model, often referred to as an ethic of care, the moral imperative is grounded in relationship and mutual responsibility. Choices are contextually bound, requiring strategies that maintain connections and a striving to hurt no one.
- The notion of a plurality of moral voices, which recognizes that perspectives of both justice and care are factors in moral decision making, is an important consideration for nursing.
- Understanding varying perspectives from which moral decisions are made enables nurses to appreciate their own and their patients' approaches to ethical dilemmas, and to avoid making inappropriate judgments about another's moral capabilities.

DISCUSSION QUESTIONS AND ACTIVITIES

1. What does it mean to say that moral values are culturally relative?
2. What factors would you consider in determining a person's phase of moral development?
3. Explore the model that you think best reflects the process of values development. Discuss it with classmates, giving a rationale for your choice.
4. Identify stages of values development of three people you know of different ages.

5. Compare and contrast the ethic of care and the ethic of justice, and discuss this topic with classmates. Which perspective do you think is most appropriate for nursing? Why?

6. Why is it useful for nurses to be aware of phases of values development for themselves, patients, and colleagues?

REFERENCES

Botes, A. (2000). A comparison between the ethics of justice and the ethics of care. *Journal of Advanced Nursing, 32*(5), 1071–1075.

Bowden, P. (2000). An "ethic of care" in clinical settings: encompassing "feminine" and "feminist" perspectives. *Nursing Philosophy, 1*, 36–49.

Colby, A., & L. Kohlberg (1987). *The measurement of moral judgment volume I: Theoretical foundations and research validation.* Cambridge, MA: Cambridge University Press.

Cooper, M. C. (1989). Gilligan's different voice: A perspective for nursing. *Journal of Professional Nursing, 5*(1), 10–16.

Cooper, M. C. (1990). Reconceptualizing nursing ethics. *Scholarly Inquiry for Nursing Practice, 4*(3), 209–221.

Davis, K. (1992). Toward a feminist rhetoric: The Gilligan debate revisited. *Women's Studies International Forum, 15*, 219–223.

Duckett, L., M. Rowan-Boyer, M. B. Ryden, P. Crisham, K. Savik & J. R. Rest (1992). Challenging misperceptions about nurses' moral reasoning. *Nursing Research, 41*(6), 324–331.

Fowler, J. W. (1981). *Stages of faith: The psychology of human development and the quest for meaning.* San Francisco: Harper & Row.

Gilligan, C. (1982). *In a different voice: Psychological theory and women's development.* Cambridge, MA: Harvard University Press.

Gilligan, C. (1987). Moral orientation and moral development. In E. F. Kittay & D. T. Meyers, eds., *Women and moral theory* (pp. 19–33). Savage, MD: Rowman & Littlefield.

Gilligan, C., J. V. Ward, J. M. Taylor & B. Bardige (1988). *Mapping the moral domain.* Cambridge, MA: Harvard University Press.

Gostin, L. O. (1995). Informed consent, cultural sensitivity, and respect for persons. *Journal of the American Medical Association, 274*(10), 844–855.

Gremmen, I. (1999). Visiting nurses' situated ethics: Beyond "care versus justice." *Nursing Ethics, 6*(6), 515–527.

Hall, E. T. (1973). *The silent language.* Garden City, NY: Anchor Press.

Hekman, S. J. (1995). *Moral voices, moral selves.* University Park, PA: Pennsylvania State University Press.

Kittay, E. F., & D. T. Meyers (1987). *Women and moral theory.* Savage, MD: Rowman & Littlefield.

Kohlberg, L. (1981). *The philosophy of moral development.* New York: Harper & Row.

Larrabee, M. J., ed. (1993). *An ethic of care.* New York: Routledge.

Leininger, M. (1978). *Transcultural nursing: Concepts, theories and practice.* New York: John Wiley & Sons.

Leininger, M. (1984). *Transcultural care diversity and universality: A theory of nursing*. Thorofare, NJ: Slack.

Little, M. (2000). Introduction to the ethics of care. Presentation at *New century, new challenges: Intensive bioethics course XXVI*, Kennedy Institute of Ethics, Georgetown University, Washington, DC, June 10, 2000.

Noddings, N. (1984). *Caring: A feminine approach to ethics and moral education*. Berkeley, CA: University of California Press.

Piaget, J. (1963). *The origins of intelligence in children* (M. Cook, trans.). New York: Norton.

Santrock, J. W. (2008). *A Topical Approach to Life-span Development*. New York, NY: McGraw-Hill.

Thomas, J. (1990). *Ethical frameworks for decision making*. Peterborough, ON: Broadview Press.

Tripp-Reimer, T. (1987). Cultural assessment. In J. P. Bellack, & P. A. Bamford, eds., *Nursing assessment: A multidimensional approach* (pp. 226–246). Boston: Jones & Bartlett.

Walker, L. J. (1993). Sex differences in the development of moral reasoning: A critical review. In M. J. Larrabee, ed., *An ethic of care* (pp. 157–176). New York: Routledge.

Woods, M. (2011). An ethic of care in nursing: Past, present and future considerations. *Ethics and social welfare*, 5(3), 266–276.

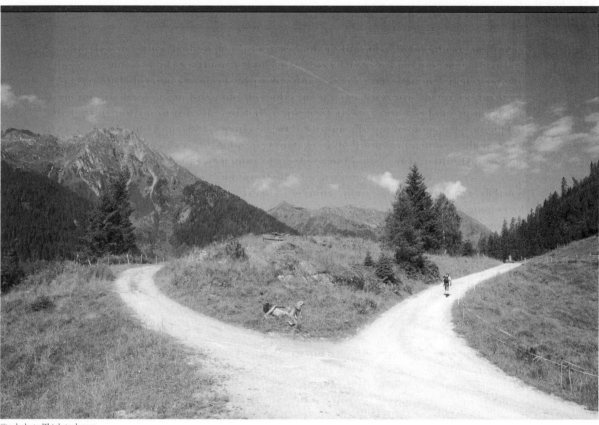

CHAPTER 6
ETHICAL DECISION MAKING
OBJECTIVES

After completing this chapter, the reader should be able to:

1. Describe and differentiate ethical dilemmas, moral uncertainty, practical dilemmas, and moral distress.

2. Describe and differentiate between the following related concepts: moral outrage, moral residue, moral disengagement, and moral courage.

3. Describe the process of making thoughtful decisions.

4. Discuss the nursing process as a decision-making model.

5. Discuss similarities between scientific process and ethical decision making.

6. Describe the role of emotions in ethical decisions.

7. Examine the process of ethical decision making.

8. Apply the ethical decision making process to clinical case situations.

INTRODUCTION

Everyone makes decisions as part of everyday living. Some decisions seem routine, such as what to have for lunch or what to wear to work. Other decisions, like where to go to college or university, which job to accept, or whether to marry, call for more deliberation. Nurses constantly make decisions. We decide matters related to patient care, institutional policy, or how to collaborate or initiate referrals. Often we make decisions without conscious awareness of the process, but have an innate sense of *knowing* what to do.

Ethical decision making may not seem as clear-cut as decisions made in other areas of life. How do we decide whether to remove life support measures for a patient, or whether to cut funding for childhood immunizations in favour of other, equally important programs? What factors are involved in an ethical dilemma that make "the right choice" either evident or obscure? Nurses, by virtue of their close proximity to patients and the amount of time they spend with patients, should be involved in decision making and working through ethical dilemmas as part of the health care team, and as advocates for patients' best interests. While much decision-making power in health care has traditionally been given mainly to physicians, the increasing scope of nurses' practice and the interdisciplinary nature of decision making in many health care settings means that nurses are more and more involved in helping to work through difficult patient concerns, especially those with ethical dimensions (Zomordi & Foley, 2009). This chapter introduces and defines the concept of an ethical dilemma, relates ethical decision making to the nursing process, and presents some guidance for ethical decision making.

MORAL/ETHICAL PROBLEMS

Jameton (1984) describes three different types of moral problems: *moral uncertainty*, which occurs when the nurse identifies a moral problem but is unsure of the morally correct action; *moral dilemma*, which occurs when two or more mutually exclusive moral claims clearly apply and both seem to have equal weight; and *moral distress*, which arises when the nurse knows the morally correct action and feels a responsibility to the patient, but institutional or other restraints make it nearly impossible to follow through with appropriate action (p. 6).

Moral Uncertainty

Moral uncertainty occurs when we sense that there is a moral problem but are not sure of the morally correct action, or when we are not sure what moral principles or values apply, or when we are not able to define the moral problems (Jameton, 1984).

At times, moral uncertainty may mean that we are simply not able to clearly know or express the moral problem (Canadian Nurses Association, 2008). This happens to us when we have a sense that something is not quite right, often called a "gut feeling." We are uncomfortable with a situation, but can't quite articulate the problem. Jameton (1984) offers the example of a nurse caring for an older patient who is somewhat neglected, with little attention being given to the patient's problem. The nurse feels dissatisfied with the patient's treatment, but is unable to pinpoint the nature and cause of the inadequacy.

Moral/Ethical Dilemmas

A dilemma exists when a difficult problem seems to have no satisfactory solution, or when all solutions to a problem appear to be equally favourable (Davis, Aroskar, Liaschenko & Drought, 2009). An **ethical dilemma** or moral dilemma occurs when there are conflicting moral claims. Dilemmas can present in at least two ways. According to Beauchamp and Childress (2008), a conflict can be experienced when there is evidence to indicate that a certain act is morally right and other evidence to indicate that the act is morally wrong, but neither evidence is conclusive. An example of this can be seen in the example of a terminally ill patient. While most would think it is morally right to preserve life, many would also believe it is morally wrong to prolong suffering. A dilemma may also occur when the person believes that one or more moral norms exist that support one course of action, and one or more moral norms exist that support another course of action, and the two actions are mutually exclusive. Health care providers face this type of dilemma, for example, when they must decide who gets the critical care bed. Should they make the decision relative to who is most deserving, who arrives first, who is younger, or who has the best chance of survival? Different people perceive or conceptualize conflicts in different ways. Conflicting moral claims can be said to occur, for example, between obligations, principles, duties, rights, loyalties, and so forth.

Let us examine different perceptions of conflicting moral claims. The nurse might perceive a conflict between adherence to two different principles, such as wishing to avoid the suffering a patient experiences as a result of hearing a bad prognosis, while at the same time respecting the patient's right to know. In this instance, the nurse might perceive a direct conflict between the principles of non-maleficence (the wish to do no harm) and autonomy (assuring that the patient is self-governing). In another instance, the nurse might perceive a conflict of duties. This type of conflict can occur, for example, when nurse managers must make decisions regarding staffing patterns. The nurse manager will recognize a duty to the institution, but will also feel a duty to meet the needs of individual patients and nurses. This will often result in a conflict, when the needs of the institution do not allow for meeting the needs of individuals.

There are instances when the nurse might feel conflicting loyalties. For example, in providing care for a patient who is HIV-positive, who admits to the nurse that she is sexually active and not using protection against transmission of the virus, the nurse may experience a conflict between being loyal to the patient and being loyal to others or society at large. In this instance, the nurse could experience a conflict between doing what seems morally right and avoiding actions that carry legal consequences. This situation can also be conceptualized as a conflict between the nurse's duty to maintain confidentiality and the duty to warn those at risk. All of these examples portray ethical dilemmas that nurses commonly experience. These moral problems offer conflicting moral claims, and the possible solutions appear to be at once favourable and unfavourable.

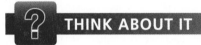

THINK ABOUT IT

Facing Ethical Dilemmas

Put yourself in the position of the nurses in the six examples noted in the discussion of ethical dilemmas in the section above.

- How would the situation present a conflict for you?
- How do you think you would respond in each situation?
- Why would you respond in that manner?
- Think about a personal experience of a moral dilemma and describe why it was a dilemma for you.

Practical Dilemmas

One must be careful to differentiate between **moral dilemmas** and **practical dilemmas**. Occasionally, situations arise in which moral claims compete with non-moral claims. Non-moral claims can often be identified as claims of self-interest (Beauchamp & Childress, 2008). Consider, for example, the nurse who must work overtime, caring for a gravely ill patient. The nurse might perceive a dilemma because she promised to take her children to the movies. Though the nurse might say that her duty to her children conflicts with her duty to care for the patient, it can be argued that the duties are not of equal moral weight. The duty to keep the promise to her children is a practical duty that is grounded in self-interest rather than having a moral claim. In decisions that involve practical dilemmas, moral claims have greater weight than non-moral claims. Differentiating moral and practical dilemmas is an important facet of decision making.

Moral Distress

Occasionally, nurses face situations that present moral problems that seem to have clear solutions, yet are unable to follow their moral beliefs because of institutional or other constraints. Nurses in these predicaments are said to experience **moral distress**

(Jameton, 1984). These situations differ from those that present moral dilemmas. When moral distress occurs, there are no conflicting moral claims. The *right* action is clear, yet institutional or other constraints make it nearly impossible to pursue this course of action. It is important to note that nurses who experience moral distress often feel a personal responsibility to the patient. The distress occurs when the nurse violates a personal moral value and fails to fulfil a perceived responsibility. For example, nurses in the hurried atmosphere of a particular hospital's same-day surgery report that they are expected to have sedated patients sign consent forms, recognizing that the physicians have often neglected to explain the scheduled procedures fully. The nurses know that this practice is one that does not respect patients' right to informed consent and thereby violates the patients' autonomy. However, they feel they have neither personal authority nor access to decision-making channels, and therefore believe themselves to be powerless to make the necessary changes. Jameton points out that in situations of this sort, it can be personally risky for staff to criticize a practice that is felt to be in the best interest of the institution at large.

Situations in which nurses experience moral distress may represent practical, rather than ethical, dilemmas. Nurses may face the choice of continuing to participate in a system that they feel is ethically flawed, resigning, or acting in a manner that they believe is correct but that could jeopardize their employment. Moral distress will undermine integrity if it is easier for nurses to comply with policies they believe are morally wrong than to pursue the ethically correct action.

Although moral problems of all types are difficult, situations involving moral distress may be the most difficult moral problems facing nurses, and can lead to devastating outcomes in some situations (Corley, 2002). Reports of the number of nurses who experience moral distress vary. Nearly fifty percent of nurses in one study reported that they had acted against their conscience while providing care to the terminally ill (Rushton, 1995). Other studies have shown that as many as thirty percent to fifty percent of nurses either leave their units or leave nursing altogether as a result of moral distress (Corley, 2002; Millette, 1994; Redman & Fry, 2000).

Other studies show that moral distress causes nurses to have physical and psychological problems, sometimes for many years. Some researchers have related "burnout" to the experience of moral distress, and suggest that many nurses leave the profession as a result. More important, there is anecdotal evidence that nurses' moral distress can affect the quality of patient care and subsequent health outcomes (Corley, 2002).

The consequences of moral distress can be profound. There is evidence that, as a result of moral distress, some nurses lose their capacity for caring, avoid patient contact, and fail to provide good physical care. Hamric (2000) calls moral distress, "a powerful impediment to nursing practice" (p. 201). Nurses may physically withdraw from the bedside, barely meeting the basic physical needs of patients, or may leave the profession altogether (Fenton, 1988; Hefferman & Helig, 1999; Kelly, 1998). Loss of nurses from the workforce is an indirect but strong threat to patient care. The nursing shortage is compounded by a health care system in which increasingly complex technology is used to care for patients who are very old, very young, or very sick. Those in society with the greatest need may be the ones who suffer most acutely when nursing care is affected.

Unrelieved moral distress over a period of time can erode a nurse's values and affect confidence and self-esteem. Unfortunately, there is no assurance that following what one considers to be the morally correct course of action will garner either employer or legal support. Nurses should view these situations as practical dilemmas. Ethical decision making assures that moral claims hold greater weight than non-moral claims. Thus, in the example offered above, the moral claim of respecting the right to informed consent constitutes greater weight than the non-moral claim of systemic efficiency. The decision-making guide described in this chapter can be used to help nurses make practical decisions when facing moral distress.

ASK YOURSELF

Have You Experienced Moral Distress?

Moral distress occurs in situations that present moral problems which seem to have clear solutions, yet institutional or other constraints prohibit morally correct action. Consider a situation in which you experienced moral distress.

- What were the circumstances?
- How did you feel?
- How did you resolve the distress?

Moral Outrage

Moral distress and **moral outrage** share the common element of feelings of powerlessness (Jameton, 1993). In cases of moral outrage, nurses do not participate in the act, and therefore do not believe they are responsible for the wrong that is done, but perceive that they are powerless to prevent it or act upon it. The nurse is more likely to be on the fringes of the moral situation rather than directly involved. For example, the charge nurse on a medical/surgical floor on the evening shift is working at the desk when the nursing supervisor comes to the floor to use the telephone to call a hospital administrator. The charge nurse overhears the supervisor describing a situation in which a patient was endangered when a physician insisted on performing a surgical procedure in the patient's room. The surgeon was in a hurry and felt the patient would be safe, even though there were violations of patient privacy, informed consent, and safety. The charge nurse has no involvement in the situation, but recognizes a grave moral problem. Whistleblowing may be a response to moral outrage but, in most cases, is considered a last resort. There are usually more constructive and meaningful ways to try to resolve issues, even those that lead to moral outrage, that can help to change institutions and practices. Whistleblowing should be considered only when all other options have been exhausted.

Moral Residue

When nurses find that they are being asked to compromise their values time and time again, this can lead to what we call **moral residue** (CNA, 2008). In situations of moral distress, we know what the right thing is that should be done, but are unable to act upon it. Being in situations like this, over and over, can result in feelings of guilt, inadequacy, and powerlessness (Schluter, Winch, Holzhauser & Henderson, 2008). Over time, having one's values compromised can take an understandable toll on one's ability to maintain a positive approach to nursing work. Moral residue, however, is not entirely negative. Carrying forth these kinds of feelings, and a strong awareness of the experiences that result in feeling compromised, may help nurses to try to approach future problems differently and attempt to avoid the compromising of deeply-held values, when possible.

Moral Disengagement

When nurses work in environments where they feel that their views, contributions, and ethical concerns are not valued by the institution or agency, they can, over time, become disengaged or far less invested in their nursing role and practice. They may become blasé or dispassionate, may express a lack of caring about outcomes and/or express lack of interest or lack of engagement in what they do. This may be due to the fact that, conceivably, they feel that they have little or no power to change or alter situations and that their engagement in difficult ethical situations or advocacy for patients has not been fruitful or worthwhile. Some of this apathy may even progress into feelings of resentment, demonstrated by being unkind or uncaring towards patients and colleagues (CNA, 2008). **Moral disengagement** is a very serious problem that can occur if the "ethical commitments" of nurses (CNA, 2008, p. 7) are repeatedly devalued or ignored.

Moral Courage

While many of the concepts that we outline in this chapter are related to the more negative sequelae of moral distress, there are also positive concepts and outcomes that we experience and can see when approaching ethical dilemmas. **Moral courage** is one such example. The concept of moral courage is somewhat similar to **steadfastness**, which we discuss elsewhere. To have moral courage is to stand up for what one believes in, even in the face of opposition or adversity. "Standing firm" (CNA, 2008, p. 7) in the face of objections or disapproval is a difficult stance to take and people who can do this are thought of as having moral courage. Often, advocating for patients and families may mean taking a stance that might be far different from those taken by others on the health care team, and doing so may present challenges or even threats to a nurse who stands up for what he or she believes is in the best interest of the patient. It may mean personal or professional hardship to take a position that is seen as unpopular or as causing "trouble" or "problems" for others. While both standing up for one's beliefs and values and advocating for a patient may be difficult in practice, we also know that nurses describe feelings of regret and guilt if they do not pursue ethical concerns or "stand up" for what they feel is right for their patients (Pavlish *et al.,* 2011).

MAKING DECISIONS

The process of making thoughtful decisions follows a similar pattern in most circumstances. This pattern includes gathering data, comparing options, using some criteria for weighing the merits of each option, and making a choice. Evaluating outcomes or circumstances surrounding the choice provides more data regarding the *rightness* of the choice. A simple example of this process is how you choose what clothes to wear today. The data you gather includes such things as where you are going, what you will be doing, the weather, what is clean or handy, your mood, the colours you prefer, and the style of clothing you anticipate others will be wearing. You may narrow the choices to several options that would be acceptable or appropriate, and you compare these based on some criteria. The criteria may be what is least wrinkled, or feels most comfortable, or makes you look or feel more confident, or is more appropriate for weather conditions, or a combination of such considerations. Using the criteria, you narrow down the options and make a choice. As you move through the day, you gather more data about the *rightness* of your decision. For example, are you comfortable? Do you feel dressed appropriately for the meeting? Are you warm enough? Does the colour seem to make you stand out? Your evaluation of whether or not you made the right decision provides information about the strength or validity of the criteria you used to guide your decision, and whether to use the same criteria to guide similar decisions in the future.

Nursing and Ethical Decision Making

As nurses we commonly use the **nursing process** model for decision making. Utilizing both logical thinking and intuitive knowing, the nursing process is a deliberate activity that provides a systematic method for nursing practice. The nursing process directs nursing practice, standardizes nursing care, and unifies nurses (Christensen & Kenney, 1995). Familiar to most nurses, the process generally includes the following interactive and sequential steps: problem identification, based on assessment of subjective and objective data; development of a plan for care, guided by desired outcomes; implementation of interventions; evaluation of the outcomes; and revision of the plan over time. Criteria used in making nursing care decisions derive from areas such as knowledge of normal anatomy, physiology, psychology, pathophysiology, therapeutic communication, family dynamics, pharmacology, microbiology, nursing and other theories, human energy fields, familiarity with standards of care and protocols, experience related to what has worked in similar situations, and intuitive knowing. The process is systematic and involves both logical thinking and intuitive knowing.

The College of Nurses of Ontario provides a structured process, "Working Through Ethical Situations in Nursing Practice" (2009, p. 15) for approaching ethical dilemmas in their *Practice Standard for Ethics.* This process is grounded in the nursing process and the steps are familiar to nurses, thus making this model easy to apply in difficult or complex situations that involve values or value conflict.

FIGURE 6–1 **WORKING THROUGH ETHICAL SITUATIONS IN NURSING PRACTICE**

The following are the four steps outlined in the College of Nurses of Ontario *Practice Standard for Ethics*:

- Assessing and describing the situation

  In this initial stage, the key priorities are identifying what the ethical problem is, the values involved, and any policies, practice standards or institutional rules that might apply to the situation. Another important step is actually identifying and articulating the problem at hand. While this may sound like an obvious first step, it may well be very challenging to describe and articulate the problem. Finally, this first step includes identifying a wide range of possible options, including those that might, at first glance, seem untenable or not feasible.

- Making plans/deciding upon an approach

  In this second stage, a plan should be formed to try to solve the problem or address the situation. Whether the plan for action involves doing something or doing nothing, consulting with others is critical throughout all the stages of this kind of a decision-making model, but especially at this point. In forming a plan, it is important to take into account the views of those who may clearly disagree with the proposal. This ensures that a diversity of perspectives are taken into consideration when making decisions.

- Implementing plans/taking action

  The third stage involves taking action. Remember that the best course of action may well involve doing nothing, and we must be clear and explicit about this, if our choice is, in fact, not to act. The document outlines the kinds of activities that must take place alongside implementing a plan, including communicating clearly and consistently, and providing ongoing support to those who are affected by the situation. This support extends not only to patients and families during this stage, but also to health care professionals, who are a pivotal part of implementation of a plan of action.

- Evaluation/Outcome

  A crucial part of implementing any kind of plan of action is evaluating the outcomes that result from the decisions that are made. Involving all stakeholders in the process of evaluation is important in order to ensure that an evaluation is thorough and relevant. It may be necessary at this point to reformulate the plan, identify new options, or propose changes to standing policies and institutional guidelines.

Adapted from *Practice Standards: Ethics* (College of Nurses of Ontario, 2009).

Scientific Process and Ethical Decision Making

The process of decision making in ethics follows a procedure that is similar to the scientific process. "A comparison between the giving of good reasons in science, which is called 'explanation,' and the giving of good reasons in ethics, which is called 'moral justification,' reveals striking procedural similarities bordering on identity" (Gibson, 1991, p. 3). Gibson notes similarities between the scientific process of explanation, which moves from *observation → hypothesis → law → theory*, and the moral justification process of ethics, which moves from *assessed ethical dilemma → rule → principle → theory*. A strong knowledge base regarding societal rules, ethical principles and theories, and professional codes and standards is as important to making ethical decisions as knowledge of principles related to physical, psychological, social, and human science is to other nursing judgments.

ETHICAL DECISION MAKING

We often approach ethical problems with a problem-solving frame of reference. Similar to both nursing process and scientific inquiry, the ethical problem-solving process generally includes the following steps: (1) defining the problem and collecting information, (2) identifying objectives to be achieved, (3) listing alternative ways to meet objectives, (4) evaluating each way of meeting the objectives, and (5) choosing the best alternative.

Differences of culture or values among the various participants involved in ethical decision making often become an important issue. In this regard, defining the problem includes both determining the ethical issue at hand and identifying the value systems of those involved. Consider, for instance, parents who wish to terminate life support for a seriously injured child who is hospitalized with no hope of recovery. The parents believe that life support is causing harm by interfering with what they refer to as the natural process of death, while the physician feels that removing life support constitutes murder. The problem includes both the issue of terminating life support and the conflicting values of physician and family. Although both parties might identify what is best for and least harmful to the child as the ultimate objective, the list of potential options would be different for the family and the physician. Determining which principles and theories guide the people involved enables the nurse to help clarify the issue and facilitate the process of coming to an ethical decision.

Emotions and Ethical Decisions

Many approaches to ethical decision making describe a primarily cognitive process in which emotions are subordinated to reason. In a holistic view of people, however, both thinking and feeling are credible ways of knowing, each having a legitimate role in ethical decision making. Callahan (2000) suggests that heart and mind should not be viewed as antagonistic in the moral arena; rather, both reason and emotion should be active and in accord as we come to an ethical decision. Noting that emotions should influence reason while reason is monitoring emotions, she describes emotions as personal signals providing information regarding both inner processes and interactions with the environment.

It is important to appreciate not only what you *think* about what is right or wrong in a situation, but also what you *feel* in relation to the circumstances and decision to be made. If you are feeling discomfort, even though reason is pointing in a particular direction, it is wise to further explore both the arguments posed through reason and your reactions to them. Callahan (2000) writes:

> In our technological culture perhaps the greatest moral danger arises not from sentimentality, but from devaluing feeling and not attending to or nurturing moral emotions. Numbness, apathy, isolated disassociations between thinking and feeling are also moral warning signals . . . the absence of emotional responses of empathy and sympathy become critical bioethical issues. (pp. 30–31)

In the same way that people may approach an issue with differing moral reasoning, their emotional responses might be quite different from your own. In such situations you might see validity in the other's response and broaden your own view. On the other hand, you may recognize that the chasm between the two is too deep to bridge. Callahan suggests that such social conflicts and challenges present new ethical problems that may require dealing with the consequences of an ethical decision by repeating the decision-making process.

? THINK ABOUT IT

The Role of Emotions in Decision Making

Consider your emotional response to the following situations and how it would affect your dealing with and caring for the people involved.

- You work in a busy urban clinic primarily serving new immigrants to the country, and you hear one of your co-workers comment that "it's a waste of time trying to do health education, because these people just don't understand, and are just a drain on the system."

- You are working in an emergency department at the local hospital, where a two-year-old child dies as a result of injuries sustained while being "disciplined" by the mother's boyfriend. The child had previously been placed in foster care due to neglect, and had been returned to the mother's care only a week prior to this event.

- You are the head nurse in a coronary intensive care unit. You receive a call from a cardiologist from another hospital who is desperate to get a bed in your unit for a young pregnant woman in congestive heart failure. An hour prior, your last available bed was taken by a forty-two-year-old chronic cocaine user, who has had another myocardial infarction.

PROCESS OF ETHICAL DECISION MAKING

The nature of the ethical problem requires a decision-making process in which key facets are revisited from evolving perspectives, even as you move toward a decision or resolution. Many models for decision making describe step-by-step processes that are linear in nature, failing to reflect the potential for an evolving perspective. The guidelines presented here provide a framework for entering a decision-making process that requires the ongoing evaluation and assimilation of information. Keep in mind, though, that no model for ethical decision making is a substitute for reflection and thoughtfulness, or a guarantee of a good decision or outcome (MacDonald, 2002). Rather, an ethical decision-making guide helps us to consider multiple views, perspectives, and important steps in the process of working through an ethical dilemma. Furthermore, no ethical decision-making guide is meant to be applied in a purely linear fashion. The decision-making process is iterative and dynamic in nature, with each step being revisited as often as is required and moulded by the dynamics of changing facts and contexts, evolving beliefs, unexpected consequences, and participants who move in and out of the process. Before we outline the steps in an ethical decision-making process, it is important to note that, on an ongoing basis, as ethical practitioners, we must always be attentive to morally problematic situations (McDonald, 2001). We must be aware of what a moral dilemma is and what a practical problem is, as well as the differences between them. Being aware and being sensitive to moral and ethical dilemmas is a key foundational attribute of ethical practitioners. Without this "moral intuition" (McDonald, 2001), we cannot begin to enter into an ethical decision-making process, as we may have difficulty identifying what kinds of situations are truly ethically or morally problematic. We must be able to recognize that the particular problem, in fact, has a moral dimension (MacDonald, 2002). The following describes the steps involved in the process of ethical decision making.

Gather Data and Identify Conflicting Moral Claims

When an ethical problem occurs, gather information or facts in order to clarify issues. Identification of the conflicting moral claims that constitute the ethical dilemma is the first part of the process. You should examine the situation for evidence of conflicting obligations, principles, duties, rights, loyalties, values, or beliefs. Additionally, data provide an understanding of the ethical components, principles of concern, and the various perceptions of issues and principles by those involved in the situation. You must pay attention to societal, religious, and cultural values and beliefs. In order to situate the problem, you must explore the not only the context of the problem but also the context of decision making. Clinical issues and the stated, inferred, or known preferences of all involved (primarily the patient, but the preferences of family members and the health care team may well be relevant) must also be considered. Often, a situation you initially think constitutes an ethical dilemma will actually turn out to be a practical dilemma. This recognition allows the participants to appropriately weigh choices and expedite decision making. One important part of this stage of decision making is to identify what you know and admit what you do not know (McDonald, 2001). You may not have the perspectives or views of all involved and it may be difficult for you to acquire them. Alternatively, you may not have enough time to gather adequate information in one area or from one perspective. In this case, we must then attend to and be as articulate and transparent about what we don't know, as we are about what we do know. In order to begin to work through the dilemma, the values, benefits, and burdens need to be identified (MacDonald, 2002). This requires actively seeking this kind of information from a number of perspectives.

Identify Key Participants

Identify the key persons involved in the decision-making process and delineate each person's role. Determining the rights, duties, authority, context, and capabilities of decision makers is a critical component of the process (Curtin & Flaherty, 1982; Husted & Husted, 1995). The focal question is, *"Whose decision is this to make?"* Identification of the principal decision maker or decision makers is sometimes all that is needed to facilitate the process. Recognition that one has the legitimate authority to make an important decision is an empowering event. Once the principal decision maker is identified, the roles of the other participants can be explicitly outlined. As MacDonald (2002) notes, examining the relationships between key participants is also an important step. For example, nurses often feel the burden of difficult ethical decisions, even though the responsibility for the decision lies with the patient or the nearest relative. In these instances, the nurse serves as a resource for information, a source of emotional support for those making the difficult decision, and a facilitator of the decision-making process. Nurses must also be carefully attuned to the dynamics of relationships between patients, relatives, friends, and caregivers.

Determine the Moral Perspective and Phase of Moral Development of Key Participants

Knowledge of moral development and ethical theory may provide a helpful framework for understanding participants and their perspectives and responses in the process. Assess how those involved fit into paradigms of moral development. It is valuable to recognize, for instance, whether the principal decision maker is at a developmental level where choices reflect a desire to please others, and is thus susceptible to choosing an alternative solely on the basis of seeking approval. (See Chapter 5 for an in-depth discussion of moral development.) It may also be worthwhile to try to reflect upon the level of moral response that each key player articulates in relation to the problem. Establishing that a response is expressive, pre-reflective, or reflective may help you gain insight into the reasons behind the moral convictions of others, as well as assist you in exploring their perspective and reasoning in a way that is relevant to them, and most facilitative for the decision-making process. In the following text box (Figure 6–2), we revisit the levels of moral response, as outlined by Thomas and Waluchow (1998) and introduced in Chapter 5.

FIGURE 6–2 **EXAMINING MORAL RESPONSES**

Thomas and Waluchow (1998) examined the way that people respond to a moral problem or question. They identify three levels of response or reflection. This is a review from chapter 5 in which we examined moral responses within the context of values development.

- At an expressive level, responses to moral problems are uncritical or unanalyzed. Usually cited in personal experience or emotions, the response may not, on its own, provide justification for the person's position on the moral problem.

  - An example of an expressive statement might be: "Withdrawal of nutrition and hydration should never happen because it is murder."

- At a pre-reflective level, reasons behind one's position are often references to rules, laws, or principles that are accepted without question or critical analysis. They may refer to the status quo, that is, a conventional community standard that is usually agreed upon by many. At this level, reference to these kinds of rules is often not done alongside critical reflection as to whether or not these rules or standards are actually good, but it is done with what may be blind acceptance of rules without question.

  - An example of a pre-reflective statement might be: "I disagree with the withdrawal of nutrition and hydration because it will directly cause death. The Catholic Church prohibits this on the basis of protecting sanctity of life and I am Catholic."

- At a reflective level of moral response, moral judgments and responses are based on "principles, rules and values to which we ourselves consciously subscribe." (Hardingham, 2001, p. 2). At this level, one is able to offer clear, thoughtful reasons about one's position on a moral problem.

  - An example of a reflective statement might be: "Withdrawal of nutrition and hydration is a difficult concept to accept for many because of the social values we place on food and water. However, in some cases, with clear consent, a careful examination of the values of the patient, a negative prognosis and a demonstrably poor quality of life, it may be carefully considered with measures taken to minimize and ease any suffering."

It is crucial to identify the participants' ethical perspectives and explicitly stated values and beliefs. For example, if one of the major participants involved in discussions relative to discontinuing life support believes that it is always wrong to take a life (see our discussion of deontology in Chapter 2), the process of negotiation with those who believe differently is likely to be frustrating. It would be more beneficial under those circumstances to begin the discussion by defining the point at which death actually occurs, thus finding common ground. When those involved present with diverse values, your role may be to facilitate their coming to a consensus around goals and the understanding of principles.

At this point, and throughout the process, we must always keep "checking in" with ourselves, to see how we are feeling about the situation, how we are responding to the views and values of others, and our kind of moral response. No one can be a completely detached ethical decision maker. We always have our own views, values, and beliefs, which may affect how we approach the problem. "Checking in" with ourselves and our "moral barometer" on a continuous basis is an important part of any ethical decision-making process.

Determine Desired Outcomes

Identifying the desired outcomes and their potential consequences is a substantial step in the decision-making process. At this point, participants will exclude those outcomes that are totally unacceptable. As with the nursing process, implementation of a plan of action cannot logically occur without explicit knowledge of the desired outcome. Likewise, evaluation of the success or failure of the plan is measured by the degree to which the outcome is met. Clarifying the outcomes and their anticipated consequences enhances the understanding of options and alternatives.

Identify Options

Having determined the desired outcomes, participants should identify possible options for action. Various options begin to emerge through the assessment process. Participants must consider legal and other consequences. They must also determine which alternatives best meet the identified outcomes and fit their basic beliefs, lifestyles, and values. In addition to attending to the basic values, lifestyles, and beliefs that are held by those most affected by a decision, one must also be able to identify which factors in each alternative are "morally significant" (McDonald, 2001). Consider an alternative in which we would be breaking an important promise previously made to a patient. Would this breach of trust significantly harm the patient? Would it exploit them or treat them in a paternalistic way, thus limiting their autonomy? Would it cause indelible damage to the fidelity that exists between you and the patient?

To help in identifying morally significant factors in proposed alternatives, we must each have a good working knowledge of ethical theories and principles. Additionally, we must be aware of the values, norms, and beliefs of our institutions, professions, and workplace cultures through review of policies, mandates, and mission and vision statements. We can use the resources around us to help identify morally important factors: clinical ethics consultants or research ethics consultants, formal ethics case conferences, research ethics boards or ethics committees, mentors, and those we have identified in our own professional life as persons of high moral integrity (McDonald, 2001). Our own judgments, along with the deliberation of those in the workplace for whom we have great deference, are also very helpful elements within the process. Remember, though, that discussing a sensitive patient care situation involves serious professional and legal responsibilities for protecting the privacy and confidentiality of others that must always be respected. This process helps to narrow the list of acceptable alternatives. It is critical to eliminate all unacceptable alternatives and begin the process of listing, weighing, ranking, and prioritizing those that are found to be acceptable. Participants must make a choice among options with both head and heart; taking time to dwell with remaining alternatives, recognizing that there is rarely a "good" solution. Remember that when considering possible options, as a nurse, you must try to bear in mind that there may be consequences of certain options that are farther reaching than one patient or one clinical situation. There may be implications for families, other professionals, institutions, or groups of patients. Many people may be affected by a decision, including yourself. As McDonald notes, we must be honest about our "own stake in particular outcomes and encourage others to do the same" (McDonald, 2001). Once an option is chosen, the decision makers must be willing to act upon the choice.

Act on the Choice

Taking action is a major goal of the process, but can be one of the most difficult parts. It can stir numerous emotions laced with both certainty and doubt about the rightness of the decision. Participants must be empowered to make a difficult decision, setting aside less acceptable alternatives. Chapters 19 and 20 discuss empowerment in more depth. It is important to be attentive to the emotions involved at this point of the process.

 THINK ABOUT IT

Before acting upon a specific alternative, we can ask ourselves a few simple but important questions. These might include questions like:

- What would get you to change your mind, and act differently from this alternative?

- Are you setting a good moral example to others?

- Are you doing what you would think a good or virtuous person would do? If not, why? And which other alternative would the good person choose, then?

- From a Kantian or deontological perspective, consider the alternative as a universal maxim for anyone in a similar situation. Would you want the alternative to be such a maxim?

- Have you breached confidentiality or caused harm to any trust relationships?

- After all these questions, are you still content with the identified alternative?

Adapted from *A framework for ethical decision making:* Version 6.0 (McDonald, 2001)

Evaluate the Outcomes of the Action

After acting upon the decision, participants begin a process of response and evaluation. As in all decision making, reflective evaluation sheds light on the effectiveness and validity of the process. Evaluate the action in terms of the effects upon those involved. Ask, "Has the original ethical problem been resolved?" and "Have other problems emerged related to the action?" As the situation changes and new data emerge, participants must identify subsequent moral problems and adjust the course of action based upon both new information and responses to the previous decision.

Figure 6–3 is a guide for ethical decision making. Questions may need to be revisited several times and may emerge at various points as the process unfolds and new data are presented. For example, information about options may begin to emerge before all the parties involved are identified, and data regarding ethical perspectives of the various parties may be clarified only at the point when options are being discussed. No matter how much information the participants gather, they may make the decision with an awareness that they would like to have still more data, although having a long list of viable options may actually make it more difficult to come to a decision.

FIGURE 6–3 **A GUIDE FOR ETHICAL DECISION MAKING**

Gather Data and Identify Conflicting Moral Claims
- What makes this situation an ethical problem? Are there conflicting obligations, duties, principles, rights, loyalties, values, or beliefs?
- What are the issues?
- What facts seem most important?
- What emotions have an impact?
- What are the gaps in information at this time?

Identify Key Participants
- Who is legitimately empowered to make this decision?
- Who is affected and how?
- What is the level of competence of the person most affected in relation to the decision to be made?
- What are the rights, duties, authority, context, and capabilities of the participants?

Determine the Moral Perspective and Phase of Moral Development of Key Participants
- Do the participants think in terms of duties or rights?
- Do the parties involved exhibit similar or different moral perspectives?
- Where is the common ground? The differences?
- What principles are important to each person involved?
- What emotions are evident within the interaction and with each person involved, including yourself?
- What is the level of moral development of the participants?

(Continued)

Determine Desired Outcomes
- How does each party describe the circumstances of the outcome?
- What are the consequences of the desired outcomes?
- What outcomes are unacceptable to one or all involved?

Identify Options
- What options emerge through the assessment process?
- How do the alternatives fit the lifestyles and values of the person(s) affected?
- What are the legal considerations or implications of the various options?
- What alternatives are unacceptable to one or all involved?
- How are alternatives weighed, ranked, and prioritized?

Act on the Choice
- Be empowered to make a difficult decision.
- Give yourself permission to set aside less acceptable alternatives.
- Be attentive to the emotions involved in this process.

Evaluate the Outcomes of the Action
- Has the ethical dilemma been resolved?
- Have other dilemmas emerged related to the action?
- How has the process affected those involved?
- Are further actions required?

APPLYING THE DECISION-MAKING PROCESS

Application of the decision-making guide in clinical situations is illustrated in the following case and discussion:

> A couple are pregnant with their second child after numerous unsuccessful attempts with artificial insemination. During a routine ultrasound at 28 weeks gestation, the physician discovers that the fetus is anencephalic. The life expectancy of an anencephalic baby is only a few days to weeks after birth. The couple struggles with the choice of whether to terminate the pregnancy at this time or to carry the child to term.

Gathering Data and Identifying Conflicting Moral Claims

One conflict relates to the principle of non-maleficence (the wish to do no harm). Terminating the pregnancy can be perceived as harmful to the baby, while carrying it to term may result in emotional or physical harm to the mother. Another conflict relates to the duty to preserve life, allowing the pregnancy, birth, and death of the baby to take its natural course, versus the duty to alleviate the suffering that carrying the pregnancy to term might impose on the mother. Some of the important facts in this situation include knowing the life expectancy of a baby born with anencephaly, knowing the parents' attitudes toward abortion, appreciating the feelings that this news brings forth, and knowing the meaning of this pregnancy to the parents.

Identifying Key Participants

Valuing input from the physician and others, both parents have the moral and legal right and the responsibility to make the decision. They may want to consult family or friends, and they may request a second opinion. Though competent, the parents may have difficulty making a decision soon after receiving the painful news. Since this is not an emergency, the nurse and others should allow time and provide support, while the parents process the information and deal with their emotions. If, for example, one parent wants the pregnancy terminated and the other is strongly opposed, participants should further explore who has the right to make the ultimate decision.

Determining the Moral Perspective and Phase of Moral Development of Key Participants

It is important to consider whether the stance of both parents is the same. Are they thinking about the rights of the infant versus the rights of the mother, or the duty to preserve the family integrity? If one parent thinks the pregnancy should be terminated and the other feels that the baby has a right to life, no matter how short it may be, can a common ground be reached? Do the parents seek guidance from those in authority, or from beliefs regarding right and wrong in this situation? Do they talk of a relationship with the baby in utero and the impact of choosing to end its life—on the baby, its sibling, or their relationship?

Determining Desired Outcomes

Through discussion of outcomes, more insight into ethical theory may emerge. In this situation, participants could describe the desired outcome as prevention of unnecessary suffering for the mother and the baby. Further exploration might reveal the sense that carrying the baby to term would create such anguish for the mother that her emotional health, and even family integrity, would be threatened. In that instance, terminating the pregnancy would be more compassionate than prolonging the suffering of the mother and allowing the inevitable, yet slow, natural death of the baby. Legal considerations would include any laws related to access to abortion.

Identifying Options

In this case, the physician presented the options at the outset: the parents could terminate the pregnancy, or allow it to go to term. One might well look at the risks for the mother involved in both choices. Participants need to clarify their beliefs regarding life, abortion, family responsibility, duties, and the like. If carrying the pregnancy to term presents a health risk for the mother, an additional dilemma would arise regarding responsibility to the older sibling and family integrity versus responsibility to the baby.

If either carrying the pregnancy to term or terminating it now is acceptable, participants have the task of determining factors that may weigh one alternative more strongly than the other. They may decide that the grieving process of the baby's death has already begun and would be only intensified if the pregnancy were carried to term. With this in mind, they might decide to end the pregnancy.

Acting on the Choice

Deciding to terminate the pregnancy, the parents move toward action. As the logistics of scheduling and preparing for the termination proceed, it is important to attend to the parents' emotional responses and to ensure that they have other needed support.

Evaluating Outcomes of Action

The parents resolved the dilemma of whether to terminate the pregnancy or carry it to term by choosing to proceed with termination. Reactions to the choice may emerge in the forms of guilt, depression, acceptance, or always wondering how things might have been different if the other path had been chosen. If the parents have long-term reactions, such as deep guilt or depression, they might come to a point of saying that, faced with such a situation again, they would decide to carry the pregnancy to term. On the other hand, they may examine issues surrounding the emotions with the awareness that the decision to terminate the pregnancy helped them deal with these issues and that, despite the pain, they made the best decision possible at the time.

 THINK ABOUT IT

Various Responses to Terminating Pregnancy

Consider which areas of the "Guide for Decision Making" in Figure 6–3 may have to be revisited in the following variations of the case presented above.

- The mother indicates that she thinks she will "go crazy" if she carries the pregnancy to term, and the father says, "no one is going to kill my child."
- The local hospital has a religious affiliation that does not permit abortions. The parents feel that terminating the pregnancy is the better decision, but the closest hospital that could perform the procedure is a four-hour drive and their parents and support network would not be present.
- The mother refuses to consider any alternatives, stating that "Allah will make the baby fine."

SUMMARY

Ethical decision making requires knowledge and attention to many factors. Determining the existence of an ethical dilemma is the beginning step in the process, which includes defining the problem, identifying desired objectives, listing and evaluating alternatives, choosing the best course of action based on one's knowledge and the current circumstances, and evaluating the outcomes of the action taken. One must consider both reason and emotion in making ethical decisions. Nurses are encouraged to utilize the decision-making process described in this chapter as a guide in dealing with dilemmas encountered in clinical settings. As with every other nursing skill, comfort and competency with ethical decision making comes with repeated practice.

CHAPTER HIGHLIGHTS

- Dilemmas exist when difficult problems have no satisfactory solutions or when all the solutions appear equally favourable.
- In decisions involving practical dilemmas, moral claims hold greater weight than non-moral claims.
- Making thoughtful decisions in any arena follows a pattern that includes gathering data, comparing options based on particular criteria, making and acting on a choice, and evaluating outcomes or circumstances surrounding the choice.
- One's value system affects how one defines and deals with an ethical issue; thus, resolution of ethical dilemmas requires determining the ethical issue at hand and identifying the value systems of those involved.
- Both emotion and reason have legitimate roles in ethical decision making.
- Ethical decision making requires ongoing evaluation and assimilation of information, with revisiting of various steps in the process as often as required by the dynamics of changing facts, evolving beliefs, unexpected consequences, and participants moving in and out of the process.
- Familiarity with and practice in applying ethical decision making enables the nurse to develop competence and confidence with the process.

DISCUSSION QUESTIONS AND ACTIVITIES

1. Search an on-line database for scholarly articles related to ethical decision making. How do other models compare to the ones presented in this text? Discuss what you like or would change about specific models.

2. Working in small groups, discuss ethical and practical dilemmas that you have experienced, then choose an example of each type of dilemma to illustrate for the class.

3. Describe a situation in which you or someone you know experienced moral distress, noting moral and non-moral claims in the situation.

4. Talk with practising nurses about their experiences of ethical dilemmas. Identify their approaches to dealing with such dilemmas, including their processes of ethical decision making.

5. Use the ethical decision-making process to revisit an ethical dilemma that you have encountered in the past, or to guide you through a current dilemma. Examine your level of comfort with each part of the process, noting areas of strength and areas needing more practice.

6. Discuss the interaction among moral development, moral perspective, and ethical decision making.

7. In a small group, share an experience in which you feel you demonstrated moral courage. Discuss some strategies that nurses can use to support the moral courage of nursing colleagues.

8. Identify some examples of environmental constraints that may lead to moral distress. What kinds of barriers or constraints have you encountered, in your professional or personal life, when trying to "do the right thing"? How did this make you feel?

REFERENCES

Beauchamp, T. L., & J. F. Childress (2008). *Principles of biomedical ethics* (6th ed.). New York: Oxford University Press.

Callahan, S. (2000). The role of emotions in ethical decision making. In J. H. Howell & W. F. Sale, eds., *Life choices: A Hastings Center introduction to bioethics.* (2nd ed.). Washington, DC: Georgetown University Press.

Canadian Nurses' Association (2008). Code of Ethics for Registered Nurses. *CNA*: Ottawa.

Christensen, P. J., & J. W. Kenney (1995). *Nursing process: Application of conceptual models* (4th ed.). St. Louis, MO: Mosby.

College of Nurses of Ontario (2009). Practice Standard: Ethics. College of Nurses of Ontario: Toronto.

Corley, M. C. (2002). Nurse moral distress: A proposed theory and research agenda. *Nursing Ethics, 9*(6), 636–650.

Curtin, L., & M. J. Flaherty (1982). *Nursing ethics: Theories and pragmatics.* Bowie, MD: Brady.

Davis, A. J., M. A. Aroskar, J. Liaschenko & T. S. Drought (2009). *Ethical dilemmas and nursing practice* (5th ed.). Norwalk, CT: Appleton & Lange.

Fenton, M. (1988). Moral distress in clinical practice: Implications for the nurse administrator. *Canadian Journal of Nursing Administration, 1,* 8–11.

Gibson, J. (1991). An introduction to the study of ethics and ethical theories. In B. R. Furrow, S. H. Johnson, T. S. Jost, & R. L. Schwartz, eds., *Bioethics: Health care, law, and ethics* (pp. 1–6). St. Paul, MN: West.

Hamric, A. B. (2000). Moral distress in everyday ethics. *Nursing Outlook, 48,* 199–201.

Hardingham, L. (2001). Reflective practice. *Alberta RN* (May/June 2001). Retrieved January 25, 2009, from http://findarticles.com/p/articles/mi_qa3929/is_200105/ai_n8941245/pg_1?tag=art Body;col1.

Heffernan, P., & S. Heilig (1999). Giving "moral distress" a voice: Ethical concerns among neonatal intensive care unit personnel. *Cambridge Quarterly of Healthcare Ethics, 8,* 173–178.

Husted, G. L., & J. H. Husted (1995). *Ethical decision making in nursing.* St. Louis, MO: Mosby.

Jameton, A. (1984). *Nursing practice: The ethical issues.* Englewood Cliffs, NJ: Prentice-Hall.

Kelly, B. (1998). Preserving moral integrity: A follow-up study with new graduate nurses. *Journal of Advanced Nursing, 28,* 1134–1145.

MacDonald, C. (2002). *A guide to moral decision making.* Retrieved January 26, 2009, from http://www.ethicsweb.ca/guide/.

McDonald, M. (2001). *A framework for ethical decision making.* Version 6.0 Ethics [Shareware]. Retrieved January 25, 2009, from http:www.ethics.ubc.cq.

Millette, B. E. (1994). Using Gilligan's framework to analyze nurses' stories of moral choices. *Western Journal of Nursing Research, 16*(6), 660–674.

Pavlish, C., D. Brown-Saltzman, M. Hersh, M. Shirk & A. Rounkle (2011). Nursing priorities, actions and regrets for ethical situations in clinical practice. *Journal of Nursing Scholarship, 43*(4), 385–395.

Redman, B., & S. T. Fry (2000). Nurses' ethical conflicts: What is really known about them? *Nursing Ethics, 7*(4), 360–366.

Rushton, C. H. (1995). The Baby K case: Ethical challenges of preserving professional integrity. *Pediatric Nursing, 23*(1), 16–29.

Schluter, J., S. Winch, K. Holzhauser & A. Henderson (2008). Nurses' moral sensitivity and hospital ethical climate: A literature review. *Nursing Ethics, 15*(3), 304–321.

Thomas, J. & W. Waluchow (1998). Well and good: A case study approach to biomedical ethics. *Ad Edition.* Peterborough: Broadview Press.

Zomordi, M., & B. Foley (2009). The nature of advocacy versus paternalism in nursing: clarifying the 'thin line.' *Journal of Advanced Nursing, 65*(8), 1746–1752. doi: 10.1111/j.1365-2648.2009.05023.x

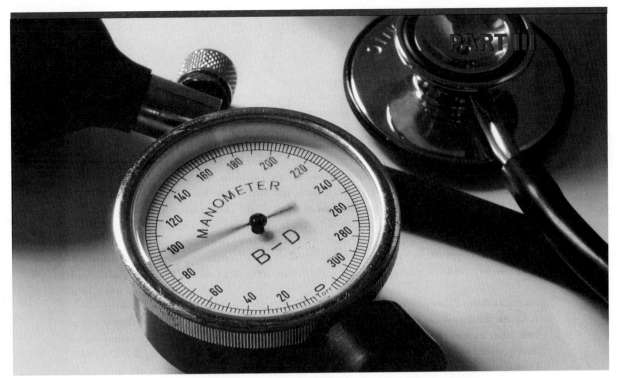

PRINCIPLED BEHAVIOUR IN THE PROFESSIONAL DOMAIN

Part III examines various categories of issues that affect the profession of nursing and the everyday practice of individual nurses. Recognizing nursing as a profession, the chapters describe the responsibilities of nurses related to ethical, legal, professional, and practice issues. These issues are examined in light of ethics and contemporary nursing. This part includes chapters discussing legal issues affecting nurses; professional issues, such as autonomy, authority, and accountability; issues related to the relationship between nurses and the health care system; issues related to technology and self-determination; and scholarship issues.

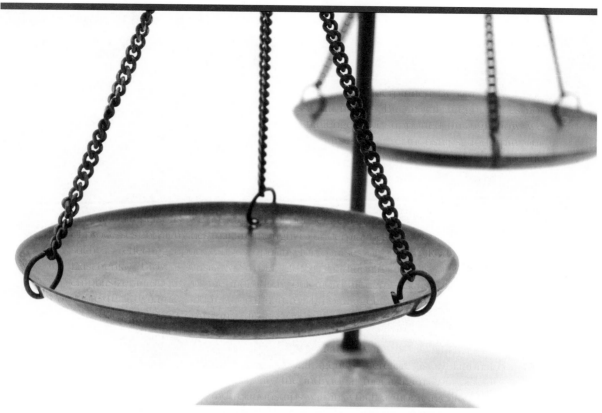

CHAPTER 7

LEGAL ISSUES

OBJECTIVES

After completing this chapter, the reader should be able to:

1. Recognize the difference between ethics and the law, and discuss the relationship of each to the other.
2. Describe sources of law.
3. Identify steps in the process by which laws are passed in Canada.
4. Distinguish between constitutional law, statutory law, administrative law, and common law.
5. Describe the difference between public and private law.
6. Define tort, and distinguish between unintentional and intentional torts.

7. Describe the importance of the right to privacy in Canada.

8. Discuss the notion of consent and important elements.

INTRODUCTION

Up to this point, the focus of this book has been upon values, morals, and ethics. You will recall from Chapter 2 that moral thinking, though influenced in great measure by prevailing cultural tradition, is essentially an individual enterprise. Ethics are rules of behaviour produced by moral thinking and may be either informal or formal rules of actions. Professional organizations, such as the Canadian Nurses Association, the American Nurses Association, and the International Council of Nurses, provide documents outlining a formal set of ethical guidelines. These guidelines offer some general rules that are intended for use as a tool to guide professional behaviour but are not, in themselves, fully enforceable. Laws, on the other hand, consist of enforced rules under which a society is governed. Many laws either directly or indirectly affect the practice of nursing. Highly publicized issues such as termination of life support and "do not resuscitate" status indicate a recent trend toward involving the legal system in issues that were previously thought to be ethical in nature. This chapter discusses the relationship between ethics and the law, general legal concepts, areas of potential liability for nurses, and recent legal trends. The legal regulation of nursing is addressed in Chapter 8.

RELATIONSHIP BETWEEN ETHICS AND THE LAW

Law is the system of binding rules of action or conduct that govern the behaviour of people in respect to relationships with others and with the government (Guido, 1997). Laws meant to reflect the moral beliefs of a given population are devised by groups of individuals serving in an official capacity. There are four basic functions of the law in society: (1) to define relationships among members of society, and to declare which actions are and are not permitted; (2) to describe what constraints may be applied to maintain rules, and by whom they may be applied; (3) to furnish solutions to problems; and, (4) to redefine relationships between people and groups when circumstances of life change (Kozier & Erb, 2007).

The law establishes rules that define our rights and obligations, and sets penalties for people who violate them. Laws also describe how government will enforce the rules and penalties. In Canada and the United States, there are thousands of federal, provincial, state, and local laws. Among others, these laws ensure the safety of citizens, protect property, prohibit discrimination, regulate the professions, provide for the distribution of public goods and services, and protect the economic and environmental interests of society.

How are ethics and laws related? Laws are intended to reflect popular belief about the "rightness or wrongness" of particular acts and are, like ethics, built upon a moral foundation. In most countries laws represent an attempt to codify ethics.

Law can serve as the public's instrument for converting morality into clear-cut social guidelines, and for stipulating punishments for offences (Beauchamp, 2001). One would expect that laws would be congruent with the prevailing moral values of a society; indeed, they usually are, at least in most democratic societies. For example, most people would agree that the murder of an innocent person is an immoral act. Laws that prohibit murder reflect this ethical standard. Murder of the innocent is both ethically and legally prohibited in every culture. As society's needs and attitudes evolve, laws emerge to reflect these changes. Occasionally, however, governments create and enforce laws that many people believe to be unjust or immoral. In a democratic society, constitutional law provides mechanisms to change or abolish unjust or unpopular laws.

Some authors of nursing ethics texts take the view that professional ethical standards are congruent with the law, that is, that which is legal is also ethical, and vice versa. These authors imply that following a set of ethical guidelines, such as those provided by the Canadian Nurses Association, the American Nurses Association, and the International Council of Nurses, provides nurses with a legal safety net. This is usually, but not necessarily, true. Laws exist that can be considered (by some at least) to be unethical. Some illegal acts are considered by many to be ethical.

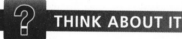

THINK ABOUT IT

Consider the following examples of situations that are illegal but arguably ethically fine:

- Breaking the speeding limit to rush a sick child to hospital;
- Breaking and entering into an isolated mountain cabin, if you are lost and suffering from exposure;
- Stealing a life preserver from someone else's boat to throw to a drowning person;
- Physically injuring someone in order to restrain them from imminently injuring someone else.

Consider the following situations or actions that are unethical but legal:

- Lying in almost any situation except in court or in advertising;
- Cheating on your spouse;
- Making sexist comments, or having views that some would consider to be racist;
- Gossiping about someone else.

What are some reasons for the possible discrepancy between what is legal and what is ethical? First, there are differences between ethical points of view. Deontology and utilitarianism, for example, offer quite opposite answers to some basic ethical questions. While the utilitarian perspective would allow consideration of euthanasia, for example, to provide for the good of many, deontological views might require that life be protected regardless of circumstances. Thus, a law thought to be ethical by the utilitarian might be considered unethical by the deontologist. Second, human behaviour and motivation are more complex than can be fairly reflected in law. Think back to Chapter 4. Individuals may consider the same act either right or wrong, depending to some extent on their stage or level of moral development. For example, acts of civil disobedience, such as those committed by Mahatma Gandhi and Martin Luther King, Jr., although considered at that time to be illegal, are generally considered to have been motivated by high ethical standards. In his letter from the Birmingham Jail, Martin Luther King, Jr. wrote, "there are two types of laws: just and unjust. I would be the first to advocate obeying just laws. One has not only a legal but a moral responsibility to obey just laws. Conversely, one has a moral responsibility to disobey unjust laws" (1996, p. 574). Third, the legal system judges actions rather than motivations. For example, nurses following personal moral convictions or professional ethical codes can find themselves at odds with the policies or practices of the institutions where they are employed. In certain instances, the legal system may determine that an employing institution has the right to dismiss or discipline a nurse for setting aside or flouting institutional policy in favour of ethical considerations. Fourth, depending upon the political climate and other variables, laws change. Recent examples of laws that have changed and evolved over time include those related to expanded roles of nurses, abortion, fetal tissue use, organ transplantation, self-determination, privacy, informed consent, suicide, and legal definitions of death. As defined in Chapter 3, integrity is fidelity in adherence to moral norms sustained over time. One should be able to predict that nurses with integrity will not alter their basic moral beliefs in response to changes in the law. Thus, there are several valid circumstances in which there may be a discrepancy between what is legal and what is considered ethical.

GENERAL LEGAL CONCEPTS

Nurses need to familiarize themselves with the law and legal system for several reasons. First, the law authorizes and regulates nursing practice. Nurse practice acts and regulatory acts of the individual provinces and territories describe both the activity of nurses and their scope of practice. Chapter 8 discusses the legal regulation of nursing in greater depth. Second, the legal system scrutinizes nursing actions and omissions. The profession is in a dynamic state of change: advanced practice nurses are expanding the traditional boundaries; critical care nurses are performing complex and vital tasks; staff nurses are caring for older and sicker patients; and many nurses are practising in new settings. Working in such a dynamic and quickly evolving health care environment, nurses must have basic knowledge about both new and long-standing laws and legal processes. This knowledge will help ensure that our actions are consistent with legal principles, and that we can advocate effectively for the profession and patients while remaining within the confines of the law. Knowledge of legal principles is a necessary component of ethical decision making. In order to make informed choices, nurses, physicians, patients, and families must be able to identify the potential or real legal implications of such choices.

Sources of Law

There are at least four different sources of law that are relevant to the practice of nursing: constitutional law, statutory (legislative) law, administrative law, and common law. The foundation of Canada's legal system outside Quebec is developed from common law (Quebec's system is based on civil law). Law can be divided into two main branches—private law and public law. Some laws are made by legislation, some by rule-making bodies, and some by judicial precedent. There is frequent overlap between the sources and branches of the law.

Constitutional Law

Constitutional law refers to formal sets of rules and principles that describe the powers of the government and the rights of the people. The principles that are set out in a constitution, coupled with a description of how these principles are to be interpreted and carried out, form the basis of constitutional law. Many times, constitutional law is noted in reference to the United States because of the strength of its written constitution. Many countries and states, in fact, have constitutions. The format of constitutions is highly variable—they may be written (as in the United States, Australia, and Japan) or unwritten (United Kingdom). They may be codified, meaning they are contained in a single document—again, the United States is a good example of a codified and written constitution—or they may be uncodified, meaning that they are contained in several documents. Israel and New Zealand have uncodified constitutions.

In Canada, our constitution is unique. It is partly written in several documents rather than one overarching constitutional document. Additionally, it is partially unwritten and partly derived from rules of common law developed by the courts. In Canada, constitutional law is highly complex. Our most important constitutional document is the *British North America Act* (1867). This act was revised many times and finally renamed the *Constitution Act* in 1982. Part one of the *Constitution Act* is the ***Charter of Rights and Freedoms***, which guarantees rights to individuals and groups and that you can read in full at http://laws-lois.justice.gc.ca/eng/charter/page-1.html. The subsequent parts of the act note other rights and powers to groups such as Aboriginal persons, as well as noting further amendments to the original act. At the same time that the *Constitution Act* was passed (1982), the *Canada Act* was also passed, which essentially severed Canada's dependence on the United Kingdom to pass legislation, a process referred to as "patriation."

The *Charter of Rights and Freedoms,* however, is the document most people are familiar with. It also is a document most people describe as a truly Canadian document—representing notions of human rights and dignity. As nurses, we should be especially familiar with the *Charter of Rights and Freedoms,* its meaningfulness in all realms of practice and professional life, and how our role as advocates for individuals and groups is supported by the kinds of values articulated in the *Charter,* which are considered by many to be values that, as a country, we embrace and embody.

Statutory/Legislative Law

Formal laws written and enacted by federal, or provincial/territorial legislatures are known as **statutory** or **legislative laws**. Parliament passes many laws each year; these are added to the volumes of federal and provincial statutes already in force. Because many people think that every problem in society can be solved by passing a law, legislatures make more and more laws to satisfy the demands of society and, in some cases, especially vocal special-interest groups. Provincial health care, professional regulatory acts, non-smoking health acts, statutory recognition of nurses in advanced practice (including prescriptive authority), and proposed health care reform legislation are all examples of statutory or legislative law. For more information on how laws are passed through legislative processes, see Chapter 14.

Administrative Law

Administrative law involves the operation of government agencies. Federal, provincial, and municipal governments set up administrative agencies to do the work of government. These agencies regulate such activities as education, public health, social welfare programs, and the professions. Administrative law consists mainly of the legal powers granted to administrative agencies by legislative bodies and the rules that the agencies make to carry out their powers. Provincial regulations bodies for nursing are examples of this type of agency. These regulatory bodies are granted the authority to execute the intent of provincial statutes by creating, implementing, and enforcing comprehensive and appropriate rules and regulations relevant to the safe practice of nursing. As administrative bodies, the role of colleges of nursing is to protect the public rather than to advocate for nurses. Rules made public by the individual provinces' regulatory bodies carry the same weight as other law.

How Laws Are Made in Canada

In Canada, there are two main ways in which laws are created, through either the judicial system (known as "common law" or "case law") or through the legislative or administrative system of the government (known as "statutory law"). **Common law** (sometimes called **case law**) developed originally in England, and is a system of laws derived from the decisions of courts and judges. This is in contrast to the laws set out by the government through acts, statutes, codes, or laws that enable, command, or enact, which is known as statutory law. Traditionally, statutory law may be seen as more important because there is less room or freedom for interpretation by judicial bodies. While there is room for interpretation in common law, the notion of precedent acts as a regulating force by establishing principles by which courts and judges make decisions in subsequent cases.

Common law is a tradition followed in all Canadian provinces except Quebec. How the common law system is set up, at a federal and provincial level, is outlined by the terms of the *Constitution Act* (1867), which divides judicial responsibility between the levels of government. Within the provincial judicial systems, courts and judges make decisions at various levels. Each level must answer to or abide by the decision of a more superior court. For example, a decision in a lower court in British Columbia may be overturned by a higher court such as the British Columbia Court of Appeals. One important thing to note, however, is that a decision made at the highest level of a provincial court is not binding in other provinces, so a decision made at the highest court in Nova Scotia would not apply to Ontarians, although it could well be considered as relevant or persuasive if the same issue were to be heard in an Ontario Court of Appeals. The highest court of appeal is the Supreme Court of Canada; the federal government decides who will serve as members of this court.

Statutory law refers to the body of law laid down by the legislature, either by the Parliament of Canada or by one of the provincial or territorial legislatures. At the federal level, bills (which eventually become laws) are passed by a complex process that involves a number of federal governing bodies within **Parliament**, which is made up of three parts: the **Governor General of Canada**, the appointed **Senate**, and the elected **House of Commons**. The governor general represents the queen and is responsible for calling Parliament together, reading the Speech from the Throne (outlining the priorities of the elected government), and approving all bills passed through the House of Commons and the Senate. The Senate (also referred to sometimes as the Upper Chamber) consists of members appointed by the governor general on the advice of the prime minister. Senators represent areas of the country and may serve until age 75. They are not replaced if and when a new government is elected. The House of Commons is made up of elected officials from various ridings (electoral areas) across Canada. Generally, a member of the House of Commons serves for the period of time that the current government is in power, which is normally no more than five years.

So how does a law get introduced and eventually passed? Usually it is introduced as a proposal or a "**bill**" in the House of Commons (or the Senate: it would then go to the House of Commons). Once introduced in the House of Commons, the proposed bill goes through a series of three "readings," which means that the proposed bill is debated, discussed, revised, and amended. At each reading, the bill is voted on by the members. At the final or third reading in the House of Commons, if the bill is voted to be passed, it moves forward to the Senate and then the governor general, who gives the bill **Royal Assent**. Until a bill is given Royal Assent, it cannot become a law. Royal Assent is a formal completion of the legislative processes and is carried out in Commonwealth countries by the representative of the sovereign. It represents the authority granted to the representative—in this country, our governor general—to act on behalf of the queen to assent to legislation. It is rare, if not unheard of, that a bill passed by a House of Commons would be met with dissention by the governor general, as she or he acts upon the advice of the prime minister. Therefore, many people view the Royal Assent to legislation as a mere formality.

Nurses should also have some basic knowledge about various types of law. **Civil law**, or **private law**, deals with the rights of individuals and may refer to issues of **contracts** and **torts** (wrongs or harms done to others). **Criminal law** refers to the system that defines particular crimes and regulates the apprehension, charging, and procedures of trying suspected offenders. Criminal law also includes the system by which decisions are made regarding the punishment of persons convicted in the courts of committing a criminal act. The ***Criminal Code of Canada*** (a federal act) is the formal articulation of all criminal offenses and procedures.

THINK ABOUT IT

In Canada, there are two main forms of legislation—**acts** and **regulations**. **Acts** are usually passed in the federal Parliament or in a provincial legislature. **Regulations** are usually made within the confines of a specific act and are often referred to as "delegated" or "subordinate" legislation for this reason. Note, though, that both acts and regulations are legally binding.

The Canadian government enacted the *Tobacco Act* in 1997. This act controls the sale, promotion, and labelling of tobacco products. It was put in place to protect the public, and specifically youth, from the proven dangerous effects of smoking on health. Some of the tenets of this act include restrictions on tobacco companies regarding how they advertise or market their products, requiring that they refrain from promoting tobacco through lifestyle ads, ads targeted at youth, or ads depicting the use of tobacco as glamorous or exciting. Furthermore, tobacco companies may not sponsor youth-related activities or lend their name (and funds) to a cultural or sports facility.

In 2008, two new provisions of the *Tobacco Act* came into effect. One prohibits the public view of tobacco products in almost all places that sell them. A second provision prohibits workplace smoking rooms.

In addition to the federal *Tobacco Act*, each province and territory has legislation governing smoking. For example, in 2002, Newfoundland passed its *Smoke-Free Environment Act*, amended in 2005 to ban smoking in all public places, including bars. Quebec's *Tobacco Act* (2006), requires a smoking ban in all indoor public places, with a ban on designated smoking rooms effective 2008. Ontario has the *Smoke-free Ontario Act,* which also bans smoking in all public and work places as of 2006. The Ontario act now also prohibits smoking in vehicles, in reserved seating in open-air stadiums, and in underground parking lots. Finally, Saskatchewan's *Tobacco Control Act* has a complete public ban on smoking, including casinos, private clubs, and bingo halls. This contrasts with neighbouring Alberta, which still allows smoking in casinos, bingo halls, and bars.

(Continued)

- What is your stand on smoking in public areas?
- Reflect on your stand and what kinds of experiences or beliefs have influenced you and your views on smoking.
- Do you think that these types of legislation limit the autonomy of persons?
- How do these kinds of laws protect those most vulnerable?
- What do you think should be more important for governments, protecting the autonomy of individuals or protecting the vulnerable? Why? Use the smoking laws to illustrate your views.

Branches of Law

Law can be divided into two different branches: public and private. Recall that law is a system of enforceable principles and processes that govern the behaviour of people in respect to relationships with others and with the government. In general, legal matters related to the relationship between people and the government are the domain of public law, and issues arising out of relationships between people are the domain of private law.

Public Law

Public law defines a person's rights and obligations in relation to the government and describes the various divisions of government and their powers. One important branch of public law is **criminal law**. Criminal law deals with crimes—that is, actions considered harmful to society. Even though a crime might be committed against a particular person, the government considers the commission of a serious act, such as murder, to be harmful to all of society. In Canada, the federal government presides over criminal law. The documents that outline and define aspects of criminal law include primarily the *Criminal Code of Canada,* but also acts such as the *Youth Criminal Justice Act* (2003) and the *Controlled Drugs and Substances Act* (1996). While these are federal documents, the provincial governments are given the power to administer the criminal justice system, enforce laws, and prosecute offenders. Laws are enforced by the police, the courts, and the penal system, all under provincial and municipal jurisdiction. Crimes range in seriousness from public drunkenness to murder. Criminal law defines these offences and sets the rules for the arrest, the appropriate procedures to ensure due process, and the punishment of offenders.

   In the course of practice, nurses can be accused of a variety of criminal offences. For example, nurses can be accused of directly injuring a patient, either intentionally or unintentionally. Nurses can also be accused of crimes related to their actual relationship with the government. These include such actions as falsifying narcotic records, failure to renew licences, and fraudulent billing. In most countries that have a common law system, as Canada does, crimes are delineated according to seriousness as either indictable offences or summary offences.

Indictable offences are serious crimes that carry significant fines and jail sentences. Examples include first- and second-degree murder, arson, burglary, extortion, kidnapping, rape, and robbery. These crimes are punishable by jail terms. Nurses are rarely accused of felonies in the course of practice. However, this can occur. For example, it is possible that those participating in the unauthorized removal of life support from a terminally ill patient could be accused of first-degree murder, because of the intentional nature of the act that resulted in death. This could occur even though the act might be viewed as beneficent by the majority of people. A nurse who unintentionally caused the death of a patient by administering a medication that a patient is allergic to could be charged with second-degree murder or manslaughter.

A *summary offence* is a less serious crime, usually punishable by a fine, a short jail sentence, or both. In the United States system, these crimes are known as misdemeanors. Examples of summary offences include disturbing the peace, solicitation, assault, and battery (assault and battery are also considered intentional torts and can be decided by private or civil law). A nurse who strikes a patient or gives an injection without consent could be accused of the summary offence of battery.

Private Law

Private law is also called **civil law**. It determines a person's legal rights and obligations in many kinds of activities that involve other people. These activities include everything from borrowing or lending money to buying a home or signing a job contract. There are a number of branches of private law, including contract and commercial law, tort law, property law, labour law, inheritance law, family law, and corporations law. Private or civil law often is representative of a society's attitudes toward such issues as family, marriage, property ownership, labour laws, small businesses, and privacy. In Canada, privacy is of particular concern, and the protection of personal information is considered an important priority of both individuals and agencies that hold our personal or private information. There are a number of federal and provincial statutes that help to protect privacy, and these will be discussed later in the chapter. The branches of private law that are most applicable to nursing practice are contract law and tort law.

Contract Law

Contract law deals with the rights and obligations of people who make contracts. A **contract** is an agreement between two or more people that can be enforced by law. Contracts may be either written or oral; however, in the presence of both a written and oral contract, the written contract takes precedence. In health care, contracts may be either expressed or implied. Expressed contracts occur when two parties agree explicitly to certain terms, as in an employment contract a nurse signs when beginning employment at a hospital or agency. Implied contracts occur when there has been no discussion between the parties, but the law considers that a contract exists (Kozier & Erb, 2007). The nurse–patient relationship is essentially an implied contract in which the nurse agrees to give competent care.

Tort Law

A **tort** is a wrong or injury that a person suffers because of someone else's action, either intentional or unintentional. The tortious action may cause bodily harm; invade another's privacy; damage a person's property, business, or reputation; or make unauthorized use of a person's property. The victim may sue the person or persons responsible. Tort law deals with the rights and obligations of the persons involved in such cases. Many torts are unintentional, such as damages that occur as a result of accidents. But if a tort is deliberate and involves serious harm, it may also be treated as a crime. The purpose of tort law is to make the person whole again, primarily through the award of monetary damages. Because it can involve negligence and malpractice, tort law is the branch of law with which nurses are most familiar. There are three types of torts (or wrongs): unintentional torts, intentional torts, and liabilities.

Unintentional torts occur when an act or omission causes unintended injury or harm to another person. The majority of lawsuits against nurses and other health care professionals are unintentional torts, usually claims of negligence. The unintentional torts of negligence and malpractice are most relevant to nursing (Hodgson, 2007).

Negligence

Negligence is the failure to provide a standard of care that is reasonable. Often the terms "negligence" and "malpractice" are used interchangeably, as negligence can imply care or treatment that falls below the standard of a reasonable and prudent nurse.

As part of ensuring the safety of citizens, the law requires that every person be accountable for behaving in a reasonable way, particularly if the welfare of others is at stake. For example, there is certainly no law against throwing rocks into the air. However, throwing rocks off a bridge into highway traffic is not the act of a reasonable or prudent person. The resultant injury that might ensue (and has, in a number of cases in Canada and the United States) would be considered to be negligent, as the person would have not acting in a reasonable way toward others.

The word "negligence" is rooted in the Latin term "negligentia," which literally means, "not to pick up," or to neglect. To neglect is not *necessarily* the same as to commit an error or be careless (although instances of careless or erroneous nursing actions might be classified as negligent) because someone might be using as much care as possible, but still have their actions fall below the standard to which we would hold them. Take, for example, a case of a nurse who has been in active practice for many years, but has not taken part in any professional development activities or continued learning activities. Within her professional practice, she may, on an individual level, try hard to provide high-quality, competent care to her patients.

However, although she may not be "careless" *per se*, her lack of updated skills and knowledge may contribute to negligent care. Most provincial regulatory bodies are now paying attention to how much continued learning and professional development licensed nurses are taking part in, and requiring it as evidence of continued competent practice.

Standards of competent care are set out by various mechanisms: nursing education and accreditation of nursing programs and curricula, up-to-date textbooks and peer-reviewed evidence-based articles outlining practices, provincial nursing certification examinations, nursing practice standards, and best practice guidelines all act to set standards of nursing care at a particular level. Individual hospitals and agencies require certification in particular skills or roles—nurses often must be certified on an ongoing basis, for example, to give chemotherapy or to insert an intravenous or a central line. If a nurse fails to meet the standard of care, either through not attending to his or her practice or by failing to ensure certification or qualification, then that nurse can be considered to be negligent.

In most cases of negligence, the injured person (also called the *plaintiff*) would likely sue the accused offender (also called the *defendant*) through civil litigation for damages or compensation. However, this would require that the case go through a court process. In order for a case of negligence to be heard by the court, the case must have four important attributes (Morris, Ferguson & Dykeman, 1999; Tingle, 2007). First, a duty to care must exist. **Duty to care** is an important overarching legal principle in nursing and it refers to the legal obligation imposed on someone to act beneficently toward another or refrain from acting in a way that would cause harm to another (Keatings and Smith, 1999; Potter and Perry, 2008). Briefly, this means that nurses have a duty to act in a way that does not harm their patients and promotes their best interests. Furthermore, they should act to prevent foreseeable harm. Second, there must be evidence that the defendant has failed to comply with that duty to care. In other words, their care must be shown to fall below the level of care required to maintain the duty of care. Third, there must be demonstrable suffering or injury to the plaintiff. Finally, the suffering or injury must be shown to be a result of the negligent conduct of the defendant.

Tort law in relation to negligence has a very specific goal—to compensate the injured party for harm. In this instance, the law does not punish the defendant. The courts, in this case, function to establish that negligence has in fact occurred, by examining each case for the four components noted above and then attaching a compensatory amount to the injury or harm caused by either intentional or unintentional negligence.

Anyone can be sued for negligence. A storeowner who fails to clear a significant amount of ice from his sidewalk may be sued for negligence if someone slips and becomes injured. A bicycle rider might sue someone for negligence who opens their car door and knocks the cyclist off the road, injuring them. Omissions can also be considered negligent—in other words, failure to do something that a reasonable person might do. Failure to warn persons that there is spilled liquid on the floor of the grocery aisle might result in a negligence suit if someone unknowingly walks through the liquid, slips, and falls, sustaining an injury. So while anyone potentially can be found to be negligent, nurses, physicians, and other health care professionals are held to higher standards. *Foreseeability* is a significant part of assessing whether negligence occurred or not, in many health care cases. Foreseeability is having the knowledge that one's actions or omissions might result in harm or injury. Nurses have special knowledge about medication administration, procedures, and treatments, which includes knowledge regarding the foreseeable potential harms or injuries of those medications and treatments. While someone trained as a car mechanic might not have knowledge of the potential harms of an improper dressing change, a nurse is expected to understand the potential harms of not maintaining sterility and cleanliness. As a more specific example, an untrained layperson caring for her bedridden elderly mother at home without assistance might not know the dangers from lying in one position all the time. However, a nurse in a long-term care setting is expected to have knowledge of properly turning and positioning patients in order to maintain skin integrity and prevent skin ulcers and serious subsequent complications. Standards of care and practice standards outline the kinds of specialized knowledge that nurses must have and that contribute to nurses' unique ability to be able to foresee potential benefits, harms, and risks of particular actions or omissions. Thus, when a nurse fails to do this, she or he can be considered to be negligent.

In 2004, a group of Canadian researchers published the *Canadian Adverse Events Study* in the *Canadian Medical Association Journal.* It was the first pan-Canadian study examining the rate of adverse events in Canadian hospitals (Baker *et al.*, 2004). Adverse events in the study were defined as those injuries or complications caused by health care management rather than the condition or disease of the patient. Notably, a number of the adverse events related to nursing care, either directly or indirectly. One out of every thirteen patients admitted to a Canadian hospital, at the time of the study, experienced an adverse event. The three main areas in which adverse events occurred were surgery, medication, and infection. Nursing care is at the front line in every aspect of hospital care, and while the researchers did not point a finger at nursing, the implied message was that nurses were responsible for much of the delivery of patient care in hospitals and could also be responsible, even in part, for some of the adverse events that patients experienced. Therefore nursing, as a profession, must be attentive to the kinds of adverse events reported and the ways they can be monitored and, eventually, completely prevented. Would increased education or continued professional development help? Could the systems of communication in the hospital be improved? Are there policies in place that are helping or hindering nurses in the delivery of care? Are the physical environments amenable to delivering competent care, or are there marked limitations, such as lack of resources or continued understaffing, that might undermine the ability of nurses to deliver competent care? Reports like this one need to be translated into close examinations of practice, environments, and institutional structures, not just individual professionals. However, noting this, each individual nurse is responsible for providing safe and competent care. Additionally, nurses in most jurisdictions have a professional responsibility to report cases of unsafe or incompetent care, negligence, or malpractice. So as nurses, we have both individual and collective responsibilities to prevent negligence.

? THINK ABOUT IT

A very common area for nursing liability involves medication errors. There are many ways that nurses can make errors of medication preparation and administration. The nurse can give the wrong medication, or the wrong dose, at the wrong time, by the wrong route, or to the wrong patient. Because of the frequency and likelihood of medication error and the potentially serious consequences that can result, nurses need to be especially careful in administering medicine. Nurses are responsible for safe and appropriate administration of medication, regardless of physician orders, workload, unusual circumstances, or institutional policy. There are many examples of medication errors cited in the literature. It is not unusual for damages to be awarded to victims or families when medication errors occur. Again, however, medication errors need to be examined from both an individual and an institutional perspective. Staffing mixes with increased numbers of higher levels of regulated nursing staff (i.e., RNs) have been shown to reduce rates of medication errors (Doran *et al.*, 2001). It makes sense that units with lower nurse-to-patient ratios might have lower rates of medication errors, because nurses can afford the proper amount of time to administer medications.

- What other factors do you see that might influence rates of medication administration errors on a nursing unit?

- How do you see technology either helping or hindering the administration of medication? Think about where you work. Are there persons who fill the medication carts or are they automatic or computer driven?

- What kinds of improvements could a nursing unit put in place to help prevent medication errors?

- Think about a medication error you might have made, nearly made, or noted another nurse making. What happened? What did you learn? How did the unit nurses and administrators handle the event? What kinds of factors contributed to that error?

Intentional torts are "wilful or intentional acts that violate another person's rights or property" (Catalano, 1991, p. 69). A tort must include three elements to be considered intentional: the act must be intended to interfere with the plaintiff or his property; there must be intent to bring about the consequences of the act; and the act must substantially cause the consequences. In some cases, it may be difficult to prove that the damages or injury actually result from the act; proof of the defendant's intention is typically sufficient (Catalano, 1991). Examples of intentional torts include fraud, invasion of privacy, assault, battery, false imprisonment, slander, and libel.

Fraud is a deliberate deception for the purpose of securing an unfair or unlawful gain. Although nurses are seldom accused of fraud, when this occurs it is usually prosecuted as a crime. Examples of potential areas of nurses' fraud include falsification of information on employment applications, false representation of health states in order to access services or secure insurance funds, and falsification of patient records to cover up an error. Fraud is a concern in Canada related to health insurance billing. The Web site for the Ontario Ministry of Health and Long Term Care has a section devoted to the discussion of health card fraud, which is an ongoing problem (Ontario Ministry of Health and Long Term Care, 2002). As with some other intentional torts, fraud can lead to both civil and criminal proceedings. Because of the deliberate nature and potential harm of fraudulent acts, court decisions tend to be harsh. Fraud is a more significant concern in the United States, where complex billing procedures and inequality of reimbursement set the stage for not only errors but also opportunities to gain funds or access to medical care through misrepresentation or other forms of deception. In the United States, an incident of fraud in health care can result in up to five years imprisonment, up to $25 000 in fines, and exclusion from reimbursement from both Medicare and Medicaid for up to five years (Mazzocco, 2000).

Privacy and Confidentiality

The **right to privacy** is the right to be left alone or to be free from unwanted publicity. Stated more generally, the right to privacy includes "the right to enjoy private space, to conduct private communications, to be free from surveillance and to respect the sanctity of one's body." (Holmes, 2006).

Individuals have the right to withhold themselves and their lives from public scrutiny. The intentional tort of **invasion of privacy** occurs when a person's privacy is invaded. In Canada, protection of privacy is now not only an individual priority, but also a governmental priority. Various complex legislations have been put in place, at both the federal and provincial/territorial levels of government, to ensure that the personal information and private health information of individuals is protected. Fiesta (1988) outlines four types of invasions of privacy: intrusion on the patient's physical and mental solitude or seclusion; public disclosure of private facts; publicity that places the patient in a false light in the public eye; and appropriation of the patient's name or likeness for the defendant's benefit or advantage (p. 160).

The terms "*assault*" and "*battery*," though usually used together, have different legal meanings. Both are intentional torts. **Assault** is defined as the unjustifiable attempt or threat to touch a person without consent that results in fear of immediately harmful or threatening contact (Bernzweig, 1990). Touching need not actually occur. **Battery** is the unlawful, harmful, or unwarranted touching of another, or the carrying out of threatened physical harm. Battery can include any wilful, angry, violent, or negligent touching of a person's body or clothes, or of anything held by or attached to the person (Guido, 1997). In the course of everyday activities, nurses have been accused of both assault and battery. For example, if a nurse threatens to give an injection to an unruly or noncompliant adult patient without consent, actionable assault has occurred. Battery is often thought of as such actions as slapping, shoving, or pinching, but the courts have upheld battery charges in actions that were much more subtle. Regardless of intent or outcome, *touching without consent is considered battery.* Even when the intention is beneficent and the outcome is positive, if the act is committed without permission, the nurse can be charged with battery. Surgical procedures that are performed without informed consent are the most common example of battery occurring in the hospital setting. Common defences to charges of battery arise from two other legal concepts: necessity and consent. **Necessity** refers to the privilege granted to a person to touch another person. A physician or a nurse may touch a person in order to provide care or direct medical aid to that person in an emergency situation. **Consent** implies express or implicit permission for another to touch you. A nurse may not ask directly each time he takes a patient's blood pressure to "touch" the patient, but by asking if he can take the patient's blood pressure, he is essentially asking for permission to touch the patient's arm. By agreeing to have one's blood pressure taken, one implicitly agrees to being touched. An example of express permission would be signing a consent form for an invasive procedure, such as a liver biopsy or a surgery.

False imprisonment is the unjustifiable detention of a person, or an act intended to result in such confinement, without consent and without authority of law (O'Keefe, 2000). Such acts can include physical restraint of the person, or acts intended to accomplish confinement, such as refusing the patient clothing or car keys. If false imprisonment is accompanied by forcible restraint or the threat of restraint, assault and battery may also be charged. There may be special cases in which persons may be detained for a limited period of time or held by authorities without explicit consent. Some examples include being detained by the police, being detained for capacity assessment or assessment of suicidal risk, and quarantine.

Defamation is any statement that represents a false claim against or a derogatory remark about an individual, group, product, company, government, or nation that would lead to a falsely negative image. Defamation tort law is designed to protect the esteem and positive image of subjects. It is, however, a difficult tort to prove and because of this, very few cases of defamation have been tried in civil courts. In a landmark 1970 case, *Murphy v. LaMarsh* (13 DLR 3d 484), the B.C. Supreme Court classified defamation as follows:

> . . . a shameful action is attributed to a man (he stole my purse), a shameful character (he is dishonest), a shameful course of action (he lives on the avails of prostitution), (or) a shameful condition (he has smallpox). Such words are considered defamatory because they tend to bring the man named into hatred, contempt or ridicule. The more modern definition (of defamation) is words tending to lower the plaintiff in the estimation of right-thinking members of society generally.

Defamation must be demonstrated to be harmful, must be aimed at the person or his or her reputation and must be conveyed to others, either verbally (also called slander) or in writing (libel). **Slander** and **libel** can occur in nursing and health care. By making value judgments or voicing that a patient is unco-operative, malingering, unintelligent, or drug-seeking, a nurse may be committing actionable slander. Nurses may also be accused of slander as a result of inappropriate defamatory remarks voiced against another professional. Nurses can risk accusations of libel when writing information in patients' charts that can be damaging. Judgmental, critical, or speculative statements made in patients' charts such as "The patient is drug-seeking" or "The patient is very unco-operative" can lead to an accusation of libel, particularly if the patient has reason to believe that the words adversely affect the care given by others.

Defences against accusations of defamation include truth telling (i.e., the remark or statement is accurate or true), statements made in good faith (i.e., with the belief that they were, in fact, true), statements provided to a third party that are negative but justified (i.e., a negative remark on a job or academic reference), privilege (i.e., statements made by a person to his or her spouse, on a legislature floor, or in a court room), and opinion (as opinion is a subjective notion and cannot be proven to be "true" or "untrue"). Furthermore, there may be a legal or moral duty to pass on defamatory information in certain circumstances. A nurse has a duty to report child abuse, a director of nursing service has the duty to report truthfully the character and qualifications of nurses seeking employment references elsewhere, and peer review disciplinary groups are required to discuss privileged information for the purpose of disciplining others and following due process. Nurses have a professional obligation to report incompetent or illegal practice of others. To avoid accusations of defamation, prudent nurses will take care to observe appropriate channels of communication when making reports of this nature. In the absence of privileged communication, truth is a good defence for defamation.

Intentional infliction of emotional distress (also called "intentional infliction of mental distress" or the "tort of outrage" in some jurisdictions) is a relatively new tort claim. This allows a claim to be made against someone who acts in a heinous, reckless, or extreme way, to bring about emotional distress in a plaintiff. This tort claim was created to allow for instances when a threat is not imminent or the threat of harm is in the future—as this could not be considered as assault. (In order for a claim of assault to be made, the threat has to be fairly imminent, causing harm.) This new tort claim allows for claims against persons who cause emotional distress to others, and for compensation to be granted to the plaintiff.

Some examples might include failing to tell an estranged spouse the whereabouts of her or his child for many years, or lying to someone about your death or the death of another person. In health care, unfortunately, we might be able to think of examples of cases in which the intentional infliction of emotional distress might be claimed by patients against nurses, especially those patients who are more vulnerable, isolated, and dependent upon visiting nurses, or institutionalized. On a positive note, this is not, at this time, a common tort claim in the general public or in health care.

THINK ABOUT IT

It is important that nurses be aware of the legal system in relation to their practice. While the rate of litigation for malpractice or negligence against nurses and health care professionals is much lower in Canada than in the United States, there are still cases in which nurses have been charged with this serious crime.

In 1998, Lisa Shore, an otherwise healthy ten-year-old girl, was admitted to the Hospital for Sick Children in Toronto, Ontario, for relief of pain due to reflex sympathetic dystrophy syndrome resulting from a leg fracture earlier in the year. This syndrome results in extreme pain and sensitivity of the affected area. On admission, Lisa was given a steady a dose of morphine and within approximately twelve hours, was found to be in respiratory and cardiac arrest, and was pronounced dead shortly after that. Her death was noted to be caused by the administration of morphine with other medications and insufficient monitoring. The coroner's report classified Lisa's death as a homicide and the nurses who were caring for her were charged with negligence in 2001. The charges of negligence were withdrawn in 2003. Two years later, the two nurses went through a disciplinary hearing at the College of Nurses of Ontario and were found guilty of professional misconduct with a suspension of licensure for a period of one month, which was suspended.

In another case at the Hospital for Sick Children, Sanchia Bulgin, a seventeen-year-old girl with sickle cell anemia, died after routine gallbladder surgery. Sanchia was given morphine post-operatively, a drug to which she had a known sensitivity. She also was inadequately monitored for signs of bleeding and shock, and hemorrhaged to death. There were a number of recommendations made by the coroner regarding prevention of any further deaths like this one, including better communication between members of the nursing and medical team; better training for nurses about vital signs, shock, and sickle cell disease; and monitoring post-operative patients.

Nurses do not go to their jobs with intentions to do harm or to make fatal errors. Incompetence, carelessness, or lack of knowledge may, unfortunately, exist in nursing and certainly may lead to errors, some of them serious. On the other hand, even well-intentioned, competent, and careful nurses can make mistakes.

(Stewart, 2002)

- Read more about the coroner's recommendations made after reviewing the Lisa Shore and Sanchia Bulgin cases. Discuss the recommendations in light of your current workplace and practice.

- Coroner's verdicts and summaries can be found at: http://www.mcscs.jus. gov.ca/english/office_coroner/verdicts_and_recs/verdicts_and_recs_intro.html

- What are your feelings as you read the cases and the coroner's recommendations?

(Continued)

- Reflect on any situations that may have made you feel that you were unable to practise safely or competently. What did you do?

- How would you react today if you were asked to do something that you considered to be beyond your level of competence or skill?

- How much should family members or patients be told about mistakes or errors that may have occurred while they were in the health care system?

CONSENT

Consent is a complex legal and ethical notion, arising from notions of dignity and autonomy. It is entrenched in the idea that persons have the right to decide what can and cannot be done to them. In law, it is often referred to as the right to be free from interference.

Before health care treatments of all kinds can be provided, consent of the patient must be obtained. An exception is made in cases of emergencies and other extenuating circumstances. However, nurses should practise with the ever-present idea that patients must consent to be touched, to have treatments administered, to undergo surgery, to be given medications, to allow testing to be done, and to have even low-risk procedures carried out. Many treatments and skills that nurses carry out on patients can arguably be considered to be low risk, such as bathing, positioning, taking vital signs, and physical assessments. Other activities, such as dressing changes, venipuncture, wound irrigation, and catheter insertions are considered as somewhat higher risk. With the increasing scope of nursing practice, more nurses are able to do higher-risk procedures, treatments, and examinations of patients. But the most important point to note is that even the low-risk procedures, such as bathing and the taking of vital signs, must be consented to by the patient before the activities can be carried out. As noted earlier in the chapter, the intentional tort of battery involves touching of a person without the person's consent. Much of nursing care involves touching, so patient consent to touch must be sought in these circumstances.

Consent falls under provincial jurisdiction and most provinces and territories have distinct statutes in place describing consent; for example, the *Health Care [Consent] and Care Facility [Admission] Act of British Columbia* (1996), Manitoba's *Health Care Directives Act* (1992), and Prince Edward Island's *Consent to Treatment and Health Care Directives Act* (2002). In Ontario, there are two pieces of legislation that deal with consent: the *Health Care Consent Act* (1996) and the *Substitute Decisions Act* (1992). The *Health Care Consent Act* helps to protect patients' decision-making autonomy by facilitating communication with health care providers and patients, and helping to include family members as appropriate when a patient is incapable of making his or her own decisions. The *Substitute Decisions Act* addresses decision making regarding personal care and care of property in the case of a person who is deemed to be incompetent (College of Nurses of Ontario, 2008).

These documents and their specific directives vary from province to province; however, for the most part, they espouse similar values, which include protection and promotion of patients' autonomy, and authority over their health care decisions. They also usually outline the necessary elements of consent. In Ontario's *Health Care Consent Act,* the elements of consent are as follows [1996, c.2, Sched. A, s. 11 (1).]:

- Consent must relate to the treatment
- Consent must be informed
- Consent must be given voluntarily
- Consent must not be obtained through misrepresentation or fraud

These elements are, for the most part, reflected in other provincial and territorial legislative acts describing consent, alongside notions of capacity to consent. In a jurisdiction where there is no specific legislation regarding consent, these elements are usually noted when defining a valid consent: The consent must be voluntary, informed, and refer to both the treatment and the provider. Furthermore, the patient must have the capacity to consent.

In most discussions of consent in health care, we are usually referring to consent of a patient to allow a treatment or procedure. For the purposes of discussion, in the following sections, while we acknowledge that consent is required in a variety of circumstances and contexts, we will refer to consent, usually, as consent for treatment.

Consent can be explicit or implied. **Explicit consent** is either verbal or written consent specifically articulating the patient's agreement to a particular treatment or procedure. Implied consent is less concrete—but quite often encountered. It is inferred from a person's presence and actions, as well as the context of the situation. In other words, a pregnant woman who admits herself to the hospital to give birth under the care of her obstetrician implies consent for the obstetrician to examine her. **Implied consent** does not mean, however, that the person's consent should be taken for granted or assumed. Just as a patient in the post-operative cardiac ward might not give express consent to have his vital signs taken every six hours, it is still important for the nurse to ensure that the patient is willing to have his vital signs taken when she enters the room to do so.

Voluntary Consent

In order for consent to be considered valid, it must be provided freely, without coercion or undue influence. In other words, it must be provided by the patient of his or her own free will, without feelings of obligation, urgency, or necessity unrelated to the treatment. This has implications regarding which member of the health care team obtains consent, when, and how. Consent should be obtained by the appropriate health care provider with a nonjudgmental, skilful, and thorough approach. Nurses are not often called upon to obtain informed consent for surgical procedures or other invasive procedures, such as wound debridement, lumbar punctures, or biopsies. Usually surgeons or physicians obtain such consent. However, nurses are often the ones patients turn to when they have questions about the consent that they provided. Some patients may voice to the nurse that they felt unable to "say no" or ask for more time to make the decision, as they didn't want to displease the physician who was providing their care. While the physician may well have approached the consent process in a facilitative, approachable, and relaxed way, patients may still feel intimidated by the role of the physician and the process of providing consent. In this case, nurses must be attuned to patients' needs and whether or not the consent was voluntarily given.

Informed Consent

Consent is informed if the person receives information about the proposed treatment that any reasonable person would want to know in the same situation in order to make a similar decision. Additionally, the person must have received answers to her questions or requests for additional information.

Information must include the condition for which she is being treated; the nature of the treatment; the expected benefits of the treatment; the known, anticipated, or foreseeable risks and/or side effects of treatment; alternative options for treatment; and the likely outcomes if no treatment is provided. Information should be provided to patients at an appropriate level, keeping in mind patients' age and developmental stage. Medical jargon and highly technical terms should be avoided as much as possible, and, if used, should be defined and explained thoroughly to patients. Opportunity should be provided for patients to think about the options provided to them, along with the risks and benefits, in order to formulate questions and recognize where they require more information in order to be fully informed.

Informed consent is not a panacea. It is impossible to list every possible risk, every potential benefit, and sometimes, every known accessible or real alternative option. Furthermore, some people quite mistakenly believe that lay persons cannot ever fully understand the implications of all the possible benefits, risks, and side effects of proposed treatments, and they conclude that the process of obtaining informed consent is, therefore, ineffective or useless. All this, however, should not deter health care professionals from providing as much accurate, appropriate, and thorough information as possible to patients and allowing them the time and freedom to make an informed, voluntary decision.

Treatment and Provider

Consent, when given, is usually specific to a treatment or procedure as well as a particular provider. This element of consent is noted to be a response to the kind of "blanket" consents that used to exist in many health care contexts. For example, patients used to sign blanket consents when entering hospital for any and all testing and investigations. Today, a patient would provide informed consent for each individual test and investigation to be carried out.

When a patient consents to have one treatment, he is not implying consent, in any way, for other related or unrelated treatments. For example, when a patient consents to have his blood taken for a complete blood count, differential, and electrolyte measurement—all common blood tests—he is not providing consent to also have a blood test for human immunodeficiency virus (HIV). Consent to have an HIV test must be taken separately, with an entirely different kind of discussion. Furthermore, in many cases, consent is attached to a specific provider. For surgical procedures, this is almost always the case. A patient signs a consent to allow a particular surgeon to perform the surgery and has, in the case of elective or urgent surgery, usually met and discussed the procedure with the surgeon already. In emergent cases, this might not be the case; however, even a signed consent in an emergent surgical situation would usually refer to a particular surgeon. So if the surgery is then performed by a less qualified person (such as a trainee or resident) or an alternative physician without seeking explicit permission, this would not be in keeping with the patients' original informed consent.

Capacity to Consent

When we talk about capacity, we are usually talking about a legal capacity to provide consent. In general, capacity refers to the ability to learn, gather, retain, and apply knowledge. In law, it is the ability to understand the significance of behaviours and the influences upon behaviours or decision-making abilities, as well as the ability to appreciate the foreseeable consequences of decision-making processes. The legal notion of capacity formally refers to the age and the mental competence of the person to understand and appreciate information provided to her, along with the risks, benefits, and value of alternatives, as well as the consequences of the decision once made (Downie and Caulfield, 2002). Since age and mental competence are the two key concepts in capacity, the two groups for whom consent becomes a more difficult or complex matter are adults with questionable capacity (due to disability or mental health issues) and children.

CASE PRESENTATION

The case of *Starson v. Swayze* (2003) involved Scott Starson, a brilliant physicist who had been diagnosed with bi-polar disorder and had been hospitalized various times for his disorder. After Starson had been found to be voicing death threats, he was held in a mental health facility in Ontario for treatment. The treating psychiatrists wished to administer medications to Starson to control his symptoms of bi-polar disorder. These medications included anti-Parkinson's medications, mood stabilizers, and anti-psychotic medications. While Starson stated that he would agree to psychotherapy, he refused the medication on the grounds that it affected his ability to think and to conduct his scientific research. A provincial Consent and Capacity Board hearing found that Starson was incapable of making treatment decisions and ordered that he undergo treatment.

(Continued)

A number of appeals followed, at the provincial and the federal level, and the Courts found, repeatedly, that the decision to deem Mr. Starson incapable was unreasonable and that he had the right to refuse treatment, because he could understand the information that was an important part of the decision and he also appreciated the consequence of the decision. Starson clearly understood that he had a mental health problem, agreed that he suffered from many of the symptoms described by the psychiatrists in the court proceeding, and also agreed that he would undergo psychotherapy. He also understood the foreseeable consequences of a decision to either take medication or not. Eventually, at the level of the Supreme Court of Canada, it was ruled that the Board's finding of incapacity was unreasonable and the decision was upheld to allow Starson the right to refuse treatment. The Court emphasized that patients such as Starson do have the right to refuse treatment, even if it is deemed by others to be in their best interests, but they must be able to demonstrate understanding of the information relevant to decision-making, as well as all the possible consequences of the decision.

Children and Capacity to Consent

Consent is not an "all or nothing" concept. Many persons have evolving capacities in many areas of their lives, and the ability to learn and retain knowledge for the purpose of making decisions is one area in which capacity may be developing. It is not the case that on their eighteenth birthday, young adults are suddenly able to make decisions for themselves that they were incapable of making the day before. Most adolescents have evolving capacity to make decisions alongside their evolving moral agency.

As children, our **values** and decisions are mostly dictated by those of our parents or guardians. The food we eat, the school we attend, the church where we may worship or the lack of religion in our lives—all these things are not usually based on autonomous choices we make as children, but on the choices our parents make for us, based on their values, beliefs, and ideas about what is in our best interests. As we grow and expand our social world, our ideas about the values and beliefs we held as children and usually attributed to our parents now include ideas from friends, teachers, mentors, and community members. Additionally, during adolescence, most young people tend to want to find their own "identity" or worldview, which may differ from that of their parents and may be more strongly aligned to that of peers and mentors. Through this process, we learn, as we reach adulthood, what our own values and beliefs are, usually influenced by a combination of those instilled in us through our parents, guardians, families, culture, environment, socioeconomic status, neighbourhood, school, teachers, religion, and community groups, and those that we find and internalize ourselves. What this demonstrates, though, is that capacity to consent is as dynamic as one's own moral agency, developing over time and with experience and exposure to decision making and different circumstances.

Some children and adolescents, however, have a more advanced level of understanding, and may be deemed to be "mature minors." Usually a mature minor is a young person above the age of thirteen; however, there have been instances in which children as young as seven or eight have been found to be mature minors. The notion of a mature minor is part of common law and not statutory law—in other words, decisions about whether a child can be considered a mature minor are not made by referring to statutes or legislation. Rather, these decisions are made by an *ad hoc* or a "case-by-case" decision by the court, taking into consideration the child's age, intelligence, education, and previous experiences.

In a 2006 Manitoba case, heard at the Supreme Court of Canada in 2008, *A.C. et al. v. Director of Child and Family Services*, a fourteen-year-old Jehovah's Witness was forced to undergo a blood transfusion to replace blood lost in complications from Crohn's disease, against her explicit and articulately stated objections to this procedure, based on her deeply held spiritual beliefs. The case focused specifically on older minors who are forced to accept treatment, even though they have the mental capacity to make treatment decisions. The Court noted that, in minors under the age of sixteen, treatments that would be considered in the "best interests" of a child could be court-ordered. For young persons under the age of sixteen, their views and opinions must be considered in a way that is appropriate, depending on the developmental age and stage of the young person. Everyone must be provided with some autonomous decision-making opportunities for decisions regarding their integrity and health. However, how much autonomy can or will be provided should, according to the Court, correspond with the level of maturity and independence that is demonstrated by each person, on a case-by-case basis. At the end of the day, even with consideration of the views and opinions of a minor, the Court can still intervene, citing the best interests of the young person.

THINK ABOUT IT

The Case of Tyrell Dueck

Tyrell Dueck was a thirteen-year-old boy diagnosed with osteosarcoma in Saskatchewan. Tyrell's parents refused to consent to traditional treatments for osteosarcoma, which include chemotherapy and surgery for amputation. In most cases of osteosarcoma, early treatment with chemotherapy can lead to a significant chance of recovery with a year. Without chemotherapy, Tyrell had a very small chance of recovery beyond a year. In many cases, children of Tyrell's age would be included in the decision-making processes, as much as their developmental stage would allow. It was noted that Tyrell was highly uninvolved in decision making for his care, as his parents made the decisions for him. This concerned the health care team, who started a legal process to assume guardianship of Tyrell. Two issues were key in this case and both have legal and ethical implications. The first important issue was determining the best interests of Tyrell. The second

(Continued)

important issue was determining if Tyrell had the developmental capacity to make decisions for his own care.

Eventually the health care team was awarded guardianship of Tyrell and chemotherapy was started. During his treatment with chemotherapy, Tyrell then voiced that he did not want further chemotherapy; however, he also did not want his leg amputated. This choice demonstrated, to some, the inability of Tyrell to understand the situation at hand because without these options, patients with osteosarcoma ultimately succumb to the disease. So the health care team returned to the court system to help determine if Tyrell was a "mature minor," in other words, could he be deemed capable of making his own decisions without parental involvement?

Adding to the concern of the health care team was the fact that they felt Tyrell's father did not allow any health care staff to approach or talk to Tyrell without his presence. In a return to the courts, it was deemed that Tyrell did not have the decisional capacity of a mature minor, that he was strongly influenced by his father, and that he likely had not obtained information about the risks and benefits of options for treatment, as much of the information he did receive was "filtered" through his father. During the court proceedings, it was determined that the cancer had in fact spread to his lungs and at this point, any further treatment was futile.

Tyrell died soon after this.

(Nelson, 1999)

- How do you think the best interests of Tyrell should have been determined? What do you think was in his best interests?

- This case involves differences in values. How should health care professionals approach persons who have different values that affect care?

- What is different about a competent adult refusing treatment for him or herself compared to an adult refusing treatment for his child?

- Discuss the notion of a "mature minor." What kinds of things should a child or young person demonstrate in order to be considered a mature minor?

Adults with Diminished Capacity

Normally, we expect that adults will have decisional capacity. However, there are many factors that can interfere with the ability of an adult to be competent to take part in decision making about their care. Disease processes, disabilities, developmental delays, dementia, and neurological injuries are some examples.

Again, remember that capacity is not an "all or nothing" concept. Persons may have diminished capacity for a temporary period, if they experience, for example, post-operative delirium or disorientation due to a medication. Furthermore, persons who have limited capacity may be able to consent to certain things, but for other kinds of decisions may require assistance, support, or a substitute decision maker.

Legislation exists in most provinces and territories allowing persons to appoint valid substitute decision makers or proxies, and create advance directives for care, in the event that they are unable to make decisions by virtue of diminished capacity. In this case, it is important that nurses and other health care providers attend to the previously stated wishes of persons as articulated through advance directive documents, as well as through proxies. Substitute decision makers are

> person or persons with the best knowledge of the patient's specific wishes, or of the patient's values and beliefs, as they pertain to the present situation. In general close relatives are preferred as substitute decision makers in the belief that they will know the patient well enough to replicate the decision that the patient would make if he or she were capable. (Lazar *et al.*, 1996, p. 1436)

In some cases, such as a person with a chronic disability or developmental delay, there are directives and substitute decision makers in place before an event or decision that requires urgency or efficiency in decision-making processes. In other words, a person who may have had limited capacity since childhood may, more often than not, have these kinds of things in place to help when care decisions must be made. However, for someone who is competent who sustains an injury, or has a stroke or neurological event that leads to diminishment of their decision-making capacity, it is ideal when their wishes have been previously documented using advance directives. This makes it much easier for substitute decision makers and the health care team to act in a way that the patient would have also wanted, if she were able to contribute to the decision. Nurses should educate patients about the advantages of having a living will or advance directive and the positive benefits of having discussed these issues with those closest to them.

If an adult's capacity is questioned, this activates a process of determining capacity that involves multiple persons, over time. Take the example of a woman found on the street late at night with some minor injuries, who is disoriented and possibly delusional. The woman is brought to the emergency room and, before treatment of her minor injuries and a full assessment of any further injury or illness, consent is sought. However, in this case, as the woman has no identification and seems to be disoriented and delusional, her capacity to consent for her own care is questioned by the health care team. Instead of a "one-off" decision being made merely for the sake of expedient treatment, a systematic and rigorous process to assess capacity must be undertaken.

CASE PRESENTATION

1. Marc is a forty-two-year old man with advanced AIDS, living at home with his partner of ten years, Charles. Charles and Marc have discussed the future and, together, have written a living will for Marc. Charles is Marc's substitute decision maker. Recently, Charles has noticed that Marc is becoming forgetful and behaving oddly. He suspects that it is the early stages of AIDS-related dementia.

(Continued)

Marc has also been investigated for AIDS-related lymphoma, as he has had frequent fevers, night sweats, and extreme weight loss with lymph node swelling.

When Marc's physician informs them that Marc does in fact have lymphoma, the physician notes that the disease may have spread to the brain, which may account for some of Marc's changing behaviours. While noting that the lymphoma has spread, the physician recommends treatment immediately, noting the burden that it will pose, but assuring both Marc and Charles that it may be possible, through timely treatment, to arrest the rate of the spread of the malignancy. Previously, Marc has clearly expressed to Charles that he would not want to have any burdensome treatment just to extend a life in which he could not participate fully. Charles isn't sure if this is what Marc meant but he is unable to get Marc to discuss this, as Marc's episodes of forgetfulness and disorientation are rapidly increasing in frequency and intensity.

2. Lucille is an elderly woman who was diagnosed with Alzheimer's disease over 15 years ago. She lives in a residential seniors' centre in Vancouver with advanced medical care. Both her daughters are listed as joint substitute decision makers. One daughter, Maggie, lives in the city and visits her mother almost daily. She is highly involved in her mother's care. Hannah, Lucille's other daughter, lives on the East Coast and gets out west twice a year to spend a few days with her mother. Recently, Lucille's physical condition has deteriorated and she has become noticeably more frail. Her ability to take nutrition and hydration by mouth has worsened and she is quickly losing weight. The medical team approaches Maggie about placement of a feeding tube. Maggie quickly agrees, but asks for time to consult with her sister. Two days later, Hannah arrives and promptly tells the medical team that her mother would never have wanted a "tube to feed her" and that they should not do the procedure as it would be in opposition to Lucille's wishes, which, she states, her mother discussed with her and not Maggie. Maggie is visibly upset and the two sisters appear to have a significant amount of tension between them.

Later in the day, Hannah again approaches the medical team, and tells them that Maggie is "too close" to the situation and she cannot make decisions in the best interest of their mother. Hannah tells them that Maggie is severely depressed, on medication, and unable to work, and that she has told Hannah her only reason for living is "to take care of mom." Without her mother, Hannah states, Maggie would have no reason for living.

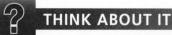

THINK ABOUT IT

Questions to Consider

1. In each of the cases, who should give consent for care?
2. What are some things that the health care team can do, in each of the above situations, to help facilitate substitute decision making?

DOCUMENTATION

Nursing documentation is an important part of practice. It communicates to others not only the care and treatment of clients but also valuable information about assessments, evaluations, progress, and concerns related to client care. Nursing notes are part of patient's health record—a document that reflects the overall interdisciplinary care of a patient during a period of time, an admission to a health care institution, or the progress of an outpatient at a clinic or family doctor's office.

Being clear, accurate, concise, and nonjudgmental is important when making nursing notes. One must ensure that any information documented in health records reflects what actually occurred or was said. Patients' own words should be labelled as such, using quotation marks. Only actual events should be noted, not speculations about what might have happened or what might happen in future. Of course, there may be exceptions. For example, a nurse may document that over a shift, a patient becoming increasingly less oriented and note the concern for the immediate future. Clarity is important—using proper language and grammar so that others reading the health record at a later time have a full understanding of the events. Being concise or brief is also important. It is necessary to document as completely as possible, so being concise does not necessarily mean that one must compromise on quality of information. Additionally, legibility is important in hand-written records. As noted earlier in the chapter, making judgmental remarks might be seen as libelous. Notations that a patient is "unco-operative," "lazy," or "unwilling" are all judgments, and there is no place in nursing notes for these kinds of remarks. If a patient is, in fact, not willing to undergo, for example, a burdensome treatment, it should simply be noted that the patient refused the treatment. A competent and discerning nurse would explore with the patient why she refused the treatment and try to help facilitate understanding about the importance of the treatment, while exploring the valid reasons the patient may have for not consenting to this particular treatment on this particular day. Those kinds of things may be noted in the nursing notes, but a quick descriptor, "unwilling," not only is judgmental, but also does not allow for any kind of intervention or support for the patient.

Further supporting the need for clear, accurate, concise, and nonjudgmental documentation is the fact that nursing notes can be introduced as evidence in court proceedings or disciplinary hearings. Health records, which may include nursing notes and legal documentation in most provinces, are also known as "business records," i.e., records relevant to the operation of hospital or agency. In many jurisdictions, a nursing record can be called as evidence; therefore, documenting in a sloppy, careless, or incomplete way demonstrates not only lack of accountability, but also a lack of professionalism.

There are many problems in nursing documentation that we see frequently. Sometimes there are significant gaps in the records, that is, periods of time not accounted for or documentation about specific shifts that might be missing. It is always difficult, later on, to verify that something was done when no documentation exists. In terms of the use of documents in courts and hearings, complete documentation provides a way for nurses to "remember" the day or the event. When documentation is complete and accurate, it serves as a more effective cue to memory and a more reliable source of information. Documentation may be messy, difficult to read, or sloppy. There may be errors in the documentation or documentation by someone other than the nurse who provided the care. *The person who provided care* must document the care accurately. In other words, a nurse simply covering for his colleague who is on a break cannot chart that the original nurse completed the morning care and gave medications. He can document only the care he gave during the relief time and nothing more. Finally, there may be cases in which documentation is falsified or facts and events misrepresented. In this case, a nurse may be considered negligent and certainly accountable for his actions.

In an important Canadian case, which originated in Ontario in 1976, *Kolesar v. Jeffries,* the Canadian Nurses Protective Society (2007) notes that a patient who had undergone a spinal fusion was returned to a post-operative surgical unit. The morning after his surgery, he was found dead. Upon review of the nursing notes, it was found that there were no nursing notes from the previous night at ten o'clock until five in the morning. According to the courts, this clearly established blame, that is, liability, as the assumption was that if nothing was charted, nothing was carried out. In other words, no documentation implied no nursing care. Yet, in an interesting subsequent case, *Ferguson v. Hamilton* (1983), the notion that no nursing notes implies no care for that time period was rejected, with two caveats. First, there must be clear evidence that there was care provided during the period of time. Second, there needs to be confirmation of a usual institutional practice not to chart for periods of time. The important message here is that, to the world outside of a hospital or agency, lack of adequate documentation leaves questions and concerns about quality of nursing care.

Technology and Documentation

Most hospitals and health care agencies now have some form of computerized documentation. Many of these programs require special training and orientation to the programs and are complex, integrated, and a key part of the patient's health record. Electronic records have many advantages—they can be easily transferred (with explicit permission) between providers and institutions with a few simple keystrokes. If a patient's primary physician is in another country or halfway across the world, electronic records can easily be shared for efficient transfer of important information. Computerized documentation is standardized in terms of legibility and where to find it. In other words, there are no problems with reading persons' writing or trying to flip through pages in a paper chart looking for a test result or notation. Furthermore, electronic documentation can help with accuracy by automatically identifying who made the entry, the date and time the entry was made, and even the computer on which the entry was recorded.

The accuracy of computerized documentation can also identify improper access to information or records. For example, a nurse cannot access the computerized personal health records of her father-in-law, who is in the hospital on another unit. Another example might include accessing the record of a friend or colleague who is also a patient in the facility where you work as a nurse. While it might seem harmless to look up their blood tests for someone you know to tell them all is fine and reassure them, if they are not directly under your care as a patient, then it is inadvisable, even illegal, to access their health records through a computer.

Nurses' use of electronic communication raises a number of legal and ethical questions. What are the legal implications of electronic communication? What is our responsibility for maintaining patient confidentiality? Does this change with the use of electronic documentation? How does electronic documentation affect or change nursing practice?

Some provinces have updated their privacy legislation to reflect the ubiquity of computerized record keeping. Nurses should be familiar not only with institutional policies and procedures around electronic record keeping but also with provincial privacy laws.

Privacy and Confidentiality

The right to privacy and the duty of confidentiality are two important concepts in law and ethics. They are often, mistakenly, used interchangeably. In health care, privacy is the right of the patient, while confidentiality is what we owe to the patient, when we have intimate knowledge of their personal or health data. Privacy is considered a constitutional right in Canada and it may affect how other laws are enacted. Confidentiality, on the other hand, is a duty of a health care professional who has an obligation to not share that information. This obligation or duty may be ascribed by an institution or it may be implicit in the relationship between the person who provides the information and the person who then receives it and is expected to keep it confidential (Slowther & Kleinman, 2008).

In Canada, both federal and provincial legislation regulate the collection, storage, and dissemination or sharing of personal information by the government and by agencies that hold or store such information. The laws prescribe how this kind of data can be collected, stored, and accessed or used.

At a **federal** level, two privacy laws exist: *The Privacy Act* (1983) and the *Personal Information Protection and Electronic Documents Act* (**PIPEDA**). *The Privacy Act* imposes obligations on how federal government departments collect, manage, use, and share personal information that they hold. It also provides individuals with the right to change or correct information held about them, and outlines mechanisms with which to do so.

PIPEDA applies to personal information about customers that is collected, used, or disclosed by all organizations involved in commercial activities, including the retail sector, the federally regulated private sector (e.g., banks, airlines, telecommunications), the service industry, and provincially regulated organizations (Office of the Privacy Commissioner of Canada, 2008). Oversight and enforcement of these laws is carried out by the Privacy Commissioner of Canada. This office also hears and investigates privacy complaints of individuals.

According to PIPEDA, personal information (e.g., identifiable information that may include your name, age, height, weight, medical records, income, purchases, spending, race, ethnic origin, skin colour, blood type, DNA, fingerprints, marital status, religion, education, address, and phone number) can only be collected by a company involved in commercial activities within the following guidelines:

- Information must be gathered with the explicit knowledge and consent of the person.
- Information must be gathered for a reasonable (relevant) purpose.
- Information must be used only for the specific purpose for which it was collected.
- Information must be kept accurate and current.
- Information must be accessible for inspection and correction by the individual.
- Information must be stored securely and destroyed appropriately.
- Policies regarding information in companies must be clear, and easy to understand and access.

Additionally, the law gives individuals the following rights:

- To know who within an organization is responsible for protecting your personal information.
- To complain about how an organization deals with or manages your personal information or if you believe that your privacy rights have not been protected.
- To be supplied with a product or service even if you refuse consent for the collection, use, or sharing of your personal information, unless that information is necessary for the transaction.

Each **province** has legislation regarding privacy as well. Currently the only province that does not have legislation is Newfoundland and Labrador: That province's legislation has been passed but is not yet active. Provincial and territorial privacy legislation functions to govern the collection, use, and disclosure of personal information gathered, held, and used by government agencies. Oversight of this is again either by a provincial commissioner or ombudsperson.

Some provinces also have specific legislation regarding the collection, use, and sharing of personal health information. Alberta, Saskatchewan, Manitoba, and Ontario have each passed laws addressing personal health information. Alberta has the *Health Information Act* (2001), as well as the *Personal Information Protection Act* (PIPA) (2004). Ontario has the *Personal Health Information Protection Act* in addition to the *Freedom of Information and Protection of Privacy Act* (FIPPA), and the *Municipal Freedom of Information and Protection of Privacy Act*. Saskatchewan has the *Health Information Protection Act*.

As you can see, privacy is a highly complex and highly legislated concept in Canada. As Canadians, we value this; privacy is entrenched in *Canadian Charter of Rights and Freedoms* and is, to that effect, a constitutionally protected value. Although the term "privacy" is not used in the *Charter* document, Sections 7 and 8 outline the following rights:

> 7. Everyone has the right to life, liberty and security of the person and the right not to be deprived thereof except in accordance with the principles of fundamental justice.
>
> 8. Everyone has the right to be secure against unreasonable search or seizure.

Inherently understood in these sections of the *Charter* is the right to privacy of individuals, unless, as Section 7 notes, there is justification for not maintaining confidentiality and protecting the privacy of individuals.

Privacy and confidentiality are highly valued in the modern world. One Supreme Court Justice, in a decision on a now well-known landmark Canadian case, noted the following:

> . . . Privacy is at the heart of liberty in a modern state . . . [g]rounded in man's physical and moral autonomy, privacy is essential for the well-being of the individual. For this reason alone, it is worthy of constitutional protection, but it also has profound significance for the public order. The restraints imposed on government to pry into the lives of the citizen go to the essence of a democratic state. [R. v. Dyment (1988), 45 C.C.C. 93d, 244 (S.C.C.), at para. 17.]

Nurses have access to patients' personal and health information on a constant basis. We refer to records with personal health information in order to complete histories and assessments. We collect information from patients regarding their personal habits, health, diagnoses, treatments, and even views on health and illness. Maintaining this information in a confidential manner is incredibly important—from both a legal and a professional perspective. Most regulatory bodies overseeing nursing practice in each province have practice standards regarding privacy and confidentiality. Hospital acts in each province also reinforce the patients' rights to confidentiality in records held in hospitals. Nurses in all sectors—not just hospitals—have a professional responsibility to maintain patient confidentiality in all aspects of care. Nurses who do not respect this responsibility can be found guilty of professional misconduct.

There are some exceptions to maintaining confidentiality. They include the following:

- The client expressly consents that her information can be shared to persons other than those named who can have access to the information.
- Situations that require mandatory reporting. These may include the mandatory duty to report child abuse or suspected child abuse, certain communicable diseases, and negligent or incompetent practices on the part of other health care professionals.
- A court order is used to obtain health records for use in a court proceeding.

The complex nature of privacy and confidentiality, added to the increased use of electronic documentation to collect and store personal data, makes patients sometimes more vulnerable than they ever have been. Many people are confused and overwhelmed by the depth and degree of legislation around privacy and confidentiality, and are unsure of how the laws apply to them, either as private citizens or as patients in a health care environment. Even some health care professionals do not fully understand the concepts of the patient's right to privacy and the duty of professionals to maintain confidentiality. This is demonstrated by the number of disciplinary hearings related to breaches in privacy and instances of not maintaining confidentiality adequately. As the laws become more and more a part of our daily lives and we learn through experiences, both positive and negative, nurses can no longer say "I didn't know" when it comes to privacy and confidentiality of patients' personal and health information. It is the responsibility of individual nurses to learn about privacy legislation in their province or territory as well as institutional policies, professional standards, and expectations, and apply these to individual accountable nursing practice.

Accountability in Practice

Accountability in practice refers to both legal accountability and to professional accountability. Recall that expertise in practice is not only one hallmark of a professional, but also a legal and ethical imperative. There have been monumental advances in knowledge and technology in the past several years. With the advent of health insurance in the post–World War II era and malpractice litigation in recent years, standards of care have become very stringent. Society's expectations of nurses' knowledge and abilities are high. Consequently, nurses must strive to maintain up-to-date knowledge and technical skills through professional development activities. Lack of knowledge is no defence in a court of law or during a professional disciplinary hearing. It is, in fact, tantamount to an admission of negligence. It is important that nurses know and uphold institutional, professional, and legal standards of practice and work within their scope of practice, never attempting to perform any task or administer any medication that is unfamiliar. Nurses' actions are examined in light of current information, professional or statutory scope of practice, and institutional and professional practice standards. Statements such as "Everyone does it that way," "it's what I learned in school twenty years ago," or "I did the best I could" will not protect a nurse from being found negligent.

Accountable practice also includes close attention to detail. Nurses make serious errors when they become over-tired or distracted, are called away from tasks, are inattentive to patients' changing health status, or do not take the time to document thoroughly. Attention to detail will prevent many of the errors that could result in charges of negligence. Ethics and the law are closely related in regard to attention to detail. Recall from Chapter 2 that deontological ethics requires that each person be seen as an end and not as only a means, and that one is compelled to fulfil one's duty to others, thus implying that nurses must focus clearly upon each patient and each task. Attention to detail will serve to improve patient outcomes and ensure that the profession continues to engender the public trust.

SUMMARY

As the enforceable system of principles and processes that govern the behaviour of people, laws reflect moral and ethical tradition. Though there is sometimes disagreement regarding the rightness or wrongness of certain laws, the laws are generally consistent with popular beliefs.

Laws can be constitutional, statutory, or administrative, and are divided into public and private realms. Public law deals with the relationship between persons and the government, and private law deals with the relationship between people. Nurses and other health care providers are most likely to be involved in liability cases related to tort law, a division of private law. Tort law includes unintentional torts, such as negligence and malpractice, and intentional torts, such as fraud, invasion of privacy, assault, battery, false imprisonment, defamation and intentional infliction of emotional distress.

Consent is an important overarching legal and ethical notion. Nurses must be aware of the four elements of consent—that it be voluntary, that it be informed, that it relate to specific providers and treatment, and that capacity to consent be assessed. Furthermore, they should be aware of consent legislation in the particular province they work in. As advocates, nurses can help patients to understand the notion of substitute decision makers or proxies, and help patients in creating advance directives, in keeping with helping patients to maintain their autonomous wishes even if they become unable to participate in decision making.

Persons are owed the right to privacy and, as professionals, we have a duty to maintain confidentiality. Numerous federal and provincial laws protect the privacy of individuals. Some of these laws specifically address the collection, use, and sharing of personal health information. Nurses must be aware of federal and provincial legislation, and of professional standards and institutional policies around maintaining confidentiality of patient information.

CHAPTER HIGHLIGHTS

- Ethics is the foundation of law; however, because laws are created by individuals and there are differences in beliefs among people, ethics and the law are not always congruent.

- Statutory law is created through the law-making process in federal or provincial legislatures; it is also called legislative law.

- Administrative law consists mainly of the legal powers granted to administrative agencies by the legislature, and the rules that the agencies make to carry out their powers.

- Common law, also known as case law, is a system of law based largely on previous judicial decisions.

- Public law defines a person's rights and obligations in relation to government, and describes the various divisions of government and their powers.

- Private law, also called civil law, determines a person's legal rights and obligations in many kinds of activities that involve other people.

- A tort is a wrong or injury that a person suffers because of someone else's action, either intentional (wilful or intentional acts that violate another person's rights or property) or unintentional (an act or omission that causes unintended injury or harm to another person).

- Consent is an important foundational ethical and legal notion.

- Nurses must take care to ensure patients' consent to care.

- Protecting the privacy of persons is a key priority in Canada.

- Federal and provincial legislation exists to help protect the privacy of individuals.

DISCUSSION QUESTIONS AND ACTIVITIES

1. Discuss with classmates their opinions about the courts becoming involved in issues that have traditionally been considered ethical in nature.

2. Read the *Canadian Charter of Rights and Freedoms*. (http://laws-lois.justice .gc.ca/eng/charter/page-1.html) How do these rights relate to patient care? How do they relate to nurses?

3. Discuss recent examples of federal or provincial legislation that create changes in the health care delivery system or in the practice of nursing.

4. In the common law system, how do previous court decisions affect the outcome of current cases?

5. Discuss instances in which nurses can be charged with crimes of public law, even though acts were committed without malice in the process of giving nursing care.

6. Discuss specific examples of unintentional torts.

7. How can you protect yourself from being accused of an unintentional tort?

8. In what instances can nurses be charged with intentional torts, even though they follow a professional code of ethics?

9. Discuss areas of potential liability for nurses and the present health care delivery system.

REFERENCES

Links to all provincial privacy legislation can be found on the following Web page from the Office of the Privacy Commissioner of Canada. Retrieved April 10, 2012 from http://www.priv.gc.ca/ resource/prov/index_e.cfm#contenttop.

A.C. et al. v. Director of Child and Family Services. Manitoba, Canada. Retrieved April 10, 2012, from http://www.scc-csc.gc.ca/case-dossier/cms-sgd/sum-som-eng.aspx?cas=31955.

Baker, G. R., P. G. Norton, V. Flinloft, R. Blais, A. Brown, J. Cox, E. Etchells, W. A. Ghali, P. Hebert, S. R. Majumdar, M. O'Beirne, L. Palacios-Derflingher, R. J. Reid, S. Sheps, R. Tamblyn (2004). The Canadian Adverse Events Study: the incidence of adverse events among hospital patients in Canada. *Canadian Medical Association Journal 170*(11): 1678–1686.

Beauchamp, T. L. (2001). *Philosophical ethics: An introduction to moral philosophy* (3rd ed.). Boston: McGraw-Hill.

Bernzweig, E. P. (1990). *The nurse's liability for malpractice* (5th ed.). St. Louis, MO: Mosby.

British North America Act, Constitutional Acts. Retrieved April 10, 2012, from http://canada. justice.gc.ca/eng/pi/const/lawreg-loireg/p1t11.html.

Canadian Nurses Protective Society. (2007). Quality documentation: Your best defence. *Info: A legal information sheet for nurses.* Ottawa: Author.

Catalano, J. T. (1991). *Ethical and legal aspects of nursing.* Springhouse, PA: Springhouse.

College of Nurses of Ontario. (2008). *Practice guidelines: Consent.* Toronto: Author.

College of Registered Nurses of British Columbia. (2003). *Nursing documentation.* Vancouver: Author. Retrieved April 10, 2012, from https://www.crnbc.ca/Standards/Documentation/ Pages/Default.aspx.

Doran, D., L. McGillis Hall, G. R. Baker, G. Pink, S. Sidani, L. O'Brien Pallas & G. Donner (2001). Nursing staff mix and patient outcome achievement: The mediating role of nurse communication. *International Nursing Perspectives, 1*(2-3), 74–83.

Downie, J., & T. Caulfield (2002). *Canadian health law and policy* (2nd ed.) Toronto: Butterworths Canada.

Ferguson v. Hamilton Civic Hospitals et al., CCLT 254

Fiesta, J. (1988). *The law and liability: A guide for nurses* (2nd ed.). New York: John Wiley & Sons.

Guido, G. W. (1997). *Legal issues in nursing* (2nd ed.). Norwalk, CT: Appleton & Lange.

Health Card Fraud. (2002). Ministry of Health and Long Term Care, Ontario. Retrieved April 9, 2012, from http://www.health.gov.on.ca/english/public/pub/ohip/card_fraud.html.

Hodgson, J. (2007). The legal dimension: Legal system and method. In Tingle, J. & Cribb, A. (eds.) *Nursing Law and Ethics.* (3rd edition). Oxford, UK: Blackwell Science Ltd.

Holmes, B. (2006). *The right to privacy and Parliament.* The Library of Parliament: Parliamentary Information and Research Service.

Keatings, M., & B. Smith (1999). *Ethical and legal issues in nursing* (2nd ed.) Toronto: Elsevier.

King, M. L., Jr. (1996). Letter from the Birmingham jail. In J. Feinberg, ed., *Reason and responsibility: Readings in some basic problems of philosophy* (9th ed., pp. 572–580). Belmont, CA: Wadsworth. (Reprinted from M. King, Jr., *Why we can't wait*, 1963, John Davis Agency.)

Kolesar v. Jeffries. (1976), 9 O.R. (2d) 41 at 48 (H.C.J.), varied 12 O.R. (2d) 142 (c.A.) aff'd (*sub nom, Joseph Brant Memorial Hospital v. Koziol*) [1978] 1 S.C.R. 491.

Kozier, B., & G. Erb (2007). *Concepts and issues in nursing practice* (8th ed.). New Jersey: Prentice Hall.

Lazar, N., G. Grenier, G. Robertson & P. Singer (1996). Bioethics for clinicians: 5. Substitute decision-making. *Canadian Medical Association Journal, 155*: 1435–1437.

Mazzocco, W. J. (2000). "Mixed" billing raises questions. *Advance for Nurse Practitioners,* 24–25.

Morris, J. J., M. Ferguson & M. Dykeman (1999). *Canadian nurses and the law.* Toronto: Butterworths Canada.

Murphy v. LaMarsh (13 DLR 3d 484). From R. Martin and G. S. Adam (1994) *A Sourcebook of Canadian Media Law*, pp. 569–573. Ottawa: Carleton University Press.

Nelson, E. (1999). Law, ethics and consent to medical treatment. *In Touch, 2*(6). Alberta: Provincial Health Ethics Network.

O'Keefe, M. E. (2000). *Nursing practice and the law: Avoiding malpractice and other legal risks.* Philadelphia: F. A. Davis.

Potter, P., & A. Perry (2008). *Fundamentals of nursing.* Toronto: Mosby.

R. v. Dyment (1988), 2 S.C.R. 417 (Supreme Court of Canada). Slowther, A., & I. Kleinman (2008). Confidentiality. In P. A. Singer & A. M. Viens, (eds.) *The Cambridge textbook of Bioethics* (pp. 43–50). Cambridge, England: Cambridge University Press.

Starson v. Swayze, [2003] 1 S.C.R. 722 (Supreme Court of Canada), (2001), 201 Dominion Law Reports (4th) 123 (Ontario Court of Appeal).

Stewart, A. (2002). Medical error—cautionary tales that leave us wondering about the system. *University of Toronto Medical Journal, 79*(2), 125–128.

The Personal Information Protection and Electronic Documents Act. (2000, with 2006 update). Retrieved April 10, 2012, from http://laws.justice.gc.ca/en/P-8.6.

Tingle, J. (2007). Nursing negligence: general issues. In J. McHale & J. Tingle, *Law & Nursing.* 3rd edition. London, UK: Elsevier.

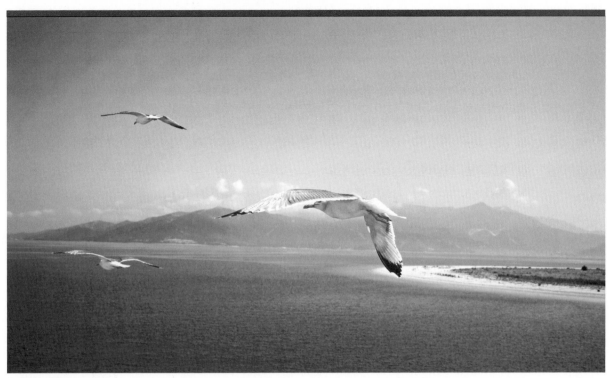

Nagy Melinda/Shutterstock.com

CHAPTER **8**
PROFESSIONAL ISSUES

OBJECTIVES

After completing this chapter, the reader should be able to:

1. Discuss what it means to be a "professional," including traits commonly associated with professional status and the historical debate regarding the professional status of nursing.
2. Discuss the relationship between codes of ethics and professional status.
3. Discuss the relationships among the concepts of expertise, ethics, and professional status.
4. Discuss autonomy in terms of both the individual nurse and the profession of nursing.
5. Discuss the relationship between professional autonomy and ethics.
6. Discuss the concept of "*accountability*," including various mechanisms of nursing accountability.

7. Explain the relationship between accountability and professional status.

8. Define the concept of "*authority*," differentiating between professional and personal authority.

9. Discuss the concept of unity and its relationship to professional status in nursing.

INTRODUCTION

The history of nursing carries a legacy of challenges to the claim that nursing is a profession. The role and image of nurses has evolved into the modern image of nurses after many iterative changes, often reflecting other historical trends. As a predominantly female profession, the image of nursing has also evolved alongside the image and status of women. This makes the history and evolution of nursing unique from other professions that have been traditionally male-dominated. Many might ask why it is important to define nursing as a profession, or to engage in the long-standing debate about whether or not it truly is a profession. In today's health care system, nurses have tremendously diverse roles and responsibilities across widely varying contexts. Their distinctive contribution to the provision of high quality care has made them invaluable—a crucial part of the health care team. Nursing's thorough academic preparation, intensive clinical training, unique body of expertise, autonomous practice, strong ethical guidelines, and sense of altruism makes nursing undoubtedly a profession, rather than what has often been labelled an "occupation." The link between ethics and principles such as autonomy, accountability, and altruism, and the foundations of the profession of nursing are clearly evident. Yet the debate over whether or not nursing is a profession continues. As practising nurses, it is imperative that we have a comprehensive understanding of the evolution of our profession, the kinds of legacies that continue to have a lasting effect on our practice today, and strategize ways to move forward as a more unified and autonomous professional group.

We will begin by examining the meaning and historical context of the term "profession," and what it means to be considered a professional. We will then discuss the professional status of nursing and the selected characteristics of expertise, autonomy, accountability, authority, and unity in nursing.

PROFESSIONAL STATUS

Professions exist to meet the needs of society. Society at large determines its needs, and authorizes certain people to meet those needs. There is a uniform process by which professionals develop the values that lead to a type of social responsibility and desire to meet the needs of society (Aydelotte, 1990). Professionals contract with society by promising to meet a set of identified needs better than any other group of people. In turn, society grants the profession a monopoly over these particular services. This has also, historically, elevated professions to higher social rankings. Traditionally, those who were in the professions were from higher social classes simply because they had greater access to higher education. While this is no longer the case, in most places there is still great "social esteem and prestige" (Sparkes, 2002, p. 481) accruing to those in professions. As a result of more open access to entering professions and reaping the subsequent social rewards, many occupations that were not previously designated as professions are now seeking professional status (Hoyle and John, 1995; Sparkes, 2002). Historically, professions have attempted to instil in their members a sombre recognition of the profound nature of their social responsibility through the recitation of pledges and oaths, such as the Hippocratic Oath for physicians and the Nightingale Pledge for nurses.

Since before the turn of the twentieth century, nurses and others have debated the professional status of nursing. Professions have been described in a number of ways, and to this day there is no single definition of a profession that is accepted by all. Gruending (1985) describes a **profession** as a complex, organized occupation preceded by a long training program. Professional education is geared toward the acquisition of exclusive knowledge necessary to provide a service that is either essential or desired by society. These attributes lead to a monopoly that provides autonomy, public recognition, prestige, power, and authority for the practitioner. Many other distinguishing attributes of professions have been proposed over the years. Among others, these can include expertise, accountability, the presence of systematic theory, ethical codes, a professional culture, an altruistic service orientation, competency testing, licensure, high income, credentialing, the description of a scope of practice, and the establishment of standards.

ASK YOURSELF

Is Nursing a Profession?

Most nursing programs have course content that is geared toward identifying the professional status of nursing through the use of identified traits or functions. While this is an important part of learning about professionalism, some approaches fail to acknowledge the other kinds of influences or conflicts that nurses and nursing students experience, along with the diversity of nurses as a group.

- Do you recall discussions in classes about the professional status of nursing? If so, what do you recall from those discussions?

- What kinds of values or traits were identified as core to the profession of nursing? Were you able to identify with these traits? Why or why not?

- What are some of the challenges in identifying "shared values" for a diverse group of professionals across different practice contexts?

- What kinds of functions do you think help establish nursing as a practice built upon a unique body of knowledge and expertise, and therefore as a profession?

(Continued)

- What (or whose) criteria should be used to judge professional status?
- Based upon what you recall, would you identify nursing as a profession, an emerging profession, a quasi-profession, or an occupation struggling to become a profession?

A classic source describing the criteria of professionals is Abraham Flexner. An educator, Flexner was well known for his 1910 evaluation of the professional state of medical schools, which at that time could be described as deplorable. As a result of these evaluations, in 1915, Flexner listed traits that he observed in the established professions of medicine, law, and the clergy. He then proposed that in order to be recognized as professions, all occupations must meet these criteria. Following are six criteria that he utilized to identify professions:

1. Professions involve essentially intellectual operations.
2. Their activities are learned in nature and based on a unique body of knowledge.
3. Their emphasis is practical, not necessarily theoretical.
4. They possess an educationally communicable technique.
5. They are well organized internally.
6. They are motivated by altruism. (Flexner, 1915, pp. 901–912)

Quinn and Smith (1987) further discuss the notion of altruism as a key attribute of a profession. They note that a profession is characterized by a commitment to the direct benefit of other human beings. While there is minimal societal control over the way that a profession carries out its responsibilities, there must be strong internal motivation and organization to ensure that the notion of the direct benefit of others is and continues to be a priority. Additionally, the unique body of knowledge that a professional embodies must be used in a way that promotes this notion of direct benefit.

Unsolicited by the nursing community, Flexner evaluated nursing according to his criteria, which had, for the most part, been developed by the examination and evaluation of male-dominated professions. He judged that nursing was not a profession, but an occupation. Optimistically, he proposed that occupations could alter their status by developing these traits. However, there was no acknowledgement of the social context in which his evaluations and recommendations were made. At that time, women were struggling to enter professions and to be considered as professionals alongside their male counterparts. This was not only a case of opportunities being denied to women on the basis of attitudes and the social norms of the time, but also an inherent acceptance of the claim that professions should reflect what were considered to be values more closely associated with males, such as objectivity, competition, autonomy, individuality, and empiricism (Davies, 1996; Sparkes, 2002). Alongside this was a belief that the more traditionally female attributes, including altruism, expression, and nurturing, were felt to belong to any member of a profession, but could also be found merely in the supportive work of women—a belief that has had a direct impact on the debate over nursing as a profession (Davies, 1996). When we look back at this now, we see that trying to evaluate nursing as a profession at that time, using criteria developed through the evaluation of much more positivist, male-dominated structures, was misguided and ineffective. While many agree that the process used to identify traits of professions was inherently flawed from the inception (Achterberg, 1990; Ehrenreich & English, 1973; Parsons, 1986), there are also those who go further and suggest that the term "professional" itself is sexist, elitist, and racist. At the beginning of the twentieth century, the three "professions" that were said to be universally accepted as such—medicine, law, and the clergy—were made up of members who were overwhelmingly male and Caucasian, and, as we have noted, usually from higher social classes. At the time Flexner wrote his report, women had been systematically excluded from both professional education and practice. Examining and describing traits of the male-dominated "professions," and subsequently using those findings as criteria to judge the professional status of other occupations worked to effectively exclude a number of predominately female groups, not just nursing.

In 1945 and 1959, two educators, Genevieve and Roy Bixler, published landmark articles in the *American Journal of Nursing* (AJN), evaluating the professional status of nursing. These articles utilized criteria similar to those proposed by Flexner. They listed the following seven criteria of a profession:

1. A profession utilizes in its practice a well-defined and well-organized body of specialized knowledge which is on the intellectual level of the higher learning;

2. A profession constantly enlarges the body of knowledge it uses and improves its techniques of education and service by the use of the scientific method;

3. A profession entrusts the education of its practitioners to institutions of higher education;

4. A profession applies its body of knowledge in practical services which are vital to human and social welfare;

5. A profession functions autonomously in the formulation of professional policy and in the control of professional activity, thereby;

6. A profession attracts individuals of intellectual and personal qualities who exalt service above personal gain and who recognize their chosen occupation as a life work; and

7. A profession strives to compensate its practitioners by providing freedom of action, opportunity for continuous professional growth, and economic security. (Bixler & Bixler, 1959, pp. 1142–1147)*

---

* Bixler, G. K., & Bixler, R. W. (1959). The professional status of nursing. American Journal of Nursing, 59(8), 1142–1147.

Predictably, the Bixler evaluations came to the same conclusion as Flexner had: nursing was, according to their criteria, not a true profession. Though both Flexner and the Bixlers had a tremendous lasting impact on the image of nursing, their evaluations were felt to be more of a product of the times when they were examining nurses, rather than a true reflection of the profession. Their approach assumes that true professions will demonstrate all of the essential attributes. In a critique of their methods, Fowler (1990) calls their lists of characteristics "an untidy aggregation of overlapping, arbitrarily chosen, or undifferentiated elements, lacking a unifying theoretical framework that explains their interrelationship" (p. 24).

Prior to the Flexner report, nurses had some security in their identity as professionals, even though nursing, at that time, was considered by many as a supportive role rather than a profession. Even some physicians and the judicial system recognized nursing as a profession. However, following the Flexner report and the subsequent Bixler articles, nurses began to question their status as professionals (Parsons, 1986). This process of examining and evaluating the status of nurses resulted in many positive changes for nursing, including strict entry-to-practice criteria and an acknowledgement of the unique science of nursing (Elzinga, 1990). Striving to meet the criteria set by Flexner and the Bixlers, nurses became involved in research to create and articulate a unique body of knowledge for nursing, to move professional nursing education to the university setting, to become politically involved, to increase the autonomy of nursing, and to make explicit and expand their scope of practice.

Nurses as Professionals

It is now generally acknowledged that nursing is a profession. Recognizing that there are a myriad of sources claiming to define the term "professional" by describing traits, attributes, functions, or characteristics, there will likely never be complete agreement about the professional status of nursing. Even though these discussions are important, for the purposes of this chapter we propose that nursing is, in fact, a profession.

In many ways nurses, as professionals, are connected to each other and set apart from others. Professionals are connected to each other by common experiences, language, and a body of knowledge. We are set apart from others by virtue of the prestige offered to members of a profession, and by the personal, intimate, and spiritual experiences surrounding the beginning and the end of life.

Beletz describes a professional as "one bound by values and standards other than those of his or her employing organization, setting one's own rules, seeking to promote standards of excellence, and being evaluated and looking for approval from one's own professional peers" (1990, p. 18). Jameton further suggests that being a professional is similar to having a calling. He describes a calling as "something one feels called upon to do, perhaps by God, by some deep need in one's being, or by the demands of historical circumstance. A calling is central to one's life and gives it meaning" (1984, p. 18). Moving the discussion further, Reed (2000) declares that nursing is a spiritual discipline. She argues that regarding a discipline as spiritual enhances the meaning of a profession. Reed writes that there is a pragmatic and normative call to action which is freely chosen by its members—one in which the person is said to be "called" or "launched outward to others" (p. 132).

EXPERTISE

Many feel that the notion of expertise lies at the very heart of a profession. **Expertise** relates to the characteristic of having a high level of specialized skill and knowledge. It is a "composite of a knowledge base, gained through long years of study in an academic setting, and superior skill. Expertise is the primary distinguishing difference between professionals and nonprofessionals" (Beletz, 1990, p. 17). Professionals must have the knowledge and functional skills required to meet the needs of society and thereby fulfill the purpose of the profession. Regarding expertise, Jameton writes:

> Professions maintain their autonomy partly through their claim to maximal competence [expertise]. So long as people believe that the professionals are the only ones who fully understand their work, it is very hard to supervise or criticize them. (1984, p. 21)*

We gain expertise in a variety of ways. Extensive educational requirements, intense guided practice, examinations for licensure, certification, and mandatory continuing education are ways that we either attain, maintain, or assert expertise. Florence Nightingale recognized the importance of an education providing depth and breadth of general knowledge, combined with a very specific nursing focus. Today we have a knowledge base that is continually expanded through research. Having completed basic nursing education and successfully demonstrated a minimum level of competence through licensure examinations, we are further required (both ethically or legally) to continue the learning process, keep our knowledge up to date, and maintain our technical proficiency. Continuing-education programs assist us in this process. Our expertise is also advanced through graduate nursing education, specialty preparation, and the certification process.

Merely claiming expertise is not enough. Through the various mechanisms of accountability, we must prove to society that we are faithful to the promise the profession makes. In response, society grants us the authority to practise with a certain measure of autonomy. Thus, the professional realms of expertise, accountability, autonomy, and authority are interrelated.

AUTONOMY

The word **autonomy** literally means "self-governing." The concept of nursing autonomy can be discussed on two levels: autonomy of the profession and autonomy of the individual practitioner. Self-regulation is the mark of collective professional autonomy. Individual autonomy involves self-determination, responsibility, accountability, independence, and a willingness to take risks. Autonomy is generally considered to be an important criterion in judging the professional status of an occupation. People who are considered to be professionals have the power and authority to control various

---

* *JAMETON, A., NURSING PRACTICE: THE ETHICAL ISSUES, 1st Edition* © 1983. Printed and Electronically reproduced by permission of Pearson Education, Inc., Upper Saddle River, New Jersey.

ASK YOURSELF

When the Bottom Line Becomes Personal

Alex is an operating room nurse in a busy urban hospital. When his elderly, independent mother becomes ill, she is taken to the emergency room of an adjacent hospital. It is suspected that she has had a stroke and needs urgent intensive care. However, there are no beds in the intensive care unit, so she is admitted into the emergency department to wait for a bed there. Because of Alex's background, he is familiar with the kinds of medical and nursing interventions that his mother urgently requires. He notes that the nurses are too busy to advocate adequately for his mother for an intensive care bed along with the necessary tests she requires, and even for help with activities of daily living that his mother requires. He has to return to work for some of his shifts and is very worried about the care his mother will get in his absence. He notes that her meals are placed out of her reach, as is her call bell. She cannot get up to go to the bathroom herself and becomes confused at night, trying to get up herself. Her room is far from the nursing station and he is concerned that no one might hear her call out in the busy, hectic atmosphere of the emergency room. He would like neurological and vital signs checked more regularly, but notes that they are being done only once or twice a shift, although his mother has frequent changes and shifts in her neurological status. She has not been washed or assisted with personal hygiene for two days and is confused and depressed.

- How would you feel if you were Alex?
- What do you think the very busy nurses' responsibilities are regarding their ability to adequately care for Alex's mother?
- What would you do if you were Alex? What are the challenges to the options available to Alex?
- In the context of this case, discuss your own beliefs about whether it is a true ethical obligation to maintain expertise in your areas of practice, as a nurse.
- An emergency room nurse has to have a broad foundation of knowledge in a number of areas. While it is not realistic to expect that every nurse knows "everything," should it not be expected that a professional nurse has the capacity for basic nursing care and skills of advocacy? Is this an ethical or professional obligation?

aspects of their work, including the goals they work toward, whether to work and with whom, details of how the work is to be done, choice of clientele, and so forth (Jameton, 1984). We continue to debate whether nurses have autonomy.

THINK ABOUT IT

Regulation

In Canada, the goal of regulation of registered nurses is protection of the public (Canadian Nurses Association, 2007b). Professions can be regulated by an external body, such as the government, or from within, as nurses are, which we call "self-regulation." In each province and territory, the regulation and monitoring of professional registered nurses is delegated to the profession itself through regulatory bodies. Nursing regulates members through provincial and territorial regulatory bodies, including the Ontario College of Nurses, the College of Registered Nurses of British Columbia, and the College of Registered Nurses of Nova Scotia. These regulatory bodies have a number of responsibilities, always with the overarching goal of protecting the public by making sure that those who are called "Registered Nurses" have met, and continue to meet, the requirements of the profession. While each college may articulate these goals and responsibilities in a slightly different way, they remain fairly consistent and include the following:

- Setting requirements for entering the profession;
- Making certain that standards for nursing practice are met, adhered to, and enforced;
- Ensuring the consistent competence of nurses and quality of care provided by nurses;
- Making decisions regarding disciplinary action for nurses who do not adhere to standards of practice.

The Colleges of nurses in each province and territory are run and governed by nurses; in doing this, the profession remains autonomous. However, in most colleges, there are members of the public who sit on the advisory boards and disciplinary boards. Part of the responsibility of a self-regulating profession is maintaining transparency, so involving community members is an important part of ensuring trust and upholding the responsibility of the profession to society at large.

The profession of nursing in Canada is self-regulating and therefore can be said to be autonomous. The notion of self-regulation is one that explicitly recognizes that professions, as unified groups, are in the most appropriate position to set standards and guidelines for practice and education, as well as to make sure that these standards are met, and to take suitable action if they are not.

At provincial and territorial levels, the government has delegated the authority to self-regulate to a number of health care professions, including nursing. Other self-regulated professionals include physicians, midwives, chiropractors, occupational therapists, physical therapists, pharmacists, social workers, and psychologists. In nursing, as with many other health care professions, the provincial and territorial governments give professional colleges and associations the authority and responsibility to regulate members of the profession.

One mechanism of regulation is the protection of the title of "registered nurse." Other protected titles in nursing in Canada include "registered practical nurse," "RN," "Registered psychiatric nurse," and "licensed practical nurse." The protection of these titles implies that anyone identifying themselves in one of these categories is registered with a regulatory body to practise nursing in the capacity identified by the title.

Jameton (1984) implies that the profession of nursing maintains autonomy through the combination of a claim to maximal competence and a continuing monopoly over their work. He writes:

> Professions also maintain their autonomy by means of monopoly over their work. In our competitive culture, people do not achieve autonomy simply by declaring it or believing in it. Professions maintain their control over their work partly by keeping people with other skills and other ideas from doing the same work. Only nurses may legally practice nursing. Licensure, educational requirements, certification of schools, and the like help nurses maintain control over nursing practice. This control is strengthened when nurses— rather than physicians and nonprofessionals—control the processes of licensure and certification. (p. 21)*

No other group has the ability to do the work of nurses; consequently, in Canada, as noted, there is a legal restriction barring non-nurses, that is, persons who do not have a title of "registered nurse," from practising nursing or using the term "nurse" to describe their role. This legally sanctioned monopoly helps to establish autonomy, and ultimately to protect the public.

Nurses are both legally and ethically required to practise autonomously. Autonomous practice serves as a safeguard for the patient, nurse, physician, and institution. Nursing codes of ethics support the nurse's autonomous decision-making and responsibility. The Canadian Nurses Association *Code of Ethics for Registered Nurses* (2008a) and the International Council of Nurses *ICN Code of Ethics for Nurses* (2006) implicitly and explicitly reflect nursing autonomy and responsibility. The purpose of autonomy as described in these codes is to protect the patient from harm, and allow for the full benefit of professional nursing care.

We often hear questions about the autonomy of individual nurses. As a nurse, do you really have autonomy? Can you say that you are autonomous, even though you are required to follow the orders given by physicians? Are you autonomous, even though you can't get to know the patients because you have too many

---

* *JAMETON, A., NURSING PRACTICE: THE ETHICAL ISSUES, 1st Edition* © *1983.* Printed and Electronically reproduced by permission of Pearson Education, Inc., Upper Saddle River, New Jersey.

patients and too much work to do? Lyon defines autonomous nursing practice as "the diagnosis and treatment of phenomena that nurses have the self-directed authority to treat" (1990, p. 270). Furthermore, she writes that nursing has a social mandate for two different scopes of practice: the medical scope that requires physician authorization to initiate treatment, and the autonomous nursing scope that requires no authorization.

Hospitals and other health care institutions require qualified and knowledgeable persons to carry out physicians' orders and the medical plan of care. When we seek employment at these institutions, we are implicitly agreeing to perform the functions for which we are hired. This includes carrying out the medical plan of care alongside the provision of unique nursing care. Accepting a position implies this contract. Nevertheless, we are legally and ethically required to use independent judgment in making nursing decisions. The exercise of independent nursing judgment is valuable to health care institutions because of the safeguards that are afforded. Nurses are in fact responsible for their own practice, both in providing independent nursing care and in collaborative roles, such as transcribing a medication order written by a physician and administering the ordered drugs to a patient. While nurses are accountable for maintaining competency in their own practice, a nurse who, for example, transcribes a drug or a dosage ordered incorrectly by a physician and then administers it, is in fact, responsible for that medication error. Competency and accountability in nursing implies responsibility for all conduct and actions—even collaborative ones. A nurse who is transcribing a medication order must have basic knowledge about the drug, dosage, safety, and side effects, as well as how all these relate to the individual patient. This is a part of competent nursing care and is also what it means to be an autonomous health care professional with unique responsibilities working in a collaborative, interdisciplinary team environment.

Autonomy does not mean that we have absolute control of every facet of practice. Although accepted as one of the three prototype professions, medicine, for example, no longer retains the measure of control it once enjoyed. Government regulations guide some facets of medical care, such as salary rates or caps and length of hospital stays. Consequently, physicians, though continuing to maintain professional status, are experiencing less absolute control over patient care than ever before. In the past, some (including Abraham Flexner) based the argument that nurses were not autonomous on comparisons between the independent decision-making capacities of medicine and nursing. That comparison no longer illustrates a great degree of distinction.

It is clear that nurses do not always feel autonomous, and, in fact, some may not practise autonomously. Certainly there are nurses who spend each workday complying with physicians' orders without question and completing various nonautonomous tasks, exercising no independent nursing functions, making no nursing judgments, initiating no self-directed interventions. In the truest sense, these nurses are only marginally practising professional nursing and cannot be said to be autonomous. When we practise in this manner, we fail in our ethical duty to make independent nursing judgments.

ACCOUNTABILITY

> "Nurses are accountable for their actions and answerable for their practice."
>
> (Canadian Nurses Association Code of Ethics for Registered Nurses, 2008a)

According to the American Nurses Association (2001), "**Accountability** means to be answerable to oneself and others for one's own actions. In order to be accountable, nurses act under a code of ethical conduct that is grounded in the moral principles of fidelity and respect for the dignity, worth and self-determination of patients" (p. 8). Safe, autonomous practice is ensured through various processes of nursing accountability. Accountability is related to both responsibility and answerability. Because of the trust accorded to nurses by society (gained through recognition of nurses' expertise) and the right given to the profession to regulate practice (autonomy), individual practitioners and the profession must be both responsible and accountable. The annual Gallup poll on Honesty and Ethics of professions in the U.S. consistently finds the public rating nurses as the most trusted of all professions (Gallup, 2011). For many of the thirteen years that nurses have been on the list, they have been named as the profession with the highest ethical standards and level of honesty. Added to the list of professions in 1999, nurses have consistently been the highest rated, with the exception of 2001, shortly after the September 11 terrorist attacks. That year, when the poll was conducted in November, firefighters were rated highest. With a rating of eighty-four percent in 2011 (which translates roughly as eighty-four percent of the public have the highest trust in nurses), nurses are followed by pharmacists (seventy-three percent), medical doctors (seventy percent), high school teachers (sixty-two percent), and police officers (fifty-four percent). The occupations at the bottom of the list include car salesmen (seven percent), telemarketers and lobbyists (both with no positive rating). A high level of accountability goes hand in hand with sustaining the high level of trust that the public has in the profession of nursing.

Related to the concepts of autonomy and authority, accountability is an inherent part of everyday nursing practice. Each nurse is responsible for all individual actions and omissions.

Mechanisms of Accountability

Accountability is based on the implicit contract between nursing and society as a whole. The Canadian Nurses Association notes that self-regulation ensures that nursing as a profession continues to be one of the most trusted professions in Canada, by making certain that the public receive "safe and ethical care from competent, qualified registered nurses" (Canadian Nurses Association, 2007b, p. 1). The profession of nursing has developed several mechanisms through which this relationship between nursing and society is made explicit, thereby acknowledging both the professional and the public areas of nursing accountability. These mechanisms include codes of nursing ethics, standards of nursing practice, nurse practice acts, nursing theory and practice derived from nursing research, educational requirements for practice, advanced certification, and mechanisms for evaluating the effectiveness of nurses' performance of nursing responsibilities (ANA, 1985). In both a professional and a legal sense, we must be familiar with various mechanisms of accountability.

Codes of Nursing Ethics. Nearly universally accepted as one criterion of a profession, a code of ethics is profoundly important to nursing. A **code of nursing ethics** is an explicit declaration of the primary goals and values of the profession that indicates the "profession's acceptance of the responsibility and trust with which it has been invested by society" (ANA, 1985, p. iii). Like other professions, nursing has developed and enforces specific obligations to ensure that members of society will find them to be competent and trustworthy. These obligations correlate to the rights of individual patients and society as a whole (Beauchamp & Childress, 2001). Upon entrance into the profession, nurses make an implicit moral commitment to uphold the values and moral obligations expressed in their code. Nurses are called upon to base professional judgment upon consideration of consequences and the universal moral principles of respect for persons, autonomy, beneficence, non-maleficence, veracity, confidentiality, fidelity, and justice (ANA, 2001). Examples of professional codes of ethics for nurses include the Canadian Nurses Association *Code of Ethics for Registered Nurses* (2008a), the American Nurses Association *Code of Ethics for Nurses* (2001), and the International Council of Nurses *Code of Ethics for Nurses* (2000).

Standards of Nursing Practice. Standards of nursing practice are written documents outlining minimum expectations for safe nursing care. Standards may describe in detail specific acts performed by nurses, or may outline the expected processes of nursing care. We use standards to guide and evaluate nursing care. As part of establishing and sustaining the public trust in nurses, standards are in place and publicly accessible in order to clearly demonstrate the commitment of the profession to transparency and accountability as self-regulated professionals (Canadian Nurses Association, 2008b). Courts look to standards of nursing practice for guidance when malpractice cases are deliberated. The two basic types of standards of nursing practice are internal and external standards (Fiesta, 1988).

Internal standards of nursing practice are developed within the profession of nursing for the purpose of establishing the minimum level of nursing care. They help to ensure that nurses are competent and safe to practise. These documents guide us in providing nursing care, and can be used as a consistent baseline to measure the practice of individual nurses. While outlining the minimum expectations for practice, standards are of vital importance. As outlined by the Canadian Nurses Association, nurses are the largest group of front-line health professionals in the country, caring for diverse groups and individuals in a variety of contexts and settings. Therefore, having standard expectations for practice assists not only nurses but also the public in having access to what kind of standards and best practices guide nurses in their professional activities and practice settings. Standards help protect the public, who are the recipients of nursing care (CNA, 2008b).

As nursing is a self-regulated practice, each province and territory has regulatory bodies that set the standards of practice and enforce professional practice and conduct. Alongside these standards is the Canadian Nurses Association *Code of Ethics,* which articulates the kinds of values that the nursing profession supports and embodies. Together, standards and codes of ethics make up the basis for a practice in nursing in Canada (CNA, 2008a; 2008b).

In addition to nursing practice standards, the Canadian Nurses Association has a number of policy statements, publications, position papers, fact sheets, and position statements that all demonstrate accountability and are publicly available. Examples of these include the Canadian Nurses Association *Position Statement on Providing Nursing Care at the End of Life* (2008c), the *Position Statement on Registered Nurses, Health and Human Rights* (2004), and the *Position Statement on Emergency Preparedness and Response* (2007a).

External standards of nursing practice consist of guides for nursing care that are developed by non-nurses, the government, or institutions. These standards describe the specific expectations of agencies or groups that utilize the services of nurses. They serve some of the same functions as internal standards, including guidance and evaluation. Examples of external standards include such documents as the *Health Professions Act* in British Columbia (1996), the *Act Respecting the Protection of Confidential Disciplinary Proceedings of Health Professions* in Nova Scotia (2008), and the *Regulated Health Professions Act* in Ontario (1991). Nurses are responsible and accountable to know and follow the standards of care for the profession, the specialty (if applicable), the geographic area, and the institution in which they practise.

CASE PRESENTATION

The "Real World" of Nursing

Erinn is a new graduate nurse working on a large medical surgical unit. She wrote the Canadian Registered Nurses Examination (CRNE), passed, and now has a licence to practice. While she worked under her temporary licence, immediately after graduation, the unit manager ensured that she had lighter assignments and was paired up with a more experienced registered nurse, in order for Erinn to learn the policies and procedures of the unit before getting used to having a full patient load on what is, traditionally, a very heavy unit.

When the unit manager and staff find out that Erinn has been successful in her CRNE and has become a licensed registered nurse, they congratulate her heartily. The next night, Erinn returns to work to find that she has a very heavy assignment and is not paired up with anyone to help her. Up until now, she has had only four patients on night shift and has been able to cover for one other nurse while that nurse goes on break. Tonight, Erinn finds that she has been assigned nine patients. One patient requires careful monitoring as she becomes disoriented at night and is at risk for falls or wandering. There is no one available to provide constant care for the patient tonight. Another patient requires administration of a chemotherapy drug via a peripherally inserted central catheter (PICC) line. The report notes that the PICC line is not working well and may require reinsertion.

Erinn approaches James, the nurse in charge, to ask for help. She isn't sure how she can provide constant care for one patient, with eight others. Erinn is also very concerned about the patient with the PICC line who requires chemotherapy. The hospital has a policy stating that only nurses who have undergone special certification may administer chemotherapeutic agents. While she has flushed PICC lines, Erinn has not been certified to insert one.

James tells her that they are very understaffed tonight, as the nursing supervisor pulled two of the unit nurses to cover in the intensive care unit. He suggests that Erinn first go and try to flush the PICC line and if it sticks, just push harder. He quietly adds that he knows the policies state not to do this, but it usually works, if you "do it just right." If it doesn't work, he adds, he'll show her how to insert one himself and she can do it. He also tells Erinn that he will prepare the chemotherapy drug but Erinn will have to give it. Finally he instructs Erinn to just try to look in on the patient requiring constant care once in a while, as often as she is able. "If something happens," he states, while shrugging, "we'll deal with it."

Erinn is well aware that her provincial regulatory body outlines seven standards of practice and that one of the standards, accountability, is demonstrated by "maintaining competence and refraining from not performing activities for which she/he is not competent" (College of Nurses of Ontario, 2009).

James sees Erinn hesitating. "This happens all the time," he says to Erinn, "Welcome to the real world!"

? THINK ABOUT IT

- What dilemmas does Erinn face?
- What are the alternatives available to Erinn?
- Can Erinn meet the standards and adhere to the policies of the institution?
- What role does James have in ensuring accountable and competent care? Has he met that standard?
- If something adverse happened to any patient on this shift, as a result of not adhering to policies and standards, who should be responsible?
- Do institutions have a role in ensuring competent, safe, and accountable care? If so, what is their role?
- Is there any way that Erinn can meet the standard of accountability, following James's advice?
- What would you do? How would you feel in this situation?
- What are the ethical implications for the institution, James, and Erinn?

Scope of Practice Statutes. Each province and territory has laws or statutes respecting the regulation of nursing. While some statutes are specific to nursing, such as the *Registered Nurses Act* for Saskatchewan (1988) or Newfoundland (2008), others are "umbrella" types of legislation, such as the *Regulated Health Professions Act* in Ontario (1991), and the *Health Professions Act* in Alberta (1999), which cover a variety of health professions and are not restricted to the profession of nursing. Scope of practice statements outline, in a general way, what members of a profession can do. They involve **controlled acts**, which can only be done by a qualified member of a designated profession. A controlled act carried out by a non-qualified person can potentially result in harm. Examples of controlled acts include: managing the labour of a pregnant woman and delivery of a baby, casting a fracture, giving a substance by injection or inhalation, or communicating a medical diagnosis.

The Canadian Nurses Association, in conjunction with the Canadian Pharmacists Association and the Canadian Medical Association, notes that the following four principles must be included in any scope of practice statement. First, the statements should *focus* on care that is highly responsive to the needs of the patients and communities and also ethical, safe, and of high quality. Second, there needs to be enough *flexibility* to allow health care professionals to practise at a level that relates to their education, skills, and competence. Third, there must be *co-operation* to engage in *interdisciplinary collaboration* as a means of providing high-quality care. *Co-ordination* and *patient choice* must always be a part of any scope of practice statement, as means of ensuring that patient care is appropriate and relevant (Canadian Nurses Association, 2003).

The statutes in each province set out how the **scope of practice** is outlined by the colleges that oversee regulation for each health profession (e.g., College of Nurses of Ontario, College of Registered Nurses of Nova Scotia, College of Registered Psychiatric Nurses of British Columbia). They provide frameworks outlining how colleges should operate the regulatory processes, as well as the disciplinary processes that must be carried out if a complaint is received regarding the conduct of a health professional who is registered with the college in that province or territory.

Nurses are responsible for following legislation that outlines their scope of practice, as part of being accountable and maintaining the trust of the public. As one example, the *Regulated Health Professions Act* in Ontario (RHPA) (1991) outlines the scope of practice for registered nurses, along with a list of thirteen specific authorized controlled acts that only qualified persons can perform (College of Nurses, 2011). Of the thirteen controlled acts, registered nurses are authorized to conduct three, and these are carefully outlined in the RHPA. Other controlled acts are outlined in the RHPA, but they are not included in the scope of practice of nurses, e.g., communicating a diagnosis, casting a fracture.

Abiding by provincial and territorial legislation governing scope of practice and regulation, maintaining requirements for entry to practice, making sure members are conducting ongoing competency evaluation, setting and monitoring standards for practice, and adhering to codes of ethics are all part of the responsibility and accountability of being a self-regulated nursing profession in Canada.

Nursing Theory and Practice Derived from Research. A frequently cited characteristic of professions is the existence of a unique body of knowledge derived from research. Recall that Genevieve and Roy Bixler's first two characteristics of a profession relate to a unique body of knowledge. The Bixlers' second characteristic calls for professions to constantly enlarge the body of knowledge by use of the scientific method (1959). In the past, authorities debated whether nursing's body of knowledge was unique to the profession, or was borrowed from behavioural and physical sciences and medicine. It seemed clear to some that nursing knowledge had been derived from the combination of experience and intuition, and by borrowing from other disciplines (Leddy & Pepper, 1989). Responding to arguments that nursing was not a true profession because of this lack of a clearly unique body of knowledge, nurses in academic and clinical settings began gathering data and doing legitimate research. The process of theory building and research in nursing continues to increase the unique body of nursing knowledge. There are many unique nursing research peer-reviewed journals, interest groups, and conferences across Canada and around the world. More and more nurses are entering and continuing into graduate school, doing doctoral and post-doctoral research. At most schools of nursing, academic nurse educators also maintain clinical and research agendas in order to maintain currency and contribute to the growing body of unique nursing knowledge and research. The benefit of this process is twofold. First, the expanded knowledge base enables nurses to respond to the needs of society more knowledgeably and skilfully. Second, the presence of a clearly unique body of knowledge aids in validating nursing as a true profession.

AUTHORITY

In terms of nursing, **authority** usually refers to the legitimate power and sovereignty of the government. The authority to practise nursing is granted by statute, based upon the contract the profession has with society. As with any self-regulated profession in Canada, the provincial and territorial governments grant authority to the professional colleges and associations of nursing that exist in each province and territory. This is done with the mutual understanding that there are clear mechanisms for public accountability, transparency of processes, and acknowledgment of the rights and responsibilities of self-regulation. Authority assumes a certain measure of autonomy. Donabedian relates authority to both autonomy and accountability:

> Society grants the professions authority over functions vital to itself and permits them considerable autonomy in the conduct of their affairs. In return, the professions are expected to act responsibly, always mindful of the public trust. Self-regulation to assure quality in performance is at the heart of this relationship. It is the authentic hallmark of a mature profession. (1976, p. 8)

In a practical sense, authority is granted by society in the form of permission for the profession to exist, coupled with the privilege granted to individuals to practise the profession. Thus, as with autonomy, authority for nurses is two-tiered. As noted, provincial and territorial regulatory bodies have statutes designed to protect the health and safety of the public. These statutes describe scope of practice and provide frameworks for regulatory processes carried out by provincial and territorial colleges or associations of nursing. Thus, the provincial and territorial regulatory bodies have the legitimate authority to regulate the practice of nursing within each jurisdiction.

Having specified requirements for entry into practice, defined nursing, and described the scope of nursing practice, nurse practice acts empower the provincial and territorial regulatory bodies to grant individual nurses the authority to practise. This authority is granted through the process of examination and licensure. Licensure benefits both the public and the professional. It protects the public from the unqualified, and it protects professionals' job territory by establishing a monopoly. The protection afforded by licensure enhances our status by authenticating the profession (Beletz, 1990). After meeting all requirements for entry into practice, we are granted the legal authority to practise nursing.

The authority given to each nurse to practise is contingent upon the nurse continuing to uphold the established standards of nursing. Provincial and territorial colleges of nursing have the power and responsibility to discipline nurses who do not follow established standards or who violate provisions of licensure law. Discipline can take several forms, including suspension or revocation of licence. Disciplinary processes must be made publicly accessible, to some degree. This is a significant part of maintaining the accountability of the profession. In order to avoid any appearance of impropriety or secrecy, disciplining members must not be seen as something that happens behind closed doors. Because the goals of disciplinary processes are to protect the public and to maintain trust in the profession, transparency and accessibility to the proceedings and outcomes are of the utmost importance. In the case of suspected incompetence or professional misconduct, most disciplinary processes involve a formal hearing. Moreover, these hearings almost always involve members of the public, who serve as members of the panel and contribute to the proceedings.

UNITY

There is general agreement that one of the defining characteristics of a profession is a sense of **unity** among its members. This unity is multifaceted and based on what Aydelotte (1990) calls moral uniformity and class ideology among its practitioners. Most nurses believe that as a profession we have shared values. Ideologies, or worldviews, are embedded in values and beliefs. While we have values and beliefs as individuals, many nurses share broad common values and ideas about what "ought" to be. These kinds of values are usually expressed explicitly in codes of ethics and mission statements. If we look at the Canadian Nurses Association *Code of Ethics* (2008a), some of the shared values expressed there include the provision of safe, compassionate, competent, and ethical care; the promotion of health and well-being; the preservation of dignity; the promotion of informed decision making; the maintenance of privacy and confidentiality; the promotion of justice; and accountability. Although these values are articulated in a Canadian context, many codes of ethics for nursing across the globe embrace similar values. Unity relates to the ability of nurses to organize for the purpose of fulfilling the profession's promises and the relationships that nurses have with one another.

Shaw and Degazon (2008) note that in discussing the shared values of a profession, we must take into account the changing face of nursing and the incredible diversity of age, ethnicity, gender, ability, lifestyle choices, country of origin, and sexual orientations that exist within the profession as a whole. In acknowledging that we are a diverse group of professionals, we imply that while we have shared values, the notion of a "collective culture" (p. 44), as Shaw and Degazon call it, is something far different than it was a few decades ago. The authors emphasize the importance of not only identifying what they label as "core professional values" (p. 44) but also teaching them as formal core competencies in nursing baccalaureate programs, as opposed to leaving it to individual educators to address them informally. The core professional values that Shaw and Degazon identify are: altruism, autonomy, integrity, human dignity, and social justice. These values, and their incorporation and integration into nursing education programs, are felt to be a meaningful reflection of the modern diverse nursing collective culture.

Through unity, the profession of nursing is able to coherently standardize professional characteristics such as competence, autonomy, leadership, authority, accountability, and social justice. Through political and policy processes, we work together to meet the health care needs of society and to continuously raise the status of the profession. The structural component of a professional community is realized through a professional association. The professional association provides a collective identity and serves as the voice of the profession to both the profession and society (Beletz, 1990). It fulfils four basic functions: to standardize services provided by its members; to provide a professional hub for members; to assist with educational needs of members; and to perform political, advisory, and policy functions. There is an expectation that professionals will be active members and leaders of their professional association. Across Canada, many professional nursing associations exist in every province and territory. Some examples include the Registered Nurses' Association of Ontario, the College and Association of Registered Nurses of Alberta, and the Association of Registered Nurses of Newfoundland. Additionally, many special interest groups exist for nurses with expertise, interest, and engagement in a particular area of practice, research, or education. Some examples are the Canadian Association for the History of Nursing, the Canadian Association for Neuroscience Nurses, and the Canadian Nursing Students' Association.

Although systematic organization of professional groups is a necessary part of fulfilling the profession's responsibilities, we also need unity among individual members and groups of nurses who work together. "Unity involves showing sympathy, care, and reciprocity to those one appropriately identifies with, working closely with others toward shared goals, keeping promises, making mutual concerns a priority, sacrificing personal interests to the relationship, and attending to these over a period of time" (Jameton, 1984).* Beletz eloquently describes this type of unity:

> The professional's bond with colleagues emanates from relationships established by shared mysteries of a common technical language, educational background, rites of passage, styles of work, attire, and a consciousness of being set apart and insisting on being set apart from other occupational categories. Colleague relationships are expected to be cooperative, equalitarian, and supportive vis-à-vis clientele and peers. (1990, p. 19)

Many people use the terms unity and loyalty interchangeably. In this discussion, we differentiate these qualities, referring to unity as an attribute of a profession, as a united whole, to articulate and embrace shared values, principles, and virtues. We refer to loyalty, on the other hand, as involving strong feelings of support or allegiance, which may be demonstrated by a commitment or dedication to someone or something. Unity is an attribute of the profession, while loyalty may be an individual attribute. We can articulate our shared values as a profession; however, individual nurses in complex situations may well find that loyalties are far more difficult to navigate. Though loyalty is considered a virtue, there are certain risks when we experience too strong a sense of loyalty to each other, as is the case with most virtues. Jameton (1984) warns that nurses must take care not to allow their loyalty to each other to not supersede their loyalty to their patients. For example, mistakes that nurses or doctors make should be reported to patients. Because of a sense of loyalty and friendship that exists between co-workers, there is a risk that our duty to patients will be neglected. We are required to examine and prioritize conflicting loyalties closely. In this context, Jameton identifies nurses' main priorities as patients, nurses and the nursing profession, physicians, hospitals, other health professions, and society. Questioning which of these priorities should be central and which should be peripheral, he suggests that the best choices for first priority are patient, nursing, and society.

ASK YOURSELF

Who Should We Be Loyal to? And to What End Should We Be Loyal?

In 1994, twelve children died while undergoing or after having undergone cardiac surgery at the Children's Hospital of Winnipeg. Throughout these events, many health professionals involved in the treatment of these children voiced concerns about the conditions of the cardiac surgery department, and about the treatment of the children. A significant number of those voicing concerns included the intensive care and surgical nurses at the hospital.

---

* *JAMETON, A., NURSING PRACTICE: THE ETHICAL ISSUES, 1st Edition* © *1983.* Printed and Electronically reproduced by permission of Pearson Education, Inc., Upper Saddle River, New Jersey.

A full review and eventual inquest was carried out to determine culpability, review processes and infrastructures that existed at the time in that hospital and department, and to avoid further deaths of children undergoing cardiac surgery.

During the inquest, it was found that while the nurses did voice their concerns to those in positions of authority, their concerns were trivialized at times and dismissed as being overly emotional reactions to the deaths of the children instead of valid concerns of knowledgeable professionals who function as part of a multidisciplinary team.

Some of the nurses were understandably hesitant and afraid to voice their concerns, as their colleagues had been treated in a dismissive and patronizing manner. While they continued to care for children undergoing surgery, they did so with grave misgivings.

Today, we have the luxury of being able to reflect on this case and others like it, by reading inquests and reports and learning from the challenges and tragedies of others. We must always remember, when reflecting on cases like this, that the individuals involved were undergoing significant challenges, conflicts, and anguish. Our own critique of these past situations must always include our own compassion and empathy for the difficulties endured by others.

To read more about this case, go to http://www.pediatriccardiacinquest.mb.ca.

- Imagine yourself in a situation where you have grave concerns about the multidisciplinary care of the patient you are responsible for. How would you feel?

- How far would you go to have your concerns or voice heard? Would you risk your job, livelihood, future employment, professional reputation?

- In cases like this, what should the role of nursing administration be? ? What about the role of regulatory bodies or professional associations? Do they have a role to play?

- Jameton (1984) discusses a priority of loyalties with the patient always coming first, and nursing and society falling after. In this case, the nurses did try to advocate for the patients by voicing their concerns. When these concerns were not heeded, what else might they have done at that point?

- Reflect on your own place of work. Do you feel that you have a voice to advocate for others or to challenge actions or decisions you do not agree with? Why or why not?

SUMMARY

Because ethics is a commonly cited criterion for judging the professional status of an occupation, the study of ethics must include a discussion of nursing's professional status. In order to discuss professional issues in nursing rationally, one must examine the meaning and historical context of the term "professional." Beginning with Abraham

Flexner's 1915 opinion that nursing did not meet his criteria for professional status, there has been continuing debate about this topic. Striving to create professional status for nursing, nurses have worked to establish themselves as autonomous, ethical professionals. There are those who believe that the original methods of determining professional status were flawed by a cultural and historical context of sexism, racism, and elitism. Though this debate will continue, there are a number of traits that are nearly universally accepted as belonging to professional groups. Of those traits, expertise, autonomy, accountability, authority, and unity were discussed here as professional characteristics of nursing.

CHAPTER HIGHLIGHTS

- Acknowledgment of professional status depends on meeting particular criteria that include, but are not restricted to, expertise, autonomy, authority, accountability, and unity.
- Historical and cultural influences have affected the definitions commonly used for the term "professional."
- A system or code of ethics is generally accepted as one trait of professions.
- Because society gives professionals a monopoly over the services they provide, ethics demands that those services must be provided with expertise.
- Because it is self-regulating, the profession of nursing can be said to be autonomous.
- There are legal and ethical imperatives for individual nurses to practise autonomously.
- Autonomy does not mean full and absolute control over every aspect of practice.
- Grounded in the moral principle of fidelity, accountability refers to being answerable to someone for something one has done.
- Mechanisms of accountability include, but are not restricted to, codes of nursing ethics, standards of nursing practice, nurse practice acts, and nursing theory and practice derived from nursing research.
- Authority for nurses to practise is granted through the legal processes of society.
- Nursing unity relates to the profession's ability to organize for the purpose of fulfilling promises made to society.

DISCUSSION QUESTIONS AND ACTIVITIES

1. Write your own definition of the term "professional." In your definition, include the characteristics of a profession.
2. List ten different occupations and compare their common characteristics. Which of the ten occupations meet your criteria for professional status?

3.   Discuss the relationship between historical and cultural influences and Flexner's method of identifying professions.

4.   Discuss the relationship between the concepts of fidelity, professionalism, and expertise.

5.   Discuss the statement, "To be less than maximally competent is unethical."

6.   Find recent examples of case law that relate to court opinions regarding autonomy in nursing.

7.   Read the nurse practice act in your province or territory. Evaluate your province or territory's law in terms of how useful it is as a mechanism of accountability.

8.   What are some ways that regulatory bodies make sure that their member nurses are competent to practice?

9.   If you were to come up with the core values you embrace in your role as a nurse or a student nurse, what would they be? Why would you choose each of those values?

10. Think about the influences on the image of women and nurses throughout modern history that we discussed in Chapter One. What impact have these influences had on the status of nurses as professionals?

REFERENCES

Achterberg, J. (1990). *Woman as healer*. Boston: Shambhala.

American Nurses Association. (2001). *Code for nurses with interpretive statements*. Washington, DC: Author. Retrieved on April 19, 2012 from http://www.nursingworld.org/MainMenuCategories/ EthicsStandards/CodeofEthicsforNurses/Code-of-Ethics.pdf

Aydelotte, M. (1990). The evolving profession: The role of the professional organization. In N. L. Chaska, ed., *The nursing profession: A time to speak* (pp. 16–23). St. Louis, MO: Mosby.

Beauchamp, T., & J. Childress (2001). *Principles of biomedical ethics* (4th ed.). New York: Oxford University Press.

Beletz, E. (1990). Professionalization: A license is not enough. In N. L. Chaska, ed., *The nursing profession: Turning points* (pp. 16–23). St. Louis, MO: Mosby.

Bixler, G. K., & R. W. Bixler (1959). The professional status of nursing. *American Journal of Nursing, 59*(8), 1142–1147.

Canadian Nurses Association. (2003). *Joint position statement: Scopes of practice*. Retrieved April 18, 2012, from http://www2.cna-aiic.ca/CNA/documents/pdf/publications/PS66_Scopes_of_ practice_June_2003_e.pdf

Canadian Nurses Association. (2004). *Position Statement: Registered Nurses, Health and Human Rights*. Retrieved on April 18, 2012 from http://www2.cna-aiic.ca/CNA/documents/pdf/ publications/PS116_Health_and_Human_Rights_2011_e.pdf

Canadian Nurses Association. (2007a). *Position statement on emergency preparedness and response*. Retrieved January 2, 2009, from http://www2.cna-aiic.ca/CNA/documents/pdf/ publications/PS91_Emergency_e.pdf

Canadian Nurses Association. (2007b). Understanding self-regulation. *Nursing Now, Issues and Trends in Canadian Nursing, (21)*. Ottawa: Canadian Nurses Association.

Canadian Nurses Association. (2008a). *Code of ethics for registered nurses*. Author. Retrieved January 20, 2009, from http://www2.cna-aiic.ca/CNA/documents/pdf/publications/Code_of_Ethics_2008_e.pdf.

Canadian Nurses Association. (2008b). *Standards and best practices*. Retrieved April 18, 2012, from http://www.cna-aiic.ca/en/professional-development/nurseone-knowledge-resources/standards-and-best-practices/.

Canadian Nurses Association. (2008c). *Providing care at the end of life*. Retrieved April 18, 2012 from http://www2.cna-aiic.ca/CNA/documents/pdf/publications/PS96_End_of_Life_e.pdf

College of Nurses of Ontario. (2009). *Professional Standards*. Revised 2002. Toronto: Author. Retrieved April 18, 2012 from http://www.cno.org/Global/docs/prac/41006_ProfStds.pdf

College of Nurses of Ontario. (2011). *RHPA: Scope of Practice, Controlled Acts Model*. Toronto: Author. Retrieved April 18, 2012 from http://www.cno.org/Global/docs/policy/41052_RHPAscope.pdf

Davies, C. (1996). The sociology of professions and the profession of gender. *Sociology, 30*(4), 661–678.

Donabedian, A. (1976). Foreword in M. Phaneuf, ed., *The nursing audit: Self-regulation in nursing practice* (2nd ed.). Norwalk, CT: Appleton & Lange.

Ehrenreich, B., & D. English (1973). *Witches, midwives, and nurses: A history of women healers*. New York: The Feminist Press.

Elzinga, A. (1990). The knowledge aspect of professionalisation: The case of science-based nursing education in Sweden. In Torstendahl, R. and M. Burrage (eds.) *The Formation of Professions: Knowledge, State and Strategy,* Sage; London; pp. 151–173

Fiesta, J. (1988). *The law and liability: A guide for nurses*. New York: John Wiley & Sons.

Flexner, A. (1915). Is social work a profession? *School Society, 1*(26), 901–911.

Fowler, M. (1990). Social ethics and nursing. In N. L. Chaska, ed., *The nursing profession: A time to speak* (pp. 24–31). St. Louis, MO: Mosby.

Gallup. (2011). Record 64% Rate Honesty, Ethics of Members of Congress Low.

Retrieved on April 19, 2012 from http://www.gallup.com/poll/151460/record-rate-honesty-ethics-members-congress-low.aspx

Gruending, D. L. (1985). Nursing theory: A vehicle of professionalization. *Journal of Advanced Nursing, 10*, 553–558.

Hoyle, E. and John, P. (1995). *Professional Knowledge and Professional Practice*. London: Cassell.

International Council of Nurses. (2006). *The ICN code of ethics for nurses*. International Council of Nurses, Geneva Switzerland. Retrieved April 19, 2012 from http://www.icn.ch/images/stories/documents/about/icncode_english.pdf

Jameton, A. (1984). *Nursing practice: The ethical issues*. Englewood Cliffs, NJ: Prentice-Hall.

Leddy, S., & J. M. Pepper (1989). *Conceptual bases of professional nursing* (2nd ed.). Philadelphia: Lippincott.

Lyon, B. (1990). Getting back on track; nursing's autonomous scope of practice. In N. L. Chaska, ed., *The nursing profession: A time to speak* (pp. 267–274). St. Louis, MO: Mosby.

Parsons, M. (1986). The profession in a class by itself. *Nursing Outlook, 34,* 270–275.

Quinn, C. A., & M. D. Smith (1987). *The professional commitment: Issues and ethics in nursing.* Philadelphia: Saunders.

Reed, P. G. (2000). Nursing reformation: Historical reflections and philosophic foundations. *Nursing Science Quarterly, 13*(2), 129–136.

Shaw, H, & C. Degazon (2008), Integrating the Core Professional Values of Nursing: A Profession, not just a Career. *Journal Of Cultural Diversity, 15*(1), p.44–50.

Sparkes, V. J. (2002). Professional and professionalisation: Part 1: Role and identity of undergraduate physiotherapy educators. *Physiotherapy, 88*(8), pp. 481–492.

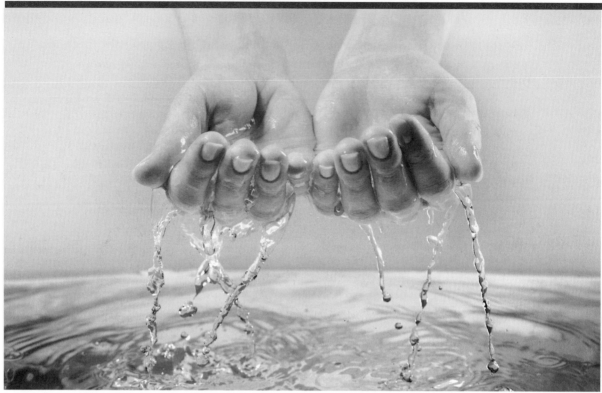

Chepko Danil Vitalevich/Shutterstock.com

CHAPTER 9
PROFESSIONAL RELATIONSHIP ISSUES

OBJECTIVES

After completing this chapter, the reader should be able to:

1. Identify relationships and potential conflicts that nurses face as professionals and team members.
2. Characterize the nature of various conflicts.
3. Examine beliefs about the relative strength of various obligations.
4. Identify the multiple and often complex obligations of nurses.
5. Discuss issues related to nurses' relationships with colleagues, institutions, and other health-care professionals.
6. Discuss strategies for maintaining moral integrity when managing conflicts within relationships.

INTRODUCTION

Armed with knowledge about the physical, psychological, social, and spiritual realms of nursing care, and proudly possessing a wide range of coveted technical and professional skills, new nurses expectantly enter the workforce. Anticipating respect for our opinions and encouragement to focus our efforts on giving excellent care, we soon realize that our attention must be divided between giving patient care and dealing with the challenges of providing care within the context of diverse teams across settings. In addition to the opportunities that teamwork provides, it can also present confusing and frustrating challenges, forcing us to examine conflicting loyalties, question previously held values, make decisions based upon both practical and moral considerations, and test our skills of negotiation, conflict management, and resolution. What is being challenged in these kinds of situations of conflict? Typically, our *moral integrity* as nurses is being challenged and, many times, the kinds of conflicts we encounter in relationships are conflicts of deeply-held values.

The nurse continually affirms that each person is a moral agent, an autonomous being worthy of respect and having the duty to pursue solutions to problems of a moral nature. It is important that solutions consistently honour the uniqueness and value of each person and faithfully adhere to ethical principles. This process requires us to critically examine our own particular values and determine an ethically sound method of conflict resolution, even before conflict arises. It also implies that we must acknowledge that valuing the uniqueness of others refers not only to patients and families, but also to colleagues, students, instructors, and other health-care professionals. Mutual respect requires that we honour the uniqueness of everyone we encounter in our role as nurses, and adhere to ethically sound principles across all our professional relationships, not just those with our patients.

Recognizing that the profession of nursing struggles to overcome contextual barriers with cultural and historic overtones, we must enter professional relationships with attentiveness and skill. A key part of sound ethical practice relates to how we, as nurses, approach and function in complex relationships. Nursing, by its very nature, is embedded within and often defined by the relationships we have with others. As the Canadian Nursing Association notes in their *Code of Ethics for Registered Nurses,* the values that underpin ethical practice are "grounded in nurses' professional relationships with individuals, families, groups, populations and communities as well as with students, colleagues and other health-care professionals." (CNA, 2008, p. 3). Rather than attempting to offer broad solutions to a comprehensive list of system-related problems, this chapter provides the opportunity to examine critically selected problems related to nurses' relationships within the health care delivery system and discuss the inherent challenges and professional opportunities for growth that these relationships provide, all from a perspective of maintaining moral integrity as professionals.

MORAL INTEGRITY AND RELATIONSHIPS

Moral integrity refers not only to good moral character but also to the sense of being whole, complete, or intact. Our moral integrity is underpinned by our values and beliefs, both as individuals and as professional nurses. But moral integrity does not exist in a vacuum. It can be enhanced, challenged, or supported through how we conduct ourselves within relationships. As nurses, our relationships underpin our professional practice. A nurse's moral integrity, within the context of therapeutic relationships, can help contribute to patient well-being and respect for others.

When we discuss moral integrity in the context of professional nursing care, we need to first recognize that, as nurses, we are moral agents. This implies that, as autonomous and rational persons, we are capable of deliberate action, and can engage in the kinds of processes and activities that are thought to underpin these kinds of deliberate actions, such as reflecting upon various options for courses of action (Rodney, Kadyschuk, Liaschenko, Brown, Musto & Snyder, 2013). Traditional models of the moral agent emphasize autonomy of the individual, but more modern discussions emphasize the contextual, dynamic, and relational nature of moral agency and the social connections inherent to examinations and discussions of moral agency (Peter, 2011). In other words, more modern ideas about a moral agent stress the fact that while a moral the context of agent must have autonomy to act, actions with moral dimensions can only exist within relationships with others. Moral agency, therefore, is a relational concept and requires thinking about not only the individual moral agent, but also about the kinds of social structures and relationships within which a moral agent exists.

So, as moral agents, nurses have relationships with many others, including patients, families, nursing colleagues, other health care professionals, institutions, communities, and groups. Often within those professional relationships, we encounter situations of conflict that evoke strong personal responses. Codes of ethics and institutional policies may offer little help when our values are tested or challenged or when we encounter strong conflicting values. Despite our professional obligations, we cannot simply put aside our own values and beliefs, but must instead be aware of the impact of these values and beliefs on our ability to provide safe and ethical care. These kinds of conflicts, therefore, are important to highlight and talk about, as they represent opportunities for us to really examine and evaluate the values and beliefs that we ourselves hold. While the focus of much discussion in ethics in on the area of patients' rights, values, and respect for such, the focus shifts to the nurse in discussions of moral integrity and professional conflict—often to the nurse whose values have been "pushed to a limit" (Yeo, Moorhouse, Khan and Rodney, 2010, p. 349). Yeo and colleagues, in their thoughtful discussion on integrity, claim that when any nursing professional value is pushed to a limit (as in a situation of conflict), this can easily become an issue of moral integrity.

PROBLEM SOLVING IN SITUATIONS OF CONFLICT

Practical and ethical dilemmas are part of everyday nursing practice. Though many dilemmas involve patient-centred issues such as self-determination, confidentiality, and the like, we frequently encounter troubling moral questions related to our professional relationships, conflicting role expectations, and patterns of interaction within institutional settings. In the long run, problems of this nature can affect patient well-being and moral integrity both directly and indirectly and are, therefore, very important to us on a professional level. These problems are often more troubling to us than problems directly involving patients. Recognizing that dilemmas of this sort are frequent and troubling, we must consider rational methods of solving problems before they occur. If we fail to try to solve conflict, we may add to the problem.

Although there is no foolproof formula for solving conflicts, there are some general guidelines or steps that can be helpful. First, we must remain attentive to personal values and beliefs. Consistent awareness of and adherence to personal values enables us to approach problems with integrity. Second, we should construct a hierarchy of loyalty or obligation, based upon both personal and professional values and beliefs. For example, do you owe a primary obligation to the physician, the institution, or the patient? Third, when conflicts arise, we should determine the nature of the problem. Is the dilemma ethical or practical in nature? Is it a conflict of loyalty, obligation, duty, values, principles? Fourth, we should consider and weigh the alternatives thoughtfully, including the degree of immediate harm or potential for harm, as well as the long-range effects that could occur with any given alternative. Fifth, it is imperative to develop solutions that recognize each person as an autonomous being, worthy of respect. Note that these steps are very similar to the steps identified in various ethical decision-making models that we discussed in Chapter 6. Thoughtful utilization of these steps will help us work through, and hopefully begin to resolve, most professional conflicts.

Step One: Remain Attentive to Personal Values

Before looking at other considerations, we must acknowledge our own personal values and beliefs. This attention to integrity is not related to self-interest; it predicates action based on coherent and integrated moral values. Integrity ultimately leads to trustworthiness and gains the respect of others. Beyond questions of loyalty or duty, we are compelled to maintain our own integrity in seeking to do the right thing. This is sometimes referred to as attention to matters of conscience. Childress (1978) distinguishes between **appeals to conscience** and appeals to self-interest or convenience, in that appeals to conscience are personal and subjective beliefs, founded on a prior judgment of rightness or wrongness. These are motivated by personal sanction, rather than external authority. Institutions, in turn, must recognize the nurse as a person and encourage ethical autonomy. This enables us to act in ways that are rational, free from coercion or manipulation, and consistent with personally held values and principles (Benjamin & Curtis, 2010).

Acknowledging your own set of values and principles is a process that takes time. As we grow and develop, so does our moral autonomy, or our ability to identify our own beliefs and hold onto them, even in the face of adversity or conflict. This is a difficult skill to develop and, like any skill, gets easier the more we practise exercising our own moral values and beliefs in everyday challenges. Institutions that encourage and facilitate our own ability to explore and hold true to our values and beliefs, while understanding and acknowledging the values of the institution, are the ones that create positive morale-enriching environments.

Step Two: Clarify Obligations

Even nurses who possess a high level of integrity do not escape a sense of conflicting loyalty on occasion. When this happens, how do we determine the best course of action? We can be prepared by examining our **obligations**, and devising a rational and consistent hierarchy. An obligation signifies being required to do something by virtue of a moral rule, a duty, or some other binding demand. Some obligations derive from a particular role or relationship (Honderich, 2005). We may believe an obligation is owed to any of the following (in no particular order, as priorities may change depending on the context and situation): the patient and support network, other patients who may be affected in the future by problems that occur in the present, the employer that the nurse has an implied or expressed contract with, the profession of nursing, peers and other co-workers, other health care professionals, society at large, family, and self. Having multiple obligations can, understandably, create the potential for conflict. In Chapter 2 we discussed Kantian deontology, which describes adherence to duty as part of our ethical obligations. However, Kant offers little advice on how to manage conflicting duties. And in reflecting upon the multiple obligations and relationships we must maintain as nurses, it is obvious that potential conflicts in values, beliefs, and duties are sure to arise. While Codes of Ethics and institutional policies may be helpful at times in approaching these kinds of complex situations of conflict, many agree that they are simply not adequate. To some degree, however, acknowledging that our primary professional obligation must always be to the patient provides a solid starting point for working through and resolving potential conflicts.

So, let's acknowledge that we have a primary obligation to patients above all others. Because nurses are professionals, we have a moral obligation to maintain fidelity—we must be faithful to the promises we have made to society, and thus give top priority to advocating for the individual needs of each patient. The International Council of Nurses *Code of Ethics for Nurses* (2006) makes it clear that the nurse's primary responsibility is to the patient. By following established professional codes of ethics and maintaining integrity and loyalty to patients, we also fulfil related obligations to the broader society, the profession, and ourselves.

The duty that nurses and other health care professionals have to their patients is often described as a fiduciary relationship. A legal term, a fiduciary refers to someone who has an ethical duty to act in the best interests of another. Simply put, it is the ethical obligation health care professionals have to act in a way that protects others, furthers their interests and their wishes, and, essentially, sets aside the agendas and competing priorities of the practitioner in favour of the patient's immediate and long-term needs. Consider an example of a nurse who is participating in the resuscitative efforts of someone in a cardiac arrest at exactly the same time he is entitled to be taking a coffee break. Clearly his fiduciary duty would dictate that he remain part of the life-saving efforts and delay his break. An obvious example, perhaps. Next, consider the nurse who is over-tired from working too many night shifts in a row, who is also the primary caregiver for her elderly mother, and is a single mother, who arrives to work to find that she has been assigned a patient who, after being cancelled for surgery, has been reported as being angry and aggressive with the nursing staff. When she enters the patient's room, she finds that he is refusing all medication and blood work. He is visibly upset, angry, and confrontational with the nurse. For a moment, she is tempted to return his anger and share with him her own frustrations, letting him know that "everyone has problems!" She is even tempted to just walk out of the room and leave him. However, realizing that, while difficult, her own frustrations must be set aside while she is in the role of nurse, she stays and voices to him her understanding of how frustrating it must be to have a surgical procedure cancelled. She asks him how she can help and after some discussion gets the patient to agree to take his medications and allow blood work to be done, in preparation for a possible surgery tomorrow. While this does not ease her own frustrations, she can be assured that she has acted in the patient's best interests, and not allowed herself an inappropriate opportunity to vent her own feelings of frustration and anger.

Step Three: Determine the Nature of the Problem

It is important for us to be able to determine the nature of the problem. Is this a problem of moral uncertainty, moral distress, moral dilemma, or moral outrage? Or is this a problem or conflict of a more practical nature?

Ethical considerations should carry more weight than matters of self-interest, though, clearly, we owe some consideration to our own needs when encountering professional conflicts. Consider the commonly-encountered example of nurses being asked to "float" to unfamiliar settings in institutions due to fluid and dynamic staffing ratios and measures of acuity. This practice redistributes the workload and often offers the promise of improved nursing care. However, nurses frequently object to the prospect of being asked to float. Some nurses complain, "I've never worked there; I would be unsafe to practise in that setting!" They are tempted to refuse to float to unfamiliar settings. These nurses are faced with a moral and professional dilemma because the nurse has obligations both to ensure the welfare of the patient and to meet the needs of the institution. In either case—in assigning a nurse to float or in accepting the assignment—one must be guided by the principles of non-maleficence and beneficence: the actions that the nurse is expected to perform must be relatively certain to do good and do no harm. In that regard, neither the nurse, the patient, nor the institution will benefit from requiring a nurse to perform tasks for which that nurse is not prepared. To do so would be unethical. When faced with situations of this sort, we can look to our codes of ethics for help. Regarding this particular situation, for example, the ICN *Code of Ethics for Nurses* (2000) is very specific about the nurse's duty: "The nurse uses judgment regarding individual competence when accepting and delegating responsibility." The Canadian Nurses Association *Code of Ethics for Registered Nurses* (2008) also addresses this type of situation: "Nurses practice within the limits of their competence. When aspects of care are beyond their level of competence, they seek additional information of knowledge, seek help from their supervisor or a competent practitioner and/or request a different work assignment. In the meantime, nurses remain with the person receiving care until another nurse is available" (p. 18). Similarly, the ANA *Code of Ethics for Nurses* (2010) states, "As the scope of nursing practice changes, the nurse must exercise judgment in accepting responsibilities, seeking consultation, and assigning activities to others who carry out nursing care." (p. 8)

Nevertheless, it could also be said that to refuse an assignment is unethical on a number of levels. As the CNA *Code of Ethics for Registered Nurses* (2008) states, we must not abandon patients in need of care. If there is no one else available to care for the patient, we are obligated to give care, albeit only the type of care for which we are prepared and competent. For example, nurses temporarily assigned to specialty units can be asked to give basic, supportive nursing care, but should not be asked to perform technical tasks for which they are unprepared. In the same regard, we should not attempt tasks for which we are not prepared: to do so will compromise fidelity. We should not, however, refuse to accept float assignments simply because we fear the unknown, because familiarity is comfortable, or for other self-interested reasons.

Step Four: Consider and Weigh Alternatives

Fourth, we should consider and weigh possible options or solutions thoughtfully, including the degree of immediate harm or potential for harm, as well as long-term effects that could occur with any given possible solution. Harm to those directly involved must be assessed as well as potential indirect harms, such as to society, or to the already-standing relationships based on trust and mutual respect. Although some alternatives may seem attractive initially, there may be long-term effects that are undesirable, which must be considered and weighed against each other. In looking at possible solutions to professional conflicts and threats to moral integrity, nurses must take into account not only the actual relationships but also the diverse values that may be held by others who are involved and that must be considered.

Step Five: Develop Respectful Solutions

Fifth, it is imperative to develop solutions that recognize each person as an autonomous being, worthy of respect. Developing mutually respectful solutions is not a one-step process, but a process that demands attention and work. Care must be taken to find solutions that are in the best interests of patients, but that may also keep relationships intact. Furthermore, this part of the process may also involve examining institutional policies or traditions that are likely to continue to contribute to potential situations of conflict and then advocating for change.

📖 **CASE PRESENTATION**

Facing a Dilemma in the Newborn Nursery

Susan is a nurse employed in the newborn nursery of a small hospital. She is working toward completing her Master's degree and has an important exam she must attend at 4:30 P.M. Susan is scheduled to leave work at 3:00 P.M., but by 4:00 P.M., Dean, the nurse for the next shift, has not yet arrived. Susan knows Dean well and knows that he commutes from out of town and is frequently late. His lateness is tolerated and the nurse manager has never addressed the situation. There is an LPN who is capable of caring for the newborns, but hospital policy requires the presence of an RN in the unit at all times. The supervisor is unable to give her any assistance. All the babies are quiet; she expects Dean to arrive soon and feels the LPN can handle the nursery for a short time. Susan is torn between honouring her duty to patients versus leaving to attend her exam.

❓ **THINK ABOUT IT**

What Should the Nurse Do?

- Is this a practical or an ethical dilemma? What factors make this either a practical or an ethical dilemma?
- Do you think Susan's duty to stay outweighs her obligation to attend her exam?
- What is the harm that could occur if she leaves before Dean arrives?
- What is the harm that could occur if she stays and misses her exam?

The situation in the above case presentation regarding the newborn nursery constitutes a practical dilemma. Moral and non-moral claims are in conflict. Based upon the principles of beneficence, non-maleficence, and fidelity, Susan has a moral obligation to the patients committed to her and to the institution. On the other hand, her obligation to attend class is a matter of self-interest and is not based upon a moral principle *per se*. There is the potential for harm to the newborns if she leaves the unit inappropriately staffed. An emergency could arise for which the LPN is not prepared. Possibly Dean will not arrive at all. If Susan utilizes Kant's moral imperative—one should do only that which could become a rule for all people—a decision to leave the unit unattended by an RN would be untenable. By leaving, she would create a situation that should not become a rule for all nurses in all situations. A rule suggesting that all nurses should leave patients improperly attended could harm many patients in the future and as a result could also harm society's faith in the profession of nursing. Based upon a comparison of moral versus practical considerations and the potential harm that could result if Susan left the unit improperly attended, it seems clear that she should not leave. This is not meant to imply that nurses should always subjugate personal needs to patient or institutional ones. Staying at work later than scheduled as a result of an occasional, unpredictable circumstance is one thing; being required to stay repeatedly is something entirely different. If nurses find that they are being asked to stay late time and time again, they should approach the manager and nursing administration to ensure that there are adequate staffing plans and coverage in place across shifts and units. Coverage and staffing are essential parts of providing safe and quality nursing care to patients. Often, if the practice of staying late goes on consistently and nothing is said, it is understandable why nothing might be done about it by managers or administrators, as long as no negative events occur and no one speaks out. However, clearly, this practice is not in the best interests of patients or nurses. It also might contribute to low morale and a difficult working environment. Supporting all nurses in being able to provide safe, quality care and not feel forced to subjugate personal needs to institutional ones is a key role of nursing leaders.

NURSES' RELATIONSHIPS WITH INSTITUTIONS

Another obligation we have as nurses is to the institution or agency in which we practice. By accepting and maintaining terms of employment and payment for services, we have both a legal and moral obligation to the institution or agency where we work. This obligation, however strong, does not suggest that we should jeopardize personal integrity or subordinate loyalty to the patient. To succeed in the age of technological advancement, competition, and litigation, institutions need the services of nurses who express the professional characteristics of autonomy, integrity, and ethically based practice. Conflicts arise when the institution's goals are focused more on "bottom-line" economics than on moral responsibility and patient welfare. Conflict is inevitable when nurses, whose primary loyalty is to the welfare of patients, are employed by institutions that set priorities in a unilateral or authoritarian manner, without seeking input from front-line workers like nurses. Some examples of these kinds of decisions, often poorly received, include the following: elimination of important programs, employment of poorly qualified staff or inadequate numbers of staff, or other decisions that have a negative effect on patients' needs.

CASE PRESENTATION

When Economy Replaces Excellence

Western District Hospital was a busy acute care centre that serviced a distinct community in a highly urban environment. There were many unique programs and services that met the needs of the ethnically diverse community surrounding the centre. For many years, the hospital maintained excellent nursing care standards. After a period of difficult financial strain, the board of the hospital decided to amalgamate with two other large urban centres in the same city, to create a corporation that would, it was hoped, strengthen each centre and provide financial stability. Each of the three hospitals had a unique personality and set of special services and programs. After much enthusiastic publicity and positive hype, the amalgamation took place.

Immediately after the amalgamation, the hospital, under the auspices of the new corporation, began restructuring the delivery of care at the Western District Hospital, in order to cut back expenses. Important and well-used services were closed and nurses who provided services in these units were moved to other programs. The most junior nurses on the other units were dismissed, after more senior nurses were forced to take their positions. New mission and vision statements were introduced and the unique, highly patient-centred care at Western District was replaced by a clear orientation toward efficiency, episodic care, and an overarching concern for the "bottom line."

It was clear to many nurses that patients would no longer be receiving the excellent nursing care that had been the hallmark of the hospital for many years. However, many nurses felt trapped, as they had worked for years in the same hospital and couldn't imagine working anywhere else, despite the current problems. They also felt powerless to change policies and priorities that were made without consideration for the best interests of the community.

THINK ABOUT IT

How Do Nurses Respond to Bottom-Line Economics?

- What kinds of dilemmas are likely to occur in this situation?
- Recognizing that a nurse's primary responsibility is to patients, how does the new hospital arrangement affect the nurse–patient relationship?
- Can nursing practice maintain a patient-centred, ethically sensitive focus in this type of setting? Discuss your thinking.
- What alternative solutions to potential problems faced by nurses in this situation can you suggest?

We enter the workforce with very different perceptions than our employing institutions. Having learned that autonomy and accountability are valuable components of the nursing role, we believe we have an overarching fiduciary duty to our patients. We also expect that our beliefs will be honoured and that our opinions and knowledge will be respected. Hospitals and other health care institutions, on the other hand, tend to be sharply hierarchical and bureaucratic institutions that expect the primary loyalty of nurses and other subordinates to be to the institution (Jameton, 1984). Institutions expect nurses' actions to be directed toward attaining the goals of the system: goals that may focus strongly upon ensuring the well-being of the institution itself and sustaining patterns of power and control with such secondary goals as "quality" patient care, defined usually by the institutions and not by individual providers. Difficulties arise when there is conflict between the goals of nurses and patients and those of the institution.

Problems arise, in part, because the institution's demands for loyalty are often inequitable (Jameton, 1984). Though requiring employees to accede to certain requests, institutions rarely reciprocate with similar loyalty to nurses. For example, due to budget constraints, most institutions are fairly rigid about nurses' work hours. We are expected to arrive ready to begin, and complete work according to a set schedule. We are sometimes directed to complete more work than can reasonably be done. Nurses, loyal to the institution and to the duty that they feel toward the patients in their care, are often willing to skip meals and breaks and complete work after "clocking out." In essence these practices, though very stressful for nurses, are financially appealing to institutions and are often overlooked by nurse managers and unit administrators, who are also under pressure to adhere to budgetary constraints.

We need to balance professional obligation and the ideal of compassionate service with basic personal commitments. Most nursing organizations and regulatory bodies support the notion of professional development, which may include, at times, attending lectures, seminars, or other learning activities on your own time, with personal sacrifice, such as free time away from work, your lunch hour, or time with family and friends. Sometimes a patient situation or unit issue may require that an individual nurse or group of nurses stay after a shift or at times outside their required working hours, to discuss the situation or attend a meeting. Furthermore, most specialty units, such as coronary care, intensive care units, or operating rooms, require nurses to have additional training and usually will provide financial reimbursement for such. The courses, however, are intense and difficult to fit into a full-time work schedule. These are the kinds of sacrifices and hardships that come along with being a professional and maintaining currency with one's profession. However, consistently repeated, self-sacrificing, altruistic behaviour on the part of nurses is self-defeating, and does not establish conditions of employment conducive to high-quality nursing care. It tends to support and perpetuate a flawed system; as long as nurses continue to work selflessly, the system (rather than the patient) benefits. Nurses willing to work in this way devalue the work of nurses and perpetuate the expectation that this type of one-sided self-sacrifice will continue. Of course, on rare occasions this sort of problem can occur in any institution, but when we repeatedly accept workloads that are unreasonable, we become complicit in continuing the wrongs. Although working extra appears to fulfil both professional obligations and the ideal of compassionate service, it may only meet obligations in a very shallow way and may result in negative outcomes for all stakeholders (Benjamin & Curtis, 2010). In the long run, this type of behaviour is potentially harmful to both patients and nurses. Jameton says:

> A basic choice is forced on those who work in hospitals by the existence of prevalent and systematic problems in health care. If one fails to resist exploitation, incompetence, and corrupt practices, one becomes responsible for them. If one resists them, one enters into conflict with conventional conceptions of behavior for employees and thereby risks reprisals. One has to choose between complicity and self-sacrifice . . . (1984, p. 289)*

Jameton's term *self-sacrifice* is related to the willingness of some nurses to risk reprisals for resisting exploitation in the health care system. He does not suggest that nurses sacrifice all issues of self-interest in favour of institutional interests. Moreover, it is important to be clear that our fiduciary duty does not imply that we should sacrifice our well-being on a consistent basis, in order to protect and further the best interests of our patients. Certainly, if that is the case, it is highly indicative of an unhealthy and problematic work environment and one in which there are significant issues of organizational ethics.

In some instances, we base the motivation for altruism on misguided beliefs about duty. Some believe that altruism is necessary to fulfil their duty to patients. Though many philosophers consider altruism and sacrifice to be virtues, Ayn Rand (1996) suggested that altruism may also have dehumanizing effect. Rand believed that those who are altruistic have a nightmare view of existence—believing that people are trapped in a malevolent universe. Using the term *self-sacrifice* in a fashion nearly opposite to that of Jameton, Rand viewed a persistent willingness to sacrifice as flowing from poor self-esteem and inappropriate priority setting. Moreover, she believed that those with poor self-esteem have difficulty valuing others. Because genuine regard is partially a product of sympathy (imagining oneself in the situation of another), one must value oneself in order to value others. Additionally, nurses who repeatedly sacrifice for the good of an institutional system fail to assume the power to change the wrongs that are committed.

CASE PRESENTATION

When Patients Suffer from Lack of Nursing Care

Tim, an RN, works weekends on the skilled nursing unit of a small rural hospital that recently underwent significant financial hardship. Forced to amalgamate with a much larger urban centre, the hospital then dismissed nearly one-third of the staff of the skilled nursing unit. Lately, when Tim comes to work, he feels

(Continued)

---

* *JAMETON, A., NURSING PRACTICE: THE ETHICAL ISSUES, 1st Edition* © *1983.* Printed and Electronically reproduced by permission of Pearson Education, Inc., Upper Saddle River, New Jersey.

totally overwhelmed. Although he always considered himself efficient, Tim is distressed because he rarely has enough time to complete his work. He knows that many of the patients suffer because of lack of attention. Those who are bedridden are not turned on a regular schedule, they often wait for assistance with eating until their food is cold, and medications are rarely given on time. Suffering from expressive aphasia and hemiplegia secondary to a CVA, Mrs. Wallace was admitted to the skilled nursing unit after two weeks in the intensive care unit. Mrs. Wallace has been on the skilled nursing unit for three weeks when her daughter, Nina, notices a large reddened area surrounding a small gray ulcer over her mother's coccyx. Concerned, Nina asks Tim what caused this problem. Even though Mrs. Wallace's nursing care plan calls for attention to activity, including frequent turning and sitting in a chair twice daily, Tim suspects that this was not consistently done the previous week. He recognizes that the reddened area is the beginning of a large pressure ulcer, a problem that might have been prevented with proper attention to activity and good nutrition. Tim hesitates to tell Nina that the problem is a potentially serious one that might have been prevented by good nursing care measures. He believes she has a right to know, but is hesitant to implicate himself or the other nurses, and he is afraid that he will lose his job if he complains.

 THINK ABOUT IT

How Do Nurses Make Decisions When Loyalties Conflict?

- What are the ethical principles implicit in this situation?
- What are Tim's conflicting loyalties?
- The remaining staff on the unit is efficient and hard-working—skipping lunch and staying overtime to complete their work. Do you believe the staff is responsible for the apparently poor nursing care that Mrs. Wallace is getting?
- Do you believe Tim should tell Nina the truth about the pressure sore?
- Should Tim risk losing his job by whistleblowing?
- Is this an ethical or practical dilemma?
- What harm can result from either option?
- What would you do?

The previous case presentation is another example of a practical dilemma. The conflict that Tim is experiencing is between the principle of beneficence (the desire to do good for the patient) and a sense of loyalty to the institution or the other nurses with whom he works. There may also be an element of self-interest—Tim may not want to be implicated in the harm that the patients are experiencing as a result of the staff cutbacks. Tim's fiduciary duty is owed to the patients—Mrs. Wallace in particular, other patients suffering from the shortage of staff, and future patients who could potentially be harmed by perpetuation of the problem. Keeping in mind that the notion of a fiduciary duty implies putting aside one's own interests or agendas, there are strong arguments that he should act to correct the situation. He may choose to take any number of actions: he can work through the administrative hierarchy to improve staffing; he can answer Nina's questions honestly; though his job will certainly be jeopardized, he can inform the media of the problems that were created by the drastic staffing shortages. In any case, if Tim fails to act to solve the problem, he will be complicit in its perpetuation and the subsequent harm to patients.

Another example related to the inequitable demands of institutions for loyalty is seen in the customary practice of requiring nurses to complete incident reports. Institutions may discourage nurses from talking to patients about mistakes that have been made. They much prefer that nurses file incident reports. These documents, geared toward institutional goals, are filed and kept for use in the event the hospital needs a legal defence, use in firing or disciplining workers, or use in reorganizing services to prevent future incidents (Jameton, 1984). Thus, patient-centred goals based on the principles of autonomy, fidelity, veracity, and respect for persons are subordinated to institutional goals of employee control and risk management.

Nurses' loyalty to the institution is an important mode of control. Without loyalty, administrators cannot manage institutions (Jameton, 1984). For this reason supervisors and administrators sometimes react negatively when nurses support and co-operate with each other to make changes. The ensuing perception of nonsupportive supervisors is a contributing factor to job stress and dissatisfaction (Moore, Kuhrik, Kuhrik & Katz, 1996). In the end, this can be harmful to nurses and patients alike. Jameton says, "Where institutions as a whole fail to serve patients well, this demand for loyalty can interfere with the nurses' expressions of loyalty to nurses and patients" (1984, p. 121).

NURSES' RELATIONSHIPS WITH OTHER NURSES

Nurses work together in close proximity, day in and day out. No other profession is so intimately connected with issues of life, death, and personal care. The knowledge gained from the intimate experiences of birth, illness, life, and death are powerful. Nurses are connected to each other and set apart from others: connected by common experience, language, and knowledge, and set apart through a perceived professional mystique. Nurses work together closely, identify with each other, and supervise or are supervised by other nurses. The practice of one affects the practice of others.

Loyalty is a natural product of long-term acquaintance and close working relationships. Some view loyalty among members as a distinguishing characteristic of a profession. Jameton defines loyalty as:

> showing sympathy, care, and reciprocity to those with whom we appropriately identify; working closely with others toward shared goals; keeping promises; making mutual concerns a priority; sacrificing personal interests to the relationship; and giving attention to these over a substantial period of time. It supports showing respect for persons. And it resolves potential conflicts in autonomy by making values and goals that I see as my own more like values and goals of those who work with me. (1984, p. 118)*

Promoting faithfulness and commitment, loyalty is very limited and exclusive in its scope. Though normally viewed as admirable, loyalty is seldom regarded as a cardinal virtue because of its inherent potential for fanaticism and blind injustice (Honderich, 2005).

In practical matters, loyalty is a productive virtue. It enhances unity, strength, and power. Facing bureaucratic, economic, and political forces, our loyalty to each other and to the profession adds strength to our call for improved patient care, public welfare, nursing autonomy, and optimum employment conditions.

While having the potential to strengthen the profession of nursing and improve the welfare of patients, loyalty among nurses can also result in negative outcomes, when not prioritized alongside other loyalties and obligations. Though our primary obligation is to patients, those of us who are overly loyal to other nurses might act in ways that are harmful to patients' health status. For example, a nurse having blind loyalty to another nurse might cover up a co-worker's incompetent practice, illegal drug use, or other actions that have the potential to harm present or future patients. For this reason, we must be careful to maintain objectivity in balancing loyalty to nurses and the profession against the obligation owed to patients. Part of being a self-regulating profession means monitoring incidents of professional misconduct. Legal definitions of professional misconduct are complex and vary between provinces, with different legislation governing the regulatory practice of nursing. However, one principle is clear. Failure to report unethical or unsafe practice of another member of the profession is clearly misconduct. As a licensed professional, you have an ethical and professional responsibility (and in most cases, a legal one as well) to report incidents of unsafe, harmful, or unethical behaviour of another licensed professional nurse. The method by which it is reported or addressed should be thoughtful, maintain confidentiality, and be directed toward the appropriate person, agency, or regulatory body (College of Nurses of Ontario, 2000).

CHALLENGES IN NURSES' RELATIONSHIPS WITH OTHER NURSES: WORKPLACE INCIVILITY

Workplace incivility encompasses a number of phenomena that are interrelated and all concerning. Horizontal or lateral violence, bullying in the workplace, harassment,

---

* *JAMETON, A., NURSING PRACTICE: THE ETHICAL ISSUES, 1st Edition © 1983.* Printed and Electronically reproduced by permission of Pearson Education, Inc., Upper Saddle River, New Jersey.

oppression, sabotage (Dunn, 2003) and "nursing eating its young" (Tunajek, 2007, p. 3) are all examples of the kinds of phenomena that are identified in discussions of nursing workplace incivility.

In nursing, the issue of workplace incivility is sometimes discussed as bullying in nursing (Randle, 2003). Bullying is defined as consistent behaviours that demean and degrade others (Adams, 1997). Randle's 2003 landmark article in the *Journal of Advanced Nursing* describes the experience of nursing students, who describe bullying behaviours from supervising nurses as "distressing" (p. 397). This phenomenon has been referred to colloquially in nursing as "eating your young" (Truman, 2004; Tunajek, 2007), an expression that refers to, at best, the inability to nurture those who are younger or less experienced than oneself and, at worst, the practice of cutting down, demeaning, or demoralizing those who are younger. It is suggested by some that the victimization or bullying of younger and less experienced colleagues has long been a part of nursing, still a highly hierarchical profession (Farrell, 2001). It is considered a kind of horizontal violence, which is defined as, "harmful attitudes, actions, words and other behaviours directed toward nurses by colleagues. Horizontal violence humiliates, denigrates, and injures the dignity of another, and it indicates a lack of mutual respect and denies fundamental individual rights." (Tunajek, 2007, p. 3)

This practice, according to Truman (2004) and others who have also discussed this phenomenon (Pugh, 2005; Randle, 2003) contributes to low rates of job satisfaction, poor self-esteem, and low retention rates for new nurses. For many nurses, this kind of workplace incivility can have physical and psychological consequences, including hypertension, irritable bowel syndrome, weight gain or loss, depression, anxiety, and post-traumatic stress disorder (Woelfle & McCaffrey, 2007). Each of these, in turn, contributes to poor patient care, and in some cases, may lead to further and continued demeaning treatment to patients and other nurses in turn. In fact, Pugh (2005) and Randle (2003) both emphasize that bullying nursing students leads to those same students bullying others, patients, and younger nursing students. In other words, without attention and dialogue about this pervasive problem, it will continue in a cyclical fashion, as victims become perpetrators.

Does bullying and demeaning of younger workers occur only in nursing? Certainly not. It occurs across professions, genders, and environments (Pugh, 2005). It may be more visible in nursing because of the expectation that nurses will always display only nurturing and caring behaviours to all around them. It also may be more visible because the work of nursing is done in the public eye. Nursing stations are out in the open, with conversations and activities visible to anyone who may walk by. Nursing care is often carried out in corridors and shared rooms. Medication rooms, utility rooms, and kitchens in hospitals are shared by a variety of allied health professionals, as well as patients and family members. However, there are also claims that this kind of workplace incivility may not be obvious to outsiders. It may be composed of "innocent" or "joking" remarks that seem innocuous to others and that may be taken ambiguously. Often, these kinds of remarks result in others pushing back with more intentional actions or remarks that, if continued, can reach a kind of tipping point, through cyclical but more serious remarks and behaviours. This, according to Tunajek (2007) can contribute to a "toxic environment" (p. 30) in which nurses must practice.

According to Pugh (2005), the vulnerability of nurses to workplace incivility may result from two things. First, it may be due to the tremendous workload that most nurses deal with on a daily basis. The stress and fatigue that go alongside this degree and intensity of work may contribute to displacement of stress and anxiety onto other nurses. With increasing technology, an aging workforce, and shortages in the profession in Canada, workload will continue to be an issue. The second factor Pugh refers to is the fact that many nurses are, in fact, excluded from the power structure of their workplace and have limited input into decision making that affects their own professional lives. This lack of power can contribute to lateral violence, as is commonly seen in other kinds of social groups who are oppressed and lack power in their daily lives (Dunn, 2003).

Other kinds of negative behaviours that may contribute to workplace incivility include oppressed group behaviours and silencing behaviours. These two types of behaviours tend to characterize groups rather than individuals and both may become cyclical. "Oppressed group behaviours" refers to a group of learned behaviours that include low self-esteem, powerlessness, frustration, and a perceived lack of mutual support that can lead individuals to believe that they cannot rely on anyone other than themselves (DeMarco and Roberts, 2003). The lack of autonomy and control acknowledged by those who exhibit oppressed group behaviours leads to feeling unsupported by others, and in turn to an inability to support those within the group. Many may feel that they have nothing left to give to others, as the demand for self-reliance is too great. "Silencing behaviours" are learned behaviours that are seen more often in women than in men. They occur when individuals are more valued or rewarded for silence and lack of expression of feelings or emotions, and so those individuals learn to avoid outspokenness or having any kind of meaningful voice. The overarching feelings of powerlessness that result from silencing behaviours can lead to a lack of assertion and denial of feelings and emotions, as well as conflict avoidance. Often, in situations where silencing behaviours are found, conflict acknowledgement or resolution is replaced by silence and avoidance. In nursing, this is often also characterized by the lack of a "public voice" (Buresh and Gordon, 2000) and a subsequent lack of appreciation among members of the public and decision-making bodies, who may not understand the work that nurses do or the impact that nursing care has.

Workplace Harassment

In law, some of the behaviours that are considered examples of workplace incivility are categorized under the label of "personal harassment." However, the term is, to some degree, poorly defined, and the problem is much too infrequently discussed in public venues. The Canadian Human Rights Commission (2006) defines "harassment" and "personal harassment" as follows:

Harassment is any behaviour that demeans, humiliates or embarrasses a person, and that a reasonable person should have known would be unwelcome. It includes actions (e.g., touching, pushing), comments (e.g., jokes, name-calling), or displays (e.g., posters, cartoons). The *Canadian Human Rights Act* prohibits harassment related to race, national or ethnic origin, colour, religion, age, sex, marital status, family status, disability, pardoned conviction, or sexual orientation.

Disrespectful behaviour, commonly known as "personal" harassment is not covered by human rights legislation. While it also involves unwelcome behaviour that demeans or embarrasses an employee, the behaviour is not based on one of the prohibited grounds named above. Nevertheless, some employers choose to include personal harassment in their anti-harassment policies. (p. 3)*

Under Canada's *Labour Code,* all employers are required to design their own policies and guidelines for workplace harassment. However, many workers are unaware that such policies exist or that they have specific rights in regard to how they are to be treated by colleagues and supervisors.

Many nurses who experience harassment or bullying, according to Pugh (2005), don't seek help or advice from their supervisors or institutions, and sooner or later leave the profession. Research demonstrates that nurses who report high rates of conflict also report high rates of burnout, which can lead many to abandon the profession altogether (Rowell, 2005).

What options are available to nurses who experience harassment or bullying? First, most institutions now have policies regarding harassment, and often have officers or employees designated to deal with harassment and discrimination issues. Universities (and some hospitals) typically have harassment and discrimination offices, which take complaints from students, faculty members, and employees, and conduct investigations.

In Ontario, Bill 168 was introduced in 2009 and passed in 2010; this legislation amends the *Occupational Health and Safety Act*, requiring every workplace in Ontario with more than five employees to create clear written policies on workplace violence and harassment that are reviewed annually, to provide training on these policies and programs, and to implement them across the institution (Legislative Assembly of Ontario, 2009). In addition, many professional organizations have developed written guidelines for addressing workplace incivility, such as the Registered Nurses Association of Ontario "Preventing and Managing Violence in the Workplace" document (RNAO, 2009).

Making managers and nurse leaders aware of these kinds of problems can help, as a start. Programs and informal support systems can be put in place to address issues like these and to create initiatives and simple solutions for addressing these kinds of behaviours, making the workplace an easier and more positive environment, and increasing satisfaction, self-esteem, and retention.

---

* Source: 1.2 Identifying Harassment. Anti-Harassment Policies for the Workplace: An Employer's Guide, March 2006, http://www.chrc-ccdp.ca/publications/anti_harassment_toc-eng.aspx Immigration and Refugee Board of Canada. Reproduced with the permission of the Minster of Public Works and Government Services Canada, 2012.

NURSES' RELATIONSHIPS WITH OTHER HEALTH CARE PROFESSIONALS

Nurses work within the context of an interdisciplinary team. We work most closely with physicians, and much of the literature on teamwork in nursing focuses on nurses' relationships with physicians. Nurses' relationships with physicians are an important factor in the quality of patient care. Ideally, the work of nurses and physicians should be complementary and synergistic. Because both professions hold claim to the primary goal of patient health, one would expect a strong sense of collegiality and collaboration between nurses and physicians. When this kind of a relationship does exist, it is rewarding and productive. When there is conflict between nurses and physicians, the relationship is stressful and damaging to nurses, physicians, and patients alike. Because nurses and physicians work in close proximity, conflict that occurs between them is a strong contributor to the lack of job satisfaction for nurses.

Nurse–physician relationships have generally reflected the prevailing gender roles in society. These roles were clearly defined for centuries. The traditional nurse was expected to obey the physician, much as the wife was expected to obey her husband. Physicians demanded obedience, and nurses hesitated to disagree with physicians, even if there was good reason to do so. Unfortunately, these attitudes have lingered, to some degree, in both professions (Benjamin & Curtis, 2010).

Given the bureaucratic nature of most health care institutions, particularly hospitals, the relationship between physicians and nurses is complex and peculiar. Generally, nurses are employees of the institutions, while physicians are independent practitioners who have the privilege of institutional practice. Physicians, who may not be employees of the institutions, have no formal chain-of-command relationship with the nurses who care for their patients. Curtin and Flaherty (1982) write, "This tradition of self-employed 'guest practitioners' in health care institutions having so much power over the large groups of 'full-time employees' of the institutions defies explanation, but it is a fact of life in health care" (p. 144). Though they issue orders to nurses directly, physicians are not employed by, subordinate to, or even responsible to the institutional administration. These dual lines of authority are confusing, and have the potential to severely limit the autonomous decision-making role of the nurse (Benjamin & Curtis, 2010). Because most nurses are employees with either expressed or implied contracts with institutions, they have an obligation to perform the tasks required by the institutions. One of the major tasks that most institutions require of nurses is the implementation of physicians' orders. When nurses question or disagree with physicians, they may feel distressed, believing they are being disloyal to both the physician and the institution.

Another contributor to conflict in the nurse–physician relationship is the rapid advent of advanced practice nursing. Having an expanded knowledge base and a unique scope of practice that includes many functions that were once the sole domain of physicians, advanced practice nursing can contribute to the tensions that exist between nurses and physicians. The outmoded tradition of the nurse who obeys the physician is in direct conflict with the autonomous nurse who thinks independently, makes nursing diagnoses, and implements independent nursing actions (Benjamin & Curtis, 2010).

What actions should be taken by the nurse who questions or disagrees with an order or action of a physician? The nurse must remember that the primary obligation is owed to the patient, not the physician. Nurses are autonomous practitioners. They have the knowledge and experience, and the legal and ethical responsibility, to make independent judgments, even when carrying out physicians' orders. Since a nurse is also responsible for patient care, carrying out orders that may be incorrect or unsafe, or against the explicit wishes of the patient, may well constitute an ethical and legal issue for the nurse as well as the physician. When deciding what action to take in situations where nurses disagree with physicians' orders, Benjamin and Curtis (2010) suggest that nurses apply the test of the **spectrum of urgency**. At one end of this spectrum are problems that are minor and may be solved at a more leisurely pace. At the other end are urgent problems that require quick solutions and immediate actions. The low-urgency end of the spectrum includes situations where there is little risk of serious harm, or there is significant time available to examine all aspects of the situation. The high-urgency end of the spectrum consists of emergencies in which lifesaving actions must be carried out at once. Nurses may have time to discuss and negotiate satisfactory solutions to problems at the low-urgency end of the spectrum, but problems at the high-urgency end of the spectrum require efficient and timely action.

CASE PRESENTATION

Making a Decision in an Urgent Situation

Ramanthy is the night-shift charge nurse in the emergency department of a small but busy hospital. She has advanced certification and twenty-five years of experience. Ramanthy works well with the other members of the emergency room staff, and is comfortable and efficient in situations of extreme urgency. The emergency department is usually staffed by emergency physicians. Because one of the regular physicians recently moved away, there have been a series of physicians with various degrees of preparation and ability moonlighting in the department, particularly on the night shift. During an unusually busy shift, an ambulance arrives with a middle-aged man having severe chest pain and dyspnoea. His condition quickly deteriorates, and after a few minutes he experiences cardiac and respiratory arrest. The physician on duty, Dr. Andrews, is a family practice physician moonlighting after his regular shift at a local community health centre. Ramanthy perceives Dr. Andrews as nervous and hesitant. During the first phase of the "code," Dr. Andrews seems uncertain of every detail. As the nurse in charge, Ramanthy begins instituting a seldom-used protocol that was

(Continued)

developed for use in the event that the nurses are faced with a cardiac arrest when no physician is present. All the nurses are trained in intubation techniques, but hospital policy prohibits them from performing that particular procedure. Ramanthy suggests to Dr. Andrews that he intubate the patient. After several clumsy attempts, Dr. Andrews angrily orders Ramanthy to call an anesthesiologist at home to come and intubate the patient. Ramanthy realizes that the patient's chances of survival are best if he is intubated quickly. She asks the unit clerk to call the anesthesiologist. Over his angry objections, Ramanthy removes the laryngoscope and endotracheal tube from Dr. Andrews's trembling hands and proceeds to intubate the patient quickly and successfully. The patient responds to resuscitation attempts and is discharged five days later.

THINK ABOUT IT

Was Ramanthy's Decision Correct?

- What is your immediate response to the situation in which Ramanthy finds herself?
- Where would you place this situation on the "spectrum of urgency"?
- What are the arguments in favour of Ramanthy's actions?
- What are the arguments in favour of Ramanthy's following Dr. Andrews's orders?
- Do you consider Ramanthy's actions to be based upon ethical principle?
- Did Ramanthy place herself at risk of reprisal, legal action, or professional disciplinary action?
- What would you have done?

Nurses are charged with making thoughtful, fair, and knowledgeable decisions in relation to questioning physicians' orders, while also being careful to consider the overall harm that can result from any given action. Recognizing that the physician's goal, like that of the nurse, is the welfare of the patient, we must be mature and objective when questioning orders. Nurses have an ethical obligation to protect the patient from medical incompetence. Nevertheless, we must be careful in this regard, keeping in mind the overall harm that can result from the practice of constantly and inappropriately questioning insignificant aspects of physicians' orders.

WORKING AS PART OF A TEAM

While maintaining an awareness of the primary obligation owed to patients, nurses must be sensitive to those who work beside them. Each person is a moral agent and must be recognized as worthy of dignity and respect. As the co-ordinator of patient care, the professional nurse is accountable for the quality of nursing care rendered to patients. This accountability includes supervision, delegation of nursing care functions, and disciplining of other health care providers. The inherent practical, moral, and legal implications of these functions are facets of the role of professional nurse that must be undertaken with sensitivity and respect.

The structure of health care delivery in some institutional settings makes the professional nurse responsible for delegating a number of nursing functions to staff members such as licensed practical nurses, personal support workers, personal care providers, and nursing students. As the co-ordinator of patient care, the registered nurse is accountable for all nursing care that patients receive, whether from the nurse directly or from other members of the nursing care team, including nursing students.

Registered nurses have a twofold responsibility. Their primary duty is to the patient, to ensure that the care provided is appropriate, high-quality, and individualized. However, an ethical duty also exists to those we work with as a team. The Canadian Nurses Association notes in its *Code of Ethics* that, as part of being accountable, "Nurses share their knowledge and provide feedback, mentorship and guidance for the professional development of nursing students, novice nurses and other health-care team members" (CNA, 2008, p. 18). Furthermore, the code goes on to note that "Nurses treat each other, colleagues, students and other health-care workers in a respectful manner, recognizing the power differentials among those in formal leadership positions, staff and students. They work with others to resolve differences in a constructive way" (CNA, 2008, p. 49).

As mentioned earlier, one discouraging phenomenon is poor treatment of and lack of mentorship for nursing students. Many students enter their clinical practice with high expectations and an overly idealistic outlook. While it is important to acclimatize them to the realities and challenges of the health care system, demoralizing them by belittling their abilities or acting in an intimidating manner serves no constructive purpose and furthers the image of nurses "eating their young." This expression describes the phenomenon of being hard on those who are more junior, in order to teach them the realities of the roles they are aiming to fulfil one day. It also refers to the practice of not supporting nursing students and novice nurses, by challenging them, leaving them on their own without adequate knowledge or resources, being unfriendly or unapproachable, or presenting professional work and skills as being behind a veil of mystique, inaccessible to novices or students not "in the know." These types of practices are counterproductive to quality patient care and the sustainability of the profession. They are also unethical and highly unprofessional, even worthy of being labelled as professional misconduct, if serious enough.

In addition to delegation, the supervisory role of professional nurses occasionally includes disciplining of others. Disciplining is a difficult task that must be done with insight, respect, compassion, and logic. The nurse must be keenly aware of the effect of disciplinary action upon others and must focus on the intended goal. The traditional methods of discipline, such as punishment and chastisement, are damaging to the spirit and counterproductive in practice.

Nurse managers' method of disciplining may set the tone for the entire nursing unit. Discussing poor leadership, Dilley says, "Nurse managers from hell can be easily identified. They use coercion—as in, 'do as I say or you'll find yourself on the night shift.' They belittle their employees in front of patients or other staff. They communicate by memo rather than face-to-face. They change policies without input from others. They are rude and thoughtless" (2000, p. 9).

A good nurse manager may also set the tone of the unit through the style of discipline. Quoting the great teacher Maria Montessori, Leah Curtin (1996) writes, "'Our aim is to discipline for activity, for work, for good; not for immobility, not for passivity, not for obedience'" (p. 51). Curtin suggests that the most meaningful method is self-discipline, which corrects the problem, strengthens the character of the worker, and improves performance. She defines discipline as a process by which the rules are internalized and become a part of the individual's personality. This process is possible only if the person knows the rules, understands their purpose, and agrees that they deserve compliance. To achieve this result, the nurse must model the expected standard daily and have few rules—all of which are applied consistently, change infrequently, and apply to all personnel equally. The nurse has a moral obligation to both patients and personnel to uphold rules that protect the health and safety of patients, other employees, the institution, and oneself as leader (Curtin, 1996, p. 51).

MOVING FORWARD

Maintaining moral integrity in the face of conflict can be challenging. Often conflict in the workplace can make us feel drained and discouraged, but it is important to realize that these conflicts are also positive opportunities for professional and personal growth and change. This growth and change, however, doesn't happen all at once. It is part of an iterative journey that we undertake as moral agents. What are some strategies for dealing with conflicts in ways that can contribute to ones' moral integrity? First, it is important to understand others' perspectives, motives, and intentions, especially those that are very different from your own. Active listening, asking questions, and acknowledgement of the importance of diverse opinions about complex problems are key activities involved in understanding the views of others. Advocating for what you feel is right is also an important part of maintaining moral integrity. Many times, students talk about how difficult the possibility of speaking up for a patient might seem, especially as less experienced and more junior members of the team. Like any virtue, advocacy, when practiced, can develop further. Advocating for small issues at first can help one develop skills for advocating for patients when more is at stake. Finally, finding and recognizing moral mentors is a key step in development as a moral agent. Having a trusted colleague or former respected teacher as a moral mentor to turn to in times of adversity or conflict, to help you work through a problem, can be an invaluable resource and can help build capacity, support networks, and trust among colleagues.

SUMMARY

In the professional realm, nurses are faced with the dichotomy of striving to meet their primary obligation to patients while dealing with problems among providers and within the institutional system. Nurses must be prepared to examine personal beliefs, prioritize obligations, and devise morally sound solutions to problems. Solutions must reflect an overall respect for persons and recognize the moral agency of individuals. Nurses are guided in this endeavour by personal values and beliefs and by professional codes of ethics.

CHAPTER HIGHLIGHTS

- As a moral agent, each person has the duty to pursue solutions to moral problems.
- Maintaining moral integrity is a learning journey, as is the development of any virtue.
- Problems or conflicts that occur related to other ethical principles can easily become conflicts of integrity.
- Solutions to practical and ethical problems in the professional realm must be sensitive to personal values and beliefs.
- Nurses must be able to identify and prioritize conflicting obligations.
- It is important for nurses to acknowledge and examine conflicts in the professional realm.
- Problem resolution requires thoughtful consideration and weighing of alternative solutions.
- In solving problems, nurses must recognize that each person is an autonomous being with unique values, worthy of respect.
- Nurses must seek solutions to moral problems related to conflicting role expectations in the institutional setting.
- Nurses must seek solutions to moral and practical problems related to relationships among nurses, physicians, and other health care professionals.

DISCUSSION QUESTIONS AND ACTIVITIES

1. Describe some potential problems that you have experienced, in the professional realm or in your personal life, that fall into each of the following categories:

- Conflicts of obligation
- Conflicts of principle
- Practical dilemmas
- Conflicts of loyalty

2.   Discuss with your classmates situations that could reasonably occur in the work setting that would constitute an appeal to conscience.

3.   More new graduate nurses are leaving the profession in the first two years of practice, than ever before. What do you think are the challenges that they face that lead them to the decision to leave? What should the nursing profession change in order to address this phenomenon?

4.   Think about moral mentors you have had in the past. What attributes have they had that made them a strong resource for helping with working through complex moral problems or conflicts?

5.   List the positive and negative aspects of loyalty. Do you feel loyalty is a virtue, no matter what?

6.   Describe what you consider to be an ideal professional relationships that can occur between nurses and physicians.

7.   Think about the practice settings you have been in previously. Have you ever witnessed a practice that has made you uneasy or concerned? Think about how you dealt with this situation and how you would deal with it if faced with the same thing today.

REFERENCES

Adams, A. (1997). Bullying at work—How to confront and overcome it. Virago Press: London.

American Nurses Association (2010). Code of ethics for nurses with interpretive statements. Washington, DC: Author. Retrieve May 2, 2012 from http://www.nursingworld.org/MainMenuCategories/EthicsStandards/CodeofEthicsforNurses/Code-of-Ethics.pdf

Benjamin, M., & J. Curtis (2010). Ethics in nursing (4th ed.). New York: Oxford University Press.

Buresh, B. G., & S. Gordon (2000). From silence to voice: What nurses know and must communicate to the public. Ithaca, NY: Cornell University Press.

Canadian Human Rights Commission. (2006). Anti-harassment policies for the workplace: An employer's guide. Ottawa: Canadian Human Rights Commission. Retrieved May 2, 2012, from http://www.chrc-ccdp.ca/publications/anti_harassment_toc-en.asp#12.

Canadian Nurses Association (2008). Code of ethics for registered nurses. Author.

Childress, J. (1978). Appeals to conscience. Ethics, 89, 316–321.

College of Nurses of Ontario. (2000). Accountability means taking action. Communiqué, 25(4). Retrieved August 19, 2008, from http://www.cno.org/pubs/mag/cmqVol25no4.pdf.

Curtin, L. (1996). Ethics, discipline and discharge. Nursing Management, 27(3), 51–52.

Curtin, L., & M. J. Flaherty (1982). Nursing ethics: Theories and pragmatics. Bowie, MD: Brady.

DeMarco, R. F., & S. J. Roberts (2003). Negative behaviours in nursing. American Journal of Nursing, 103(3), 113–116.

Department of Justice Canada. (1985). Canada Labour Code. Ottawa: Department of Justice. Retrieved May 2, 2012, from http://laws.justice.gc.ca/en/L-2/.

Dilley, K. B. (2000). Out from under their thumbs. *American Journal of Nursing, 100*(5), 9.

Dunn, H. (2003). Horizontal violence among nurses in the operating room. AORN Online. 78(6).

Farrell, G. A. (2001). From tall poppies to squashed weeds: Why don't nurses pull together more? *Journal of Advanced Nursing, 35*(1), 26–33.

Honderich, T., ed. (2005). The Oxford companion to philosophy. 2nd edition. New York: Oxford University Press.

International Council of Nurses (2006). The ICN code of ethics for nurses. International Council of Nurses, Geneva, Switzerland. Retrieved May 2, 2012 from http://www.icn.ch/images/stories/documents/about/icncode_english.pdf

Jameton, A. (1984). Nursing practice: The ethical issues. Englewood Cliffs, NJ: Prentice-Hall.

Legislative Assembly of Ontario. (2009). Bill 168: Occupational Health and Safety Act Amendment (Violence and Harassment in the Workplace) 2009. Retrieved on May 3, 2012 from: http://www.ontla.on.ca/web/bills/bills_detail.do?locale=en&BillID=2181

Moore, S., M. Kuhrik, N. Kuhrik & B. Katz (1996). Coping with downsizing: Stress, self-esteem and social intimacy. *Nursing Management, 27*(3), 28–30.

Peter, E. (2011). Fostering social justice: The possibility of a socially connected model of moral agency. *Canadian Journal of Nursing Research, 43*(2), 11–17.

Pugh, A. (2005). Bullying in nursing: Building a culture of respect combats lateral violence. Cross Currents (Winter) (n.p.).

Rand, A. (1996). The ethics of emergencies. In J. Feinberg, ed., Reason and responsibility: Readings in some basic problems of philosophy (9th ed., pp. 541–545). Belmont, CA: Wadsworth.

Randle, J. (2003). Bullying in the nursing profession. *Journal of Advanced Nursing. 43*(4), 395–401.

Registered Nurses Association of Ontario. (2009). Preventing and Managing Violence in the Workplace. Toronto: RNAO. Retrieved on May 3, 2012 from: http://www.rnao.org/Page.asp?PageID=122&ContentID=2972

Rodney, P., S. Kadyschuk, J. Liaschenko, H. Brown, L. Musto & N. Snyder (2013). Moral agency: Relational connections and support. In J. L. Storch, P. Rodney & R. Stazomski , eds. Toward a Moral Horizon: Nursing ethics for leadership and practice. 2nd edition. Toronto: Pearson.

Rowell, P. (2005). Being a "target" at work: Or William Tell and how the apple felt. *Journal of Nursing Administration, 35*(9), 377.

Truman, K. M. (2004). Education enhances recruitment and retention in the emergency department. Don't eat your young, nurse them. *Nursing Management, 35*(7), 45–48.

Tunajek, S. (2007). Workplace incivility – Part 1: Anger, Harassment and Horizontal Violence. AANA News Bulletin. March.

Woelfle, C. Y., & R. McCaffrey (2007). Nurse on nurse. *Nursing Forum, 42*(3).

Yeo, M., A. Moorhouse, P. Khan & P. Rodney (2010). Concepts and Cases in Nursing Ethics. 3rd edition. Toronto: Broadview.

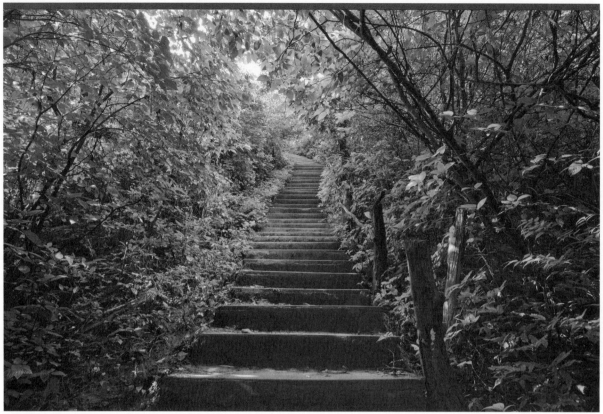

CHAPTER **10**

PRACTICE ISSUES RELATED TO END-OF-LIFE CARE

OBJECTIVES

After completing this chapter, the reader should be able to:

1. Discuss the impact of technology on nursing and health care at the end of life.
2. Apply beneficence and non-maleficence to decisions about technology.
3. Discuss issues and dilemmas related to current technology and to life-sustaining interventions.
4. Relate the concept of medical futility to health care decisions.
5. Relate economics to decisions regarding health technology and medical futility.

6. Discuss considerations in decisions about cardiopulmonary resuscitation and artificial sources of nutrition for patients.

7. Describe legal issues associated with end-of-life care.

8. Describe palliative care nursing.

9. Discuss the general principles behind, and effective nursing strategies for, having a palliative care family conference.

10. Describe nursing considerations for patient care in the midst of technology at the end of life.

INTRODUCTION

Nursing care, in a variety of environments and contexts, will inevitably involve care of patients who are at the end of their lives. As nurses, we provide care throughout the entire trajectory of a life, and end-of-life care is a significant responsibility of nurses within a multidisciplinary team. At the very end of a life, it is, more often than not, the nurses who are with the patient at all times and play a major role in *how* patients' lives end. This awesome responsibility brings with it significant challenges and ethical concerns. The use of technology, quality of life, medical futility, and decision making are important concepts in all aspects of health and nursing care, but become paramount in the context of providing nursing care at the end of a life.

THE USE OF TECHNOLOGY AT THE END OF LIFE

The term *technology* includes a vast range of scientific advances that affect health and health care. Technology has become an integral part of how patient care is provided. While many of us are accustomed to technology as a constant presence in health care, it can create complex ethical dilemmas. Technology can alter the way we communicate and provide care. Issues of technology, patient self-determination, futility, and feasibility are very much intertwined and, as nurses, we must be aware of our values and beliefs about what constitutes a humanistic caring role and what detracts from that role. Rapidly evolving technologies present the challenge of dealing with new kinds of ethical issues, and nurses in all practice settings must be prepared to face this challenge.

The Benefits and Challenges of Technology

Scientific advances in the past hundred years have been phenomenal. These advances include medications, surgical techniques, machines and equipment, diagnostic procedures, specialized treatments, expanded understanding of the causes of disease and the progression of disease, gene diagnosis and therapy, and greater insight into what is required for people to stay healthy. New interventions have saved lives, improved quality of life, alleviated suffering, and significantly decreased the incidence of some diseases. Before the advent of many modern health-related technologies, people experienced illness and death as an inevitable part of the cycle of their lives. Although death was not necessarily welcomed, it was expected as the natural outcome when the body could no longer ward off the effects of certain diseases or injuries. If someone was born with, or developed, a deformity or disability, it may have been seen as a bad stroke of luck or even a curse, but was also considered part of who the person was. Life began when the infant started breathing, and life ended when the heart and breathing stopped.

In all practice settings, nursing care is inextricably intertwined with ever-expanding advances of scientific knowledge and technology. However, the many benefits brought to the health care arena by technology are often accompanied by serious dilemmas for both practitioners and patients. Technology brings to the fore many questions related to issues of living and especially dying, and the changing definitions of both that are brought on by scientific advances. While not all questions and issues result in ethical dilemmas, many can and do. These kinds of dilemmas may include the availability of and accessibility to technologies, which patient situations warrant the use of available technologies, and who decides when to initiate and when to withdraw particular interventions. The rising cost of providing accessible technological advances also raises issues in the realms of priority setting and distributive justice. Additionally, nurses must be concerned about the amount of nursing energy and attention that technology requires. As much as we say that nursing focuses on holistic caring for the patient, nurses are faced with increasing demands to focus their attention on technology rather than on their patients.

Current technology makes it possible to restart arrested hearts, use machines to breathe for people, assist the body in dealing with the final stages of disease through use of medications and other interventions, eliminate diseased parts through surgery, and even to replace malfunctioning or diseased vital organs. The ability to prolong life, or at least to extend the functioning of the physical being, has prompted the necessity of dealing with some very important issues related to the use of technology at the end of life. One dilemma relates to questions of quality of life, and whether physical existence is synonymous with *living*. Another issue relates to whether the availability of certain technologies means they should always be used. Still another issue relates to the process of decision-making regarding the use of technology at the end of life. While the use of high-tech interventions to sustain life is welcomed by many patients, others worry that these same technologies may keep them alive against their wishes, or with a poor quality of life (Breitbart *et al.*, 2000; Valente, 2004). This fear arises out of concerns that prolonging a poor quality of life also implies, for many people, a prolongation of suffering, pain, and the associated cost and burden of extending life in this way (Valente, 2004). As we see, many concerns at the end of a life relate to decisions about how and for whom technologies will be used, and the subsequent quality of life.

Principles of Beneficence and Non-maleficence

When dealing with issues of technology at the end of life, the principles of **beneficence** and **non-maleficence** are relevant to consider and may, in fact, be in conflict. A particular technology, which may be implemented with the intention of *doing good* (beneficence), may result in much suffering for the patient. Inducing such suffering is counter to the maxim of *doing no harm* (non-maleficence). In some circumstances this is accepted as part of the treatment process, such as pain associated with surgery or the side effects of chemotherapy. We are willing to endure the discomfort because there is an expectation of a positive outcome such as recovery, and that we will ultimately be or feel healthier. In circumstances where there is little or no expectation of recovery or improved functioning, an essential question is whether the harm imposed by technology outweighs the good intended by its use. Suffering associated with technology may include physical, spiritual, and emotional elements for both patient and family. Making decisions regarding the use of technology may cause pain, and there is suffering in living with unknown results of these ongoing decisions. Relief of suffering, a goal of healing from its earliest days, needs to be addressed in all patient encounters.

Current Issues in the Use of Technology

Current technologies related to organ and tissue transplantation, genetic engineering, reproduction, and sustaining life have profound potential for affecting our lives and health in positive ways. Their use also presents dilemmas for patients, families, professionals, and society. Nurses generally do not make the decisions regarding implementing or withdrawing particular technologies (except perhaps in situations like initiating cardiopulmonary resuscitation following specific protocols), yet we are involved as the caregivers of those receiving interventions and in many levels of patient care that involve technology. In most health care environments, nurses function as part of an interprofessional team, providing key information for, and contributing to, decisions regarding patient care and the use of technology. One of nursing's primary responsibilities is to help patients and families deal with the purposes, benefits, and limitations of the specific technologies. The withdrawing or withholding of treatment is a prime example of a dilemma related to technology at the end of life and will be a focus throughout the chapter. Other issues related to technology and the end of life will be discussed briefly, and the reader is encouraged to further explore particular areas as the need or interest arises.

QUALITY OF LIFE

The ability to keep people alive and physically functioning through use of technology has led to much reflection and discussion about what constitutes life and living. Some people believe that biological life must be preserved, regardless of the effect on the person whose body is being kept alive. This belief is sometimes referred to as the "**sanctity of life**" position. Someone who believes strongly in a "sanctity of life" perspective would posit that all human life should be valued, no matter what, and at all costs. Preservation of human life is of the utmost importance, often even if that life is thought by others to be of poor quality or that life involves no sentience or awareness of self and others. This position is often cited in the "pro-life" position in political or ethical arguments about life-and-death issues such as abortion, contraception, stem cell research, euthanasia, and assisted suicide. Others suggest that living implies a quality that goes beyond physical existence or simply, *living*. **Quality of life**, a subjective appraisal of well-being and the factors that make life worth living and contribute to a positive experience of living, means different things to different people. It is difficult to find a clear and concise definition of quality of life, because of the multidisciplinary usage and variable cultural understandings, making it a very subjective notion that is widely used across a variety of contexts. Farquhar (1995) points out that definitions of quality of life derive from both lay and "expert" sources, and range from global understandings of the concept, such as satisfaction with life, to focused definitions used for research; for example, health or functional ability. Ideas incorporated in understandings of the concept include fulfilment, satisfaction/dissatisfaction, conditions of life, happiness/ unhappiness, experiences of life, and factors such as comfort, functional status, socio-economic status, independence, and conditions in one's environment.

Farquhar (1995) suggests that deciding what weight to give different dimensions of the concept presents problems in defining quality of life. For instance, when evaluating personal quality of life, which does a person rank as more important: happiness, or functional status, such as the ability to get around and care for oneself? Nurses need to understand patients' diverse and dynamic perspectives on what constitutes quality in their lives in order to incorporate these factors into goal setting and care planning. How each person defines quality of life can change over time. For example, persons with debilitating health concerns may rate the quality of their lives quite positively, although others might feel that they could never live with such limitations. As another example, a person might think that, at the end of their life, they would utilize any and all means in order to prolong their life, but in reality, when they are eventually faced with their imminent death, they opt instead for fewer interventions in order to experience what they view as a more peaceful death. Furthermore, perceptions of quality of life can change with age and specific life experiences. At the end of life, patients may define quality of life in a far different way than we would expect. A definition of quality of life, at that point, may include simply being pain-free, or enjoying everyday kinds of activities, being able to have control over decisions or still being able or allowed to help others, spending time with loved ones, experiencing positive relationships, and a supportive and caring environment (Gourdji, McVey & Purden, 2009).

Cella's definition of quality of life acknowledges two dimensions: the subjective dimension and the multidimensional perspective (Cella, 1992; Gourdji, McVey & Purden, 2009). The subjective dimension refers to the fact that quality of life is, as we have noted, highly personal and tied to deeply-held values and notions of what is meaningful. The second dimension acknowledges the multidimensional view of self each one of us holds, based on our ideas of what constitutes well-being, and related to our physical functioning, and our social, emotional, and spiritual lives.

When patients and families are confronted with technological options at the end of life, nurses need to help them clarify their perceptions regarding quality of life, and discuss not only how life might be extended, but also how quality of life may be affected by various options. Nurses should also be vigilant about exploring patients' values and beliefs regarding perceived quality of life in order to help them make healthcare decisions that will enhance and contribute to their quality of life.

Treating Patients: When to Intervene and to What End

One of the most controversial bioethical topics of recent years centres on withholding or withdrawing life-sustaining treatments when they are deemed to have poor outcomes or offer no benefit. Decisions about withholding or withdrawing medical treatment are generally made by physicians in consultation with patients and family members. Approaches to dealing with these decisions reflect varying attitudes and concerns and may be confusing for all involved. A brief look at history sheds light on current attitudes about dealing with contemporary medical treatment. Questions related to the ethical limitations of medical care date back to the time of Hippocrates, when physicians were taught that the goal of medicine was to relieve suffering and reduce the effects of disease by lending support to natural processes. Medicine was not intended for situations in which the body was overpowered by disease, since interventions might merely prolong the suffering. The accepted ethical stance recognized the limitations of medicine, and withheld treatments that held little potential for healing (Jecker, 1995).

The scientific era that began emerging in the seventeenth century fostered a change in this ethical stance. Rather than revering and working with natural processes, conquering and dominating nature became the goal of science. In the nineteenth century, as medicine began to align more with science and biological causes for diseases were discovered, the goal of medicine became the conquest of disease by exercising power over nature. Jecker notes that ethical problems involving aggressive medical treatments where there is little likelihood of success, or poor quality of expected outcomes, "are the outgrowth of a scientific tradition whose mission is to control and dominate, whose proving ground is nature, and whose means is an unfailing faith in the scientific method" (1995, p. 144). Within this narrow focus of curing disease, ethical issues of personal quality of life and dimensions of suffering are often unrecognized and neglected. With their attention to healing and caring, nurses play an important role in calling attention to concerns that go beyond the narrow focus of curing, and broaden perspectives to attend to issue such as quality of life.

Issues of Life, Death, and Dying

Ethical dilemmas faced in health care settings at the end of life often relate to issues of and attitudes toward living and dying. When technology is involved, these ethical dilemmas become even more complex. Important questions that are deliberated by those involved include, "When does life end?" "How can we be sure that someone has died?" and "Who decides?" Technology has stretched the boundaries and clouded the waters surrounding how and when lives end. Perspectives vary from the belief that life ends when the heart stops but brain activity continues, to the view that life only ends after all brain activity has ceased. Technology makes this discussion even more complex and raises questions such as, *"What happens when a person requires technology in order to keep them alive?"* and *"Must a person in an irreversible coma be kept alive at all costs?"*

In our society, death has become an unnatural event, frequently associated with hospitals and other institutions, surrounded by tubes, machinery, and what are often labelled as heroic efforts. Determining when life ends has become a critical issue related to use of technology, prompting the involvement of courts in decision-making. The general attitude, especially among health care providers, is that death is the enemy to be overcome or kept at bay for as long as possible, regardless of the age or health condition of the person. Thus death is often viewed as a failure on the part of the health care provider. It is understandable, therefore, that many health care providers have difficulty dealing with death as a possible outcome for patients, and find it a difficult topic to discuss. However, we must remember that dying is more than a medical occurrence; it is a spiritual process that involves the individual, family, and community. Although medical interventions can assist and support those in the dying process, current technologies can prolong suffering by prolonging the dying process, and separate people from their families by actual physical barriers and institutionalization.

Another reason that the topic of death may be avoided is that discussing death requires us to face issues of meaning in life and anxieties and fears regarding our own mortality. However, lack of discussion of death as a possible outcome may lead families and patients to have unreasonable expectations and false hopes of what the system can offer. Demands for inappropriate interventions, or accusations that not enough was done, may arise from such situations. Patients and families need support in recognizing and honouring their responses, beliefs, and fears regarding death. By facing our own issues about death, we are better able to facilitate this process with patients and their families.

ASK YOURSELF

What Are Your Views on Death and Dying?

What many people fear most regarding death is suffering and dying alone.

- What has your experience been related to death, what has shaped your attitudes regarding death, and what are your fears related to death?
- How might the use of technology at the end of life contribute to this concern or attitude?
- How can nurses minimize or deal with the effects of technology on patients in the dying process?
- How can nurses support patients and families in recognizing and honouring their own responses and beliefs regarding death?

- If machines and medication are keeping a body functioning, even if the person is apparently unaware, is that person still alive? Think carefully about it and discuss your response.
- Do you think that brain wave activity in the midst of severe deterioration of major systems constitutes living?

Personal attitudes prompt different expectations and scenarios when we are faced with decisions about heroic efforts and life-sustaining technologies. We must be aware of our own attitudes concerning living and dying, as well as the beliefs and expectations of patients, families, and other health care providers. Such awareness alerts us to situations in which there are differing attitudes among the parties involved, and provides an opportunity for opening lines of communication before a serious dilemma arises. Consider, for example, the patient who tells the nurse that he feels that his body is just giving up in spite of all the medications and treatments he is receiving, and he would like to go home to die peacefully, yet the physician is considering another surgery that is helpful about 30 percent of the time. In such a situation it would be important for the nurse to explore this area further with the patient, and either communicate his wishes to the physician or facilitate the patient's talking with the physician about his wishes.

Relieving suffering and supporting what the patient considers to be a dignified death are important elements of the nursing role. Nurses also can be instrumental in helping negotiate different views as to what constitutes quality of life, and dignity in death, for individuals, families, and the medical and multidisciplinary team. Certainly, nurses play a significant role in helping patients and families understand the impact of technology on life and death as patients make decisions in a very difficult time.

Palliative Care

Two primary obligations that we have to people who are dying are comfort and company (Moss, 2001). When life-sustaining or more aggressive interventions are no longer of benefit or are not desired by the patient, the focus of care becomes palliative, that is, directed toward comfort, support, and symptom relief. **Palliative care** is comprehensive, interdisciplinary, and total care, focusing primarily on comfort and support of patients and families who face illness that is chronic or not responsive to curative treatment (Billings, 2000; Critchley *et al.*, 1999; Moss, 2001). Palliative care focuses on the best quality of life for patient and family through meticulous control of pain and other symptoms, a personalized plan to optimize quality of life as defined by patient and family, and spiritual and psychosocial care. Palliative care requires delivery of co-ordinated and continuous services in home, hospice, skilled nursing facilities, or hospital, and includes support for families in bereavement. Members of a palliative care team can include nurses, physicians, spiritual support persons, pharmacists, and persons in social services, mental health services, and pain services. The World Health Organization defines palliative care as:

> An approach that improves the quality of life of patients and their families facing the problems associated with life-threatening illness, through the prevention and relief of suffering by means of early identification and impeccable assessment and treatment of pain and other problems, physical, psychosocial and spiritual. (WHO, 2003)

The backbone of palliative care is good nursing care that continues to support the dignity and self-respect of patient and family. Palliative care nursing is a growing specialty across the globe. Originally, palliative care nurses' main responsibilities were to provide physical care to patients and support to families, but now this role has evolved into a nursing specialty that also includes teaching, consultation, research, and leadership (Johnston & Smith, 2006; Skilbeck & Payne, 2003). In addition to these roles, nurses often co-ordinate palliative care teams. Still, the main responsibilities of many palliative care nurses are tied to their clinical roles and the provision of holistic care to patients and families at the end of life in order to both improve the quality of life of patients and help to ensure a dignified death in which patients' wishes are respected.

As we have discussed, there is often a lack of consensus on what constitutes a good death, or a "dignified death" and the subsequent practical decisions embedded in these concepts, such as the provision, withholding, or withdrawal of treatment. At times, families may disagree about when it is time to stop other interventions and focus on palliative care, or time to consider withdrawal of treatment, and the nurse's ability to communicate effectively with and facilitate communication among those involved is crucial. Families often need time to see what we see regarding the patient's condition and the expected outcomes of various interventions. We have to be willing to take as much time as necessary and be available as often as needed to explain and negotiate care decisions. One way that nurses can be most effective in end-of-life care and palliative settings is by maintaining open and clear communication with patients and families. Often a family conference is needed in order to discuss end-of-life care. Family conferences are an important way to help meet the needs of families and patients at the end of life and often serve as the key process by which difficult decisions are made about limiting or stopping life-sustaining therapy (Curtis *et al.*, 2001; Lautrette *et al.*, 2006). In many cases, patients who are at the point where recommendations are being made to withhold or withdraw treatment, are no longer able to communicate their own wishes and, therefore, the views of family members and substitute decision-makers are of the utmost importance. Nurses play a key role in family conferences by facilitating communication, advocating for family and patient wishes, and leading difficult discussions.

Here are some ways that nurses can facilitate a family conference regarding end-of-life care (adapted from Curtis *et al.*, 2001):

- Make sure that everyone involved in the patient's care can be present and has the time and energy to take part.

- Make sure everyone present knows everyone else in the room, and their roles in end-of-life care of the patient.

- While everyone will be aware that the purpose of the meeting is to discuss end-of-life care, it can be difficult to initiate the discussion. One effective method is to clearly note that the discussion is one that occurs with every patient's family at the end of life.

- Set clear goals for the conference and make sure everyone agrees that these are the goals.

- Review what the family actually knows and understands regarding the patient's condition and prognosis.

- Discuss the patient's condition, prognosis, and proposed treatments or withdrawal of treatments using straightforward language, avoiding medical jargon, complex terms or colloquial terms. Don't purposefully avoid the words "death" or "dying" or use colloquial terms or jargon in place of these terms.

- Three key things to acknowledge include: uncertainty, the wishes of the patient, and any expectations of hope.

- Expectations of hope may need to be redirected away from cure or recovery towards a death with dignity and respect for the wishes of the patient.

- Be very clear that if there is a proposal to withdraw or withhold treatment, this does not mean that care or attention to needs will be withheld or withdrawn.

- Discuss directly what the patient's death may be like, and acknowledge any uncertainty or worry about this.

- Ensure that, after listening to the family, a recommendation is explicitly provided by the health care team.

- Acknowledge emotions and reactions of the family to proposed recommendations.

- Summarize the important or key points in the discussion and allow for clarification or correction.

- Make sure questions are answered and that there is a follow-up plan for next steps and further clarification of the discussion.

While family conferences are utilized in a variety of settings for many different reasons, they are of the utmost importance at the end of life for a number of reasons: to make sure that health care professionals and families are "on the same page" in terms of treatment and moving forward, and to make sure that the wishes of the patient and/or those of a substitute decision maker are respected in end-of-life decision making.

Palliative care can be difficult for some settings and health care teams to provide, and the literature emphasizes that there is much room for improvement in end-of-life care in many health care settings in Canada (Heyland *et al.*, 2010). Fast-paced acute care settings and long-term care settings are two areas where providing high quality palliative care may be difficult. In acute care, there is often an emphasis on recovery and cure, a push to free up beds for new patients, and patient caseloads for nurses are often based on the patient's acuity and physical condition. A nurse with eight patients in an acute care medical ward may have difficulty spending adequate time with one palliative patient. In long-term care settings, the challenges are somewhat different. With the move of less acutely ill but still palliative patients out of hospitals and into the community and long-term care settings earlier and more frequently, patients are more often remaining in long-term care settings until the end of their lives, whereas in the past, they might have remained in hospital. Palliative care in long-term care settings may not be ideal, due to high workloads, a limited capacity to provide quality palliative care, and few opportunities for education of nurses and allied health workers. The literature notes that problems associated with the provision of palliative care in these settings include: poor communication, inadequate pain management, unnecessary interventions and hospitalizations, poor advance care planning, and little to no attention paid to patient and family wishes regarding end-of-life care (Gill, Hillier, Crandall & Johnston, 2011). With increased awareness of the importance of high quality palliative care and the evolution of palliative care nursing as a recognized specialty, more can be done to advocate for quality end-of-life care in all settings. Groups like the Canadian Hospice Palliative Care Association, a strong national advocacy group, are active advocates for more public awareness and policies, research, resource allocation, national standards and support for palliative care. Their vision is for "all Canadians [to] have access to quality end-of-life care." (Canadian Hospice Palliative Care Association, 2012).

How the end of life is managed is not a concern relevant only to elderly adults, as some might think. Today, many low-birth-weight infants and those with certain serious or life-threatening birth defects, who would not have survived in earlier eras, survive with the support of machines, medications, and surgical procedures. In the

ASK YOURSELF

Technology and Seriously Ill Infants

- How should decisions be made regarding situations such as extremely low birth weight infants or infants born with serious intractable conditions?

- Who should have a say in these kinds of decisions?

- How should diverse values be considered? Whose opinion counts? Who has the responsibility for the final decision, and why? Should parents' views and values always be considered the most important? Why or why not?

- If an infant will die without technology and the technology is withdrawn, do you consider that a natural or unnatural end of life? Why?

process, however, some babies are kept alive only to die after months of invasive and burdensome treatment. Others survive to face chronic health problems, with their associated financial, emotional, and physical strains on families and the health care system. There is no definitive way to predict which infants will have problems as they grow and develop. Dilemmas arise regarding how much effort to invest in "saving" a few infants who have a high probability of living only a short time or with significant health problems.

MEDICAL FUTILITY

Ethical and legal arguments for initiating or discontinuing life-sustaining treatments are based primarily on the relative benefits and burdens for the patient. "Although many health care professionals feel reluctant to discontinue life-sustaining treatments, most philosophical and legal commentators find no important ethical or legal distinction between not instituting a treatment and discontinuing treatment already initiated" (Rushton, 1994, p. 517). Withholding or removing life-sustaining treatments in situations in which the burden or harm has been determined to outweigh the benefits is, in essence, allowing the person to die as a result of the natural progression of the illness process. This is different from **euthanasia**, which is causing the painless death of a person in order to end or prevent suffering, which is currently illegal in Canada. Curtin (1996) suggests that it is not reasonable to say that the removal of artificial interventions causes death; rather, it is the condition (such as disease or accident), in response to which artificial interventions were initiated, that causes death.

In deliberations regarding withholding, initiating, or withdrawing life-sustaining interventions, **medical futility** related to the patient's situation has been discussed as a major factor. Medical futility refers to situations in which interventions are judged to have no medical benefit, or in which the chance for success is low. The Canadian Nurses Association defines futility as "a medical treatment that is seen to be non-beneficial because it is believed to offer no reasonable hope of recovery or improvement of the patient's condition" (Canadian Nurses Association, 2001, p. 1). Traditional views of medical futility have considered primarily the perspective of the physician in determining what constitutes a futile measure. Others have challenged or broadened this view by offering that the physician alone should not be the only one who can define an intervention, treatment, or outcome as futile or not (Somerville, 2000; Taylor, 1995; Weijer, 1998). Taylor (1995, p. 301) suggests that futility can be considered in four different ways:

1. Not futile; beneficial to both physical and overall well-being;
2. Futile; non-beneficial to both physical and overall well-being;
3. Futile from the patient's perspective; medically indicated but not valued by the patient;
4. Futile from the clinician's perspective; valued by the patient but not medically indicated.

The fourth category, according to the Canadian Nurses Association, has sparked the most debate. Treatments and requests for treatments that fall into this category are those that are most difficult to negotiate and rationalize, when requested of the medical team by the patient or family. Understandably, a physician may be reluctant to agree to provide treatment that is, from her or his perspective, futile. Lo (1995) suggests that there are *strict* definitions of futility that would justify unilateral decisions by physicians to withhold or withdraw interventions, and *loose,* value-laden definitions of the concept that would not justify such unilateral decisions.

Loose definitions of futility include situations that prompt variable interpretations and thus are more confusing—for example, situations in which the likelihood of success is very small; no worthwhile goals of care can be achieved; patient quality of life is unacceptable; and the prospective benefit is not worth the resources required. In these situations, the meaning of futility must consider perceptions of the patient and family and judgments of the health care team. In the absence of clear external guidelines, these less clear situations require skilful nursing care, as the people involved draw on their own understandings and resources, shaped by personal beliefs and cultural values.

Somerville (2000) and others might respond to Lo's claim, stating that there should never be a situation in which a health care professional alone makes a decision regarding futility without consideration of the views of those mostly closely involved, the contexts of the situation, and the values and beliefs of the patient and family or support network. Making difficult decisions regarding the futility or utility of proposed or available medical treatments in complex health care situations calls for significant discussion and negotiation, with particular emphasis on articulation of values and beliefs and negotiation of diversity.

In its 1999 publication, *The Joint Statement on Preventing and Resolving Conflicts Involving Health Care Providers and Persons Receiving Care,* the Canadian Nurses Association acknowledged the challenges of such negotiations, as well as the key advocacy and educational roles that nurses play in such processes.

 ## CASE PRESENTATION

A Child with Leukemia

Lucia, a twelve-year-old child with leukemia, has relapsed again in spite of routine chemotherapeutic interventions. This child has suffered the side effects of the treatment, including nausea, hair loss, and frequent hospitalizations with infections, and is deteriorating physically. She says she feels as if she is being tortured with all the needles, spinal taps, and bone marrow samples; that she has no friends; and that this kind of life is not worth living. She states that she feels none of the treatments are "really helping" her and that she doesn't want any further interventions. She calls the treatments "no use anymore" and acknowledges to one of her nurses that she knows she probably won't get better. A bone marrow transplant (the only hope for a cure at this point) would mean subjecting her to intensive chemotherapy, total body irradiation, and weeks in isolation following the transplant. When Lucia is told about the bone marrow transplant, she refuses it immediately, saying, "It won't make me better and it will make me even sicker. I don't want it – it's no use! Why should I do it? Tell me, why?" The family is told that there is a thirty percent chance that the transplant will be effective.

THINK ABOUT IT

Factors Influencing Choices Regarding Medical Technology

- What factors do you think need to be considered in making the decision about having the bone marrow transplant?

- How do percentages of risk and benefit affect your decision-making?

- In this situation, do you think a thirty percent chance of success is enough to go ahead with the transplant? What if it were sixty percent? What about twenty percent?

- Consider a similar situation, but in the case of an elderly patient. Would you then think a thirty percent chance was worth it? Why or why not? What has changed in your contemplation of the case?

- How can you help patients and families use statistical information in deliberating over their decisions? What other factors would you help them to consider?

- Who should be involved in making this decision?

Futility is often discussed in relation to cardiopulmonary resuscitation (CPR), but it relates as well to interventions that preserve patients in persistent vegetative states or dependent on the technology of tertiary care settings. One difficulty associated with medical futility is that there is no set definition of the concept, only suggested parameters that vary greatly in guiding health care providers and the public. The notion of futility can be highly subjective. If a treatment does not achieve the desired goal and is not making a patient better, many would arguably claim it is then futile. Others might feel that even if a treatment offers a remote or small future chance of achieving the desired goal (e.g., cure or recovery), then it cannot be deemed as futile.

ASK YOURSELF

What Constitutes Medical Futility?

- Discuss what you consider to be the main ethical dilemmas involving the notion of futility.

- Would you consider an expensive treatment that works 20 percent of the time to be futile? What if it works only 5 percent of the time? Explain.

- Should medical futility be an issue when treatments are not expensive? Explain. If so, then is the issue really one of simply expense?

- Do you think a decision about futile treatment should be different with children and younger adults than with the elderly? Discuss your response. Consider the values and beliefs you may hold about age and quantity or quality of life.

Because personal values come into play, health care providers, patients, and families may have differing views as to what is a benefit or burden. Because of the difficulty in defining and developing clear guidelines for medical futility, recent literature focuses less on the concept of futility, and more on the process of working with the patient and family to explain the medical circumstances fully, and negotiate care that is in the best interest of the patient. *The Joint Statement on Preventing and Resolving Conflicts Involving Health Care Providers and Persons Receiving Care* focuses on this very important process, emphasizing the roles that nurses can play (Canadian Nurses Association, 1999). For example, a patient or family may find hope and be willing to consider a treatment that has a 5 percent likelihood of success, while the health care providers see this as a futile effort. When considering quality of life, the perspective of the patient and family is essential in any determination of futility. Deciding when it is not worth continuing life-sustaining treatment is another circumstance in which the views of the parties involved may differ.

CASE PRESENTATION

Mr. Mason and His Son

Mr. Mason is a seventy-eight-year-old retired, widowed auto worker. He has had a distant relationship with his adult son, an only child, for many years: they do see each other, but not often. Mr. Mason was recently diagnosed with advanced lung cancer. Recognizing that he needed to make some plans for his immediate future, so he contacted his son and appointed him power of attorney for personal care/substitute decision maker. Mr. Mason has now been admitted to your unit in severe pain. He is somewhat confused, and you are unable to elicit information from him about his wishes regarding life-sustaining measures. You note that his most recent chart entry indicates that he does not have a written advance directive or a "living will" prepared. You carefully begin discussing this difficult subject with his son, as it is your hospital's policy that everyone admitted to your oncology unit be informed about advance directives. Following are three possible twists this case could take, each one based on a real-life situation.

Ending 1. Mr. Mason's son begins to sob uncontrollably, saying, "I was never a very good son. I left home when I was barely nineteen and didn't even write or call for many years. I am just getting to know my dad, and now this happens. I want as much time with him as possible. He told me a few days ago that he was ready to die and didn't want to be kept alive on machines. But it is so unfair to me. I want him alive and to have more time with him. Please, do everything you can to keep him alive. I need some more time with him. I need for him to forgive me."

Ending 2. Mr. Mason's son seems impatient, continually looking at his watch as you talk to him. Finally, seeming exasperated, he says, "Look, I know he's going to die. I've worked through it already. I know he wouldn't want to suffer, but that's about it. After all, I don't think anyone in their right mind would choose to suffer, would they? Listen, I don't mean to sound cold, but we haven't been close over the years and I can't pretend to be upset. It isn't fair to me or to him. We've talked a bit about the financials and I am in the process of selling his house, so I'll make sure his wishes about his money are respected. I've told my kids that basically, he's gone, and I have no intention of bringing them in to see him. Anyways, he can't talk to anyone in this state. I'd like to just clean this up today, let him go in peace, and move on."

Ending 3. The son quickly acknowledges that he understands the question. Without hesitation he says, "Look, I know you don't need to hear all this but we have been estranged for many years, mainly because of how horrible he was to my mother and me. He was barely around during my childhood, and when he was, he was a tyrant. He's never apologized, never even tried to make it up. So I'm not sure why, now, I should be asked to be merciful to him. He has never showed us an ounce of mercy. So keep him alive. I'd like to give him some time to suffer and think about the things he has done."

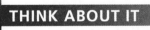

THINK ABOUT IT

Family Reactions to Medically Futile Situations

- How would you respond to the son's statement in each of these scenarios? Include both your thinking response and your feeling response.

(Continued)

- How would your feelings lead you to advise one option over another?
- How do you think the nurse should react to each response?
- What values and dilemmas are evident in each scenario?
- Identify your personal and professional values related to each scenario.
- Who should make the decision? Do you feel conflicting loyalties?
- How would you respond to the son's decision and offer him additional support?

Economics and Medical Futility

The cost of health care, particularly in relation to technology and sustaining life, has brought economic factors into discussions of futility. Some suggest that the principle of justice indicates that if a particular intervention is judged to be of limited or no benefit for one person, it should be discontinued so it is available for another patient who can make better use of the scarce resource. Lantos (1994) notes that political and economic developments in medicine in recent years, particularly in models such as the U.S. medical system, have prompted physicians and hospitals to look more closely at futile treatments. In Canada, with decreasing health care transfer payments from the federal government to each province and territory, institutions are forced to allocate resources and set priorities in all areas. Lantos suggests that it is ethical and justifiable for physicians to limit access to treatments that are expensive while offering limited benefits, and that, given limited health care resources, such decisions are socially responsible. Such an argument is consistent with utilitarian ethics, a perspective often used by government agencies when deciding about distribution of goods and services.

ASK YOURSELF

How Are Economics and Decisions About Medical Futility Related?

- Under what circumstances do you believe physicians or institutions should be able to limit a patient's access to expensive treatments?
- How do you think economics affects decisions about medical futility?
- How might patient care be affected by these decisions?

Do Not Resuscitate Orders

Cardiopulmonary resuscitation (CPR) is an area where nurses have an active role in initiating or withholding life-sustaining treatment. Considering whether to initiate CPR with a patient requires attention to professional, ethical, legal, and institutional considerations. Principles utilized to justify decisions regarding resuscitation include autonomy, self-determination, non-maleficence, and respect for persons.

The general practice regarding CPR is that ***it must be initiated*** unless (1) it would clearly be futile to do so, or (2) the practitioner has specific instructions not to do so. The legal definition of **do not resuscitate (DNR)** is not to initiate CPR in the event of a cardiac or pulmonary arrest. **DNR orders** are written directives placed in a patient's medical record indicating that the use of cardiopulmonary resuscitation is to be avoided. *The Joint Statement on Resuscitative Interventions* (CNA, 1995, p. 1) states that "unless a specific order to the contrary (do not resuscitate [DNR] has been recorded on the person's health record by the responsible physician [CPR] has come to be used as a standard intervention in virtually all cases of sudden cardiac or respiratory arrest, whether unexpected or not." DNR orders should be documented immediately in a patient's health care record, noting the reason the order was written, who gave consent, and who was involved in the discussion, whether the patient was competent to give consent, or who was authorized to do so, and the time frame for the DNR order (Thibault-Prevost, Jensen, & Hodgins, 2000). In situations of the strict definitions of medical futility noted above, Lo (1995) suggests that decisions to withhold or stop CPR are appropriately made by physicians and that, in such situations, resuscitation need not be offered as an option for patients. Some suggest that nurses are as well qualified as physicians to write DNR orders. Because nurses are the professionals who are in close and continuous contact with patients, they are perhaps better able to help patients and families articulate their views regarding end-of-life care and concerns, as well as negotiate terms of care with the multidisciplinary team. (American Nurses' Association, 1992a; Canadian Nurses Association, 2008; Martin & Redland, 1988; Thibault-Prevost, Jensen, & Hodgins, 2000). DNR decisions require open communication among the patient or surrogate, the family, and the health care team. This communication needs to include explicit discussion of the efficacy and desirability of CPR, balanced with the potential harm and suffering it may cause the patient. In addition to clear communication with the health care team and an understanding of the risks and benefits of CPR, patients must be attuned to their own values around resuscitation, and be aware of or inquire about existing institutional policies regarding CPR, as well as their right to refuse such interventions. Their health care team must be clear about the fact that refusing CPR does not mean that other treatments, including palliative care, will be withdrawn or not available. These other treatments must be discussed, offered, and negotiated with patients, as they decide about CPR and/ or DNR orders (Canadian Nurses Association, 2008). People often overestimate the effectiveness of CPR, and do not understand that CPR is not always medically indicated. Many people derive their concept of CPR from what they see in the media. In their study of how CPR is portrayed on television, Diem, Lantos and Tulsky (1996) discovered that rates of survival after CPR in television dramas were much higher than the most optimistic survival rates in the medical literature. In order to make informed decisions regarding CPR, patients and families need to understand their clinical condition and prognosis. People rarely appreciate that CPR is a harsh and traumatic procedure, and that patients with multiple, severe, chronic health problems who receive CPR rarely survive to discharge (Quill, 2000; Moss, 2001).

Tomlinson and Brody (1988) note that the relevance of considering the patient's or family's values in justifying DNR orders may vary, depending on the rationale given for the decision. In situations in which there would be no medical benefits, patient autonomy and consent may be considered less relevant. However, when the rationale for the decision is based on the patient's quality of life, either after or before CPR, determination of whether the benefit of continued life outweighs the risk of harmful consequences, such as debility or suffering, must flow from the values of the patient or patient's proxy or substitute decision maker (SDM). Competent patients have the right to refuse CPR and may request DNR orders after they have been informed of the risks and benefits involved. Good communication is the most critical key factor in assuring that any DNR decision is acceptable to all parties involved.

 ## CASE PRESENTATION

Mistaken Resuscitation

Jacob has had a chronic lung condition for the past ten of his thirty-two years. The condition causes some restrictions on his life, but he has kept up with a regular job and is very involved in his church. He is currently hospitalized with a severe respiratory infection. Although his condition did not seem to be that serious, when he was admitted he made sure that there was a DNR order in his chart. Because of a staff shortage, Lashanda, a registered nurse who usually works on another unit, has been assigned to Jacob's unit. Although she has been working on the other side of the unit, she is currently covering the whole unit while other staff are at lunch. As she answers a call light from Jacob's roommate, she notices that Jacob is not breathing and has no pulse. Since she is unfamiliar with Jacob's DNR request, she immediately calls a "code" and initiates CPR, figuring that there would be no question that this would be the appropriate action for someone of this age. Although Jacob is successfully resuscitated with no serious sequelae, he is intensely angry, saying that the resuscitation, while successful, violated his rights.

> ### ? THINK ABOUT IT
>
> ## *Decisions Regarding Resuscitation*
>
> - What do you think about Jacob's request for a DNR order? What ethical principles are involved in his choice?
> - What do you think about Lashanda's response in the situation? Do you think she acted appropriately under the circumstances? What principles may have guided her actions?
> - How do you think you might respond in a similar situation? What principles would guide your actions?
> - Imagine yourself in Jacob's situation. How would you feel and why?
> - What other strategies might a hospital unit use, in cases like these, in order to ensure patient's wishes are always followed?

DNR orders typically apply only to resuscitation situations. The fact that CPR might be considered futile does not necessarily imply that other life-sustaining interventions are futile or that other treatments will not be used. Health care providers often fail to make this distinction explicitly, thus causing confusion for patients as well. Many institutions require more specific instructions regarding what is and is not to be done for a patient. These interventions might include treatment of physiological abnormalities like fever or cardiac arrhythmias, nutrition and hydration, provision of antibiotics, or use of mechanical ventilation. Plans for and parameters of DNR orders need to be discussed with all members of the health care team so that the goal of care and the patient's wishes are clear. The presence of DNR orders requires nurses to become even more focused on providing supportive and comfort interventions, and to ensure that there is no reduction in the level of care for the patient and family. A DNR order means only that, in the event of cardiac or respiratory arrest, there are to be no attempts to resuscitate. Presuming no arrest occurs, the patient may recover from the problem necessitating hospitalization and return home.

At a more philosophical level, Scofield suggests that decisions not to resuscitate ask us "individually and collectively, to arrive at a consensus on how to integrate death and decisions about it into the legitimating values of our moral universe. Deciding what kind of life we want involves deciding what kind of death we can face" (1995, p. 184). He notes that death, which was once considered fate, is now often a matter of a choice that we do not want to have to make. This is the dilemma faced by those involved in DNR decisions.

Nursing Considerations Related to DNR Orders

Although it is generally considered the domain of the physician to write a DNR order, nurses need to be aware of the parameters surrounding such orders. Nurses need to know which patients under their care have DNR orders, and these orders need to be documented clearly in a patient's chart, and perhaps at the bedside, and reviewed periodically as the patient's condition changes and in adherence with institutional policies. If a patient or a designated SDM indicates to the nurse the desire not to be resuscitated and there is no order in the chart, the nurse should document the request in the patient's chart and bring this to the immediate attention of the health care team. The nurse may wish to explore the request with the patient or proxy, and may need to facilitate discussion of the issue between patient and other members of the health care team. Orders should specify which interventions are to be withheld, and considerations regarding the circumstances in which they are to be withheld. All persons involved in the care of the patient need to know about the orders. Since attitudes affect one's approach to others, nurses need to reflect on their own attitudes toward decisions regarding withholding of interventions, both in general and in particular patient situations, remembering that their priority should be to advocate for the patient's best interests.

Artificial Sources of Nutrition

Maintaining nutrition is a natural life-sustaining measure and a common part of the nursing role. Once a person has difficulty with functions associated with nutrition, such as chewing or swallowing, or is not conscious enough to participate in these activities, decisions about artificial sources of nutrition must be made. Ethical dilemmas arise concerning whether to classify such interventions as feeding or as medical treatments, as ordinary or extraordinary measures.

Utilizing artificial sources of nutrition may present dilemmas in situations involving persons in persistent vegetative states or end-stage dying processes for whom this intervention is maintaining physical life. We know that withholding food will eventually lead to starvation and death and, under most circumstances, is not considered an ethical action. However, it is considered appropriate to withhold or discontinue life-sustaining medical interventions when they are not benefiting the patient or are contrary to the patient's wishes. There are fewer complexities surrounding decisions to withhold artificial sources of nutrition than there are regarding decisions to withdraw medical interventions. However, as nutrition and hydration are considered by many people to constitute basic needs and are considered in a highly emotional and value-based way through a desire to provide basic nourishment when other kinds of withdrawal may be occurring (such as withdrawal of treatments), these kinds of decisions can be especially difficult for patients, families, and SDMs (Hughes & Neal, 2000).

As with any such decision, we must consider the wishes of the patient or SDM. Quality of life is an important factor, and if interventions contribute to, more than relieve, a patient's suffering, the principle of non-maleficence may sway one toward a decision of not implementing or of discontinuing such therapies. Evidence suggests that tube feeding does not improve outcomes, and has substantial risks in some patients, particularly those with dementia or multisystem illness (Finucane, Christmas & Travis, 1999; McCann, 1999; Moss, 2001). Curtin reflects that if a person is willing and able to eat and drink, even when death is imminent and the patient is suffering, attempts to quicken death by withholding ordinary nourishment is morally repugnant. However, "in situations in which death is inevitable and the conditions of living intolerable (involve extensive technological isolation from human touch, futile pain and pointless extensions of dying), highly sophisticated means of feeding are not in a patient's best interests and may be withheld or withdrawn" (1996, p. 82). Once artificial measures have been implemented, it is psychologically more difficult to decide on their removal. Curtin suggests that, unless a rational adult refuses them, such measures should be continued as long as sentient life is a reasonable expectation, but that they may be terminated when there is a reliable prediction of permanent unconsciousness. With any technological intervention, we must consider whether its use is prolonging living or prolonging dying. When competent patients refuse food or fluid, respect for persons directs nurses to honour this refusal. Nurses need to help family and other caretakers understand that people who are dying often have a decline in appetite, and that the care of keeping the person comfortable does not need to include efforts to maintain nutrition. Various involved parties may view the use of such interventions from different perspectives.

DECISION MAKING AT THE END OF LIFE

As has been noted, there are many factors involved in making decisions about withholding or withdrawing life-sustaining treatments and utilizing other technologies at the end of life. Nurses need to determine who should be involved in making the decision, and how the nurse fits into the scenario. Using the decision-making process described in Chapter 6 may assist in this process. Nurses need to be aware of institutional policies and protocols regarding various technologies in general, and at the end of life. Such policies should include approaches to reaching decisions about particular patients; ways of dealing with conflicts that may arise; protection of patient rights; description of roles of those involved in the decision-making process; and directions for documenting decisions in the patient's chart. In most situations, the patient or the patient's SDM has the ultimate authority to decide which interventions to use or withhold.

The Importance of Communication

Because nurses are in close and continual contact with patients, they are often perceived as being more available and more approachable than physicians. Patients or family members may discuss their concerns about interventions more readily with the nurse, seeking information or advice. It is important to know what they have been told by the physician, determine the patient's and family's level of understanding about the situation, and whether they have the information they need to make an informed decision. If information is needed in such areas as risks, discomforts, side effects, potential benefits, likelihood of success, or treatment alternatives, advocating for the patient in this regard is an expected nursing response. Nurses are in a key position to utilize conversations with patients and families to discover areas of confusion and to elicit information about the patient's wishes regarding interventions.

Sometimes people just need to talk out their concerns and sort through what might be perceived as conflicting messages. Providing a listening presence can help people vent emotions, speak their fears, and clarify their concerns. At times the concern may be such that the nurse must advocate for the patient by facilitating communication with the physician or other support persons, such as family members, a patient representative, the palliative care team, or a member of the ethics committee. Collaboration among all involved is important to ensure an informed choice. Effective communication can be facilitated by providing an environment that is not rushed; using terms and language that are understood by the other person and avoiding "medical-ese"; allowing time for and encouraging questions; practicing attentive listening; and offering a caring presence. Much of the palliative care nursing literature supports the claim that the most important skills that palliative care nurses have are skills related to communication, active listening, and advocacy.

Legal Issues Related to Technology Use at the End of Life

As noted in Chapter 7, what some consider to be an ethical decision may not be upheld as a legal action. In the area of health care technology, the courts have intervened in some decisions related to withholding or withdrawing life-sustaining treatments when there has been disagreement among the involved parties. Legal precedents regarding issues such as what constitutes clear evidence of a person's wishes related to these treatments and what is considered standard practice have been set in the process. Examples of two such cases are presented here. When one looks at dilemmas faced by families, health care providers, institutions, and the legal system in situations such as these, the importance of having advance directives becomes evident. **Advance directives** are instructions that indicate one's wishes regarding health care interventions or designate someone to act as a surrogate in making such decisions in the event that one loses decision-making capacity. The Canadian Nurses Association defines an advance directive as "a document prepared by a competent person intended to direct the kind of treatment that a person will receive if he or she later becomes incompetent. The two basic forms of advance directives include instructional directives about particular treatments and directives that name a substitute decision maker" (Canadian Nurses Association, 2000, p. 3). Based on a respect for the autonomy of individuals, and the acknowledgment that individuals have the right to consent, an advance directive makes it possible for people to have their authentic and autonomous wishes known, even if they cannot articulate them (Canadian Nurses Association, 1994). Advance directives, when contained in a comprehensive document such as a living will, can provide health care teams with clear directions while ensuring that family members are not conflicted over not having a clear idea of the patient's authentic wishes at the end of life (Singer, 1994, 2002). These directives are discussed further in Chapter 11 in the context of patient self-determination.

Although the following two cases took place in the United States, they remain fundamental "benchmark" cases for discussions of the notion of the use of advance directives. Note the use of the term "guardian *ad litem*." This term refers to a person who is appointed by a court to protect the best interests of another, in a very specific context only. In these two cases, a guardian *ad litem* acted to speak for these two women's best interests related to health care decision making.

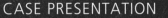

CASE PRESENTATION

Karen Quinlan

The well-known case of Karen Quinlan (Devettere, 1995; Pence, 1995) is a story of a twenty-one-year-old woman who, in 1975, was found to have suffered cardiopulmonary arrest at home alone after having been drinking at a local bar. After the ambulance crew restored heartbeat through CPR, she was admitted to the local hospital and placed on a ventilator. Within a few days she was transferred to a larger hospital, where she was kept alive with the assistance of a respirator and feeding tube. Over months she lost weight, developed contractures, and was given no hope of regaining awareness. After much deliberation, the family asked that the respirator be discontinued, but the hospital indicated that it could not grant the request unless her father was named as her guardian. When her father asked the court to appoint him guardian with authority to make decisions to discontinue extraordinary interventions, the court appointed him guardian of her property, but not of her person, and appointed a **guardian *ad litem*** to represent Karen. The guardian *ad litem* felt responsible for preserving Karen's life, and opposed removing the respirator. The physician's lawyer argued that removing a respirator from a living person was not standard medical procedure, and the judge sided with this view. When the family appealed the ruling to the New Jersey Supreme Court, the decision of the lower court was reversed and the father was appointed as her guardian. When her father requested that the respirator be removed, the physicians initiated a process of weaning her from it, resulting in her being able to breathe without the machine. Totally unconscious with severe contractures, she was transferred to a nursing home, where she died ten years later.

CASE PRESENTATION

Terri Schiavo

In another more recent case, Terri Schiavo collapsed and suffered a cardiac arrest and severe hypoxia due to hypokalemia brought on by an eating disorder (Perry, Churchill & Kirshner, 2005; Quill, 2005; Weijer, 2005). It was 1990 and Terri was 26 years of age, without a formal living will or substitute decision maker identified. Her husband, Michael, was appointed as her legal guardian.

(Continued)

After a period of several months, Terri was confirmed to be in a persistent vegetative state, characterized by eyes-open unconsciousness, sleep and waking cycles, and a lack of awareness of self or others. Michael, along with Terri's parents, Robert and Mary Schindler, provided her with a barrage of standard, experimental, and innovative rehabilitation treatments, which resulted in no change or improvement in her status. After three years, her husband accepted her diagnosis and prognosis. Once he realized this was an irreversible state, and recalling a statement that his wife had once made about not wanting her life to be maintained through technology, he stated that she would have asked to have her feeding tube discontinued as the tube was sustaining her life, through providing her with nutrition and hydration. Terri's parents adamantly opposed the removal of the feeding tube and a fierce and lengthy legal battle began over end-of-life guardianship, the role of a surrogate, respect for autonomy and how to protect and promote the best interests of a patient who could not communicate or advocate for herself. Terri's feeding was stopped twice and, each time, restarted through orders from the court as a result of appeals put forth by the Schindlers. After a number of trials, appeals, intense media coverage, and intervention by the state (through the hasty passing of the controversial "Terri's Law," which allowed the governor to intervene to order the resumption of discontinued treatment), Terri's feeding was stopped for the third time in 2005 and her feeding tube was removed, after which she died about two weeks later.

? THINK ABOUT IT

When the Courts Intervene

- As you reflect on these two cases and the markedly different positions of those involved, which position do you support in each case, and why?

- In each case, which court decisions do you think are justified or not justified? Defend your position.

- Describe the ethical dilemmas and principles involved in these situations.

- If one of your family members was in a similar situation, how do you think you would respond? Would you expect solidarity or disagreement with this position from other members of your family?

- Consider that you are a nurse caring for a patient like Karen or Terri at various stages in her situation. How would you respond to the various parties involved as decisions about her care are being discussed? What do you think the nursing role might be in interacting with families and guardians in cases where there is disagreement?

- What do you think about the role of the legal system in decisions regarding use of technology in sustaining life?

Organ and Tissue Procurement and Transplantation

There are other kinds of decisions that also involve technology at the end of life, which can be difficult and can involve the nurse in communication and advocacy. One example is the procurement of organs and tissues from patients who are dying or who have been declared as dead. Organ transplantation is no longer considered as extraordinary or uncommon a health care event as it was in the not-too-distant past. As techniques become more refined and technologies evolve for keeping patients alive in vegetative states, the possibility of a transplant becomes a hope for more and more people afflicted with the failure of a vital organ. Because the demand for organs is great and the supply limited, dilemmas related to allocation of scarce resources emerge. Questions arise regarding eligibility of recipients for organ transplant. Should these determinations be made based on a potential recipient's expectation of survival post-transplant, or power and prestige, or some combination of these and other factors? Transplantation may involve organs from dead or living human donors, animals, or artificial appliances, and there are dilemmas associated with each. Our discussion focuses on human donor issues.

Because transplantation requires well-nourished organs, procurement must occur as soon after death as possible. Thus, having criteria for determining when death occurs is imperative. Irreversible cessation of cardiopulmonary functioning is one such criterion. If a person has been maintained on life support technology, brain death is the most likely criteria to be used, which leads to issues regarding what constitutes brain death. Some suggest that the current criteria for brain death, which indicate that all functions of the entire brain must cease, are more stringent than necessary, and that irreversible cessation of higher brain functions would be sufficient criteria. Additionally, adherence to a strict brain-death-only donation criteria has often been blamed for the lack of available organs for donation. Currently, the percentage of hospital deaths resulting from brain death are estimated at one to three percent. Using other criteria, such as cardiac death, has been a subject of much debate in Canada. After the criteria for brain death was published in 1968 (Ad Hoc Committee of the Harvard Medical School to Examine the Definition of Brain Death), all organ donations in Canada were from persons who met this criteria. However, in 2006, the Ottawa Hospital announced that it had carried out an organ donation from a patient following cardiac death, or donation after cardiac death (DCD), formerly known as non-heart-beating organ donations (NHBD). This is, as Doig (2006) notes, "a major change in end-of-life practice and poses significant ethical problems for end-of-life decision-making in intensive care units (ICUs)" (p. 206). Worries over the lack of definitive criteria for cardiac death and the notion of reversibility of cardiac death have fuelled the debate and contributed to the reluctance of some provinces and institutions to carry out DCD.

The topic of DCD has been debated actively at a number of forums sponsored by the Canadian Council for Donation and Transplantation, which has publicly noted that the option of DCD should move forward in particular contexts with significant ethical guidance and intensive education (2005).

The scarcity of available organs combined with the long waiting lists of potential recipients raises the possibility that people may be declared dead prematurely in cases of both DBD and DCD. This scarcity of organs also affects organ procurement from living human beings. With living donors, issues related to voluntary informed consent and the buying and selling of organs are of concern. There are places in the world where organs are taken from people who are living in extreme poverty, or from prisoners, without their knowledge or against their will, and sold to procurement centres in more affluent countries. Desperate straits have prompted some individuals to sell an organ to raise money for personal or family needs, raising a question about whether there can be true voluntary informed consent under such circumstances.

In cases of sudden accidental death, family members may be asked to consider donation of viable organs. Consider whether there can be true voluntary consent when the family is in the midst of crisis and shock. With the urgency for a decision due to time factors for harvesting organs, coercion could be a factor. In many settings, nurses function as transplant co-ordinators and are asked to approach patients or families about considering organ donation. In such situations, these nurses are often trained to be clear about their own feelings regarding organ procurement and transplantation, and to attend to the needs of the families while also considering the constraints of organ harvesting.

NURSING PRACTICE IN THE MIDST OF TECHNOLOGY

Nursing practice continues to evolve with expanding knowledge and scientific advances in many arenas. As technology has been developed and refined, related nursing responsibilities have expanded. In end-of-life care, nursing roles vary from clinical responsibilities to patient and family advocate and palliative team leader. In the midst of all these changes, the essence of nursing remains the human focus of caring for patients and families—being attentive to the needs of persons whose lives are affected by the technology at any point. Integrating caring and technology, and juggling the demands of both, presents challenges for nurses in any area of practice, but this challenge becomes even more apparent in end-of-life care, as the human focus of nursing becomes even more paramount in the lives of patients. As new technologies become available, they will bring with them associated issues of concern, and as technology for sustaining life continues to advance, new worries about how we should live and die well will emerge. Regardless of the technology, important considerations for nursing always relate to attitudes and values, communication, and maintaining the human focus of care.

Attitudes and Values

The importance of self-awareness related to values, beliefs, and reactions is especially significant when dealing with end-of-life care intermingled with issues related to technology. The process of being more attentive to personal perspectives regarding such issues as quality of life, living, dying, medical futility, and allocation of scarce resources may be facilitated by pondering the kinds of questions posed throughout this chapter. Such awareness enables the nurse to differentiate personal values from those of patients and others involved in the situation. Principles of respect for autonomy and diversity direct the nurse to understand that individuals may judge the possible benefits of an intervention from varying perspectives. Recognizing where personal values may be different enables nurses to be more attentive to fostering good communication, encouraging others to make their own decisions, avoiding judgment about the rightness or wrongness of the decision based on personal values, and accepting those decisions if they are different from what the nurse would do.

As the various examples presented in this chapter suggest, many dilemmas that emerge surrounding technology and its use at the end of life relate to differing values among the parties involved. Facilitating discussion of values among patients and families may help them to clarify their own perspectives. Nurses also need to be alert to situations in which there may be differences in values among the patient, family physician, or other health care team member. Encouraging timely communication may avert a major dilemma, or facilitate a more effective resolution of the concern. Nurses who cannot reconcile their own values with a particular situation need to take the necessary steps to remove themselves from that situation so as to not compromise patient care or personal integrity. In so doing, it is essential to avoid abandoning the patient by ensuring that there are others who will provide the needed care for the patient.

Caring: The Human Focus

In the context of expanding scientific and technological knowledge, nurses have a responsibility to help patients and families benefit from what technology offers, while always remembering the human focus of care. This is especially important at the end of life, when that human focus of care becomes a key part of the life of a person who may be dying. Davis (1991) suggests that when medical treatment is deemed futile, nursing care in its fullest meaning is most essential. This is evident in nursing's significant role in palliative care. However alert, and in whatever stage of living and dying, an individual has a life story that continues to unfold, a story that continues to intertwine with lives of others. In the midst of the technology, nurses can encourage family and loved ones to talk with, touch, and be in touch with the patient. In this way nurses acknowledge the primary importance of relationships, even in a health care setting filled with machines, noises, and other evidences of advanced technology.

Attention to the human focus includes helping patients and families become more comfortable with the sometimes formidable array of machines and equipment, and make sense of the large amounts of clinical data that are generated. Incorporating family members in caring for the patient provides time for connecting and observing the patient in both good and bad moments, and engenders a more realistic view of the patient's condition. Rather than engendering anxiety and mistrust by shutting the family out of the patient's life, experiences, or dying processes—all critical moments—nurses should encourage them to share directly in the patient's journey. This provides families with more experiences that they can use to base difficult decisions on.

The nursing role of providing care and comfort is paramount in any health care setting, and has many facets. It may take the shape of explaining, as often as necessary, the purpose and problems related to interventions. Caring requires that the nurse see the experience from another's point of view, so that questions, fears, concerns, and frustrations may be addressed appropriately. Providing care and comfort also requires that the nurse support and encourage behaviours that enable patients and families to choose in accordance with their own beliefs and values. Being proficient in technical skills with the intent of doing what is best for the patient is part of human care, as is the ability to be with and wait with persons as they struggle through the most difficult situations.

SUMMARY

Many of the major ethical dilemmas encountered by nurses and other health care providers today are associated with advances in scientific knowledge and technology. To be able to recognize and to deal with such dilemmas, nurses need to clarify their own values, and to appreciate differences in values among the various people involved in making patient care decisions. The potential of technology has raised very deep questions about life and death that must be addressed on individual, professional, and societal levels. Issues of quality of life, relief of suffering, and futility of interventions are some facets of these questions. Decisions about when to intervene, and reasonable goals of interventions, are made more difficult because of varying perceptions of the value of such interventions, non-definitive outcomes, and issues related to availability of interventions. Principles of beneficence, non-maleficence, justice, and autonomy provide the basis for arguments on different sides of issues related to technology. Nurses must take into account their responsibilities to patients and the profession, as well as their own personal integrity, when dealing with ethical dilemmas engendered by technology. Nurses must remember that, in the midst of the technology with its associated dilemmas, there are persons who need the human focus of care that is basic to nursing practice.

CHAPTER HIGHLIGHTS

- The use of technology in health care has prompted the need to address important ethical questions regarding life, death, and allocation of resources.
- Utilization of health care technology may give rise to conflicts between the principles of beneficence and non-maleficence.
- Appropriate utilization of health care technologies requires that health care providers, patients, and families understand the purposes, benefits, and limitations of specific technologies.

- Attitudes and beliefs concerning life and death affect how health care providers, patients, families, and the legal system approach issues related to health care technology. Ethical dilemmas may arise when there are differing opinions related to the use of technology among the parties involved.

- Determination of medical futility is an important consideration in decisions to withhold or withdraw life-sustaining interventions. Ethical decisions regarding these measures require consideration of whether they are prolonging living, or prolonging dying.

- Economics may factor into decisions related to medical futility, availability of technology, and accessibility to many interventions.

- Withholding or withdrawing life-sustaining treatments in situations where the burden or harm has been determined to outweigh the benefits constitutes allowing a person to die, and is not euthanasia. Dilemmas may arise regarding whether to classify the use of specific interventions as ordinary or extraordinary measures. The courts have sometimes been involved in making this determination.

- Patient self-determination and distributive justice must be considered in decisions regarding technology. Vigilance is required to ensure that people are not harmed, exploited, controlled, discriminated against, or excluded from care by the use of health care technologies.

- Nurses are in a key position to help patients and families articulate their preferences regarding technological interventions, and to facilitate communication with other health team members in this regard. This role requires familiarity with patient and family decisions and institutional policies regarding life-sustaining interventions, and awareness that when medical care is deemed futile, nursing care in its fullest meaning is most essential.

DISCUSSION QUESTIONS AND ACTIVITIES

1. Develop advance directives for yourself, considering interventions you would choose and parameters regarding these choices. Discuss and compare your directives with classmates.

2. Go on line and download a living will from the Joint Centre for Bioethics at the University of Toronto (www.jointcentreforbioethics.ca/tools/livingwill .shtml). Critically examine the document to see if it addresses all your wishes and choices, were you completing it.

3. Discuss your beliefs regarding determinants of the beginning and end of life.

4. Describe quality of life as it relates to health care decisions.

5. Plan and engage in a debate in your class focused on economic and justice issues related to health care technologies and medical futility.

6. Observe several patients who are receiving technological interventions, and note how the technology is affecting them and their families; issues surrounding

its use; the focus of nursing care; and your reaction to the situation. Describe strengths of the nursing care you observe, and aspects that you might do differently if you were providing care. Talk to nurses and patients regarding the impact of technology on their health and care.

7. Discuss your view about nurses writing DNR orders.

8. How would you handle a situation where you feel the physician's decision regarding life-sustaining interventions was inappropriate for your patient?

9. Choose one of the topics discussed in this chapter and explore the Web sites of the CNA and the ICN regarding policies or positions statements on this issue. You may include information from other disciplines as well. Compare and contrast the positions of the various organizations. Discuss your views about this issue, and how they compare to the positions of the professional organizations.

CNA—http://www.cna-nurses.ca

ICN—http://www.icn.ch

10. Role-play a palliative care conference with students in the class, using a real or hypothetical patient case situation.

REFERENCES

Ad Hoc Committee of the Harvard Medical School to Examine the Definition of Brain Death. (1968). A definition of irreversible coma. *Journal of the American Medical Association, 205*, 337–40.

American Nurses' Association (1992a, April 2). *Position statement: Nursing care and do-not-resuscitate decisions.* Author. Retrieved January 7, 2001, from http://www.nursingworld.org/readroom/position/ethics/etdnr.htm.

Billings, J. A. (2000). Palliative care: Recent advances. *British Medical Journal, 321*, 555–558.

Breitbart, W., B. Rosenfeld, H. Pessin, M. Kaim, J. Funesit-Esch, M. Galietta & C. J. Nelson (2000). Depression, Hopelessness, and Desire for Hastened Death in Terminally Ill Patients With Cancer. *JAMA 284*(22), 2907–2911.

Canadian Council for Donation and Transplantation (2005). *Donation after circulatory death: A Canadian forum.* The Canadian Council for Donation and Transplanatation: Edmonton, Alberta. Retrieved July 19 from http://publications.gc.ca/collections/Collection/H14-2-2005E.pdf

Canadian Hospice Palliative Care Association. (2012). *Mission and vision.* Retrieved May 28, 2012 from http://www.chpca.net/about-us/mission-and-vision.aspx

Canadian Nurses Association. (1994). *Joint statement on advance directives.* Retrieved January 2, 2009, from http://www.cna-aiic.ca/CNA/documents/pdf/publications/PS20_Advance_Directives_Sept_1994_e.pdf.

Canadian Nurses Association. (1995). *Joint statement on resuscitative interventions.* Approved by the Canadian Healthcare Association, the Canadian Medical Association, the Canadian

Nurses' Association, the Catholic Health Association of Canada, and in collaboration with the Canadian Bar Association. Ottawa: Authors.

Canadian Nurses Association. (1999). *Joint statement on preventing and resolving conflicts involving health care providers and persons receiving care.* Ottawa: Author.

Canadian Nurses Association. (2000). *End-of-life issues.* Retrieved January 2, 2009, from http://www.cna-aiic.ca/CNA/documents/pdf/publications/PS43_End_of_Life_Issues_Nov_2000_e.pdf.

Canadian Nurses Association. (2001). *Futility presents many challenges for nurses.* Ethics in Practice series paper. Ottawa: Author.

Canadian Nurses Association. (2008). *Standards and best practices: CPR.* Retrieved January 2, 2009, from http://www.cna-aiic.ca/CNA/practice/standards/cpr/default_e.aspx.

Cella, D. F. (1992). Quality of life: the concept. *Journal of Palliative Care, 8*(3), 8–13.

Critchley, P., A. R. Jadad, A. Taniguchi, A. Woods, R. Stevens, L. Reyno & T. J. Whelan (1999). Are some palliative care delivery systems more effective and efficient than others? A systematic review of comparative studies. *Journal of Palliative Care, 15*(4), 40–47.

Curtin, L. (1996). *Nursing: Into the 21st century.* Springhouse, PA: Springhouse.

Curtis, J. R., D. L. Patrick, S. E. Shannon, P. D. Treece, R. A. Engelberg & G. D. Rubenfeld (2001). The family conference as a focus to improve communication about end-of-life care in the intensive care unit: Opportunities for improvement. *Critical Care Medicine, 29(2) [Suppl.]*:N26–N33.

Davis, A. J. (1991). Ethical issues in nursing research: My own experience. *Western Journal of Nursing Research, 13,* 414–415.

Devettere, R. J. (1995). *Practical decision making in health care ethics: Cases and concepts.* Washington, DC: Georgetown University Press.

Diem, S. J., J. D. Lantos & J. A. Tulsky (1996). Cardiopulmonary resuscitation on television. *New England Journal of Medicine, 334*(24), 1579–1582.

Doig, C. J. (2006). Is the Canadian health care system ready for donation after cardiac death? A note of caution. *Canadian Medical Association Journal, 175*(8), 905–906.

Farquhar, M. (1995). Definitions of quality of life: A taxonomy. *Journal of Advanced Nursing, 22,* 502–508.

Finucane, T. E., C. Christmas & K. Travis (1999). Tube feeding in patients with advanced dementia. *Journal of the American Medical Association, 282*(14), 1365–1370.

Gill, C., L. M. Hillier, J. M. Crandall & J. Johnston (2011). Nursing guidelines for end-of-life care in long-term care settings: Sustainable improvements to care. *Journal of Palliative Care, 27*(3), 229–237.

Gourdji, I., L. McVey & M. Purden. (2009). A quality end of life from a palliative care patient's perspective. *Journal of Palliative Care, 25*(1), 40–50.

Heyland, D. K., D. J. Cook, G. Rocker, P. M. Dodek, D. K. Kutsogiannis, Y. Skrobik, X. Jiang, A.G. Day, & R. Cohen for the Canadian Researchers at the End of Life Network (CARENET). (2010). Defining priorities for improving end-of-life care in Canada. *Canadian Medical Association Journal, 182*(16), E747–E752.

Hughes, N., & R. D. Neal (2000). Adults with terminal illness: A literature review of their wishes and needs for food. *Journal of Advanced Nursing, 32*(5), 1101–1107.

Jecker, N. S. (1995). Knowing when to stop: The limits of medicine. In J. H. Howell & W. F. Sale, eds., *Life choices: A Hastings Center introduction to bioethics* (pp. 139–148). Washington, DC: Georgetown University Press.

Johnston, B., & L. N. Smith (2006). Nurses' and patients' perceptions of expert palliative nursing care. *Journal of Advanced Nursing, 54*(6), 700–709.

Lantos, J. D. (1994). Futility assessments and the doctor-patient relationship. *JAGS, 42*, 868–870.

Lautrette, A., M. Ciroldi, H. Ksibi & E. Axoulay (2006). End-of-life family conferences: Rooted in the evidence. *Critical Care Medicine, 34[Suppl.]* S364–S372.

Lo, B. (1995). *Resolving ethical dilemmas: A guide for clinicians.* Baltimore: Williams & Wilkins.

Martin, D. A., & A. R. Redland (1988). Legal and ethical issues in resuscitation and withholding of treatment. *Critical Care Nurse, 10*, 1–8.

McCann, R. (1999). Lack of evidence about tube feeding: Food for thought. *Journal of the American Medical Association, 282*(14), 1381.

Moss, A. H. (2001). *What's new? Progress in palliative care, CPR, and advance directives.* Seminar at Raleigh General Hospital, Beckley, WV. January 18, 2001.

Pence, G. E. (1995). *Classic cases in medical ethics.* New York: McGraw-Hill.

Perry, J. E., L. R. Churchill, H. S. Kirshner (2005). The Terri Schiavo Case: Legal, Ethical and Medical Perspectives. *Annals of Internal Medicine, 143*(10), 744–748.

Quill, T. E. (2000). Initiating end-of-life discussions about seriously ill patients: Addressing the "elephant in the room." *Journal of the American Medical Association, 284*(19), 2502–2507.

Quill, T. E. (2005). Terri Schiavo – a tragedy compounded. *New England Journal of Medicine, 352*(16), 1630–1633.

Roberts, D. (2000). Race, gender, justice, and reproductive health policy. Presentation at *New century, new challenges: Intensive bioethics course XXVI,* Kennedy Institute of Ethics, Georgetown University, Washington, DC, June 9, 2000.

Rushton, C. H. (1994). Guidelines on forgoing life-sustaining medical treatment. *Pediatric Nursing, 20*, 517–521.

Scofield, G. R. (1995). Is consent useful when resuscitation isn't? In J. H. Howell & W. F. Sale, eds., *Life choices: A Hastings Center introduction to bioethics* (pp. 172–187). Washington, DC: Georgetown University Press.

Sinclair, S. (2011). Impact of death and dying on the personal lives and practices of hospice and palliative care professionals. *Canadian Medical Association Journal, 183*(2), 180–187. DOI: 10.1503/cmaj.100511

Singer, P. A. (1994). Advance directives in palliative care. *Journal of Palliative Care, 10*(3), 111–116.

Singer, P. A. (2002). *Living will.* Toronto: University of Toronto Joint Centre for Bioethics.

Skilbeck, J, & S. Payne (2003). Emotional support and the role of Clinical Nurse Specialists in palliative care. *Journal of Advanced Nursing, 43*(5), 521–530.

Somerville, M. A. (2000). *The ethical canary: science, society and the human spirit.* Toronto: Viking.

Taylor, C. (1995). Medical futility and nursing. *Image: Journal of Nursing Scholarship, 27*(4): 301–306.

Thibault-Prevost, J., L. A. Jensen & M. Hodgins (2000). Critical care nurses' perceptions of DNR orders. *Journal of Nursing Scholarship, 32*(3), 259–265.

Tomlinson, T., & H. Brody (1988). Ethics and communication in do-not-resuscitate orders. *New England Journal of Medicine, 318*, 43–46.

Valente. S. M. (2004). End-of-life challenges. Honoring Autonomy. *Cancer Nursing, 27*(4), 314–319.

Weijer, C. (1998). Cardio pulmonary resuscitation for patients in a persistent vegetative state: Futile or acceptable. *Canadian Medical Association Journal, 158*(4), 491–493.

Weijer, C. (2005). A death in the family: Reflections on the Terri Schiavo case. *Canadian Medical Association Journal, 172*(9), 1197–1198.

World Health Organization (2003). *WHO Definition of Palliative Care*. Retrieved from http://www.who.int/cancer/palliative/definition/en/ on 25 February 2012.

FURTHER SUGGESTED READINGS AND RESOURCES

British Columbia Ministry of Health (2012). My voice – expressing my wishes for future health care treatment. Retrieved May 28, 2012 from http://www.health.gov.bc.ca/library/publications/year/2012/MyVoice-AdvanceCarePlanningGuide.pdf

Buckley, J. (2008). *Palliative care: An integrated approach*. Chichester: Wiley-Blackwell.

Canadian Hospice Palliative Care Association (2009). *Canadian Hospice Palliative Care Nursing Standards of Practice*. Ottawa: CHPCA. Retrieved on February 24 from http://www.chpca.net/palliative_care_nursing_standards

Devettere, R. J. (1995). *Practical decision making in health care ethics: Cases and concepts*. Washington, DC: Georgetown University Press.

Green, A. (2006). A person-centered approach to palliative care nursing. *Journal of Hospice and Palliative Care*, 8(5), 294–301.

Hester, D. M. (2010). *End of life care and pragmatic decision making: a bioethical perspective*. New York: Cambridge University Press.

Heyland, D. K., P. Dodek, G. Rocker, D. Groll, A. Gafni, D. Pichora, S. Shortt, J. Tranmer, N. Lazar, J. Kutsogiannis, M. Lam, for the Canadian Researchers' End-of-Life Network (CARENET). (2006). What matters most in end-of-life care: perceptions of seriously ill patients and their family members. *Canadian Medical Association Journal, 174*(5), 627–633.

Howell, J. H., & W. F. Sale, eds. (2002). *Life choices: A Hastings Center introduction to bioethics*. 2nd Edition. Washington, DC: Georgetown University Press.

Jonsen, A. R., R. M. Veach & L. Walters, eds. (1998). *Source book in bioethics: A documentary history*. Washington, DC: Georgetown University Press.

La Porte Matzo, M. & D. Witt Sherman (eds.) (2010). *Palliative care nursing: Quality care to the end of life*. 3rd Ed. New York: Springer Publishing Company.

Loitman, J. E., C. T. Sinclair & M. J. Fisch (2010). *Palliative care: A case-based guide*. New York: Humana Press.

Lynch, M., C. Dahlin, T. Hultman & E. E. Coakley (2011). Palliative care nursing: Defining the discipline? *Journal of Hospice and Palliative Nursing, 13*(2), 106–111.

Pence, G. E. (2003). *Classic cases in medical ethics*. 2nd Ed. New York: McGraw-Hill.

Pfund, R. (2007). *Palliative care nursing for children and young people.* Oxon: UK: Radcliffe.

Sibbald, R.W., P. Chidwick, M. Handelman & A. B. Cooper (2011). Checklist to meet ethical and legal obligations to critically ill patients at the end of life. *Healthcare Quarterly, 14*(4), 60–66.

Singer, P. A., & N. MacDonald (1998). Bioethics for clinicians: Quality end-of-life care. *Canadian Medical Association Journal, 159,* 159–162.

Speak Up. (2012). *About Advance Care Planning.* Retrieved May 28, 2012 from http://www.advancecareplanning.ca/health-care-professionals.aspx

World Health Organization (2003). *WHO Definition of Palliative Care.* Retrieved from http://www.who.int/cancer/palliative/definition/en/ on 25 February 2012.

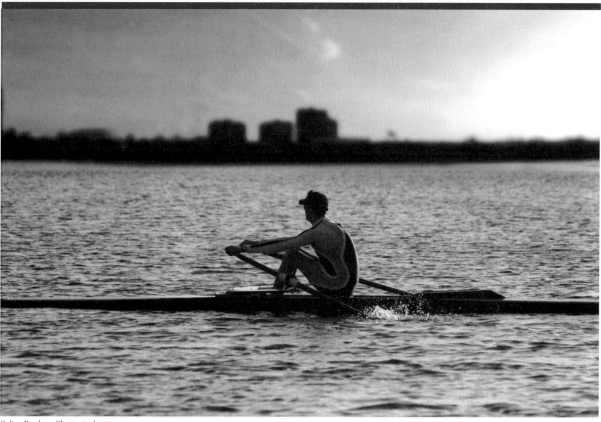

Galina Barskaya/Shutterstock.com

CHAPTER **11**

PRACTICE ISSUES RELATED TO PATIENT SELF-DETERMINATION

OBJECTIVES

After completing this chapter, the reader should be able to:

1. Discuss autonomy and paternalism as they relate to patient self-determination.
2. Describe factors that may threaten autonomy in health care settings and situations in which autonomy may be limited.
3. Examine the interaction of justice and autonomy.
4. Discuss informed consent as it relates to patient self-determination.
5. Examine legal and ethical elements of informed consent.

6. Describe the nursing role and responsibilities related to informed consent.

7. Discuss the place of advance directives in health care decisions.

8. Discuss patient autonomy related to choices for life and health.

9. Describe the nursing role and responsibilities related to patient lifestyle and health choices.

10. Describe confidentiality in relation to health care choices.

INTRODUCTION

The role of the patient and the role of the health care practitioner, and the implied responsibilities of each, have varied throughout history and in different cultures. In some cultures, decisions regarding "what is best" for the patient are deferred to the health care practitioner, who is presumed to know what will bring about healing. Indeed, until recent years, the physician was often viewed in this light. Such paternalism, even when well meaning, has been challenged in recent years, and greater emphasis has been placed on the role and rights of patients in making health care decisions. This chapter focuses on practice issues related to patient self-determination. Discussion of these issues includes both ethical and legal components, and is intertwined with issues of technology and economics.

AUTONOMY AND PATERNALISM

Self-determination derives from the principle of autonomy. **Autonomy**, which is discussed in detail in Chapter 3, denotes having the freedom to make choices about issues that affect one's own life and to make decisions about personal goals. Autonomy, which means self-governing, implies respect for persons, their ability to determine personal goals and decide on a plan of action, and their freedom to act on the choices made. The value placed on the primacy of the individual implicit in autonomy is primarily a western concept, and may not be fully accepted in other cultures. Sherwin (1992) suggests that the notion of autonomy is more than a sense of an isolated self, and must include an appreciation for the self in relation to others, recognizing that choices are made in the context of community. This view of autonomy in the context of health care leads to viewing patients as members of a social world, whose health care decisions affect others and are made in conjunction with trusted persons.

Factors that may threaten autonomy in health care settings include a prevailing paternalistic attitude that promotes the dependent role of the patient; assumptions that a patient's values and thought processes are the same as those of the health care provider; failure to appreciate a difference in levels of knowledge regarding health matters; and a focus on technology rather than caring. Persisting paternalistic attitudes have contributed to increased numbers of patients and families struggling with health care providers over control of health care decisions. **Paternalism** "derives from the privileges associated with the patriarchal family, where fathers are granted the right and responsibility to use their supposedly superior knowledge and judgment to make decisions on behalf of other family members" (Sherwin, 1992, p. 138). Paternalism implies well-intended actions of benevolent decision making, leadership, protection, and discipline. In the health care arena, paternalism is manifested in the making of decisions on behalf of patients without their full consent or knowledge. Although the principle of beneficence suggests that such decisions are focused on the patient's well-being, the power inherent in such a hierarchical arrangement can be abused, and the decisions made may reflect the interests of those other than the patient. Consider, for example, many elderly patients in nursing homes who are routinely sedated "for their own protection" because of "agitation and confusion." It is worth pondering whether medication used in this way is for the benefit of the patient, or to make life easier for the staff.

CASE PRESENTATION

Who Should Decide What Is Best?

Maureen is a thirty-eight-year-old woman with a diagnosis of multiple sclerosis (MS). She has had MS since her early twenties and has managed her life with the progressive disease, getting married, having a child, and establishing herself in a career as a counsellor at a local youth shelter. She is also actively involved in her local MS Society, and is a strong advocate for living independently with the disease.

Over the past two years, her condition has markedly worsened. She can no longer carry out her activities of daily living, nor can she drive or work. She has a daily caregiver in her home to assist her with self-care as well as the care of her four-year-old child. Her mother also helps out a great deal, but finds that it is difficult, as she is seventy-two and has advanced arthritis herself. Maureen's husband, John, a financial planner, works long hours and is feeling the strain of caring for her when her respite worker is not present. In the past two weeks, she has had episodes of forgetfulness and has had one serious fall. She has had to call her husband to come home early from evening meetings to help her with the care of their daughter. The caregiver has told Maureen's husband that she no longer considers the situation to be a safe one, for either Maureen or her daughter.

Maureen's neurologist has informed her that the disease is especially aggressive in her case and that she is no longer eligible, because of the progression, for a new experimental drug, which she was hoping she could try as part of a clinical trial, which offers a great deal of potential hope for those with MS.

Maureen's husband, John, and her mother, approach her along with her neurologist to discuss the option of being in a residence. They assure her that it would be better for her, her daughter, and her husband. He would not be worried about her when he was at work. Her daughter would be cared for by a nanny, her grandmother, and her father, and would be brought frequently to visit with Maureen. The residence that they have researched caters to younger clients and

(Continued)

is close to her home. They could decorate the unit to Maureen's taste and, they emphasize, she would be able to receive twenty-four-hour care there.

Maureen is very upset when they discuss this with her. She accuses them of "conspiring" against her and tells them that she is "not dead yet" nor is she "unable to make her own decisions." She adamantly refuses to consider this option, stating that she wishes to be home with her daughter and that there is nothing wrong with the current situation, with a few adaptations. She states that it appears that they have not considered other options. She is also angry that her physician is part of the discussion and appears to have already discussed it with her husband and mother, out of her presence.

THINK ABOUT IT

- Are John and Maureen's mother being paternalistic? Why or why not?
- Is Maureen's neurologist being paternalistic? What are the implications for his involvement in the discussion, from an ethical perspective?
- What ethical issues are evident in this case?
- What ethical issues do you think are relevant to the discussion of this case?
- Are there any other options that might be possible in this case?
- What do you think should happen next?
- What kinds of things should be considered in the discussion of Maureen's immediate future?

Inherent in the more traditional medical models is the belief that lay persons do not have the appropriate skills or knowledge to make health care decisions (Sherwin, 1992). What this attitude does not address, however, is that decisions about health require more than scientific expertise. Such decisions must take into account many factors, including the patient's values, culture, spiritual and other beliefs; evaluation of risks, benefits, and economic considerations; and effects on lifestyle and role. All the factors need to be considered within the context of the patient's life. For this to occur, patients must be engaged in the decision-making process as autonomous agents in relationships with others who can facilitate the decision-making processes.

How Far Does Autonomy Go?

Although the principle of autonomy has become a key consideration in health care ethics, it does have limits. Practitioners are not obligated to honour requests from patients or families for interventions that, in the best judgment of the practitioner, are outside accepted standards of care or that are contrary to the practitioner's own ethical views. Autonomy may also be limited by the availability of resources and by economic circumstances.

In discussions of patient self-determination, the principle of justice needs to be considered along with that of autonomy. **Justice** implies fair, equitable, and appropriate treatment in light of what is due or owed to persons, recognizing that giving to some may deny receipt to others who might otherwise have received these things. In determining who deserves what portion of finite health care resources, autonomy and justice may conflict where needs or demands for health care by autonomous patients outweigh available resources. Having finite resources implies necessarily that the rights of family members and of society must be considered in relation to the needs of individuals. Hardwig (2000) suggests that the medical and non-medical impact of treatment decisions on both the patient and the family needs to be considered. He reflects that patient autonomy implies the responsible use of freedom, which means considering the needs of family and society as well as our own desires. The limited availability and expense of many medical interventions bring such questions to the fore. Since people can be maintained on highly technological treatments (which are costly to the health care system) for prolonged periods of time, justice requires us to ask not only who deserves an intervention, but also who will gain the most benefit from it. Justice also requires that we are clear and explicit about the criteria we consider when making such decisions. Although the moral relevance of considering the interests of the family and society at large is not well addressed in current ethical theory, dilemmas faced by patients, families, and practitioners include these issues, and it is well worth pondering their implications.

ASK YOURSELF

What Is the Relationship between Nursing and Patient Autonomy?

- How would you describe nursing's role regarding the evolution of an emphasis on patient autonomy?

- How have you experienced paternalism in the health care system, as a nurse, patient or family member?

- How do you feel about the claim that the physician is most qualified to make health care decisions? What have you experienced in this regard?

- As nurses, how can we best support patients making autonomous health care decisions and facilitate decision-making processes?

INFORMED CONSENT

Informed consent provides protection of a patient's right to personal autonomy. The concept of informed consent is one that has come to mean that patients are given the opportunity to autonomously choose a course of action in regard to plans for health care. The choice includes the right to refuse interventions or recommendations about care, and to choose from available therapeutic alternatives. This is usually discussed in relation to surgery and complex medical procedures, but also includes consent to more common interventions that may have undesirable side effects, such as immunizations and medications. Even in a simple intervention such as the provision of a bed bath or insertion of an intravenous line, the consent of the patient must always be sought. Exceptions to informed consent include emergencies in which there is no time to disclose the information, situations in which a person is deemed not competent to provide an informed consent, and waivers by patients who do not want to know their prognosis or risks of treatment. Consent is considered to be informed when information is given to the person that any reasonable person might wish to have in the circumstances, in order to make such a decision, and when the person has also received answers to any questions or concerns that he or she may have (College of Nurses of Ontario, 2005). We will discuss in greater detail the necessary elements of an informed consent process below.

The emergence of informed consent *as we know it* has been affected by several factors. One factor has been the institutionalization of health care in hospitals, with their associated technologies and life-prolonging techniques, over which people are often assumed to have little control and limited understanding. However, with the availability of sophisticated medical information as easy to access as the Internet, patients often do have knowledge about technology, treatments, and techniques. In the days when health providers visited in the home, informed consent was not as necessary, because people had more control and better understanding of traditional remedies (Devettere, 2002). The courts, however, have exerted the most significant influence on shaping the doctrine of informed consent as we know it today.

Ethical and Legal Elements of Informed Consent

We must remember that, although the informed consent doctrine has foundations in law, it is essentially an ethical imperative. According to Williams (2008), "the notion of consent is grounded in the fundamental ethical principles of patient autonomy and respect for persons. Autonomy refers to the patient's right to make free decisions about his or her healthcare. Respect for persons requires that healthcare professionals foster patients' control over their own lives and refrain from carrying out unwanted interventions." (p. 12)

Information

The information component of informed consent includes both disclosure and understanding of the essential information. Figure 11–1 lists the information that must be included in an informed consent. People need access to sufficient information to help them understand their health concerns and make decisions regarding treatment. The information provided need not be "textbook" detail, but does need to offer enough explanation for the person to have a clear picture of the situation, what is being offered, and the alternatives and their risks, benefits, and consequences. Determining the adequacy of information disclosed in an informed consent is based on one or more standards: (1) *the professional practice standard*—the disclosure is consistent with the standards of the profession; (2) the *reasonable person standard*—the disclosure is what a reasonable person in similar circumstances would need in order to make an informed decision; and (3) the *subjective standard*—the disclosure is what the particular person wants or needs to know. Again, the challenge is to provide accurate and clear information in keeping with the standards, which, when considered separately, imply very different obligations of disclosure. Informed consent implies that the person has received the information and understands what is provided. Verification of understanding can be accomplished through discussion, in which patients have an opportunity to ask questions and are asked to describe their understanding of the nature of the intervention, alternatives, risks, and benefits. Although many people associate the informed consent process with a consent form, such a form is simply a representation that a clear, informed discussion took place and that the patient had an opportunity to hear, understand, and reflect upon the options available and the full information that needs to be provided in such a process. The most important part of the process is not the form *per se*, but the actual discussion that must take place, in a timely, unhurried, and thoughtful manner.

FIGURE 11–1 **ELEMENTS OF AN INFORMED CONSENT**

- A description of the health concern, diagnosis, and prognosis.
- Details about the consequences/prognosis associated with each option for treatment/intervention, as well as with no treatment.
- A description of the treatment or intervention.
- Details about potential risks for harm (physical, emotional, psychological, social, financial, etc.)
- Details about strategies in place to ameliorate potential risks for harm.
- Information about potential benefits, both to the individual and, in the case of consent for participation in research, benefits to society.
- Information about the voluntary nature of consent.
- For research participation, information about the voluntary nature of participation and the right to withdraw.
- For research participation, information as to how confidentiality and privacy will be maintained.
- Consent information should be provided at a level of understanding appropriate to the patient, with limited use of medical or legal terms and full explanation, in lay language, of any such term.
- Consent processes should not be rushed or hurried (except for cases of urgent or emergent health situations), with adequate time for reflection and informed decision making.

Voluntariness

Consent to something implies the freedom to voluntarily accept or reject it. This means that consent to health care interventions must be voluntary, without coercion, influence, force, or manipulation from health care providers or family. Force entails making someone do something against his or her will. Influence, coercion, and manipulation may be overt or subtle, and may include threats or a suggestion of threats, rewards, deception, or inducing excessive fear. The voluntary nature of consent does not prohibit health care providers from making recommendations or attempting to persuade patients to accept their suggestions. However, we must be alert to situations in which persuasion takes on the qualities of coercion or manipulation.

 CASE PRESENTATION

Language and Informed Consent

Christopher is a sixty-seven-year-old deaf man who was admitted to the hospital with atrial fibrillation. The nurse notes that he is alert, apparently oriented, and able to follow simple directions that she acts out, although he does look apprehensive as she cares for him. Christopher's social history indicates that he was brought into the hospital by a community worker who looks in on him because he is deaf and illiterate and has no family in the area. The worker had indicated that he came to the area as a new immigrant a number of years ago, along with a brother, who died the previous year. She had also noted that two of his five siblings were also deaf, and they had developed a type of sign language that was understood only by family members. At the interdisciplinary care conference, the medical resident in charge of the case voices frustration because of the need to get the patient's permission to do a stress test and to talk to him about medications and risk for stroke. The resident suggests that they should just get the patient to make an X on the form so they can go ahead with the treatment protocol because it is in the patient's best interest to do so. The social worker suggests that they get an interpreter for the deaf to come in and try to talk to him through sign language, although she is not sure he will understand.

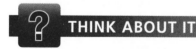 **THINK ABOUT IT**

Obtaining Informed Consent When There Is No Common Language

- What ethical dilemmas are evident in this case?
- What do you think about Christopher's decision-making capacity?

- Do you think it is possible to obtain an informed consent from Christopher? Support your position with discussion of elements of informed consent and decision-making capacity.

- In a situation such as this, it is evident that the patient has capacity for language and comprehension, although it is not understood by the health care providers, and that he has been able to care for himself with some assistance. How should these factors enter into determination of his decision-making capacity?

- How can the inability of the health care provider to communicate with a patient affect determination of the patient's decision-making capacity?

- What are the implications of denying Christopher important services because of a lack of common language and subsequent inability to ensure informed consent?

Nursing Role and Responsibilities: Informed Consent

While the practice of documenting informed consent for a procedure usually ends with the signing of a consent form, the actual process is much more complex. Following the rules laid out previously, informed consent must include explicit verification that the patient is aware of all options, the possible outcomes of each option, and the likely outcome with non-treatment. The patient must also recognize the implications that each option will have for his or her lifestyle. The nurse must be sensitive to the fact that the very act of asking a patient to sign a form giving permission for a particular treatment may constitute a form of coercion. It is the nurse's responsibility as advocate for the patient to ensure that all criteria for autonomous decision making are met. If the nurse believes that the patient does not understand the implications of any part of the process, including non-treatment and alternative options, or that the patient is unable to deliberate and to reason out the various choices, the nurse is ethically obligated to intervene or speak up on a patient's behalf. The nurse must act if it becomes apparent that the patient is not informed. Actions may include notifying the physician and requesting further information for the patient, or stopping the process until it is ensured that the decision can be made autonomously. The primary concern of the nurse is to ensure that all criteria for autonomous decision making are met. Remember, a consent form is a representation of a process, in which a patient is fully informed and volitionally able to make decisions autonomously.

Witnessing a patient's signature on a consent form implies accountability on the part of the nurse. Sullivan (1998) notes that the nurse's signature attests that the patient is giving consent willingly, is competent in that moment to give consent, and that the patient's signature is authentic. She cautions nurses who are not present when the treatment is explained to the patient to verify the patient's understanding of the procedure, inquire whether there are any questions that need to be discussed with the physician, and not to let a patient sign a consent form if there is any indication of coercion. She also stresses the importance of nurses documenting their communication with the patient and with the physician regarding any questions, concerns, or teaching related to the informed consent. Any special circumstances, such as the patient's inability to read or write, or the use of an interpreter if the patient speaks a different language, should also be documented.

ADVANCE DIRECTIVES

Given the dilemmas that can arise regarding the use of technology, we must encourage and assist people to make their wishes known concerning the use of such interventions. For those who are mentally alert and capable of making decisions, informed consent is needed prior to initiating any life-sustaining interventions. To ensure that our wishes regarding treatment are followed in the event that we have lost decision-making capacity, advance directives are needed. **Advance directives** are instructions that indicate which health care interventions to initiate or withhold, or that designate someone who will act as a surrogate or proxy in making such decisions in the event that we lose decision-making capacity. Such directives can also be considered a kind of informed consent for future interventions. Advance directives support people in making decisions on their own behalf, and help to ensure that patients have the kind of end-of-life care they want. In order to help patients be as clear as possible about their choices, the various life-sustaining measures that may be considered in end-of-life care should be discussed openly and clearly. Patients should be encouraged to express verbally, or in writing, their wishes about specific interventions such as tube feedings, breathing machines, cardiopulmonary resuscitation, antibiotics, withdrawal of food and/or fluids, and dialysis. Consideration of interventions should include how long they might want to stay on an intervention if it is initiated and their condition continues to decline or is not improving. In addition to enabling people to have choices in their dying process, the presence of clearly understood advance directives can alleviate stress on family and clinicians when dealing with end-of-life concerns.

Perhaps the most important factor in making decisions regarding end-of-life care is clear and open communication between the patient, or the surrogate/proxy, and health care providers. We need to do more than merely seek to know which potential life-sustaining technology a person does or does not want. We need to see and get to know the person who is making these decisions, along with the values and beliefs that clearly underlie the more pragmatic decisions. Eliciting a clear statement of personal values is basic to this process. What does the person value in life? What constitutes quality of life for the person? What are his or her personal beliefs and concerns about dying? We must recognize the influence of cultural, societal, spiritual, and family norms and perspectives on personal values. For example, in some cultures, speaking of death and dying is believed to bring bad luck. Family wishes may influence personal choices, and in some cultures the patient may defer decisions about end-of-life care to the family. When discussing different interventions, we need to ensure that patients understand what the procedure is and what it involves. They also need to appreciate that the risks and benefits of life-sustaining interventions vary with age, health condition, and whatever circumstances prompt the consideration of the intervention. For example, the literature shows no evidence that tube feedings prolong life or improve quality of life for patients with dementia or multisystem illness (Finucane, Christmas & Travis, 1999; McCann, 1999). We need to understand *why* the patient or family wants a particular intervention, and *what* it is that they think it will do for them.

Advance directives include **living wills** and **durable powers of attorney**. Living wills are legal documents that give directions to health care providers related to withholding or withdrawing life support if certain conditions exist. Statutes regulating living wills vary from province to province, so nurses must be familiar with their own provincial laws and statutes. In addition, nomenclature varies between provinces. Living wills guide decisions by indicating a person's desires regarding life-sustaining interventions; however, they also raise issues of concern. Directives in living wills may be vague, and may address only the interventions a person does not want. Ideally, a living will should achieve two ends. First, it should articulate the patient's clear wishes regarding specific health care interventions and decision-making processes, based on authentic values. Second, it should clearly identify a proxy or substitute decision maker who will communicate and enact the patient's wishes if she or he is unable to do so.

Part of an advance directive is indicating who it is you want to be your proxy or Substitute Decision-Maker (SDM), in the case that you are unable to make your own decisions. This person, in his or her role as proxy, would be responsible for ensuring that your wishes about health and personal care, as articulated in a living will or proxy directive, are carried out in the event of your incapacity. As noted, in different provinces, this role is called by different names. The term "attorney for personal care" is used in Ontario, while other provinces, such as Nova Scotia, New Brunswick, Manitoba, and Alberta, use the term "proxy." No matter what the label, the fundamental roles and responsibilities are the same—to make decisions on behalf of another person who can no longer do so autonomously, in keeping with their wishes, values, and beliefs. In effect, an advance directive and identification of an SDM essentially extends one's autonomy when one can no longer exercise it directly.

An important part of identifying a proxy decision maker is to make sure that there is a thoughtful and thorough discussion between the two parties, about values, beliefs, and wishes regarding health, illness, and personal care. While it isn't necessary to have values completely aligned, it is key to ensure that the proxy decision maker has both an understanding of the values of the person creating an advance directive and the motivation and will to keep the best interests of that person in mind.

Decision-Making Capacity

Conscious adults are presumed to have decision-making capacity, unless there is evidence to the contrary. **Decision-making capacity** is a medical determination relating only to the issue at hand, as people may have the ability to make decisions about some areas and not others. For example, a person may be able to make decisions about health, while being unable to make reasonable decisions about household or financial matters. Persons may have decision-making capacity at some times and not others, and in each specific situation, there must be a determination of whether they have, or do not have, the capacity. The fact that a person makes a decision that seems unreasonable to the health care provider does not necessarily indicate a lack of decision-making capacity; it may merely reflect a difference in values. If the decision seems unreasonable, or not in keeping with the patient's previously stated authentic values and beliefs, however, it is then wise to explore the patient's rationales and/or capacity regarding decision making.

Elements of Decision-Making Capacity

When evaluating a patient or surrogate decision maker (SDM) for decision-making capacity, several elements must be present. These are listed in Figure 11-2. First, the patient must be able to understand all relevant information, including the nature of the health care problem, the prognosis, treatment options and recommendations, and the risks, benefits, and consequences of each. Second, the patient must be able to communicate this understanding and her or his choices. Third, the patient must possess a set of values and goals that make it possible to evaluate whether this health care decision will be of benefit in terms of personal goals. Fourth, the patient must have the ability to reason and to deliberate over the available choices; this includes the ability to grasp notions such as risk and percentage, cause and effect, and chance and probability. Although it is not unreasonable to see some indecision, or even a change of mind once a choice has been made, a great deal of vacillation between choices may suggest the need to re-evaluate decision-making capacity. It may also indicate a lack of understanding, necessitating education or intervention by the nurse. Nurses are in a key position to observe patients and families for the presence of these elements of decision-making capacity. As patient advocates, nurses need to assess, document, and communicate to appropriate members of the health care team any concerns in this regard.

FIGURE 11–2 **ELEMENTS OF DECISION-MAKING CAPACITY**

The Patient Must:

- have the ability to understand all information.
- have the ability to communicate understanding and choices.
- have personal values and goals that guide the decision.
- have the ability to reason and deliberate.

Physicians usually have the legal authority and responsibility to determine decision-making capacity. Determining incapacity is best done in consultation with family or others who have the patient's best interest in mind. We must make a distinction between decision-making capacity and competence. Decisions about **competence**, which is the ability to make meaningful life decisions, require a legal action and always require more than simply one person to evaluate and assess competence. Legally, persons are considered competent unless there is a ruling by a judge that they cannot make meaningful life decisions.

When a patient lacks decision-making capacity, someone else must be identified as an SDM to make decisions for the patient. In the case of children, the surrogate is usually a parent or legal guardian. With adults, the SDM may be a spouse, parent, adult child or children, other relatives, or another person named as SDM in the patient's advance directives. In situations where a patient has no advance directives, or has not named a surrogate to make decisions in the event of incapacity, health care providers should work with family and others to identify an SDM. The legal process for choosing an SDM varies from province to province and you need to be familiar with the process in your province. The person chosen as SDM should be someone willing to serve in this role and able to make health care decisions that are in accordance with the patient's wishes, or that are consistent with the patient's best interest if these wishes are not known or cannot be reasonably discerned. Whenever possible, the SDM should demonstrate care and concern for, and have regular contact with, the patient. In addition, the surrogate should be willing and able to participate fully in the decision-making process, and engage in face-to-face contact and communication with caregivers. Close family members, such as parents, adult children, adult siblings, and adult grandchildren are often considered first if the patient has not designated an SDM. However, close friends or neighbours may at times be better qualified to make these decisions. The decisions made by the SDM should reflect the patient's values, including cultural and spiritual perspective, to the extent that these are reasonably known.

As noted earlier in the chapter, in different provinces, surrogate or substitute decision makers are referred to by a variety of labels and names (Singer, 2002). Furthermore, in each province, the roles are articulated and enacted somewhat differently. It is up to the nurse in each jurisdiction to have a working knowledge of the law as it pertains to advance care planning.

Nursing Role and Responsibilities: Advance Care Planning

Advance care planning refers to a communication process that may involve the creation of a living will, along with identification of a person to make health care or personal care decisions for you if you become incapacitated and unable to advocate for yourself. The goals of such a process are to ensure that your authentic choices, thoughtfully made while competent, can be carried out in the case that you are unable to articulate such wishes. Writing a living will allows you to maintain your autonomy, even when unable to directly enact choices or articulate preferences.

A living will is a document that allows you to clearly articulate advance directives. These are instructions, made in advance, that instruct others on how to provide your health care or personal care, or make choices for you and in your best interest. Best interest, in the case of a living will, means maintaining integrity of the choices made by the person.

There are two parts to an advance directive: an instruction directive and a proxy directive. A proxy directive identifies a person who will make decisions on your behalf when you are no longer able to do so. A proxy must be carefully chosen, and should have a clear idea of your authentic choices, wishes, values, and beliefs. Together, you should have thorough discussions of your wishes and values as you construct your living will.

An instruction directive is a set of instructions for the proxy to carry out. These instructions may pertain to health care decisions such as treatment, diagnostic care, or interventions, or they may be related to personal care decisions involving hygiene, nutrition, and hydration. Again, clearly, the values and beliefs that underlie such decisions should be articulated in such a document, to further guide decision making (Singer, 2002).

Living wills are legal documents and should be respected as such by health care teams and family members. In different provinces, however, they do have different roles and vocabulary, along with different understandings of how advance directives can be carried out under varying provincial legislation regarding the use of living wills. Most provinces have legalized the use of living wills. The Canadian Medical Association has a policy clearly endorsing the use of living wills and the Canadian Nurses Association's *Code of Ethics* for Registered Nurses identifies "promoting and respecting informed decision making" as an ethical principle (Canadian Nurses Association, 2008b, p. 11). The Code of Ethics states that nurses have a responsibility to "consider and respect the best interests of the person receiving care and any previously known wishes or advance directives that apply . . . " (Canadian Nurses Association, 2008b, p. 12). As well, the Canadian Nurses Association, in the 2008 publication entitled *Providing nursing care at the end of life*, outlines the responsibilities of health care practitioners and agencies to facilitate the use of advance directives, underpinned by principles of autonomy, self-determination, and rights (Canadian Nurses Association, 2008a).

What is the nursing role and responsibility regarding advance directives? Whatever the work setting, nurses have a key role and responsibility in ensuring that patients have an opportunity to complete advance directives, and in interpreting and following through with patients' wishes as expressed through these directives. As nurses, we need to be aware of legislation and institutional policies that guide and govern advance directives. We also need to be aware of the policies and procedures regarding advance directives where we work. Tilden (2000) urges us to complete our own advance directives. Doing so helps us to reflect on our own values, beliefs, and concerns associated with end-of-life issues, to learn more about the specific forms and processes involved, and ultimately to have more empathy with patients going through this process. Information concerning advance directives is often provided to patients on admission to a facility by a clerical worker; however, in many cases, a nurse completing an initial assessment, upon admission, should be asking about advance directives, living wills, and substitute decision makers. Nurses can use this as an opportunity to stress the importance of having such directives, and to advocate for patients who may need assistance in developing advance directives. This is also a beginning opportunity for us to help patients explore personal values, their understanding of themselves in the context of their current situation, and significant cultural or other issues that may influence decision making. The one realistic constraint on having this kind of thorough and thoughtful discussion is lack of time. Nurses often cite heavy patient loads, limited time to conduct thorough assessments, and multiple competing priorities as preventing them from having meaningful discussions with patients about issues such as these. As nurses, we need to be familiar with our patients' directives for care, and ensure that care is consistent with the patient's wishes as expressed in the advance directives. We also need to ensure that we make the time to promote meaningful discussions on advance directives, or at the very least, direct interested patients toward helpful resources on creating advance directives. Nursing's advocacy role includes informing other health team members of the presence and content of advance directives, alerting appropriate team members to changes in patient wishes or to evidence of changes in the patient's decision-making capacity, and intervening on behalf of the patient when wishes expressed in advance directives are not being followed. As nurses, we have an important role in increasing public awareness about advance directives through patient and community education, through research, and through education of nurses and other health care providers. It may well be that one of the most important parts of increasing awareness is to begin by creating your own living will and assisting your family and friends to do so as well. Encouraging patients to create an advance directive and emphasizing the importance of having a clear articulation of your wishes in place is much more effective if you have also done so. Having the experience of thinking through your own wishes, values, and beliefs about health, illness, and personal care, as you create your own advance directive and include those around you in the discussion, also helps to increase your own comfort with discussing similar kinds of issues in an open way with patients who may feel uncomfortable, ill at ease, or frightened by the idea of discussing or creating an advance directive.

CASE PRESENTATION

The Absence of Advance Directives

Ninety-year-old Mr. Moshe did not have advance directives when he was admitted to the hospital with Alzheimer's disease and renal failure. Although he was coherent at times and could converse with caregivers, the doctor determined Mr. Moshe did not have decision-making capacity and named his daughter Zelda, with whom he had been residing, as his SDM. At this point, Zelda approached the nursing manager to request that any inquiries about Mr.

(Continued)

Moshe's health status, from his other children, be directed to her and that her siblings should not be given access to Mr. Moshe. As Mr. Moshe's health began to deteriorate rapidly, the nursing staff asked the attending physician, in rounds, if a DNR status had ever been discussed with the patient and family. The physician agreed to find out, and spoke with the patient and his family about Mr. Moshe's resuscitation status. Although Zelda's two siblings called frequently inquiring about their father, Zelda continued to refuse to inform them about their father's condition, nor did she allow them access to him. One evening when Zelda was not present, Mr. Moshe's son called the nursing station to ask why he was not being provided with information about his father. He told the nurse that he and Zelda had been estranged for many years and that she had effectively "shut him out" of his father's life. Because of this conflict and the continuing discussion regarding Mr. Moshe's DNR status, the nurses notified the physician about the son's phone call and requested an ethics committee consultation to determine the best interests of the patient.

The ethics committee representative convened a family meeting that included Zelda, Mr. Moshe's sons, the physician, Mr. Moshe's primary nurse, and two members of the multidisciplinary team providing care to Mr. Moshe. After explaining that the purpose of the meeting was to discuss the type of care that would be in the best interests of their father, not to resolve family issues, the physician was asked to discuss Mr. Moshe's current health status and prognosis. Each of his children were given the opportunity to ask questions of the physician and primary nurse. Then each family member was asked to voice what their father valued in life, and what they believed to be his wishes regarding end-of-life care. Even though Zelda and her brothers had not spoken in nearly ten years, they each stated the same thing: that their father had told them he would never want to be on life support. The two brothers also requested that they be allowed to visit their father and to call and check on him. When they were informed that there currently was no legal SDM for their father, they agreed to have Zelda continue in that role, providing she allow them access to him. They stated that even though they were upset with her, they believed she loved him and provided good care for him. To close the meeting, all family members were invited to go and join together at their father's bedside, where they shared prayer and family stories. Mr. Moshe died that night.

 ## THINK ABOUT IT

Considering the Patient's Best Interests

- Because Mr. Moshe was coherent at times, do you think the health care team should have asked him what he would want regarding life support?

- What do you think of the choice of a surrogate for Mr. Moshe? What factors do you think were considered in appointing Zelda as surrogate? Are there factors you think should have been considered that were not?

- As the nurse caring for Mr. Moshe, what would be your concerns regarding his situation? How do you think you would have responded in this situation?

- How did the process of the family meeting address the communication that is needed for making end-of-life decisions?

- What kinds of roles can nurses play in family meetings? And in family conflict that involves patients?

- Reflecting on this case, think about your own choice if you have identified a substitute decision-maker. What factors did you consider in your choice and why?

CHOICES CONCERNING LIFE AND HEALTH

Although discussions of patient autonomy frequently focus on issues of informed consent and end-of-life decisions, issues related to self-determination can arise in any area of nursing practice. In every area of practice, nurses must deal with the effects of lifestyle choices on patients' health and healing. Many people who come into our care are suffering from the ill effects of such things as overeating; tobacco, drug, or alcohol use; risky or unprotected sexual activity; or work-related stress. These factors are considered by many to be lifestyle "choices." By virtue of this label, the implication is that some people make good choices, while others do not. Our job is to deal with the present health concern, while encouraging change toward healthier living. However, patients are often not willing or able to follow the treatment plan and make the changes needed for healthier living. Dealing with patients whose health problems are clearly related to lifestyle choices, yet who are not willing or able to change their behaviours, may present ethical or moral dilemmas for nurses. Although nurses may acknowledge that the autonomous person has the right to choose healthy or unhealthy behaviours, it may be difficult to be as caring toward those who are perceived to have brought problems on themselves.

This is another area where the principle of justice may temper the bounds of autonomy. In situations where resources are limited, questions arise regarding whether it is ethical to put resources into treatments for people whose health problems are brought on by unhealthy life choices. This is countered by the question of whether it is ethical to refuse treatment or provide a lesser level of care to someone because the provider does not agree with the lifestyle choices. It can also be countered by the argument that for some, what may appear to be "poor choices" are not in fact, choices at all. Consider the example of a woman who drinks excessive amounts of alcohol. There may be multiple factors that have an effect upon whether or not this behaviour is truly a choice: her genetic predisposition, her past experiences and support, her level of education, and her ability to enact choices in other areas of her life. As another example, think of the mother who makes very poor nutritional choices for her children. She chooses food that is quick, highly processed, and easy, instead of nutritional, complex, and vitamin-rich. At first glance, she may appear to be making poor choices. But if we care to look deeper, we may see that she is a single mother, working two jobs, and unable to spend time preparing food. She also has never had any education on nutrition and making healthy food choices. Furthermore, she feels tremendous guilt at not being home enough for her children and finds that giving in to their wishes for junk food is one way she can demonstrate her love. Finally, think of the patient who has an ongoing peptic ulcer related to extreme stress at work and home. While some of us may think that the obvious choice is to change jobs or leave the current job, it may not be a choice that is easy for that patient to make. He may be the sole supporter of a family. Others may voice trite solutions to stress at home such as *"Make time for yourself"* to the patient. It is likely far more helpful to discuss the patient's family situation and see if there are available resources that might offer the patient assistance, such as counselling or respite care for elderly parents or children with disabilities.

So while we might view "poor" health and lifestyle choices as, in fact, choices, it is important to look more deeply into the contextual situations of persons in an attempt to discover why they are making these choices before judging harshly or assuming that they have no interest in making healthier or different choices.

CHOICES REGARDING RECOMMENDED TREATMENT

What are nurses to do when patients are well informed and apparently able to follow plans of care, yet do not? Certainly one hears of physicians who refuse to continue to care for patients who do not comply with instructions—smoking cessation, for example. In a climate of limited resources, this is a question worthy of contemplation. In the most recent iteration of its *Code of Ethics for Registered Nurses,* the Canadian Nurses Association states that, as part of promoting and respecting informed decision making, "Nurses respect the informed decision-making capability of capable persons, including choices of lifestyles or treatment not conducive to good health" (Canadian Nurses Association, 2008b, p. 12). Further, quality of nursing care must not be affected by the patients' individual differences in background, customs, attitudes, and beliefs. Health care practices are an integral part of patients' backgrounds, customs, and beliefs. Therefore, it is clear that refusal to participate in a plan of care, regardless of the outcome, is the prerogative of the patient, and must not affect the caring attitude of the nurse. Unhealthy life practices are part of the whole person, and should be taken into consideration when revising plans of care.

ASK YOURSELF

How Should We Think About Lifestyle Choices When Making Allocation Decisions?

Autonomy implies that persons have the right to make choices about things that affect their lives, whether these choices have a positive or negative effect, unless these choices infringe on the rights of others. There is an argument that the societal and financial burden of resultant health problems by those persons who make "poor" lifestyle choices (such as smoking, overeating, or taking illegal drugs) may in fact infringe upon the rights of others.

To make the point clearer, let's consider an example. Queues exist for access to particular diagnostic or therapeutic interventions, such as CT or MRI scans. Some might feel that those who have a problem related to a genetic or acquired problem should be in the queue ahead of those who have a problem related to a lifestyle "choice."

This is commonly and quite dangerously implied in many discussions of those who are diagnosed with HIV and AIDS. Many feel that those who may have contracted the virus through blood transfusions should be considered or treated differently than those who contracted it through unprotected sexual contact. The implication, of course, is that those who contracted HIV through a blood transfusion were not making a choice and are "innocent victims" while the concomitant assumption is that unprotected sexual activity is always an informed choice.

Other places where these kinds of discussions surface is in the area of organ transplantation and eligibility for surgery. Consider the decision of the health care team who must choose between two clearly viable candidates for a liver transplant: one of whom has a congenital or acquired liver disease, such as primary biliary cirrhosis, and the other of whom is a self-identified lapsed alcoholic. While many believe that factors such as these should not play a part in the decision as to "who may receive the liver" or "who may receive the liver first," it is clear that they can and do play a part in such assessments and decisions.

While these decisions may be framed as purely "clinical" decisions, they often do, realistically, include judgment, by clinicians, about the "goodness" or "badness" of a patient's decision to smoke, drink alcohol, take illegal drugs, overeat, or engage in risky sexual behaviour (Walton *et al.*, 2007).

- What factors do you think should be considered when organizing patients into a queue, say, for hip replacement surgery or cardiac surgery?
- What factors should not be part of the decision, and why not?
- Is it fair that taxes are paid by all persons to support health care services that are used more often by those who might be overweight, smokers, or sedentary individuals? Why or why not?

(Continued)

- What kinds of personal values, beliefs, or biases are you identifying as you think about these questions?
- If you were making choices about allocation of health care resources, how would you consider, if at all, factors we call *lifestyle choices* (smoking, overeating, drinking alcohol, exposure to stress, drug use, etc.)?
- What kind of consequences, for patients, do you foresee if they know that they are being "judged" by health care professionals to whom they turn for advocacy, support, and holistic care?
- Have you encountered a patient who has disclosed what you consider to be a "poor" lifestyle choice? How did you feel toward that patient? Did it change your approach to her or him?
- Reflect on your own lifestyle choices and habits. Are there any that others might think are "unhealthy" or a "poor" choice? How does that make you feel? What if you had to disclose this to a health professional? Would you feel hesitant to do so?

Ultimately, choices about health care practices belong to patients. If allowed to choose, patients should not be labelled in a negative way for choices that nurses do not agree with. It is not appropriate for professionals who express the belief that all competent patients have the right to autonomous choice to then make value judgments about the choices that are made, and subsequently to label patients as noncompliant, unco-operative, or difficult. In fact, it is worth pondering whether the term "noncompliant" even belongs in nursing vocabulary. The notion of compliance relates to the paternalistic view that health care providers know what is best for patients and that, providing patients follow these directions, they will get well. Nurses should speak more appropriately in terms of motivation to follow a mutually agreed upon plan of care that incorporates patient and family values and beliefs. We must remember that patients have a right to refuse interventions, and they have a right to seek therapies other than those offered by conventional western medicine.

CASE PRESENTATION

A Challenging Patient

Rochelle, a thirty-six-year-old woman who is a known cocaine addict, presented to the emergency room (ER) with severe left leg pain and swelling. The triage nurse reviewed her chart and presenting problem, noting that she had been seen two days prior for chest pain and left leg pain. Assuming these complaints were evaluated then, the nurse sent her to the "fast track" area to be seen by the nurse practitioner (NP). The NP noted that her chart was flagged regarding her cocaine addiction and that the physician who had seen her at the previous visit, after doing an EKG, CBC, electrolytes (which were normal), and a urine drug screen (which was positive for cocaine), discharged her with diagnoses of atypical chest pain and drug use. The NP's assessment revealed no shortness of breath, cough, or chest pain; severe swelling and skin tightness of the left leg, with exquisite tenderness and positive Homan's sign, were suggestive of deep vein thrombosis. When the NP went to the ER physician saying that the patient needed to be evaluated by him, she was told to keep the patient over there and do the workup because he had a patient with a "more serious" problem in the ER.

When the ultrasound confirmed extensive deep vein thrombosis, the NP told the patient the situation and that she needed to be hospitalized. The patient immediately said that she could not stay because she had no one to watch her nine-year-old-daughter, and she began to put on her shoes to leave. The NP told her that she could choose to leave but that the reason for the insistence on her staying was that this was a very serious problem from which she could die. Rochelle's response was to start crying, saying that she thought she would go home anyway, because she had nothing to live for since her husband had died, so she would go home to die. When the NP called Rochelle's primary physician to alert him to the situation, he responded that he would come in to see her only if Rochelle agreed to stay; otherwise, it would be a waste of his time. After considerable effort, the NP contacted Rochelle's mother, who reluctantly agreed to keep her granddaughter when the NP explained the situation, and Rochelle agreed to stay.

THINK ABOUT IT

Dealing with Patients Who Make Apparently Unhealthy Choices

- What issues of patient self-determination are evident in this case?
- How do you see lifestyle choices affecting Rochelle's care? What ethical issues must be considered here?
- Take an honest look at how you think you might react to Rochelle, knowing that she frequently shows up in the ER and is a cocaine addict.
- As the nurse in this situation, how would you deal with the patient's saying she could not stay? What do you think of the way the NP handled it?
- Evaluate ethical issues involved in the responses of the various health care practitioners in this case.

Complementary and Alternative Medicine (CAM)

Many people utilize therapies that may be termed **complementary** or **alternative** in contrast to more conventional medical therapies, which may also be called allopathic or Western medical therapies (Eisenberg *et al.*, 1998). Conventional medical treatments are provided by physicians, registered nurses, and other allied health care professionals, such as psychologists and respiratory therapists. These conventional medical therapies are, for the most part, regulated by federal bodies such as Health Canada, after being tested for safety and efficacy. Examples of complementary and alternative medicine (CAM) may include acupuncture, herbal and nutritional interventions, healing touch, massage, meditation and guided imagery. While the terms complementary and alternative are sometimes used interchangeably, they have quite different meanings. Complementary therapies refer to those that are used alongside conventional therapies. An example might be a cancer patient who is receiving chemotherapy and radiation to treat her cancer, but also utilizes acupuncture and herbal remedies to help control her nausea and pain. On the other hand, alternative therapies refer to the use of those therapies instead of conventional treatment. An example might be the cancer patient who decides not to receive chemotherapy or radiation to treat cancer, but only utilizes herbal and nutritional therapies provided through care from a homeopathic doctor. Most therapies used as alternative therapies are considered to be scientifically unproven. The regulation of the providers of CAM therapies varies from province to province and this can contribute to potential risk for patients seeking these kinds of therapies. For example, the practice of homeopathy is not regulated in any province, and the practice of traditional Chinese medicine is regulated only in one province (Andrews & Boon, 2005). While there may be risks inherent in seeking some CAM therapies, the use of and interest in CAM is increasing. As of 2005, it was estimated that approximately 3.8 million Canadians (or about twelve percent) have reported going to a CAM therapist (Millar, 2001; Andrews & Boon, 2005). Rates of anywhere between twelve and twenty percent of the population in Canada using CAM therapies has been cited, and this is typical of many other Western countries (Andrew & Boon, 2005).

Several issues regarding the use of CAM need to be considered. First, people have a right to use other modalities to address their health care needs that they may feel are not being met by conventional medicine. Many people cite needs such as improving quality of life, preventing illness, and gaining control over an illness, as reasons they have for seeking CAM therapies (Willison & Andrews, 2004).

Second, nurses and other health care practitioners need to develop at least a talking knowledge, and better yet a working knowledge, of such therapies in order to be better able to discuss their use with patients. Many therapies work as an adjunct to medical interventions, some may interact in unhealthy ways, and the efficacy of many modalities is not yet known. Nurses need not be practitioners of other modalities in order to discuss them with patients any more than they need to be able to do surgery in order to discuss it. Nurses should create an atmosphere that encourages nonjudgmental discussion of all modalities being considered or employed, with a goal of using whatever is beneficial for the particular patient. Transcultural considerations (which are discussed in Chapter 18) may influence a person's choice of treatment modalities.

Third, CAM should not be discounted merely because they are not understood within the conventional medical framework; however, it is also important to counsel patients to explore the validity of claims made about a particular therapy.

Fourth, as research continues and expands in the area of CAM, the question of whether informed consent will need to at least acknowledge these therapies as treatment options must be addressed.

Fifth, nurses who are skilled in CAM need to be clear about what is within their scope of practice according to their provincial regulatory body. The ethical stance with CAM, as with other interventions, requires offering an explanation of the intervention and receiving permission from the patient or family prior to initiating the therapy. Because many of these therapies can affect conventional interventions, practitioners should apprise other health team members of their use and document both the treatments and their effects.

Controversial Choices

The value of patient self-determination is cited to support two decisions that have been the focus of much controversy in this country for many years: abortion and active euthanasia. Both of these choices are embedded in many people's fundamental values and beliefs regarding life and death. Abortion in particular is an example of an issue in which legal answers have been sought for ethical dilemmas. As well, the potential for transmission of HIV infections within health care settings raises controversial issues regarding testing and disclosure. This discussion presents some of the arguments on both sides of these three issues.

Nurses need to be very clear about their own values regarding each of these issues, and find a balance between personal values and professional obligations to patients and families. Nurses must sort out their own beliefs about what is right and wrong, so that they can differentiate between tasks and roles that are consistent with their ethical stance and those that are not, and make responsible practice decisions accordingly. Davis, Fowler & Aroskar (2009) suggest that in the process of reasoning through dilemmas such as those involved with these issues, the least that can be expected is that the nurse not abandon the patient. In fact, it is ethically problematic to ever abandon a patient and, in all cases, care must be in place and assured to all patients, regardless of what choices or decisions they make. The authors note that a nurse should view the rights and interests of others in a way that she might wish her own rights and interests considered by others, while also being mindful of a nurses' responsibilities to not only herself and the patient, but also the institution and the profession of nursing.

Abortion

The abortion debate sparks passionate, emotion-laden arguments in political, social, legal, religious, and moral arenas. Issues of self-determination arise regarding the mother's right to control her body and her life (right to choose), in contrast to rights of the unborn fetus to a chance at life (right to life). Those in the right-to-life camp believe that abortion constitutes murder of an unborn person, suggesting that it is a legal as well as an ethical matter. This has raised questions about the role of government in dealing with this ethical concern. Those who hold to the right to choose maintain that the right to privacy regarding health care decisions includes a woman's reproductive choices, implying that governmental regulation is an infringement on this privacy.

Values in relation to life are fundamental considerations in regard to abortion. Such values include beliefs about when life begins, considerations regarding quality of life for children who are unwanted, and concerns about the mother's life and health. Some believe that life starts at conception, while others hold that life begins only when a fetus is viable outside the womb. Discussions regarding viability continue to change as technology enables the survival of babies of lower and lower birth weights, and results in saving some imperiled newborns at a gestational age not much more advanced than some aborted fetuses.

Opponents of abortion hold the position that because a fetus possesses humanity and the potential for viable life, it must be accorded all human rights, including the right to life. Proponents of choice argue that, based on autonomy, a woman has a right to her own body, and that no woman should be forced to bear a child that she does not want. Because abortion is a situation in which many feel that two lives are involved, dilemmas arise regarding who has rights, and whose rights take precedence.

CASE PRESENTATION

A Conflict of Values

Emilia is a new nursing graduate who is looking for a full-time position in an acute care hospital. She has envisioned, in her career planning, that she would like to be an operating room (OR) nurse, once she has some experience. One downtown hospital is hiring new graduates to work in the OR recovery room, and she jumps at the opportunity, knowing that a position in a recovery room is an excellent stepping stone to one day working in an OR. At the end of her job interview, Emilia has a chance to ask questions. She asks the nurse manager, who is the interviewer, what kinds of patients are cared for in the recovery room, and what types of day surgeries they may have undergone. The nurse manager tells her that many patients undergo colonoscopies and uroscopies, as well as breast biopsies and tonsillectomies. She also notes that there are also quite a few patients who undergo dilatation and curettage or uterine scraping (D and C) and therapeutic abortions. When a look of concern crosses Emilia's face, the manager asks her directly, "Emilia, would that be a problem for you to care for those patients?" Emilia responds by saying, "Well, I don't agree with abortion and my religion forbids it, but I know I would be able to provide good care to all patients as a nurse."

Later that night, Emilia sends a quick text to her friend from school, Padma, to let her know how the interview went. She tells Padma that she feels uncomfortable about being asked to care for women who have undergone a therapeutic abortion, but didn't tell the nurse manager. When she asks Padma what she should do, Padma tells Emilia that she should talk to the manager about this or decline the position, if offered. Emilia considers Padma's advice. First thing in the morning, she calls the nurse manager and tells her that, upon further reflection, she feels uncomfortable providing care for patients undergoing therapeutic abortion and couldn't continue the application process. The nurse manager thanks Emilia for her honesty and confirms that a position in that recovery room would not be a good option for her, as nurses are not allowed to "pick and choose" their patients. However, she adds that there is a part-time position in the recovery room for the coronary catheterization lab and that she would consider Emilia for that position, if she wished. Finally, she gently tells Emilia to think seriously and carefully about her future career plans to work in an operating room.

? THINK ABOUT IT

- Should Emilia have said something different to the nurse manager in her interview? Was it reasonable that she went home to think about it?

- What kinds of problems might Emilia and her patients have encountered if Emilia had ignored her feelings and simply accepted the position?

- Are there any situations in which you know that you might be uncomfortable caring for patients who have made particular choices? Have you thought about how you will deal with this in your nursing practice and career planning?

There is no agreement about the morality of abortion in our society. It is a complex issue with many facets to consider. Although debate generally focuses on areas related to rights of the woman or the fetus, Mahowald (2000) suggests that it is also important to consider the morality of circumstances that provide fertile ground for abortion. She notes that immoral conditions that sometimes occasion abortion include: poverty, lack of social and medical supports for pregnancy and parenthood, stereotypical views of sex roles and biological parenthood, and a eugenic mentality that welcomes only "premium babies," those babies that meet the parents' desired specifications (p. 200). She stresses the need for society to direct more effort into rectifying these conditions.

Active Euthanasia

As discussed in Chapter 10, technology has caused death to become an unnatural event in the lives of many people. In Canada, active euthanasia and assisted suicide are both illegal, and taking part in either of them is a criminal act, even if carried out with merciful intentions or the goal of relieving suffering. Section 14 of Canada's *Criminal Code* states "No person is entitled to consent to have death inflicted on him, and such consent does not affect the criminal responsibility of any person by whom death may be inflicted on the person by whom consent is given." Additionally, section 241 refers to suicidal behaviour, indicating that "Everyone who counsels a person to commit suicide or aids or abets a person to commit suicide, whether suicide ensues or not, is guilty of an indictable offence and liable to imprisonment for a term not exceeding fourteen years." In Canada, euthanasia and assisted suicide are considered criminal conduct.

Because there is a worry that health care providers will not adhere to their personal wishes regarding end-of-life issues, and/or they have fears about prolonged suffering resulting from prolongation of dying, and about the lack of control that each of these engenders, many people consider the possibility of active euthanasia or assisted suicide. **Active voluntary euthanasia** is an act in which the physician both provides the means of death and administers it, such as a lethal dose of medication. With **assisted suicide** the patients receive the means of death from someone, such as a physician, but activate the process themselves. Justification offered by proponents of these acts include respect for the person's autonomy in choosing to end his or her life if it is deemed intolerable due to conditions of a lingering terminal illness, and compassion exhibited in relief of the patient's suffering. Opponents argue from a stance of the sanctity of life (defined and discussed in more detail in Chapter 10), saying that any such act violates the prohibition against killing human beings. They hold that suffering can almost always be relieved, and they voice concerns about potential abuses, such as **involuntary euthanasia** to contain health care costs, if such acts were permitted (Lo, 1995).

It is particularly important to consider the reason for a patient's request for assisted suicide or euthanasia. When the patient indicates that life has become intolerable, we must determine why this is so. Often, inadequate pain management and depression are factors that enter into this perception, which, when treated appropriately, may change the patient's perspective. This may not always be the case, however, and nurses need to be able to support patients and families as they struggle with questions regarding whether natural death is always the best and most loving choice (Hooks & Daly, 2000). Attending to the nature and cause of a person's suffering and providing comfort care throughout the dying process are important components of the nursing role that may influence choices regarding active voluntary euthanasia or assisted suicide.

Issues Related to HIV/AIDS

We know that human immunodeficiency virus and acquired immunodeficiency syndrome (HIV/AIDS) is a major worldwide health concern, and that the virus is generally contracted through unprotected sexual contact. The virus can also be spread through maternal–infant transmission and intravenous drug use via shared needles.

Because of the risk of exposure to HIV in health care settings, questions arise regarding issues of autonomy and confidentiality in relation to HIV testing and status. One issue relates to whether patients can be required to submit to HIV testing in situations of potential or actual percutaneous exposure of health care workers to their blood. In order to protect persons from potential discrimination, confidentiality of HIV testing and status is generally assured by law; thus, it is generally illegal to perform HIV testing or for that matter, many other kinds of tests, without a person's clear written consent. "Ethically speaking, HIV testing over the patient's objections violates the patient's autonomy and privacy as well as the spirit of informed consent . . . consent for HIV testing is important because stigma and discrimination may occur if other people know that the patient is seropositive" (Lo, 1995, p. 332).

Because of concerns about potential stigma in work or home settings related to having a documented HIV test, regardless of its result, patients may refuse a test even if they are sure it will be negative. In order to assure confidentiality and to encourage patient agreement to testing in the event of exposure of a health care worker to a patient's blood, Lo (1995) suggests an approach of anonymous testing of the patient. In this way the health care worker could know if he or she is at risk, while protecting the patient from potential stigma resulting from the test.

Another issue that has become a public concern relates to potential exposure of patients to the blood of a seropositive health care worker. Questions arise whether HIV testing among health care workers, or at least those involved in certain invasive procedures, should be mandatory; whether seropositive health care workers should have restrictions on their practice; and whether the HIV status of health care workers should be made known to patients. Some argue that if it becomes mandatory for health care workers to be tested, then it should be mandatory for all patients as well. Principles of autonomy, confidentiality, and non-maleficence become part of this discussion. Health care workers, as well as patients, have a right to autonomy and confidentiality regarding health matters, particularly where discrimination could result from disclosure. At the same time, non-maleficence directs them to do no harm to patients, and the doctrine of informed consent requires advising patients of potential risks related to interventions being considered. Economic factors enter into the discussion as well. At the present time, presuming health care workers follow universal infection control precautions, the risk of a patient contracting HIV from a seropositive health care worker is low, in contrast to the high cost of mandatory testing. Requiring such testing could well divert money from other, more effective, areas of health promotion and protection. Resources might be better used and result in more sustainable changes if they were directed toward making sure all health care professionals practise universal precautions.

Current issues related to HIV/AIDS may become less of a concern as technology advances toward more effective prevention and treatment of the disease. However, ethical concerns surrounding these issues apply to other health problems of a similar nature. Nurses and other health care workers must be aware of any factors in their own health that might put their patients at risk, and take necessary precautions to protect patients from harm. It is also essential that nurses follow universal precautions aimed at protecting themselves and others from harm. If behaviours on the part of health care workers are observed that might put patients at risk, the imperatives of beneficence and non-maleficence direct nurses to do what is necessary to protect the patient. Actions may include approaching the person involved, reporting the situation to appropriate persons within the agency, and working with groups to institute changes to prevent similar situations from occurring.

Although cases of HIV/AIDS must be reported, as with other infectious diseases, caregivers cannot disclose a person's HIV status (or any kind of personal health information) without consent. The legal and ethical right to confidentiality regarding HIV/AIDS raises an ethical issue related to protection of others when the infected individual continues behaviours that may expose others to the infection. In some circumstances, physicians are allowed limited disclosure without consent, such as to the patient's spouse. In such situations the imperative of confidentiality must be weighed against the duty to warn others in order to protect them from potential harm. At the present time there are no clear directives in this area for health care providers.

Confidentiality

The imperative of **confidentiality** in health care, which is discussed in detail in Chapter 3, can be traced at least as far back as the Hippocratic vow not to reveal secrets. In order to care for people with health concerns, nurses must be privy to very personal, and sometimes secret, information. Without the assurance of confidentiality, many people would not disclose information that is important for the diagnosis and treatment of, and caring for, health concerns. This is especially true in situations where there is stigma attached to the information disclosed, or other risks for social repercussions from it. Nurses must remember that a patient's trust is sacred, and any breach of confidentiality, no matter how small it might seem to the nurse, is a violation of this trust.

 CASE PRESENTATION

When Patients Request Confidentiality

Paige is a nurse in a busy suburban emergency room (ER). Tonight, Roger is brought in with a history of increasing shortness of breath, a worsening cough, and chest pain. This morning, when he awoke with sharper chest pain and could not stop coughing, he found he was coughing up blood. Paige admits Roger, assesses him, and cares for him during the day while he undergoes blood work, a chest

X-ray, and a CT scan, and has a sputum sample taken. The medical team in the ER request an oncology consult. Later in the evening, the consulting oncologist, after asking Paige to accompany her, asks Roger if any family members or friends are on the way. Roger says he doesn't want to bother his son right now and insists on knowing the news now. The oncologist tells Roger that she is quite sure that Roger has lung cancer from the results of the tests so far. She informs him that he needs to undergo a lung tissue biopsy the next day in order to stage the cancer but that she suspects the lung cancer may be somewhat advanced, as Roger's left lung is partially collapsed, and she recommends that he begin treatment as soon as possible. She tells Roger that it would be good to contact someone who could support him through this and to help him at home for the immediate and longer term. Roger says he will cope fine at home and doesn't require help.

When the physician leaves, Roger asks Paige what kind of support she thinks he'll need. Paige tries to explain some possible kinds of emotional and physical support that Roger may need in the immediate future. She asks Roger about his current living situation. Roger tells her that he lives on a very limited income, but "gets by," and he only talks a little to his neighbours. He has a few close friends, but they are all married, retired, and "living their own lives." Roger is a widower with one son, Thomas, who lost his job last year and just went through a difficult divorce. Roger tells Paige that he is close to his son, but doesn't want to tell him about his diagnosis. Paige reassures Roger that she will maintain his confidentiality, but suggests that Thomas might want to know. But Roger is adamant: he does not want his son to know that he has lung cancer.

An hour later, Thomas arrives at the ER after hearing from his father's neighbour. He spends some time with his father and after his visit comes out to talk to Paige. He asks her if there is anything his father needs right now. Paige responds by saying she isn't sure, and that the best person to ask would be Roger. Thomas responds, "Oh, he's so independent and he'd never tell me if he needed something. I mean, with the flu he likely won't be in long, but you never know, right? If he needs anything, I should get it in the next day or two because I've just gotten a new job. It's across the country and I'm leaving in a few days. I won't be back in town for about six to eight months and so I won't see him for a while. He's excited for me and hopefully he'll be able to visit when he gets rid of this flu bug. I will miss him so much."

Paige realizes that Roger will not tell Thomas about his diagnosis. She also knows that the oncologist suspects Roger's lung cancer is at an advanced stage and that he will need help and support. She feels badly for Thomas, who is leaving without knowing that his father is so ill. She feels very uncomfortable not informing Thomas, but realizes her duty is to protect the confidentiality of her patient, even though she thinks that telling Thomas would be in both of their best interests.

THINK ABOUT IT

- Paige is in a difficult position, although she knows that her primary duty is to protect Roger's confidentiality. How would you feel if you were Paige?

- How should Paige respond to Thomas tonight? What should she tell him tomorrow? Is there anything she could tell him, without disclosing confidential information, that might trigger him in some way to talk more with his father?

- Paige observes that Roger is very independent. He also has expressed that he does not know very much about what kind of support he might need. Should Paige recommend or even insist that Roger tell his son? How insistent should Paige be, if at all, in this regard?

- Can Paige help Roger seek support in other ways? Would there be other health care professionals that might be consulted at this point? How might she help him most, at this time?

Protecting confidentiality is not just about formal processes and policies that are in place. It is also relevant to how we, as nurses, conduct ourselves in the workplace. There are many situations in which patient confidentiality can be breached inadvertently, such as discussing patients in an open nursing unit, a hallway, or a shared patients' room, having conversations about patient care in an elevator or cafeteria, leaving documents or charts open on counters or desks, or not properly logging off after documenting on the computer. Being aware of the kinds of things we can do, as part of our everyday nursing practice, to help protect the confidentiality of patients, is an important part of being accountable and responsible.

As with so many other areas, there are situations where other factors override confidentiality. In circumstances such as court cases, the law might require disclosure. In situations where secrets entrusted to the nurse suggest potential harm for the patient or others, the duty to warn may take precedence over confidentiality. For example, if a patient tells a nurse about suicide plans that the nurse believes are genuine, and the patient is not willing to be hospitalized, protection of the patient may require the nurse to initiate the process of involuntary hospitalization. Other examples of situations that may require mandatory reporting are situations in which child abuse or neglect are suspected, situations in a long-term care setting in which elder abuse is suspected, and imminent harm to self or others. Legislation and policies are in place that carefully outline what situations require mandatory reporting and nurses must be aware of these in the context of their own practice.

SUMMARY

This chapter discussed considerations for nursing practice related to patient self-determination. The concept of self-determination derives from the principle of autonomy, and denotes the right and freedom to make choices about issues that affect one's life. Principles of justice, beneficence, and non-maleficence may temper the bounds of autonomy in some circumstances. The doctrine of informed consent is both a legal and an ethical imperative for protecting a person's right to self-determination in health care decisions. Informed consent implies the right to accept or reject recommended treatment plans. As patient advocates, we need to be alert for situations where patient autonomy may be limited, or where the patient or family do not have enough information to make informed decisions. Nurses have a particular responsibility for facilitating informed decision making regarding patient choices for end-of-life care. Nursing's professional code directs nurses to provide services with respect for the rights and dignity of the patient, regardless of a person's background or the nature of the health concern. If professional responsibilities expected of a nurse in a patient care situation are inconsistent with the nurse's ethical stance, integrity, and accountability, she should remove herself from that situation, after ensuring that there are others to assume care for the patient. A nurse's attention to the many-faceted issues surrounding patient self-determination may be the factor that ensures the patient's involvement in important health care decisions.

CHAPTER HIGHLIGHTS

- Self-determination derives from the principle of autonomy, and implies having freedom to make choices about issues affecting one's life, an ability to make decisions about personal goals, and an appreciation for self in relation to others.

- Autonomy may be threatened by factors such as paternalism; presumptions that a patient's values, knowledge level, and ways of dealing with issues are consistent with those of health care providers; and greater attention to technology than caring. In some situations, principles such as justice or non-maleficence may temper the bounds of autonomy.

- Decisions about health care require attention to patient values, culture, and beliefs; the effects of lifestyle and role; others who are affected by a patient's choices; and evaluation of risks, benefits, and economic considerations.

- Practitioners may not be required to honour requests for interventions that are outside accepted standards of care or contrary to the practitioner's ethical views. However, patients cannot be abandoned.

- Informed consent provides legal and ethical protection of a patient's right to personal autonomy regarding plans for health care, including the right to refuse interventions and to choose from available alternatives. Information necessary in an informed consent includes the nature of the concern and the prognosis if nothing is done; a description of treatment options; and the benefits, risks, and consequences of treatment options or non-intervention.

- Decision-making capacity, which is a medical determination and essential for informed consent, includes evidence of the ability to understand information, to communicate understanding and choices, to evaluate decisions in relation to personal values and goals, and to reason and deliberate. Conscious adults are presumed to have decision-making capacity unless there is evidence to the contrary.

- Nursing responsibility regarding informed consent includes verifying that the patient is aware of the available options and the implications of each, and advocating for patients to make sure that criteria for autonomous decision making are met in situations where the physician has not attended to these criteria. Nurses in advanced practice must obtain informed consent for interventions that they initiate within their scope of practice.

- Advance directives, which include living wills and durable powers of attorney, provide instructions regarding health care interventions in the event that one loses decision-making capacity.

- In dealing with patient lifestyle choices, nurses must remember to provide quality nursing care with respect for human dignity and to avoid value judgments related to differences in background, customs, attitudes, and beliefs.

- Nurses need to examine their own values and beliefs regarding various lifestyle and health care choices, and reflect upon how these values affect might their nursing practice.

- Nurses must recognize the patient's right to use complementary and alternative therapies, become more knowledgeable about other modalities, and create an atmosphere that encourages nonjudgmental discussion of such interventions.

- Ethical codes direct nurses to maintain confidentiality regarding patient health status and choices, except in special circumstances where the information suggests potential harm for the patient or another.

DISCUSSION QUESTIONS AND ACTIVITIES

1. Discuss your understanding of patient self-determination, including its ethical and legal basis, and nursing practice considerations.

2. Describe dilemmas that nurses may face related to patient self-determination and suggest approaches for dealing with such dilemmas.

3. Explore how practising nurses in your institution perceive their role regarding informed consent. What dilemmas related to consent have they encountered and how did they deal with these issues?

4. Analyze your own values regarding active voluntary euthanasia. How would you respond to a patient under your care who was deliberating such a choice?

5. Explore your provincial legislation regarding advance directives, HIV testing and disclosure, euthanasia, assisted suicide, and abortion. What are the implications of these regulations for nursing practice in your province?

6. What is the process for obtaining support and guidance for dealing with ethical concerns and dilemmas in your institution? If there is an ethics committee, how

are referrals made? Who is on the committee, and how are members chosen? Talk with a member of an ethics committee, and discuss how she or he sees the role and the effectiveness of the committee.

7. Select a case situation in which there are ethical concerns that warrant referral to the ethics committee. With classmates, role-play the ethics committee discussion, decisions, and actions regarding the case. Explain why you take the position that you do, and how you feel about the outcome.

8. Choose one of the issues discussed in this chapter and explore the Web sites of the CNA, the ANA, and the ICN regarding policies or position statements on this issue. Compare and contrast the positions of the various organizations. Discuss your views about this issue and how they compare with the positions of the professional organizations.

CNA—http://www.cna-nurses.ca/cna

ANA—http://www.nursingworld.org

ICN—http://www.icn.ch

REFERENCES

Andrews, G. J., & H. Boon (2005). CAM in Canada: places, practices, research. *Complementary Therapies in Clinical Practice, 11*, 21–27.

Canadian Institutes of Health Research, Natural Sciences and Engineering Research Council of Canada, Social Sciences and Humanities Research Council of Canada. *The council policy statement: Ethical conduct for research involving humans, 1998* (with 2000, 2002, 2005, amendments).

Canadian Nurses Association. (2008a). *Providing nursing care at the end of life.* Retrieved May 8, 2012 from http://www2.cna-aiic.ca/CNA/documents/pdf/publications/PS96_End_of_Life_e.pdf

Canadian Nurses Association. (2008b). *Code of ethics for registered nurses.* Ottawa: Canadian Nurses Association. Retrieved January 2, 2009, from http://www.cna-nurses.ca/CNA/practice/ethics/ code/default_e.aspx.

College of Nurses of Ontario. (2005). *Practice guideline: Consent.* Toronto: Author. Retrieved January 2, 2009, from http://www.cno.org/docs/policy/41020_consent.pdf.

Davis, A. J., D. Fowler & M. Aroskar (2009) *Ethical dilemmas and nursing practice.* Pearson Canada: Toronto.

Department of Justice, Government of Canada. (1985). *Criminal Code* (R.S., 1985, c. C-46).

Devettere, R. J. (2002). *Practical decision making in health care ethics: Cases and concepts.* (2nd ed.). Scholarly Book Services Inc: Toronto, Canada.

Eisenberg, D. M., B. D. Rogers, S. Ettner, S. Appel, S. Wilkey, M. Van Rompay & R. C. Kessler (1998). Trends in alternative medicine in the United States, 1990–1997. *Journal of the American Medical Association, 280*(18), 1569–1575.

Finucane, T. E., C. Christmas & K. Travis (1999). Tube feeding in patients with advanced dementia. *Journal of the American Medical Association, 282*(14), 1265–1370.

Hardwig, J. (2000). What about the family? In J. H. Howell & W. F. Sale, eds., *Life choices: A Hastings Center introduction to bioethics,* (2nd ed.) (pp. 145–159). Washington, DC: Georgetown University Press.

Hooks, F. J., & B. J. Daly (2000). Hastening death. *American Journal of Nursing, 100*(5), 56–63.

Lo, B. (2000). *Resolving ethical dilemmas: A guide for clinicians.* (2nd ed.) Baltimore: Lippincott Williams & Wilkins.

Mahowald, M. B. (2000). Is there life after *Roe v. Wade?* In J. H. Howell & W. F. Sale, eds., *Life choices: A Hastings Center introduction to bioethics* (pp. 188–203). Washington, DC: Georgetown University Press.

McCann, R. (1999). Lack of evidence about tube feeding: Food for thought. *Journal of the American Medical Association, 282*(14), 1381.

Millar, W. J. (2001) Patterns of use – alternative health care practitioners. *Health Reports 2001, 13*(1), Statistics Canada, Catalogue 82-003.

Sherwin, W. (1992). Paternalism. In *No longer patient: Feminist ethics and health care* (pp. 137–157). Philadelphia: Temple University Press.

Singer, P. (2002). University of Toronto Joint Centre for Bioethics. *Living will.* Toronto: University of Toronto Joint Centre for Bioethics.

Sullivan, G. H. (1998). Getting informed consent. *RN* (April), 59–62.

Tilden, V. P. (2000). Advance directives. *American Journal of Nursing, 100*(12), 49, 50.

Walton, N., D. K. Martin, E. Peter, D. Pringle & P. A. Singer (2007). Priority setting and cardiac surgery: A qualitative case study. *Health Policy, 80,* 444–458.

Williams, J. R. (2008). Consent. In P. A. Singer and A. M. Viens, eds., *The Cambridge textbook of bioethics.* Cambridge: Cambridge University Press.

Willison, K. D., & G. J. Andrews (2004). Complementary medicine and older people: past research and future directions. *Complementary Therapies in Nursing and Midwifery, 10,* 80–91.

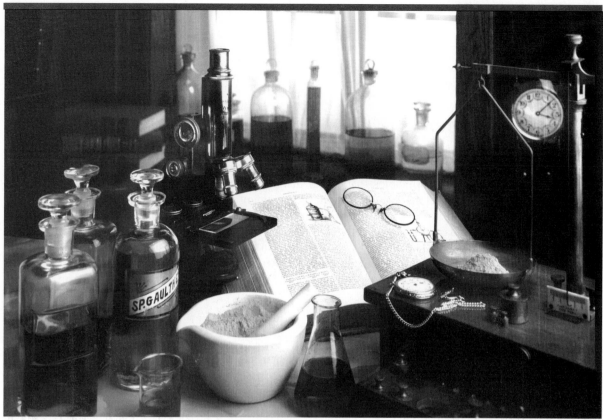
Mitchell Barutha/Dreamstime.com

CHAPTER **12**

SCHOLARSHIP ISSUES

OBJECTIVES

After completing this chapter, the reader should be able to:

1. Describe scholarship issues encountered by nurses in academic, clinical, and research settings.
2. Discuss principles basic to academic and research integrity.
3. Describe principles and standards underpinning the protection of human rights in research.
4. Explain why informed consent is mandated for research involving human participants, and describe the elements required for this consent.

5. Discuss the nursing role regarding protection of participants' rights in research.

6. Describe principles guiding personal response to dilemmas regarding nursing scholarship.

INTRODUCTION

Students, teachers, researchers, and clinicians face scholarship issues from the moment they enter a nursing program and throughout their professional careers. This chapter discusses principles that are at the heart of ethical behaviour in academic matters, in conducting research, and in the treatment of data both during the research process and in presentations or publications. Respect for all persons, including for ourselves, is basic to ethical behaviour regarding scholarship. Personal values affect how we approach situations that present ethical dilemmas. It is essential that nurses be knowledgeable about the principles that guide their ethical conduct, whether they are dealing with academic assignments, research data, or research with human participants.

ACADEMIC HONESTY

Integrity in upholding the principles of veracity and fidelity is expected of nurses in any setting, and is at the core of academic honesty. Veracity refers to telling the truth, which is an essential ingredient for trust among humans. Husted and Husted (2007) suggest that true interaction and communication cannot occur where there is no trust. These authors describe fidelity as keeping our promises, suggesting that it is the form that truth takes in any agreement between persons, such as nurse–patient, researcher–participant, or student–teacher. Integrity implies respect for oneself and others, and a personal commitment to principled behaviour over time in our personal and professional lives. When integrity is present, there can be an implicit trust that we are representing ourselves in a truthful way. Honesty and integrity are key considerations in both academic and clinical situations. Personal values such as honesty serve as the basis for professional integrity.

Students at all levels face many stresses in regard to academic performance, and nursing students are no exception. Pressures may come from many areas, such as family expectations, personal goals of being accepted into graduate school, needing a certain grade to receive tuition reimbursement, or self-expectations that say "I always get good grades." When pressures become intense, values such as honesty and integrity may be challenged.

Issues of academic integrity include plagiarism, cheating, misrepresentation of personal performance, and submission of false information. **Cheating** refers to dishonesty and deception, which may include the use of other people's work without authorization or without citation, the use of unauthorized information that is shared by or received from others, and manipulating situations in which testing or evaluation is being carried out (Cizek, 1999; Cox, 2003).

Plagiarism occurs when a person submits the work or part of the work of another and claims this work as his or her own (Simon Fraser University, 2009). **Misrepresentation of personal performance** includes submitting work that has been taken from another and representing it as your own, allowing someone else to write an exam using your name, or not being forthright about your academic records or credentials. Finally, **submission of false information** could take the form of submitting a false statement such as a medical certificate to avoid completing an assignment or writing an exam, submitting false academic records, or altering official academic documents (Ryerson University, Office of Academic Integrity, 2012).

ASK YOURSELF

What Are Your Perspectives on Academic Honesty?

- One of your closest friends is in a different section of the same course, and his section meets two days after yours. You know he has been very stressed because of his mother's illness and that he needs good grades to keep his scholarship. You have just taken the mid-term exam, and he asks you to give him an idea of the topics covered so he can focus his studying. What would you do? How do you feel in this situation? What principles would guide your decisions?

- During an exam you notice two students passing what appear to be notes between them. You are fairly sure that the instructor has not seen this. How do you feel in response to this? What would you do, and why?

- You are struggling with an assignment that is due in just a few days. A classmate says she has a paper that her cousin did for this same course three years ago that she is using as a guide, changing the text so that it seems like her writing. She offers to let you see her cousin's paper to do the same. What do you think about her plan? How would you respond? What would guide your decision?

- You are studying for an important final exam. You note that the professor has indicated that, on her Web site, the teaching assistant has provided a set of practice questions to complete to prepare for the exam. You work through them carefully, as do your colleagues. While in the final exam, you notice that the exam questions are the same as the practice questions. Everyone around you notices the same thing, but no one tells the professor. What would you do? What principles would influence or guide your decision making?

- You are writing a long paper that you are finding particularly difficult. Remembering that you did a paper on a similar topic two years ago, you

(Continued)

find it and decide that you will simply "cut and paste" sections from your previous paper into this paper. You are sure that this isn't plagiarism and that since the paper is your own work, you can do this without feeling uneasy about it. Is that true? Should you feel uneasy about this decision? If so, why?

- At the end of term, you have a number of important assignments due all at once. In addition, you have an on-line discussion that you must participate in. When preparing for posting a response to the on-line discussion, for participation marks only, you research your topic on the Internet. You find a great deal of good non-scholarly, lay resources on the topic, and decide that you will just cut the sections of text, paste them into the on-line discussion and change a few words. You do this, complete your on-line discussion quickly, and receive full participation marks. Since they weren't scholarly resources and the marks were simply for participation and not really for merit of work, you are fairly sure that this was acceptable. Later on, you are feeling that perhaps this wasn't the best way to approach the work. Why do you think you are uneasy? What would you do?

Implicit in academic honesty is a trust that work submitted by a student, whether papers, projects, or exams, is indeed the work of that student. When material from other sources is included in papers, students must utilize appropriate referencing so as to avoid plagiarizing. The breach of trust and potential consequences within a student–teacher relationship that academic dishonesty engenders are self-evident. Litigation is another potential consequence in severe situations. Because of the value of honesty, academic institutions frequently have written policies that may carry consequences as serious as the student's being suspended or expelled for dishonest practices.

 CASE PRESENTATION

Suspicions of Dishonesty

Sabrina and Jude have been close friends and study partners throughout their nursing program. They discuss their readings and class notes and frequently choose the same topic, sharing articles between them when writing papers. After a recent submission of papers, the instructor called them in and noted that their papers were almost identical, including mistakes in grammar, and said that it appeared that one had copied the other's paper. They each denied copying from the other.

THINK ABOUT IT

Considering Consequences for Academic Dishonesty

- What ethical issues are involved in this situation?
- How do you feel about incidences of academic dishonesty?
- How do you think this situation should be handled? What consequences would you consider?
- In light of the standards that guide nursing practice, what is your position on allowing a student who has violated academic honesty through plagiarism, cheating, or forgery to continue in a nursing program?
- Should nursing students be held to a higher standard for academic honesty than students in non-professional or non-health care programs, such as arts or history? Why or why not?

RESEARCH ISSUES AND ETHICS

Nurses must be accountable for the quality of care they deliver, and research is one way of documenting the efficacy of nursing practice, as well as furthering the profession and disseminating innovative approaches to practice. Both the art and science of nursing are expanded through research. Research is necessary for the ongoing development of the unique body of knowledge that undergirds the discipline of nursing, and provides an organizing framework for nursing practice. Research is an integral part of practice and education in nursing.

Participating in research can be exciting and encourage professional growth. It can also present some dilemmas for the nurse and nurse researcher in the academic and clinical realms. Seeking new knowledge and understanding is the expected motivation for conducting research. However, personal or institutional gains related to rewards like grant funds, prestige, the need to succeed, or promoting a product can be other motivating factors that may challenge principled behaviour in regard to research.

Underlying the nurse–patient relationship is the notion of trust. Trust arises out of the **fiduciary duty** that nurses, and all health care professionals, have toward their patients or clients. A fiduciary duty is one in which the nurse sets aside his or her own agenda, needs, or feelings, in order to place the patient in a position of priority. A **fiduciary** is a legal term, referring to someone who is entrusted to act in another person's best interests. It is a special responsibility, given to someone because of that person's relationship to another, or by virtue of his or her profession, as in the case of nurses, physicians, and other health care professionals.

The fiduciary responsibility that nurses have to their patients underlies the profession and nursing practice. That ability to act in another's best interest extends to all facets of patient care. Health care research, however, presents unique challenges to protecting that relationship of trust. As nurses become more and more involved in health care and nursing research, they take on new roles in which the fiduciary role looks markedly different. As nurse researchers, the goals of maintaining our fiduciary responsibilities are often intermingled with the goals of seeking new knowledge, obtaining grants, publishing, and presenting our own work. This intermingling of goals can often create conflicts of interest or role confusion.

In any case, nurses must always protect the autonomy and self-determination of the individuals for whom they provide care or involve in research activities. Care must always be taken to ensure that patients understand where the therapeutic relationship ends and the researcher–participant relationship begins. Whether the nurse is providing therapeutic care or is involving a patient in research, there exists a strong ethical obligation to protect the rights of all patients and participants, no matter what the context.

The rights of patients that we protect are the same rights as those of participants in research activities. *How* we protect these rights may differ between these groups, but in some cases, protection of these rights looks very similar. For example, we protect patients' autonomy by ensuring that they are fully informed about therapeutic procedures before they provide an informed consent. We also protect research participants' autonomy by making certain that there are clear, thoughtful, and non-coercive informed consent processes in place for research projects.

It is important to remember that there may be overlap in our clinical or therapeutic activities and our research involvement. This overlap, while unavoidable to some degree, does not change our responsibilities toward others: to protect their trust and autonomy, to make sure that we minimize any harm to them, and to act in their best interests.

Ethical Issues in Research

Many research texts focus their discussions of ethical issues in research primarily on protection of human rights. This emphasis is understandable because of violations that have occurred. Some of the most cited violations of human rights in research are those that were perpetrated by the Nazis during the Second World War and that came to public awareness during the Nuremberg Doctor trials. International efforts to provide guidelines for protection of human rights have subsequently been documented in the **Nuremberg Code**, which was developed as a set of principles for the ethical conduct of research against which the experiments in the concentration camps could be judged. This Code emphasizes the importance of informed consent for any participant/subject who is taking part in research. While the principles of autonomy and informed consent are the backbone of the ethical conduct of research, many academic researchers tend to distance themselves from the *Nuremberg Code,* favouring more recent guidelines and documents that are not associated in any way with the atrocities of the War. The **Declaration of Helsinki** was issued by the World Medical Assembly in 1964, and has been revised numerous times; the most recent iteration dates from October 2008 with the World Medical Association's General Assembly in Seoul, Korea. The *Declaration of Helsinki* differs from the *Nuremberg Code* in emphasizing notions of peer review for academic research. The *Declaration* is highly responsive to modern-day occurrences in the context of research. For example, one iteration of the *Declaration of Helsinki* includes statements that object to the phenomenon of researchers who "parachute" into developing countries to conduct research, then abandon the participants after completion of the research. Over the past few decades, this has become a problem, most notably with researchers carrying out drug trials for Human Immunodeficiency Virus (HIV) and AIDS in parts of Africa, only to leave their participants without any therapy after completion of the trial. In any kind of research, participants are giving of their time and often exposing themselves to a certain degree of risk of harm. Therefore, it is considered to be ethically problematic to carry out research on individuals who are vulnerable or less fortunate without commensurate compensation at the very least.

Canadian guidelines for the ethical conduct of research can be found in the *Tri Council Policy Statement* (TCPS 2) (Canadian Institutes of Health Research, Natural Sciences and Engineering Research Council of Canada, Social Science and Humanities Research Council of Canada, *Tri Council Policy Statement: Ethical Conduct for Research Involving Humans,* 2010). This guiding document was created in 1998 and was revised in 2010 to reflect greater attention to issues such as qualitative and social science research, research involving Aboriginal persons, and the use of vulnerable populations in research activities.

The TCPS is a federal document that provides clear guidelines on the ethical conduct of research and the fair and ethical treatment of participants involved in all types of research. In order to receive federal funding, academic and clinical institutions that conduct research must adhere to these guidelines, and an institutional Research Ethics Board must review all research prior to its being conducted. Health Canada also provides strict oversight on all clinical trials. The mandate of both the *Tri-Council Policy Statement* and Health Canada's oversight of clinical trials is to protect participants. A new version of the TCPS was released in 2008, and there are a number of changes that help to ensure protection of participants. For example, new and timely guidelines on research involving Aboriginal persons and participants in qualitative research are included in the new version.

In the U.S., federal regulations, rather than guidelines for the ethical conduct of research, exist and in order to oversee and enforce these regulations pertaining to research with human subjects, the United States Department of Health and Human Services formed an Office for Human Research Protection. Efforts to bolster protections for human research participants focus on education and training of clinical investigators and institutional review board members, auditing records for evidence of compliance with informed consent, improved monitoring of clinical trials, managing conflicts of interest so that research participants are appropriately informed, and imposing monetary penalties for violations of important research practices, such as informed consent (Spicer, 2000).

Despite these policies and guidelines, ethical lapses continue to occur in research with human participants (Hilts & Stolberg, 1999; Kaplan & Brownlee, 1999; Maloney, 2000a, 2000b). These and other concerns raise questions about whether current regulations adequately protect the rights and welfare of research participants (Moreno, Caplan & Wolpe, 1998).

THINK ABOUT IT

The following are examples of significant and well-known ethical lapses in the conduct of human-participant research:

1. Between 1932 and 1972, a group of physicians decided to observe the effect of untreated syphilis in a large group of about 400 mainly African-American migrant workers in Tuskegee, Alabama, in a study known as the Tuskegee Syphilis Study (Reverby, 2009). At the time of the inception of the study, treatments for syphilis were questionable and often toxic, until 1947, when penicillin became the standard and successful treatment. Mainly illiterate, the workers were not informed that they had the disease. They were told that they had problems with their blood and were also told that they were receiving free medical treatment, were provided with rides to and from the medical institutions, and were given funds to cover the costs of eventual funeral and burial rites. They did not receive medical treatment, even after 1947 when the standard proven treatment was widely available. They underwent a great deal of medical testing, had samples of their blood taken, and many understood, mistakenly, that this was a method of "treatment." After the introduction of penicillin to treat syphilis, this study continued for another quarter-century and the men were never offered treatment. Many continued to be observed and without knowing it, spread syphilis to others, until their eventual deaths, usually from complications of the disease.

2. Stanley Milgram, a social psychologist, carried out a study at Yale University in 1963 examining human responses to authority. In this study, he recruited participants to take part in an experiment in which they were required to deliver electric shocks to another participant in an adjoining room. The participant receiving shocks was actually an actor hired by the researcher, who did not receive shocks but instead cried out in pain at each "delivered shock." The recruited participants could not see the actor, but could hear the cries of pain and anguish. As the study progressed, participants were instructed to increase the level of volts of delivered electricity, to a point that was clearly potentially fatal. While obedient to the authority figure, as participants were asked to deliver more and more electricity to another person, they became clearly distressed and markedly affected by the level of deception involved in this experiment.

3. In the book *The Tearoom Trade* (1970), sociologist Laud Humphreys documented his doctoral ethnographic research, in which he followed men into public bathrooms to observe male–male sexual acts, colloquially referred to as

"tearooming." He would then follow the men to their cars, record their licence plates and, with the help of the local department of transportation, access their addresses. Armed with their contact information and knowledge of usually illicit and secretive sexual activity, he would confront the men in their homes and ask that they consent to be interviewed about their sexual behaviour, using false pretenses and strong coercive influence.

Each of these examples illustrates significant risks, coercion, and explicit deception, without safeguards for the participants or a reasonable balance of risk and benefits.

- What are your thoughts on these research studies?
- Do you find it shocking that they occurred so recently?
- Do you think that the policies and guidelines in place today are enough to avoid similar ethical lapses?

The three core principles of **respect for persons**, **concern for welfare**, and **justice** underlie the ethical conduct of research (Canadian Institutes of Health Research, Natural Sciences and Engineering Research Council of Canada, Social Science and Humanities Research Council of Canada, *Tri Council Policy Statement: Ethical Conduct for Research Involving Humans,* 2010). Throughout the international research community, there are also common ethical principles more specific to research and the rights of participants that have been articulated and well documented.

Respect for Persons

Implicit in the principle of **respect for persons** is the right to self-determination, which acknowledges the autonomy of the potential participant in research. This means that persons have the right to choose whether they wish to participate in the research; that is, participation is voluntary and free from undue influence or coercion of any type. **Undue influence** may refer to the fact that if there are power differences between those who are recruiting and potential participants, this may cause potential participants to feel obligated to take part or constrained in their choices. More seriously, **coercion** includes threat of harm or penalty for not participating in the research, or an offer of excessive rewards for participation. The right of self-determination means that the person has the right to withdraw from participation in the study at any time without imposed consequences, such as denial of health care or benefits. Voluntary participation requires **full disclosure**, that is, that the potential participant be fully informed of the nature of the study, the anticipated risks and benefits, the time commitment, what is expected of the participant and the researcher, and the right to refuse to participate. This is addressed through the process of informed consent, which is discussed below and visited in Chapter 11.

The *Declaration of Helsinki* (World Medical Association, 2008) states

> It is the duty of physicians who participate in research to protect the life, health, dignity, integrity, right to self-determination, privacy, and confidentiality of personal information of research subjects. (Article B: 11)*

Concern for Welfare

The balance between potential risk of harm and potential benefit is of the utmost concern in evaluating the ethical soundness of proposed research. This means that researchers need to design and conduct studies so as to protect the participants from potential harms. Harm may include physical, emotional, economic, psychological, behavioural, or social harm. Risk is assessed in a twofold fashion: assessing the magnitude or seriousness of the potential harms, as well as the likelihood that they might occur. The notions of harm and risk can certainly be subjective. In other words, researchers must pay attention to the perspectives of the participants and what they might consider to be harmful. Potential harm may be permanent or transient, and may be differently considered by different persons and groups. Moreover, potential harm may occur on a spectrum, from less severe to very serious. For example, asking new immigrants without legal status questions about the services they can access may be of significantly more risk than asking permanent residents the same kinds of things. Potential harms may be related to the research activity or to the attributes or special situations of the participants. More vulnerable participants may be subject to greater potential harms, by virtue of their health status, age, or social or economic status.

Physical harms are not necessarily related to only potential injury or serious adverse effects. They may include fatigue or physiological symptoms related to stress. Emotional or psychological harms may refer to triggering unpleasant or distressing memories without support or adequate trust in place in the research situation, being anxious or embarrassed, or feeling deceived or unduly coerced to take part in research activities. Social harms may include being exposed to others, being misrepresented, having one's reputation harmed, or having one's privacy or confidentiality breached. Financial harms may include lost earnings for time taken for participation in research activities or, more seriously, loss of employment if the confidentiality of sensitive or negative information is not maintained.

In all research activities, the burden of responsibility lies with the researcher to assess potential for harm and risk of harm and to enact all possible strategies to mitigate these harms. Most importantly, the foreseeable risk of harm must be balanced with the potential or anticipated benefits. Participants must have full information about the potential risks of harm as well as anticipated benefits, which should not be overstated, promised, or guaranteed. While it is noted that research endeavours involve a certain degree of uncertainty, there are steps that can be taken by researchers, as well as processes that can be put in place, that address ethical obligations around balancing foreseeable risks and anticipated benefits (Canadian Institutes of Health Research, Natural Sciences and Engineering Research Council

---

* *The Declaration of Helsinki,* 2008 Seoul, Korea: The World Medical Assocition.

of Canada, Social Science and Humanities Research Council of Canada, *Tri Council Policy Statement: Ethical Conduct for Research Involving Humans,* 2010).

Traditionally, research has been designated as either less or greater than minimal risk. The standard of minimal risk implies that participants are not being subjected to a greater probability of harm than they might encounter in a typical day. This, of course, relates directly to the participants and their unique everyday life. Someone living in an area of civil war, extreme poverty, or strife is subject to a greater daily risk or harm than a person living in a peaceful, democratic, and socioeconomically stable environment.

If a person, by virtue of taking part in a research activity, is potentially being subjected to a risk that is greater than what they might encounter in their daily life, then this would be considered greater than minimal risk. Greater scrutiny of research processes and safeguards, as well as enhanced protection for participants, would be defensible in this case (Canadian Institutes of Health Research, Natural Sciences and Engineering Research Council of Canada, Social Science and Humanities Research Council of Canada, *Tri Council Policy Statement: Ethical Conduct for Research Involving Humans,* 2010).

Since our role as nurses compels us to protect those in our care from unnecessary harm or risk of harm, if the risks of research potentially or clearly outweigh the benefits, the study should be redesigned or discontinued.

Justice

The principle of **justice** includes fair and equitable treatment. The **right to fair treatment** is related to the right to self-determination. Equitable treatment of participants in the selection process, during the study, and after the completion of the study is the basis of this right. Factors to consider in fair treatment include selecting participants based on the research needs and goals, not on the convenience or compromised position of a group of people; equitably distributing the risks and benefits of the research among participants regardless of age, gender, socioeconomic status, race, or ethnic background; honouring any agreements made or benefits promised; treating participants with respect, providing access to research personnel or other professionals as needed; treating persons who decline to participate or withdraw from the study without prejudice; and debriefing as needed to clarify issues or when information had been withheld prior to the study. Finally, fair and equitable treatment, while not referring to "equal" treatment of all participants, implies an obligation for the researcher to pay attention to issues of potential vulnerability or marginalization of participants. Those who may be more vulnerable, oppressed, or marginalized may well deserve special attention in order to be treated fairly within the context of the research.

The nature of research is to gather information about whatever is being studied. When persons are the focus of study, the **right to privacy** is a critical issue. Attentiveness to privacy means the participant determines when, where, and what kind of information is shared, with an assurance that information, attitudes, behaviours, records, opinions, and the like that are observed or collected will be treated with respect and kept in strict confidence. Privacy is maintained through anonymity, confidentiality, and informed consent. If even the researcher cannot link information with a particular participant, then **anonymity** exists. **Confidentiality** refers to the researcher's assurance to participants that the information provided will not be made public or available to anyone other than those involved in the research process without the participant's consent. Confidentiality is maintained by using codes rather than personal identification on data collection forms and restricting access to raw data to those on the research team who need to use the data.

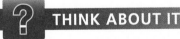

CASE PRESENTATION

Protecting Patients Who Are Research Participants

Parvati is a charge nurse in a women's health clinic. David is a close colleague, who is completing his Masters in Nursing. For his thesis, David hopes to examine the experiences of women who present to the clinic reporting domestic or spousal abuse. He hopes to eventually contribute to improving both the direct services and the referrals that the clinic provides for the women, and knows that in order to do this, their experiences and views must be sought. When Parvati asks him about recruiting his participants, he tells her that he will contact any previous clinic patients who have reported potential domestic abuse, after going through the clinic files, as he will have complete access to them, once Parvati approves. He will ask them if they are interested in being interviewed one on one, privately, at a time convenient to them. He'll tell them that it is for his thesis, which is very important both for his own professional advancement and for the clinic population. He is sure that they will wish to cooperate, as many are patients known to him and he feels that they have a good therapeutic relationship, underpinned by mutual respect and trust.

Parvati asks him if the Research Ethics Board at his university reviewed his proposal and David replies that he is in the process of putting his proposal together to submit to them, but is fairly sure that there won't be any ethical problems with the proposal. He is so sure of the project being approved that he thinks he may begin looking through the charts now, before getting explicit approval.

THINK ABOUT IT

What principles guide the ethical conduct of clinical research?

- What ethical principles are involved in this situation?
- What dilemmas do you foresee arising with David's research proposal?

- If you were a member of the university Research Ethics Board reviewing this proposal, what would you recommend and why?

- David wants to begin looking at charts right away. Should Parvati allow him to access the charts for this purpose? What principles would underlie her decision-making process in this situation?

Informed Consent

As noted above, voluntary participation in a research study requires full disclosure. Informing potential participants of the research purpose, expected commitment, risks and benefits, any invasion of privacy, and ways that anonymity and confidentiality will be addressed are included in the process of **informed consent**. The researcher must make sure that the person who is agreeing to participate in the study comprehends the information included in the consent, and has a chance to receive clarifications and additional information when needed. Written consent forms should be written in plain, everyday language without using high-level medical or legal terms, at approximately a grade seven reading and comprehension level. The literacy level of the person signing the informed consent should be determined and recorded, and the person agreeing to participate in the research must be mentally and emotionally competent to make the decision. In addition to having the cognitive capability to understand and provide consent, participants must also have the volitional capacity to make informed consent decisions. In other words, consent must be both "free, informed and ongoing" (Canadian Institutes of Health Research, Natural Sciences and Engineering Research Council of Canada, Social Science and Humanities Research Council of Canada, *Tri Council Policy Statement: Ethical Conduct for Research Involving Humans*, 2010; Chapter 1, Article 1.1, page 9).

While Munhall and Boyd (2010) suggest that the process of informed consent provides a way of including the person as a collaborator in the research rather than as a mere "subject," we must always be acutely aware of coercion or undue influence that may alter a person's ability to voluntarily provide informed consent. Pre-existing relationships, hierarchical relationships, or the use of managers, employers, or those in any kind of "power-over" relationship to recruit participants may result in people feeling coerced or unduly influenced to participate. In other words, any kind of pressure that is exerted, either explicitly or implicitly, by virtue of a pre-existing relationship, is what may be referred to as coercion. Any kind of coercive factor in recruiting and obtaining consent from potential participants in research projects must be addressed and strategies put in place to mitigate the effects of these factors. One review of nursing research protocols found more ethical concerns arising from the relationship between the researcher and study participant than from physical harm (Olsen & Mahrenholz, 2000). When the nurse who cares for the patient is on the research team and the one obtaining the informed consent, determining whether the patient is giving consent to the "nurse" or to the "researcher" can be somewhat tricky. The nurse–researcher must determine whether the patient truly feels free to refuse to participate.

Article 3.2 of *The Tri Council Policy Statement: Ethical Conduct for Research Involving Humans* (2010) lists twelve specific elements that need to be provided as part of a process of obtaining informed consent. Nurses who are assisting with research or who work on units where research is being conducted must be familiar with these elements of informed consent. If consent processes and forms do not contain these elements, nurses should bring this lack to the attention of the investigators or the institutional Research Ethics Board.

 CASE PRESENTATION

Juanita is a registered nurse, working in a large urban hospital in a thoracic surgery step-down unit. Today, she notices that two of her patients have been enrolled in a new study, in which they may receive one of the traditional pain medications for post-operative pain or be randomized into a group that receives a new type of analgesic. When Juanita looks up the new drug on the Internet, she notes that it has been used in a limited number of other contexts, but never in post-operative pain management. Juanita knows that pain after thoracic surgery can be excruciating and she is concerned.

She calls the study nurse listed on the patients' consent forms for more information. It turns out that the study nurse is Wayne, a friend from nursing school. When Juanita voices her concern to Wayne more about the study drug, he reassures her by reminding her that it isn't an experimental drug any longer, but one that is being used in a new way. He also says to Juanita that she likely knows as much as he does about the drug, as he hasn't researched it too much but does know that it is safe in the limited contexts in which it has been previously used.

He recruits patients for the study on top of his work in the cardiac unit, on his days off. He tells Juanita, "The drug company pays me one hundred dollars for each patient who is enrolled, followed up, and completes the study. It only takes a few minutes to sign them up, put a randomization number on their chart, notify the pharmacy, and get the data after surgery. It's pretty easy. You should do it too!"

 THINK ABOUT IT

- What issues of concern do you identify in this case situation?
- What ethical principles are being violated or potentially violated?

- Why is Juanita concerned? Is her concern justified? What ethical principle or principles underlie her concern?

- What kinds of potential consequences or conflicts of interest might affect the outcomes of this situation?

Special Considerations: Vulnerable Populations

Nurses must be especially attentive to protection of human rights in research with vulnerable populations. These populations may include physically, developmentally, or mentally challenged persons; young children or elderly persons; those without full legal status or refugees; persons who are living at extremely low socioeconomic levels or who are homeless; those who are dying, sedated, or unconscious; persons who are institutionalized, incarcerated, or highly dependent on agencies; pregnant women, and fetuses. Because people in these populations are potentially more vulnerable to deception and coercion, and may have decreased ability to give informed consent, advocates or guardians who clearly and explicitly have the person's best interest in mind must be involved in decisions regarding their participation in research. An important consideration for research with vulnerable populations is that the less able the person is to give informed consent, the more important it is for the researcher to protect the person's rights (Wilson, 1992). Nurses who work with these populations need to be especially cognizant of their roles as advocates, particularly when research is proposed or being conducted in their settings.

While research on vulnerable persons requires more stringent oversight and monitoring, it also is imperative to allow vulnerable persons to participate in research. Not allowing vulnerable persons access to new and innovative therapies, or to have their experiences documented or voices heard, may be thought of as a form of discrimination and may lead to further marginalization (Mastroianni and Kahn, 2004). For example, conducting research on the kinds of services accessed by persons in Canadian cities without full legal status is essential in order to gain insight into the kinds of services that they might require and the critical needs that they have. As an additional example, consider that without allowing pregnant women to participate in research, we would not have made the advances in obstetric care that have been documented nor would we have knowledge about the effects of particular drugs and treatments upon pregnant women and fetuses. As a final example, it is clear that the health, physical, and emotional needs of persons who are homeless may differ from the needs of those living in relative comfort. Therefore, by allowing those who are homeless to participate in research, their experiences are articulated and specific services that may address their needs might be put into place as a result of the evidence that such research would present.

More than Protection of Human Rights

Although protection of human subjects is a very important consideration in nursing research, other issues deserve equal attention. Wilson (1992) discusses characteristics of ethical research that go beyond the protection of human rights. These include ensuring scientific objectivity; meeting the ethical and legal requirements for the protection of participants; protecting human participants from harm, invasions of privacy, or deceit; maintaining integrity and truthfulness; treating data respectfully and impeccably; disseminating knowledge for the benefit of broader communities of learning; ensuring integrity in authorship; forthrightness in declaring intellectual contributions; and, finally, using courage to publicly question or clarify any distorted research claims made by others.

When nurses are working in agencies or institutions where research is being conducted, whether or not they are directly involved in the research, they must be aware of standards for ethical research in order to guard against violations of these standards.

Nurses who participate in conducting research may at times experience role conflict. A nurse is held to standards of professional practice that delineate the nurse's concern as safeguarding the health and well-being of the patient. A researcher is focused on processes and outcomes of a study in which patients may be used as sources of data. A responsible researcher is guided by humanistic values of moral concern in decisions regarding research participants (Fry, 1981). Thus, when there is a question of potential harm to a patient involved in a research study, the nurse's fiduciary duty, advocacy role, and therapeutic imperative take precedence over the integrity of the research protocol (Fowler, 1988a; Munhall & Boyd, 2010; Namei, King, Byrne & Proffitt, 1993). Incomplete knowledge of ethical and legal guidelines related to research is no excuse for a nurse failing to be a patient advocate in research situations. Although research is necessary for the development of scientific and therapeutic knowledge, the balance between principles guiding scientific inquiry and those guiding nursing practice must be maintained.

When nurses are employed, particularly in institutions that are research-focused, they need to clarify what is expected of them with regard to research. Nurses should know before accepting a position whether they will be required to gather data or administer treatments as part of research protocols, and whether such treatments may carry potential risk of harm to patients. Nurses in such settings need to know whether their positions will be jeopardized if they refuse to participate as part of a research team. When participation in research is expected as part of a nurse's job, the nurse must know the protocol, whether it has been approved by the institutional Research Ethics Board, and whom to consult regarding any concerns about the research process and its effect on patients.

ASK YOURSELF

What Takes Precedence — Research or Nursing Care?

Fowler (1988b, p. 354) poses some questions that are worth pondering:

- Is the good of the patient ever subservient to the acquisition of nursing knowledge?

- Does the therapeutic imperative of clinical care and the good of the patient always pre-empt the mandate to enlarge the nursing profession's body of knowledge?
- At what point must a nurse stop a specific nursing research project?
- When must a nurse intervene to halt a specific medical research project?
- Are there conditions under which a nurse should not include a specific subject in a study, even though consent has been secured?*

ETHICAL TREATMENT OF DATA

Scholarship issues regarding data include how the data is handled during the collection and analysis process, and how the data is reported. **Ethical treatment of data** implies integrity of research protocols and honesty in reporting findings. The honesty and integrity of the researcher are of the utmost importance in the ethical treatment of data. Taking care to ensure that only those who are involved in the research process have access to the data and to maintain confidentiality were mentioned previously. A critical ethical obligation of qualitative nursing researchers is to present and describe the experiences of others as authentically and faithfully as possible, even when they run contrary to our own aims (Munhall & Boyd, 2010). The imperative to report the findings as accurately as possible is an ethical obligation in quantitative studies as well.

CASE PRESENTATION

Protecting Patients Who Are Research Participants

A classmate and good friend is in the process of doing a research project required for graduation. You know she is frustrated because the on-line survey has not been completed by enough participants. She has sent out many reminders to potential participants but her response rate remains low. She needs to do well on this project in order to pass the final course of her degree and graduate. In order to have a large enough sample, she tells you that she is going to log onto her own survey and fill it in several times herself. She asks if you will do the same, noting that the surveys are anonymous and that several other friends are "helping out" in the same way. She says that, after all, the objective of the project is simply to demonstrate that one can collect and analyze data. It isn't really, she notes, about the actual data at all, but about the processes. You are aware that the best studies are chosen for presentations at the university Research Day, and have, in the past, been published.

---

* "Ethical Issues in Nursing Research: A Call for an International Code of Ethics for Nursing Research," Marsha D. M. Fowler, *Western Journal of Nursing Research* 10, pp. 352–355, © 1988. Reprinted with Permission of SAGE Publications.

THINK ABOUT IT

Honesty in Nursing Research

- What is your reaction to your friend's plan and request?
- Discuss the ethical issues involved in this scenario.
- What would you do in this case and what ethical principles would guide your actions or decisions?

Nurses involved in research are accountable to professional standards for reporting findings. The principles that guide academic honesty apply equally to nurse researchers in reporting outcomes of studies. It is dishonest to exaggerate results or adjust the facts of a study in order to maximize or minimize particular outcomes or hypotheses. When information from someone else is included in a report without appropriate referencing, this is plagiarism. In recent years, scientific misconduct has become a concern within the scientific community. Articles have been published in professional journals reporting studies that were never conducted, findings that were fabricated, or findings that were intentionally distorted by researchers (Burns & Groves, 2008; Chop & Silva, 1991; Friedman, 1990; Hawley & Jeffers, 1992; Parascandola, 1999). Although these reports have related more to biomedical studies than to nursing research, such reports present problems for disciplines in which clinical practice may be changed based on research findings. They also serve as a reminder to nurses to be vigilant regarding the ethical reporting of research findings.

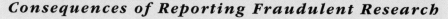

ASK YOURSELF

Consequences of Reporting Fraudulent Research

Pause and think about the havoc rendered by publication of fraudulent research.

- How might this affect how others view the integrity of the profession?
- How might this affect a reader's response to other research published in the same journal?
- How would this affect your ability as a nurse to determine whether you should adjust your practice based on reported research?
- Imagine that you have just read the report of a research project for which you gathered data and discovered that the process described was quite a bit different from what you had done, making the results take on a different meaning. How would you react and what would you do?

SUMMARY

Nurses are expected to exhibit principled behaviour in all situations. This chapter has focused on principles related to scholarship issues facing nurses. Nursing students face decisions related to academic honesty before they ever encounter a patient. Because personal values affect professional behaviour, choices made in the academic arena concerning actions such as plagiarism, cheating, or forgery may foreshadow values used to guide future professional decisions. Nurses must be familiar with principles guiding ethical practices in research and in the reporting of research findings. These principles guide nursing decisions about research protocols, participation, and advocacy for patients related to research issues. Ethical practices regarding scholarship are essential to the integrity of both the individual professional and the profession as a whole.

CHAPTER HIGHLIGHTS

- Veracity and integrity are core principles related to both academic honesty and ethical treatment of research data.

- Nursing research and researchers must adhere to nursing standards regarding the ethical conduct of research that affirm a participant's right to freedom from intrinsic risk of injury, right to privacy, right to anonymity, and the right to choose to participate or not.

- Protection of human rights, a prime focus of research ethics, is based on principles of beneficence, respect for human dignity, and justice. These principles imply protection from physical, psychological, social, or economic risk of harms; voluntary participation in research; assurance of privacy and confidentiality; and equitable treatment of all research participants.

- Informed consent for research studies, which helps to ensure that a participant's rights are protected, must include the elements promulgated in the *Tri Council Policy Statement (TCPS 2)*.

- When there is a question of potential harm to a patient involved in a research study, the nurse's advocacy role and therapeutic imperative takes precedence over the integrity of the research protocol. Nurses need to be especially attentive to protecting the rights of vulnerable groups in clinical and research settings.

DISCUSSION QUESTIONS AND ACTIVITIES

1. Review your school's policy regarding academic integrity, and discuss the ethical principles that are violated in cases of academic dishonesty.

2. Describe the realistic factors that persons reviewing cases of academic dishonesty or misconduct should consider when making decisions.

3. Think about the various roles that nurses may have in research activities. What are the responsibilities and concerns that nurses may have, when their patients are also participants in research?

4. Give examples of situations in which the nursing roles of patient advocate and researcher might be in conflict. Which role takes precedence and why?

5. Interview a nurse researcher regarding how human rights are protected in the study. Have all the required elements been included in the informed consent?

6. Discuss the potential overarching effects of unethical treatment of data on patient care.

7. Compare and contrast what the American Nurse's Association (http://www .nursingworld.org), the Canadian Nurses Association (http://www.cna-nurses .ca/cna), and the International Council of Nurses (http://www.icn.ch) say about participants' rights in research and in nursing practice.

REFERENCES

Burns, N., & S. K. Groves (2008). *The practice of nursing research: Appraisal, synthesis and generation of evidence.* (6th ed.). Philadelphia: Saunders.

Canadian Institutes of Health Research, Natural Sciences and Engineering Research Council of Canada, Social Science and Humanities Research Council of Canada, *Tri Council Policy Statement: Ethical Conduct for Research Involving Humans,* December 2010.

Chop, R., & M. C. Silva (1991). Scientific fraud: Definitions, policies, and implications for nursing research. *Journal of Professional Nursing, 7,* 166–171.

Cizek, G. J. (1999). Cheating on tests: How to do it, detect it and prevent it. New Jersey: Lawrence Erlbaum Associates.

Cox, D. H. (2003). Academic integrity: Cheating 101—a literature review. *The News about Teaching and Learning at Memorial, 6*(2). Newsletter of the Instructional Development Office.

Fowler, M. D. M. (1988a). Ethical issues in nursing research: Issues in qualitative research. *Western Journal of Nursing Research, 10,* 109–111.

Fowler, M. D. M. (1988b). Ethical issues in nursing research: A call for an international code of ethics for nursing. *Western Journal of Nursing Research, 10,* 352–355.

Friedman, P. J. (1990). Correcting the literature following fraudulent publication. *Journal of the American Medical Association, 263,* 1416–1419.

Fry, S. T. (1981). Accountability in research: The relationship of scientific and humanistic values. *Advances in Nursing Science, 4,* 1–13.

Hawley, D. J., & J. M. Jeffers (1992). Scientific misconduct as a dilemma for nursing. *Image, 24,* 51–55.

Hilts, P. J., & S. G. Stolberg (1999). Ethics lapses at Duke halt dozens of human experiments. The *New York Times,* May 13, A26.

Humphreys, L. (1970). Tearoom Trade: Impersonal Sex in Public Places. Aldine Transaction: Piscataway, USA.

Husted, G. L., & J. H. Husted (2007). *Ethical decision making in nursing: The symphonological approach.* (4th ed.) New York: Springer.

Kaplan, S., & S. Brownlee (1999). Duke's hazards: Did medical experiments put patients needlessly at risk? *U.S. World and News Report, 126*(20), 66–68, 70.

Korn, J. (1997). Illusions of Reality. A History of Deception in Social Psychology. State University of New York Press: Albany New York, USA.

Maloney, D. M. (2000a). Federal agency has all the legal authority it needs to suspend human subjects research. *Human Research Report, 15*(1), 1–2.

Maloney, D. M. (2000b). Court says state agency avoided usual way of reporting problems with human subjects: *T. D. v. New York State Office of Mental Health (Part III)*. *Human Research Report, 15*(2), 7–8.

Mastroianni, A., & J. Kahn (2004). Swinging the pendulum: Shifting views of justice in human subjects research. In *Health Care Ethics in Canada,* Second edition. F. Baylis, J. Downie, B. Hoffmaster & S. Sherwin (eds). Toronto, Canada: Thomson Nelson.

Moreno, J., A. L. Caplan & P. R. Wolpe (1998). Updating protections for human subjects involved in research. *Journal of the American Medical Association, 280*(22), 1951–1958.

Munhall, P. L., & C. O. Boyd (2010). *Nursing research: A qualitative perspective* (5th ed.). New York: National League of Nursing Press.

Namei, S. K., M. O. King, M. Byrne & C. Proffitt (1993). The ethics of role conflict. *Journal of Neuroscience Nursing, 25*, 326–330.

Olsen, D. P., & D. Mahrenholz (2000). IRB-identified ethical issues in nursing research. *Journal of Professional Nursing, 16*(3), 140–148.

Parascandola, M. (1999). Investigator fraud in clinical research. *Research-Nurse, 5*(2), 1–9, 20–21.

Reverby, S. M. (2009) Examining Tuskegee: The Infamous Syphilis Study and its Legacy. University of North Carolina Press: North Carolina, USA.

Ryerson University Office of Academic Integrity. (2012). Academic Integrity: A Student Guide. Ryerson: Toronto. Retrieved May 15, 2012, from http://www.ryerson.ca/academicintegrity/Undergraduate/index.html.

Simon Fraser University. (2009). Code of academic honesty and good conduct. Retrieved May 15, 2012 from http://www.sfu.ca/policies/gazette/student/s10-01.html.

Spicer, C. M. (2000). Federal oversight and regulations of human subjects research: An update. *Kennedy Institute of Ethics Journal, 10*(3), 261–264.

Wilson, H. S. (1992). Introducing research in nursing (2nd ed.). Redwood City, CA: Addison-Wesley.

World Medical Association. (Oct. 2008). *The Declaration of Helsinki.* Seoul, Korea: World Medical Association.

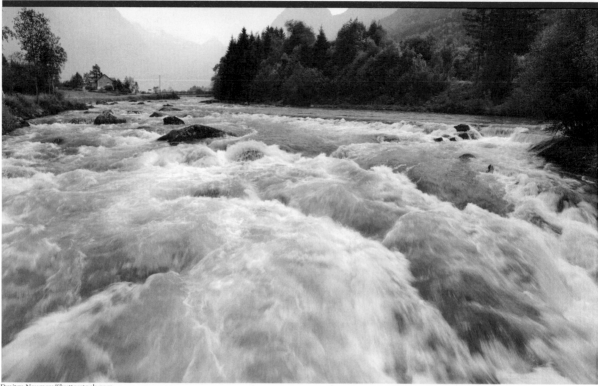

Dmitry Naumov/Shutterstock.com

CHAPTER **13**

THE FUTURE OF CANADIAN HEALTH CARE: CHALLENGES AND PRIORITIES

OBJECTIVES

After completing this chapter, the reader should be able to:

1. Identify the current challenges and future priorities in health care delivery in Canada.

2. Compare the responsibilities of the federal and provincial governments in the delivery of health care.

3. Discuss historical events that have helped to shape our current Canadian health care system.

4. Describe challenges facing other nations in the delivery of health care.

5. Identify challenges related to comprehensive coverage and accessibility in Canadian health care.

INTRODUCTION

Our health care system and how it is funded has a direct effect on how health care is delivered by physicians, nurses, and other providers. Questions about the effectiveness of delivery systems and therapies, alongside difficult decisions about how to set priorities in health care are understandably of great concern to all. Why is so much attention paid to health care and funding? The simple answer is that we will all need health care at some point in our lives, and we hope that it will continue to be a responsive, comprehensive, and accessible system. A more complete answer to why health care and funding is so important is twofold. First, as Canadians, we take great pride in our health care system, which is linked, powerfully, to our values and our identities as Canadians. Second, current spending on health care costs Canadians just over eleven percent of our total GDP (CIHI, 2012a). With rising costs, an aging population, and a seemingly unending need for more and better health care, there are concerns about the sustainability of our already-expensive system, and the challenges of continuing to be able to innovate, and able to provide highly technical care alongside comprehensive and equitable primary health care.

Alongside the ever-increasing costs of health care, the government must take into account how to sustain the current system, while ensuring equitable and fair access to high quality, safe, and efficient care. There are many questions and concerns about prioritizing health expenditures in Canada. What should we spend our health care funds on? Should health promotion and primary health care be a priority in terms of health care spending? If so, we must also ensure, then, that we can meet the current and future health care needs of an aging baby boom population, the largest aging population in recent history (CIHI, 2012b). What about technology and innovation? Should Canada be spending less on delivering health care and more on health research and innovation? If technological advances and innovation drive health care spending, many are understandably worried that those most vulnerable, such as those living in poverty, will be further disadvantaged by a lack of attention to basic health care needs of those living at the margins of our society. There are many diverse and competing needs in health care and just as many opinions on how we should prioritize health care spending to meet these diverse needs. If resources were infinite, of course, we would not have to worry about prioritizing. However, with a finite amount of resources and seemingly limitless need for health care resources, priority setting is a key challenge in the Canadian health care system today.

Our health care system must address the challenge of setting priorities and making difficult decisions about how funding will be allocated if the health care system Canadians have is to survive and flourish. The topic of how to reform our health care system in order to continue to evolve is one that has gained much attention and

interest throughout the country. Health care reform, however, is not simply a financial issue. It is an ethical issue. Setting priorities for health, deciding how health care
dollars should be spent, and deciding what and how health care will be provided to
individuals and communities is a moral activity, not simply one of adding up the col-
umns on a financial spreadsheet. What we decide are priorities reflect our values and
beliefs as Canadians, especially in the area of health care—something that we already
hold up to the world as reflective of "who we are" as Canadians.

In order to gain an understanding of this challenge and the context in which difficult decisions of prioritization and reform must be made, we first need to understand
the values that underpin Canadian health care and how these values have helped to
shape the evolution of our system as we know it today, with its strengths and challenges. To help provide context, we must also examine historical events and legacies
that have had an influence on our contemporary Canadian health care system, the
funding structures that are in place now, and then examine where we are today and
the challenges in moving our health care system into the future.

ASK YOURSELF

- What kinds of values do you think underpin our health care system in
  Canada? Try to think of four one-word values that are clearly evident as
  foundations of our health care system.

- Do you see significant differences in the values that underpin our health
  care system compared to health care systems in other countries, such as
  the United States or the United Kingdom?

- In the modern world, do you see challenges to these values as fundamental, or do you think that they are still relevant, no matter how much
  the world changes?

FEDERAL AND PROVINCIAL RESPONSIBILITIES IN HEALTH CARE DELIVERY

Our modern Canadian health care system has developed extensively over the last
century as Canada, like many other major nations, evolved through influences of
trends like industrialization, urbanization, and immigration. In 1867, when Canada
set out the *British North America Act*, the federal and provincial roles for health care
were defined in terms of very basic responsibilities. While the terms and complexities of these responsibilities have been further clarified over many years, what this
Act did was set up in very general terms the responsibilities for how the relationship
between the federal government and the provincial governments would be actualized in terms of the provision of and payment for health care services (Storch, 2005).
While provinces and territories were given jurisdiction over the provision of health

care, this couldn't possibly be done with the limited resources they had, and as their mandate to provide services increased, so did the need for assistance from the federal government. Over time, much has been done to elucidate and differentiate the federal and provincial roles and responsibilities for the provision of health care. Here is a summary of the current key responsibilities of the federal, provincial, and territorial governments in terms of health care.

FIGURE 13–1 **A REVIEW OF THE FEDERAL AND PROVINCIAL RESPONSIBILITIES FOR HEALTH CARE**

How the Work of Health Care Is Divided between the Federal and Provincial or Territorial Governments

The federal government is responsible for the following:

1. Deciding upon the principles for health care, outlined in the *Canada Health Act*.
2. Ensuring that provinces follow the set principles for the delivery of health care and adjusting federal to provincial payments based on this.
3. Assisting with the financing of provincial health care delivery of services.
4. Delivering direct health care services to veterans, native Canadians, persons living on reserves, military personnel, inmates of federal penitentiaries, and RCMP officers.
5. Some roles, such as health protection, disease prevention, and health promotion, are shared responsibilities, but the federal government plays an important role.

The provincial and territorial governments are responsible for the following:

1. Delivering and managing insured health services such as hospital and physician care.
2. Planning, financing, and evaluating hospital and physician care.
3. Managing some public health and prescription care.

(Sources: Health Canada, 2004; 2009.)

It's important to remember that while all Canadians are covered by our publicly funded health care system, it is not the case that there is one single plan that covers every Canadian from coast to coast. Instead, the health care system is really a collection of provincially-managed systems that comply with the federal guidelines or principles that are outlined in the *Canada Health Act*: Public administration, comprehensiveness, universality, portability and accessibility (Government of Canada, 1984; LaPierre, 2012). In order to continue to receive federal funding for health, provinces must demonstrate that they are abiding by the five guidelines, but there exist some differences between provinces in terms of how the guidelines are interpreted, in more specific ways (LaPierre, 2012). The model has evolved over the twentieth century, and there have been differences between the provision of care between provinces and territories (some provinces and territories have had citizens pay deductibles and co-payments in the past), but the system, at the federal level, has been built upon the principle that health care, and the care provided in hospitals, is a basic right or need that should not be provided based on the ability to pay.

Individual provinces and territories can decide what they deem to be medically necessary services and, therefore, services that are covered by the provincial health care plans (Romanow, 2002a, 2002b). If you compare the lists of covered health care services between provinces, you will see many similarities. For example, services of an optometrist or ophthalmologist are covered for most Canadians under the age of 19 to 20 and over the age of 65, unless deemed medically necessary. In most provinces, vasectomy reversals are not covered by the provincial plans, nor are cosmetic surgery procedures that are not deemed medically necessary. These are all examples of similarities in coverage between provinces. As an example of differences in terms of what is covered, the services of a chiropractor are not covered by the insurance plans of British Columbia and Ontario, while residents of Manitoba have 12 visits a year to a chiropractor covered by their provincial health plan (British Columbia Ministry of Health, 2012; Manitoba Health, 2012; Ontario Ministry of Health And Long Term Care, 2005).

Each province and territory has the responsibility for providing care to the citizens of its jurisdiction and for doing so in a way that complies with the guidelines set out by the federal government. Differences in provincial demographics and landscape account for the subsequent differences in setting priorities. A province like Ontario, with much larger urban populations and a total population of about 12 million persons, has arguably quite different kinds of priorities and needs from those in Prince Edward Island with a total population of about 140,000 persons, many of whom live in more rural settings (Ontario Ministry of Finance, 2012; PEI, 2011).

Historical Influences on Our Modern Health Care System

After the passing of the *British North America Act*, Canada continued to evolve. During the late 1800s and early 1900s, the increase in urbanization and industrialization had predictable effects on the health of Canadians. Poor living conditions and a lack of well-established health services in urban environments contributed to poor health for many, and the need for public health initiatives was recognized. Canadian nurses took the lead and the role of the public health nurse expanded as it became apparent that the environment in which we live, not simply our genetic predisposition, had a significant effect on our health and well-being. Further to this was a realization that these kinds of environmental factors could best be addressed by nurses, in what was then a somewhat independent community health nursing role (Hastings and Mosley, 1980). In addition, the influenza pandemic and a political climate that was open to progress meant that there was an increased recognition of the importance of public health (Mill, Leipert & Duncan, 2002). Alongside the rather innovative notion (for that time) that the environment in which we live has a marked effect on our health and that a public health focus was necessary, was a realization that communities needed to organize to provide help to those less fortunate, and the charitable movement that underpins much of our health care system was strengthened as charitable and volunteer-based organizations began to flourish and provide much-needed health and social services to those most in need. Group such as Children's Aid Societies and the Canadian Mental Health Association provided advocacy and support and many of these kinds of organizations continue to exist today.

With the two World Wars and the Great Depression, Canada, like other countries, needed to provide social and health care assistance to those returning from war injured or disabled, as well as provide social and welfare programs for those who had lost loved ones. Pension, welfare, and social assistance programs were developed to help those most in need. These programs, deemed to be part of the "social safety net" of Canada, were originally introduced as a "last resort" for those who truly required help to meet their most basic needs (Torjman, 2007, p. 1). Two wars and the Depression had resulted in a great deal of social need and poverty, and for many people, the services of physicians were prohibitively expensive, and for the most part, with the lack of hospitals, these services, where affordable, were provided in private homes or physicians offices.

During this same era, there were significant breakthroughs, innovations and discoveries, such as the use of anesthesia in surgery and the recognition of bacteria as a causative factor in many widespread diseases, provided helped to provide the momentum that led to the development of the modern hospital within the health care system as it exists today. In addition, with significant population increases and a greater influx of immigrants, there were diverse needs for health care and social services that health providers needed to attend to. With the widespread use of new technologies such as X-rays, and the development of antibiotics and surgery, came increased costs to the system. Many physicians could no longer afford to simply provide these services in their offices or in private homes. The move towards the hospital for the location of physician services was initiated. Hospital clinics that could provide outpatient services became the primary site of health care for many patients. Physicians provided these outpatient services and, in return, were able to participate fully in the hospital system, where the latest in knowledge and technologies was being introduced and provided.

Nurses began to take a more active role in managing the hospital environments and began to have more responsibility for technical management of patient care through duties such as taking the patient's pulse, temperature, and blood pressure, alongside physicians (Stevens, 1999). Patterns, roles, and professional relationships that developed in the health care delivery system in the early part of the century can still be seen in hospitals today. (Stevens, 1999).

Prior to the First World War, public health nursing was an elite area of nursing, with nurses at the forefront of campaigns for healthy communities and prevention of illness and disease. The war, however, emphasized the fast-paced and dynamic hospital environment for nursing, and by 1920 many general hospitals had schools of nursing attached to them. Most nursing students learned about providing hands-on care for persons with acute injuries and illness, and little about health promotion or illness prevention (Mill, Liepert & Duncan, 2002). Hospitals had also realized that classes of student nurses were a good source of free, moderately skilled labour, and many students spent long hours in the hospitals, providing care to patients with a focus on learning skills, and usually living within the hospital until graduation. Eventually, with the realization that graduate nurses were the mainstay of the front-line labour force in hospitals, many nursing schools were supported to extend their nursing education program to three years. As early as 1909, it was noted that almost all of Canada's nursing schools had extended their programs to this length of time, with a strong emphasis on in-hospital training.

At the same time, the field of public health nursing was growing alongside a realization that this was, in fact, a specialized area of nursing that required special training and preparation. Public health nurse positions had already been created in both governmental and non-governmental agencies, including the Victorian Order of Nurses and the Canadian Red Cross (Mill, Liepert & Duncan, 2002). This realization that public health nursing required special education and training helped provide a strong social force to move nursing education from being situated in hospitals to being based in universities. In 1919, the first nursing degree program in Canada was established at the University of British Columbia (University of British Columbia School of Nursing, 2012) and additional university nursing degree programs were established in other provinces soon after. Nursing education transformed from being situated in hospitals and primarily skill-based to being carried out in the classroom with a stronger theoretical base and complemented by clinical practice in hospitals and communities.

In 1948, the federal government introduced the Hospital Construction Grants Program, a program funded by both the federal and provincial governments to build more hospitals and continue to provide physician services within the hospital setting, across the country. At that time, there was already a great deal of focus on Saskatchewan, where Tommy Douglas, the young leader of the Cooperative Commonwealth Federation (a precursor of the NDP party) and Saskatchewan's premier, was advocating for good health care, available and affordable for all (Gelber, 1966). With all eyes on Saskatchewan, Tommy Douglas managed to put a program of insurance in place for health and hospital care in 1947 that, in turn, provided a model for a national system, which became a national reality in 1966 with the passing of the *Medical Care Act*, which enabled provinces and territories to set up universal health care plans and formed the foundation for Medicare, as Canada's publicly-funded health care system is also known (Gelber, 1966; McIntyre & McDonald, 2009; Taylor, 1973). With the passing of the *Canada Health Act* in 1984, the conditions for the transfer of federal funds to the provinces for health care insurance plans were made explicit. The *Canada Health Act* legislation also prohibited extra fees or billing for medically necessary services (Government of Canada, 1984).

ASK YOURSELF

How Do Historical Influences Continue to Affect Our Current Health Care System?

- Public health was emphasized in health care until the 1920s, when post-war health care became more institutionally based. How do you see this trend today? Should the focus of health care continue to be responsive, institutional, and episodic? Is this a sustainable way to manage the kinds of modern health care problems we face in Canada?

- Throughout the twentieth century, the "face" of Canada has markedly changed, with many more persons from around the world immigrating to Canada. What do you believe some current health care challenges might be, related to the changing demographics of our country?

- What kinds of challenges and concerns do you think a nurse had in 1912 compared to a nurse in 2012?

- Think about the five criteria outlined in the *Canada Health Act* that provinces must adhere to in order to receive federal funding. Are these five criteria still relevant today? Are there areas that require clarification or updating?

The following is a summary of some of the significant events that have influenced health care in Canada since Confederation.

FIGURE 13–2 **SELECTED SIGNIFICANT EVENTS IN HEALTH CARE HISTORY IN CANADA**

1867—*British North American Act:* Defined Canada as a country. This was renamed the *Constitution Act* in 1982. In this act, provinces have authority over health care, but the federal government has a responsibility to fund health care. Public health nursing is on the rise.

1928—The discovery of insulin by Frederick Banting and Charles Best, with their colleagues J. J. R. Macleod and J. B. Collip at the University of Toronto. They would later go on to be awarded a Nobel Prize for this discovery that would change health care as well as modernize front-line care for soldiers in the Second World War.

1935—The title "Registered Nurse" was protected by making registration mandatory for its use. At the same time, standards for both the education of nurses and the practice of nursing were established.

1940s—Shift from public health toward institutionalization of health care. Initiation of widespread public immunization programs.

(Continued)

1946—The Saskatchewan Government, led by provincial Premier Tommy Douglas (premier from 1944–1961 and often referred to as the "Father of Medicare" in Canada), introduces the first provincial hospital insurance program in Canada, called the *Saskatchewan Hospitalization Act.*

1957—Paul Martin, Sr., Minister of National Health and Welfare from 1946 to 1957, played a key role in the passing of the *Hospital Insurance and Diagnostic Services Act.* The five "pillars" of this act eventually became the five principles of the *Canada Health Act* (comprehensiveness, universality, public administration, accessibility, and portability).

1962—Saskatchewan's doctors' strike. Physicians in the province went on strike for twenty-three days to oppose government involvement in health care, the same day that the NDP government introduced the first public health care program, the *Saskatchewan Medical Care Insurance Act.*

1964—A Royal Commission on Health Services headed by Justice Emmett Hall (a Supreme Court justice) recommends a universal and comprehensive national health insurance program, based in part on Saskatchewan's program, in existence from 1946.

1966—Parliament creates a national Medicare program (the *Medical Care Act*) under a Liberal minority government with NDP support, with Ottawa paying 50 percent of provincial health costs. Keep in mind that as of circa 2005, the federal government funding now covers less than 20 percent of the total costs of health care in the provinces and territories.

1974—Marc Lalonde (Minister of Health) publishes *A New Perspective on the Health of Canadians* (also called the *Lalonde Report*). This report clearly cited that factors other than one's biological or genetic "luck," such as social status, environment, education, access to health care, literacy, nutrition, and lifestyle choices such as smoking or alcohol intake, were responsible for health states. This report emphasized that the determinants of health did not simply exist within the health care system, but also in other sectors, such as education and welfare systems.

1977—Liberal government under Trudeau passes the *Federal–Provincial Fiscal Arrangements* and the *Established Programs Financing Act* (also known as EPF), which represented a change from 50:50 cost sharing between the provinces/territories and federal government to new block funding. While this change provided the provinces with more freedom as to how funds were spent, they were still required to comply with the federal guidelines for provision of health care.

1982—The *Constitution Act* is passed. The first part of this act is the *Canadian Charter of Rights and Freedoms.* Preceded by the *Canadian Bill of Rights* (1960), the *Charter* is seen as an explicit articulation of national values and a document that has helped to shape national identity. It outlines the civil and political rights of all Canadians and is recognized as a fundamental document of national unity, declaring freedom as a national core value.

1984—The *Canada Health Act* is passed unanimously by parliament. This document outlines, specifically, the conditions that the thirteen provinces and territories must adhere to, in order to receive federal funding for health care. It is imperative that the provinces provide universal coverage (i.e., to all "insured" citizens) for all "medically necessary" hospital, physician, and allied health services. Ability to pay must not be a barrier to accessing health care, in any way. The five tenets of the *Canada Health Act* include universality, accessibility, public administration, portability, and comprehensiveness.

1996—Paul Martin, Jr. creates an amalgamation of two programs, the Established Programs Funding (EPF), established in 1977 (supporting health care and education) and the Canada Assistance Plan, established in 1966 (supporting social assistance) and introduces the Canada Health and Social Transfer payment system (CHST), a system of block payments from the federal governments to the provinces and territories. This coincides with massive cuts in the total transfer payments from the federal governments to health and social programs in the provinces and territories.

1997—National Forum on Health releases its report. This forum was established in 1994 to advise the prime minister on ways to reform the ailing health care system and improve the health of Canadians. The report calls for Medicare to be more strongly "evidence-based," with improvements in integrated decision making and health information systems.

1998—Marked decrease in Canada Health and Social Transfer payments to provinces and territories.

1999—Marked increase in private-sector expenditures on health care, as noted by Gratzer (2002), who cites an increase in private funding from ~23 percent in 1975 to 30 percent in 1999. These monies go toward the kinds of health care services not covered by provincial health plans, such as laser eye surgery, psychological services, in vitro fertilization, and dentistry. Most people pay for these kinds of services partially out of pocket and partially through private insurance companies, usually provided by their employer.

1999—Health care spending is ~9 percent of Canadian GDP, with a total cost of $C 95 billion annually. The majority of the funds are spent on hospital and physician care. Worries about sustainability (which initially began in the 1970s) become more pronounced (Martin and Singer, 2003).

1999—Social Union Framework Agreement carried out between Prime Minister Jean Chrétien and the premiers of the provinces and territories, except Quebec. This agreement, while not health care–specific, emphasizes the importance of social programs, equality of opportunity for all, and a reduction in barriers due to ability or mobility issues.

(Continued)

1978—In the *Declaration of Alma-Ata* (World Health Organization, 1978), the World Health Organization calls for "Health for all by the year 2000," with a call to all countries to improve primary care and health promotion along with ensuring that essential health services for all persons are provided, e.g., safe water, adequate sanitation, maternal and child health care, immunization, control of infectious disease, adequate nutrition, and safe environments. This Declaration reiterates the WHO definition of health as "a state of complete physical, mental and social well-being and not merely the absence of disease or infirmity." (WHO, 2006).

2000—First ministers announce the Primary Health Care Transition Fund (an investment of $C800 million to improve primary health care, increase health promotion and injury prevention programs, increase the number of services offered on a 24/7 basis, establish more interdisciplinary teams, and facilitate intersectoral collaboration, with the goal of helping those in the health care sector work with those in other sectors to improve the health of citizens and address issues of basic health promotion: education, social services, labour, sanitation, and so on.

2000—Alberta Premier Ralph Klein introduces legislation to allow private hospitals and a resultant two-tiered system in Alberta, with the goals of improving efficiency, reducing wait times, and delivering health care in innovative ways.

2002—The Royal Commission on the Future of Health Care in Canada conducts cross-country public hearings, led by Commissioner Roy J. Romanow, Q.C. The final report, titled *Building on Values: The Future of Health Care in Canada* was tabled in Ottawa on November 28, 2002.

2002—Senator Michael Kirby publishes a document on health care reform initiatives titled *The Health of Canadians: The Federal Role*, tabled in October 2002.

2003—First Ministers' Health Accord announced. The commitments of this accord include a significant increase in health care funding over the next three to five years. Programs such as primary health care, home care, and catastrophic drug coverage are targeted as key areas for reform and increased funding. Accountability and transparency are emphasized, along with a proposed change to the way that the federal government transfers funds to the provinces and territories, called the Canada Health Transfer, effective in April 2004. The accord also calls for better methods of reporting back to Canadians on how their tax dollars are spent on health care, by means of an annual report.

2007—The Canadian Medical Association releases a report in support of private health care as a means to improve a non-sustainable health care system.

2008–9—Canada Health Transfer payments from the federal government to the provincial and territorial governments total about $C 37 billion, roughly 20 percent of the total health care expenditures of the provinces and territories.

2012—The Drummond Report is published in Ontario. Along with the Maritime provinces, Ontario has the highest ratio of debt (~35%); only Quebec has more (50%). In order to curb the increasing debt ratio, Don Drummond was asked to lead the Commission on the Reform of Ontario's Public Services. Privatization of health care and education is discouraged, as are tax increases. Health care, the biggest expenditure in Ontario's budget, is the focus of the report, which highlights the following relevant concerns: an acute care focus, a lack of physicians, rapidly increasing drug costs, and the high cost of mental health and addiction services. The Commission suggests the following strategies to make the health care system more sustainable: increasing the focus on chronic care, spending more on health promotion and illness prevention, shifting the emphasis from hospitals to individual patients, and a better co-ordination of care across sectors.

Source: Compiled by author from information provided by Ministry of Health and Long Term Care, Ontario; Ontario Ministry of Finance; Department of Finance Canada; Health Canada; Canadian Nursing Association; Canadian Institute for Health Information; Canadian Broadcasting Corporation Archives; and World Health Organization.

CHALLENGES IN OUR CURRENT HEALTH CARE SYSTEM: PERSPECTIVES

For many Canadians, our health care system is what defines us and is deeply entrenched in our values and beliefs. Canadians take great pride in a universal health care system, and support the idea that it is the best way to provide care, for reasons related both to economics and to social justice. But our system, as it exists today, exists with serious problems, challenges, and inequities. Canada spends much more on health care (approximately C$5800 per capita in 2011) than many other comparable countries with similar systems (CIHI, 2012a). As of 2010, only Switzerland and Norway spent more per capita on health care, with many countries, such as Italy, Japan, Spain, Sweden, and France, providing some form of universal health care for far less (OECD, 2011). The United States spends far more than any country with universal health care and continues to be the country with the highest health care costs, paired with serious inequities and severe problems with access to basic health care (OECD, 2011).

Since before the Romanow Commission, there has been great concern in Canada that the health care system Canadians have today is not sustainable without significant reform. A system built mainly around the provision of acute care and problem-based care, the focus of our system is on hospital-based and physician care. Health promotion, public health initiatives, better primary health care, improved home care, and the effective maintenance of chronic diseases remain less important in terms of priorities, even though we know that putting resources into health promotion and illness prevention can, over time, help people live healthier lives. However, to shift the focus of the system from reactionary and problem-based to a system that prioritizes health prevention and effective management of chronic illnesses implies a great deal of serious change and reform to many parts of health care systems. As a basic example of where change needs to be initiated, it is the reality that for many people in both rural and urban areas, access to a family doctor or nurse practitioner is difficult, especially after regular clinic hours, and they often seek help for minor or chronic problems in urgent care clinics and emergency rooms (Schoen *et al.*, 2009).

With an aging population, and Canadians living longer with chronic illnesses, the shift towards providing better quality care that truly meets the needs of today's Canadian population means adopting strategies like providing more primary health care, spending more on prescription drugs, providing more and better out-of-hospital, after-hours, and home care, and putting programs in place for people with special vulnerabilities related to social disadvantages. This also means paying closer attention to the social determinants of health and the unique needs of those who may be marginalized or vulnerable due to poverty, illiteracy, poor housing, lack of access to healthy foods, or a lack of quality education. Our health is determined by many factors other than a presence of illness or a genetic predisposition to disease (Mikkonen and Raphael, 2010). Providing social support systems for those most affected by poverty and lack of access to basic needs, such as housing and nutrient-rich food, is one way to better sustain a health care system, by essentially addressing serious social problems before they can develop into even more serious health concerns. One way to do this is through effective primary health care. Primary health care can be defined as an approach to the provision of essential health care that focuses on equity among populations and societies, with a progressive approach to distribution of comprehensive health care resources that are scientifically sound, affordable for and supported by communities (Starfield, 2011 World Health Organization, 1978;). The goal of primary health care is usually health for all in a community, and the involvement of individuals and groups in communities is key to delivering health care. Additional key elements of primary health care include intersectoral collaboration, in which those in different sectors (e.g., education, road safety, water, health, sanitation) work together to ensure that communities can flourish. The *Romanow Report* emphasizes the need for a primary health care reform in Canada (2002). Primary health care is seen by Romanow and many others as not only a way to save health care dollars and provide more effective, relevant, and appropriate health care, but also as the foundation for building healthy communities.

Our current health care system, while effective in many ways, is still seen as lagging behind in providing effective and high-quality health care to those who are weakest and most vulnerable: the poor, the elderly, and those with chronic illnesses (Romanow, 2002a). For many elderly persons, prescriptions drugs cost more than they can afford realistically, and few options exist other than acute care settings for managing chronic problems. For those affected by homelessness, not having an address potentially means not being able to access basic health care. Many people living with chronic illnesses or disabilities pay significant amounts of money out of their own pocket for necessary therapy from health care professionals such as physiotherapists, occupational therapists, or any number of ancillary health care providers other than physicians. Our current system is set up to provide coverage for hospital and physician services—episodic care—yet many needs exist that cannot be met by this model. Critics agree that further privatization of our system is not the answer to providing these other kinds of services more efficiently (Romanow, 2002a).

Accessibility of Health Care

Problems in the delivery of health care to Canadians occur in a number of ways. While it is not be the case that the health care system lacks expensive or effective technologies, or that individuals cannot access care because they cannot pay, it is a reality that there are geographic and contextual barriers to accessing health care. Accessibility is one of the five principles outlined in the *Canada Health Act* (Government of Canada, 1984). In this section, it is noted that "reasonable access" to health care must exist for citizens without financial barriers (which might include extra billing or user fees in this context). However, the *Act* does not directly address geographical accessibility.

As urban populations continue to grow, much of the acute care services are focused on these populous areas and often affiliated with universities located in larger cities. Small local hospitals often cannot afford the expensive technology and qualified staff. Often patients from rural areas who require surgeries, transplants, or procedures such as MRIs or CT scans are taken to larger teaching hospitals in urban centres for specialized care. This is expensive and time-consuming, contributing to increased morbidity and long waits for care. Rural populations in Canada often have to do without services because of lack of providers and facilities within a reasonable distance from their homes. Accessing health care for people in rural areas often requires taking a day off work for travel and waiting in crowded waiting rooms. Many rural areas lack health care personnel, and emergency or after-hours care is often nonexistent. Many rural areas do not have 911 services available or, if they do, may face long waits through difficult terrain or seasonal challenges, such as snow or heavy rains that may make roads impassable. In the far north, in areas that are accessible only by small planes, waits for basic medical supplies have an effect on physician and nursing care. Certainly a patient living in the north of Canada will face a longer and more difficult wait for open heart surgery than a patient waiting in a downtown Montreal or Toronto hospital, simply by virtue of their geographic location. Patients may delay treatment or not become involved with prevention, health education, or rehabilitation programs because they require so much effort and time to accomplish.

The urban poor face similar kinds of access problems, not because care is geographically distant, but because access may require trips to busy centres, often with long waits for care. While there may be more centres and providers in urban areas, queues for care and long waits at appointments may result in a different kind of burden for the urban poor. Like their rural counterparts, the urban poor may be required to take time off from work in order to see a provider. For someone working at a job with a minimum hourly wage, it is much more difficult to leave work for a number of hours or a day in order to wait to see a health care provider, compared to a person in a better paid or more autonomous position. Prescribed care, such as psychology, dental care, physiotherapy, or occupational therapy, not covered by provincial insurance plans, may be unaffordable to those working in minimum wage jobs or who are self-employed with no health benefits.

Large immigrant populations live in overcrowded situations in some urban settings and, in some cases, persons living without legal status may be unable to access care or make use of a strong community network. In addition to financial constraints, there may be language and cultural barriers, as well as lack of knowledge about how to access a highly complex health care system.

Medically Necessary: Who Decides?

One of the five guiding principles of the *Canada Health Act* is comprehensiveness. This principle states that provincial and territorial health insurance plans must cover all services deemed to be "medically necessary" (Romanow, 2002b). However, the term "medically necessary" is one that has not been defined and is highly subjective. From what we know about our health care system, most services of physicians and hospital care are defined as medically necessary and are covered by provincial insurance plans. But what about everything else? Many would say that basic dental care, which is not covered by most provincial health care plans, is medically necessary. Most of us would agree that the insulin for a patient with diabetes is medically necessary and that antibiotics for a child with a fever due to a bacterial infection is also necessary, yet prescription drugs are not covered by most provincial or territorial plans, except in some special circumstances. While it's relatively easy for rational people to agree that life-saving cardiac surgery or trauma care to a victim of a catastrophic car accident should be covered by health insurance plans, it is everything else between that leaves room for disagreement and debate. Should cosmetic surgery be fully covered? What about ambulance transport? And long-term and home care? Who should be the ones to decide? For many patients recovering from a stroke, continuing physiotherapy and occupational therapy are keys to regaining function and quality of life (Legg, 2004), but these services are not usually fully covered by provincial plans outside of therapy provided in hospitals and rehabilitation settings When there are limited physiotherapy services provided by provincial health insurance plans, there are typically long waits for access to limited providers or supplemental out-of-pocket costs for assessments or consultations. For children with autism spectrum disorder, accessing early intervention either through behavioural therapy, play therapy, or occupational therapy may hold an important key to future quality of life and high functioning (Boyd *et al.*, 2010). Again, many of these services are not provided through the provincial health care insurance plans; however, in provinces such as British Columbia, funding is being provided for these children through the provision of "Autism Funds" (British Columbia Ministry of Children and Family Development, 2012). The lack of clear definition about what "medically necessary" creates inequities between provinces, as some provinces may define services as medical necessities while other provinces do not.

HEALTH CARE SYSTEMS AND SUSTAINABILITY: GLOBAL CONCERNS

The challenge to provide health care for populations across the globe requires increasing effort and creativity. Canada is not the only country worrying about challenges such as limited resources, increasing costs, and the sustainability of a health care system. Many variables play a part in these challenges, including economics, cultural factors, epidemics, environment, war, and national crises. The problems are further compounded by the relationship, or lack of relationship, between modern medicine and traditional healing systems, and preventive methods of health promotion contrasted with curative methods of treating illness. One way to assess the health of countries is to look at the rates of infant mortality. While the numbers in some countries since 2004 have not changed markedly, others have changed drastically, reflecting crises such as civil wars, political unrest, and severe environmental changes. On very broad levels, the changes or lack of changes you see in these rates over time may reflect differences in the available resources in different countries: financial, natural and human, that all affect how individuals and populations can access the basic determinants of health.

Infant mortality is expressed as the number of infants per 1000 live births who die under one year of age. As of 2012, Canada's rate of infant mortality was 4.85. This can be compared to the United States (5.98), the United Kingdom (4.56), and the European Union (4.49). Monaco has the lowest infant mortality rate, at 1.8, while currently the highest rates are found in Afghanistan (121.63), Niger (109.98), and Mali (109.08) (Central Intelligence Agency, 2012).

While some countries are grappling with decisions about the provision of high-tech care and innovative new surgical treatments, others are simply trying to provide their citizens with access to the most basic health care, in an attempt to reduce the impact of factors such as severe poverty, political unrest, and conflict on the health and well-being of those who live there. The activity of priority setting or rationing is something that health policy makers in all countries are faced with. With increasing possibilities for medical treatment and the effect of globalization, governments must make difficult decisions about how to fund health care systems, what trade-offs to make, and how to spend their health care dollars most wisely and effectively. With different kinds of priorities and challenges facing different countries, it is easy to see that no two countries face the same kinds of challenges. In Canada, we are struggling with sustaining a current system while staying true to the values that underpin the system and also ensuring that we are responsive to the changing demographics of our country and the diverse evolving needs of our populations. An additional challenge is trying to enact change while effectively adhering to broad overarching national values for health care, in not one system, but ten provincial and three territorial health care administration systems.

While there are many who champion systems such as we have in Canada, there are others who criticize it, worrying about the sustainability of the system we have. Some critics of Canada's health care system cite that the system sets up a system of rationing because of insufficient funds for specialized health care. It has been said that the waiting times for some procedures and access to specialty care can be extremely long, and even dangerous for your health. It is true that access to certain procedures and technologies is limited. Waiting lists reached crisis points in Canada in the 1980s and 1990s in areas like cardiac surgery and orthopedic surgery (Korcok, 1997). Waiting lists still exist and some of the most recent data on waiting for care in Canada demonstrates that Canadians still wait longer than they feel is reasonable for elective treatment. Waits are noted, in one report, to be longest to undergo plastic surgery and the shortest for medical oncology treatment (Barua, Rovere & Skinner, 2011). Data from surveys of specialists across Canada report an average wait time between the referral from a general practitioner and an elective procedure to be about 19 weeks, the longest reported waiting time for such a procedure in many years (Barua, Rovere & Skinner, 2011). There are also differences reported between provinces in terms of waiting for care. Critics agree that there is unequal access to health care from province to province, depending on the affluence of the province (Romanow, 2002a, 2002b). Even within provinces, inequalities abound between persons living in resource-rich urban centres versus those who live in remote rural areas. Some Canadian citizens who can afford to pay out-of-pocket go to the United States for specialized care and surgeries, and some provinces have even developed contracts with American providers to manage long waiting lists (Barer & Lewis, 2000; Korcok, 1997). In all instances, the increase in health care spending due to the high cost of technologies and research is having an impact on these systems in much the same ways as it is across the globe (Katz, Verilli & Barer, 1998; Walker, 1992).

ASK YOURSELF

Health Care — A Right or a Privilege?

- In your own clinical practice, what kinds of challenges to accessing health care do you see individuals, groups, or communities struggling with?

- Do you consider health care a basic right? As rights create obligations for others, what then are our obligations to provide everyone with access to this basic right?

- Some people view health care as a *privilege* instead of a *right*. What is the difference between these two terms? Think of yourself and those you care about who live in Canada. What does health care and access to health care mean to you and your family? What would you do if you lived in a different place, where health care was inaccessible or unaffordable to you? How would you feel?

- Nurses often act as advocates for individual patients and groups of patients. Do you see one role of nurses as being advocates for health care as a right for all?

- What kind of health care problems do you see, in your practice or your community, that arise from sectors other than health care?

SUMMARY

The current system in which health care providers function in Canada is rapidly changing. There are many questions and worries about the sustainability of our current system in light of skyrocketing costs and increasing demands for health care. Access to basic health care services has not typically been considered to be a problem in Canada, but there are problems with access to basic and specialized health care in remote or under-served areas. The needs of the Canadian population are changing as our demographics change, as patterns of immigration and settlement evolve, as the baby boomers age, and as more people are living longer with chronic illnesses.

It remains a reality that many people in the world have limited or no access to the simplest health care, something that we consider to be a basic right. While many admire the Canadian health care system and the values that provide the foundation for the system, the reality is that our health care system is suffering. As a nation, we have serious priority-setting problems that we must grapple with if our health care system is to be sustainable.

As we move forward in the 21st century, significant health and social reform must occur in order to address the inequities and realities of our system, and ensure a sustainable system that can provide high quality, appropriate care to a diverse Canadian population.

CHAPTER HIGHLIGHTS

- The provision of health care is affected by many social forces. How health care is valued and provided can be influenced by cultural, historical, sociopolitical, economic, and scientific forces.

- Increased urbanization and scientific breakthroughs, alongside the movement towards the hospital as the main location for the provision of health care, have influenced how our health care system is structured today. Social forces, such as the women's movement, the public health movement, and increased immigration to Canada, have also had an influence upon how our health care system is structured and on the priorities that have been set.

- Expansion of hospital and other health care services, alongside concerns about sustainability, have reached a point where proposals for reform must be considered.

- Many countries have structures and processes to provide basic health care services for their citizens; however, many people in these countries still have significantly limited access to these basic services.

- There are serious problems related to how to define medical necessity in Canada. This lack of a clear and explicit definition can contribute to, among other problems, further inequities between provinces.

DISCUSSION QUESTIONS AND ACTIVITIES

1. Go online and search the Canadian mass media for critical perspectives on health care. What seem to be the main issues that the media present? Do these align with what is said in the scholarly literature on sustainability in health care?

2. Review historical documents from health care agencies such as the Victorian Order of Nurses, the Canadian Red Cross, or the Canadian Nurses Association on the role of the nurse in health care in the early twentieth century. What were the main roles, responsibilities, and concerns of nurses at that time, and how do these differ from the roles, responsibilities, and concerns of a nurse today?

3. Imagine yourself thirty years in the future, being asked to come and speak to a first-year nursing class. What would you tell the students about the main health care issues in your time as a nursing student?

4. When people claim that access to health care is a "right," this implies an obligation on others to provide health care that is accessible. What do you think are some of the real barriers to providing access to very basic health care to everyone, in our high-tech, globalized world where anything seems possible?

5. Describe what you consider to be the main impact of health delivery and financing on patient care and outcomes. Identify potential ethical dilemmas related to current systems of delivery and financing, in Canada and other countries.

REFERENCES

Barer, M. L., & S. Lewis (2000). *Waiting for health care in Canada: Problems and prospects.* Toronto: Atkinson Foundation publication, University of Toronto. Retrieved September 5, 2012 from http://www.utoronto.ca/hpme/dhr/pdf/Barer-Lewis.pdf

Barua, B., M. Rovere & B. J. Skinner (2011). *Waiting your turn. Waiting times for health care in Canada. 2011 report of the Fraser Institute.* Retrieved September 12, 2012 from http://www. fraserinstitute.org/uploadedFiles/fraser-ca/Content/research-news/research/publications/ waiting-your-turn-2011.pdf

Boyd, B. A., S. L. Odom, B. P. Humphreys & A. M. Sam (2010). Infants and toddlers with autism spectrum disorder: Early identification and early intervention. *Journal of Early Intervention, 32*(2), 75–97.

British Columbia Ministry of Children and Family Development (2012). *Autism funding programs.* Retrieved September 5, 2012 from http://www.mcf.gov.bc.ca/autism/funding_programs.htm

British Columbia Ministry of Health (2012). *Medical and health care benefits.* Retrieved September 2, 2012 from http://www.health.gov.bc.ca/msp/infoben/benefits.html#notcovered

Canadian Institute for Health Information. (2012a). Health spending to reach $200 billion in 2011. Retrieved September 6, 2012 from http://www.cihi.ca/a-ext-portal/internet/en/document/ spending+and+health+workforce/spending/release_03nov11

Canadian Institute for Health Information. (2012b). Health care cost drivers: The facts. Retrieved September 6, 2012 from https://secure.cihi.ca/free_products/health_care_cost_drivers_the_facts_en.pdf

Central Intelligence Agency. (2012). Rank order—infant mortality rate. *The World Factbook.* Retrieved June 1, 2012, from https://www.cia.gov/library/publications/the-world-factbook/rankorder/2091rank.html

Gelber, S.M. (1966). The path to health insurance. *Canadian Public Administration*, 9, pp. 156–165.

Government of Canada (1984). *Canada Health Act.* Ottawa: Government of Canada. Retrieved September 1, 2012 from http://laws.justice.gc.ca/eng/acts/C-6/

Gratzer, S. (ed.) (2002). *Better medicine: Reforming Canadian health care.* ECW Press: Toronto.

Hastings, J. E. R., & W. Mosley (1980). Introduction: The evaluation of organized community health services in Canada. In C. A Meilicke & J. Storch (eds.) *Canadian health and social services policy: History and emerging trends* (pp. 145–155). Ann Arbor, Michigan: Health Administrative Press.

Health Canada. (2004). *Health care system: Federal role in health.* Retrieved January 25, 2009, from http://www.hc-sc.gc.ca/hcs-sss/delivery-prestation/fedrole/index-eng.php

Health Canada. (2009). *Health care system: Provincial/territorial role in health.* Retrieved June 1, 2012, from http://www.hc-sc.gc.ca/hcs-sss/delivery-prestation/ptrole/index-eng.php

Katz, S. J., D. Verilli & M. L. Barer (1998). Canadians' use of U.S. medical services. *Health Affairs, 17*(1), 225–235.

Korcok, M. (1997). Excess demands meets excess supply as referral companies link Canadian patients, US hospitals. *Canadian Medical Association Journal, 157*, 767–770.

LaPierre, T. A. (2012). Comparisons of the Canadian and US systems of health care in an era of health care reform. *Journal of Health Care Finance, 38*(4), 1–18.

Legg, L., & Outpatients Service Trialists (2004). Rehabilitation therapy services for stroke patients living at home: Systematic review of randomized trials. *The Lancet, 363*(9406), 352–356.

Manitoba Health (2012). Are you covered? Questions and answers about health care coverage. Retrieved September 2 from http://www.gov.mb.ca/health/mhsip/#5

Martin, D. & Singer, P. A. (2003). Canada. In Ham, C. & Roberts, G. (Eds.) *Reasonable Rationing: International Experience of Rationing in Health Care.* Philadelphia, PA: McGraw-Hill Press.

McIntyre, M., & C. McDonald (2009). *Realities of Canadian Nursing: Professional, Practice, and Power Issues.* (3rd ed.) Philadelphia, PA: Lippincott, Williams and Wilkins.

Meilicke, C. A., & J. Storch (1980). Introduction: an historical framework. In C. A. Meilicke & J. Storch (eds.) *Canadian health and social service policy: history and emerging trends* (p. 1–18). Ann Arbor, Michigan: Health Administration Press.

Mikkonen, J., & D. Raphael (2010). *Social determinants of health: The Canadian facts.* York University School of Policy and Health Management: Toronto.

Mill, J.E., B. D. Liepert & S. M. Duncan (2002). A history of public-health nursing in Alberta and British Columbia from 1918–1939. *Canadian Nurse, 98*(1), 18–23.

Ontario Ministry of Finance (2012). *Ontario Fact Sheet 2012.* Retrieved September 2, 2012 from http://www.fin.gov.on.ca/en/economy/ecupdates/factsheet.html

Ontario Ministry of Health and Long Term Care (2005). *OHIP Change to coverage for chiro-practors*. Retrieved September 2, 2012 from http://www.health.gov.on.ca/english/public/pub/ohip/chiropractic.html

Organization for Economic Co-operation and Development. (2011). *OECD Health Data 2011*. OECD: Paris.

Prince Edward Island Statistics Bureau (2011). *Prince Edward Island Population Report, 2011*. Retrieved September 2, 2012 from http://www.gov.pe.ca/photos/original/pt_pop_rep.pdf

Romanow, R. J. (2002a). *Building on Values: The future of health care in Canada – Final Report*. Ottawa: Commission on the Future of Health Care in Canada. Retrieved September 5, 2012 from http://publications.gc.ca/collections/Collection/CP32-85-2002E.pdf

Romanow, R. J. (2002b). *Medically necessary: What is it, and who decides?* Ottawa: Commission on the Future of Health Care in Canada. Retrieved September 5, 2012 from http://publications.gc.ca/collections/Collection/CP32-78-1-2002E.pdf

Schoen, C., R. Osborn, S. K. H. How, M. M. Doty & J. Peugh (2009). Experience of patients with complex health care needs, in eight countries, 2008. *Health Affairs*, pp. W1–W16.

Starfield, B. (2011). Politics, primary care and health: Was Virchow right? *Journal of Epidemiology and Community Health*, *65*(8), 653–655.

Stevens, R. (1999). *In sickness and in wealth; American Hospitals in the Twentieth Century*. John Hopkins University Press: New York.

Storch, J. (2005). Country profile: Canada's health care system. *Nursing Ethics*, *12*(4), 414–418.

Taylor, M. G. (1973). The Canadian health insurance program. *Public Administration Review*, *33*, 31–39.

Torjman, S. (2007). *Repairing Canada's social safety net*. Ottawa, ON: The Caledon Institute of Social Policy.

University of British Columbia School of Nursing (2012). *History*. Retrieved September 11, 2012 from http://www.nursing.ubc.ca/AboutUs/History.aspx

Walker, M. (1992). How they don't do it in Canada. *Reason*, 35–42.

World Health Organization (1978). *The declaration of Alma-Ata*. Retrieved January 25, 2009, from http://www.wpro.who.int/rcm/en/archives/rc32/wpr_rc32_ro5.htm.

World Health Organization (2006). *Constitution of the World Health Organization*. Retrieved September 7, 2012 from http://www.who.int/governance/eb/who_constitution_en.pdf

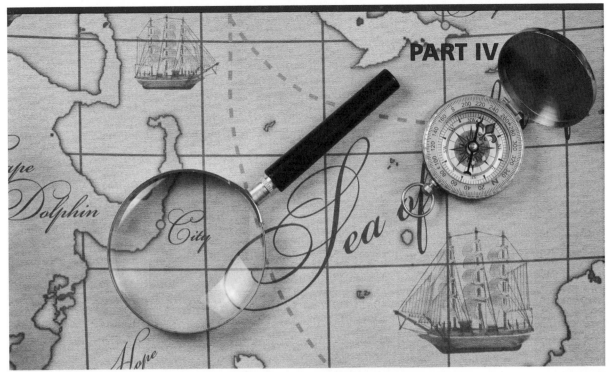

Laborant/Shutterstock.com

NURSING IN TODAY'S WORLD: CHALLENGES AND OPPORTUNITIES

Part IV recognizes that every person is affected by social, economic, political, and cultural issues. Our ability to achieve, maintain, and improve our health status is highly dependent upon the world around us. As nurses, we work with individuals and groups from diverse backgrounds, life experiences, and cultural groups. In this last section, we acknowledge that nurses today must be aware of, and sensitive to, the multitude of factors that have an impact upon the health of individuals, communities, and populations. First, we address challenges and changes in the health care system and the political environment in which we practice. We then will explore the economic aspects of health care delivery and the allocation of health care resources. We also explore important social factors and structures that have an impact on health and the provision of nursing care, framed by a discussion of the social determinants of health. Following this is a chapter addressing issues of gender and culture, and a discussion of how these are relevant to nursing practice. Our new chapter in this edition is our chapter on rural and Aboriginal nursing, which addresses unique contemporary challenges and opportunities in these areas for Canadian nurses. To end his section, we encourage nurses to consider the complex factors and issues identified in these chapters as they advocate for, and help to empower, individuals and communities through responsible and ethical nursing practice.

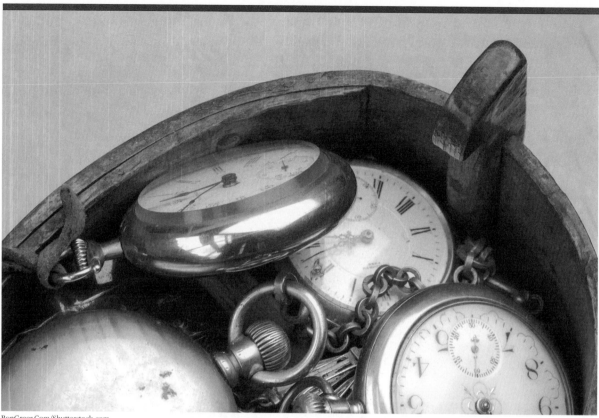

RonGreer.Com/Shutterstock.com

CHAPTER **14**
HEALTH POLICY ISSUES

OBJECTIVES

After completing this chapter, the reader should be able to:

1. Understand what makes an issue "political."

2. Distinguish between politics and policy.

3. Identify basic legislative processes that affect health policy in Canada.

4. Give examples of specific political issues related to health care.

5. Discuss your personal stand on various political issues in relation to ethics.

6. Describe the health policy process.

7. Discuss the role of ethics in policy making.

8. Explain the role of nurses in the policy-making process.

9. Describe various methods of influencing public policy.

INTRODUCTION

We can view health policy and politics in a number of different ways. Some perceive health policy as a political process, strongly influenced by ideology and party politics. Others see the health policy-making process as a thoughtful one, with decisions based on data and on the rational analysis of needs, outcomes, and costs (Donley, 1996). In reality, the health policy process is a combination of both informed rational judgments and ideological partisan politics.

Over time, nurses have become more involved in the political process, particularly in the realm of health policy. Nurses view health, at least in part, as depending on various environmental factors that can be altered by health policy decisions. Recognizing our role as advocates for patients' health, and acknowledging the importance of being involved in regulatory processes, we are assuming more responsibility in the political arena. This chapter features examples of selected political issues in the discussion of the process of creating health policy, and describes specific methods that nurses can use to influence policy.

POLITICS

Politics, political action, political issues, policies—what do these terms mean, and how are they different? Furthermore, why are they important to consider in nursing and health care? Whether you are a nurse at the bedside in an intensive care unit or a rural visiting home care nurse, your work, your scope of practice, and the structures you practise in, are all affected by politics and government policies.

Politics refers to anything that involves groups of people making decisions or influencing how decisions are made or how resources are allocated. The term implies both action and thought. It is, essentially, a neutral term although many people use the term with a negative connotation, e.g., "She is too caught up in the politics of all this." Certainly, politics and the activity of being political can be seen in a negative light, but this depends on your experience, your biases, and how invested you are in the issue or end. Typically, people tend to act in a "political" way when the issue is one that will have an effect upon their own personal or professional lives. Otherwise, they tend not to pay attention to many political issues.

Policies are plans of action that guide actions—of governments, institutions, corporations, communities, and other groups and organizations. Policies often reflect the values and beliefs of the majority, or of those directly responsible for creating the policy. Many times, when governments put policies in place, they reflect the overarching values of the government in power and may be altered when a different governing body comes into power. In Canada, our political parties hold very different views on many issues; for example, social policy issues like welfare and education, the environment, and gun control. Different political parties may take different stands on an issue because they understand the available evidence differently, or have different priorities, or have different moral or ideological points of view.

Many types of policies exist. We can have *social policies, public policies,* or *institutional/organizational policies.* The process of creating different policies may be similar; however, their jurisdiction and enactment might be markedly different. Some policies may be formulated by governmental bodies as legislation, while others may be mandated by institutions or communities. A good example of a social policy would be setting an age of consent, or having an age limit on the purchase of alcohol or tobacco. Our non-smoking policies across Canada would be good examples of public policies. One major topic for social, public, and institutional policies is health. Health policies are any policies related to health care, health promotion, or health research. Health policies of special interest to nurses include those related to the provision of physician and hospital treatment in Canada, along with province-specific decisions on coverage of related services, such as eye care, chiropractic care, nursing services, home care, and long-term care. Institutional or organizational policies are those that refer to workplace, professional, or association issues. For example, hospitals may have a policy on the nurse–patient ratio on a particular unit (institutional policy) that affects how many shifts a nurse might work in a designated period of time, while the professional nursing union has specific policies on how many shifts in a row any nurse can work (organizational policies).

HEALTH POLICY

Because health plays a critical role in the physical, psychological, and economic condition of individuals, it affects society in general. The central purpose of health policy, therefore, is the improvement of the overall health of the population. Health policy is far reaching; it influences the behaviour and decisions of people in relation to their environment and living conditions; it affects lifestyle and personal behaviour; and it affects availability, accessibility, and quality of health care services. Health-related issues receive considerable attention in the policy-making forum.

Different people define health in different ways. Different definitions of health include notions of normality, and of illness, and the factors affecting these notions. The most popular definition of health affects the kinds of investments and the degree of investment that society is willing to make in health care and social programs, and what programs are eventually funded. For example, if our society defines health narrowly in terms of illness, policy makers might choose to fund programs that focus on treatment of illness, but neglect programs that support health-promoting behaviours. In contrast, a society that defines health positively, in terms of wellness, would place more emphasis on funding programs to prevent illness or maximize health potential.

Health policies are formal and authoritative decisions centred around health. Health policies are made in both the legislative and judicial branches of government, and are intended to direct or influence the actions, behaviours, and decisions of others. Policy comprises a very large set of decisions. Examples of health policies include legislation, rules and regulations designed to guide decision-making for the government, and various governmental programs related to health. **Statutes or laws** are pieces of legislation that have been enacted by legislative bodies and approved by the government. **Rules or regulations** are policies that are established to guide the implementation of laws and programs. **Judicial decisions** are authoritative court decisions that direct or influence the actions, behaviours, or decisions of others.

Although there is significant potential for overlap, health policies fit into two basic categories: allocative and regulatory. **Allocative policies** determine how priorities are set; that is, where resources are allocated. Resources may be financial resources, human resources, or time. Here is where we see distributive justice in practice. In most countries, including Canada, special attention is given in these policies to facilitating access to goods and services for the disadvantaged, marginalized, or vulnerable. Allocative policies are based on fundamental beliefs about which distinct group or class of individuals or organizations should receive the benefits. Policy makers realize that some will receive benefits, some will not, and others will bear the expense. Ideally, these decisions are based upon public objectives (Longest, 1995). In Canada, with a publicly funded health care system (often called "medicare"), we are not forced to make decisions about how health care, specifically physician and hospital care, is allocated. However, decisions about where to build hospitals, what programs to offer at specific hospitals, and how many physicians to put into place at centres, are all decisions about allocation that affect health care. A person living in a particularly underserved rural area does not have the same access to physician care, specialty care, or acute care services that a person living in downtown Toronto or Montreal would have. This is a direct result of resource allocation decisions.

Similarly, while physician and hospital care is covered under the *Canada Health Act*, medications are not (except for inpatients in hospitals). Each province decides on a prescription drug benefit plan and these vary between provinces, as do requirements for co-payments by individuals. Many provinces have plans with some coverage for prescription drugs for the elderly or those on social assistance. Many persons who have chronic illnesses or devastating acute health care events must pay for their own medications. The way that provinces decide how they will cover prescription drugs is also an example of an allocation decision.

Regulatory policies are those designed to direct the actions, behaviours, and decisions of individuals or groups of people. Examples of regulatory policies include acts that regulate the practice of health care professionals, such as physicians, nurses, midwives, dietitians, pharmacists, physiotherapists, and chiropractors. Here are a few examples: In Ontario, there is the *Regulated Health Professions Act* (1991); Manitoba has the *Regulated Health Professions Statutes Amendment Act* (1998) and Alberta has the *Health Professions Act* (1999). Workplace regulations aimed at safe workplaces and procedures are also examples of regulatory policies. Examples include the *Occupational Health and Safety (OHS) Regulation Act* in Alberta and the *Occupational Health and Safety Act* in Ontario. There are many acts in Canadian health care that might be considered regulatory policies. Figure 14–1 provides a brief description of a few of these regulatory acts.

FIGURE 14–1 **EXAMPLES OF FEDERAL REGULATORY ACTS IN CANADA**

Assisted Human Reproduction Act
- This act is concerned with the health and safety of women involved in and children born as a result of assisted reproduction; it may include or restrict technologies and activities such as in creation of embryos in vitro, surrogate mothering, or sale of fertilized embryos or gametes (ovum or sperm).

Controlled Drugs and Substances Act
- This act is concerned with the production, sale, export, and import of narcotics (e.g., heroin, morphine, methadone) and controlled substances (e.g., ketamines, fentanyls).

Food and Drugs Act
- This act concerns the manufacturing, sale, labelling, and safety of food, natural health products, drugs, and medical devices in Canada.

Quarantine Act
- In the event of an outbreak of an infectious or highly contagious disease, this act allows the Minister of Health to quarantine persons, set up quarantine stations, and designate quarantine officers as required.

Canadian Environment Protection Act
- This act addresses issues pertaining to environmental and human health protection along with sustainability of environmental development.

As with all policies, the purpose of regulatory policy is to make sure that public objectives are met. Many nurses do not realize the impact that regulatory policies have on nursing practice. Following are selected examples of recently debated regulatory policies: policies that would allow women unrestricted access to their choice of obgyn providers, including advanced practice nurses; policies to require health records privacy; and policies to protect workers from accidental needlestick.

The Health Policy Process

Health policies are those that affect health in any way, either directly, as with immunization programs, or indirectly, as with statutes that describe the scope of practice of health care providers. The process of making health policy includes three distinct phases. These phases are both consecutive and circular. The first phase is that of **policy formulation**. This phase includes such actions as agenda setting and the subsequent development of legislation. The second phase is that of **policy implementation**. This phase follows the enactment of legislation, and includes taking actions and making additional decisions necessary to implement legislation, such as rule making and policy operation. The final stage is **policy modification**. The purpose of this stage is to improve or perfect legislation previously enacted. This might entail only minor adjustments made in the implementation phase, or it may involve major changes or the elimination of particular statutes (Longest, 1995).

Policy Formulation

The first phase of policy making is policy formulation. This phase is divided into two distinct, sequentially related, sets of activities: agenda setting and legislation development (Longest, 1995). At any point in time, there is a complex mix of three variables: health-related problems, possible solutions and alternatives, and diverse political interests. As agenda setting progresses, the emerging issues can proceed to the development of legislation.

Problems. The existence of real or perceived health-related problems is the impetus for the policy formulation phase of policy making. Problems may become evident in a number of ways. Some problems occur as the result of the interaction of certain variables related to previous policy. In the late 1980s and early 1990s, long waiting lists for cardiac and orthopedic surgical procedures across Canada resulted in a number of new policy initiatives related to resource allocation, triage of patients, and the management of queues. Other problems may gain attention as they reach unacceptable levels. Growth in the number of HIV-positive persons and the rate of spread of the virus is an example of such a problem. Other problems emerge as a result of some specific event that forces public attention. In 2003, there was a global outbreak of Severe Acute Respiratory Syndrome (SARS). While there were reported and suspected cases across Canada, a total of 44 persons died in the Greater Toronto Area and significant policies were put into place (quarantine, hospital visiting) on an emergent basis during the epidemic and afterwards as precautionary measures in the case of possible future outbreaks. Nevertheless, the mere existence of problems is not always sufficient to ensure the formulation of legislation. There must also be feasible solutions to the problems and the political will to enact legislation.

Solutions. Someone must come up with an idea to solve a problem before legislation can be initiated. The process of offering solutions to problems involves generating ideas for solving the problems, refining the ideas, and selecting from among the options (Longest, 1995). A significant example of generating ideas to solve real and potential problems in health care would be the Commission on the Future of Health Care in Canada (Romanow, 2002).

Political Circumstances. Even if we identify a serious problem and offer feasible solutions, we may not be able to influence legislation. Legislation can progress through the process only with the sponsorship and support of influential policy makers who believe in the issue and invest time and energy. Potential sponsors are sensitive to political will. Factors that influence political will include public attitudes, concerns, and opinions surrounding an issue; the preferences and relative ability of sponsors to influence political decisions; the positions of key political leaders on the issue; and other competing items on the policy agenda. Longest (1995) believes that creating a political thrust forceful enough to cause policy makers to formulate and implement new policy is often the most difficult problem. Nurses are a significant percentage of the voting population. We are in a good position to influence political decisions collectively and enhance the political will essential to formulate health policy.

Policy Implementation

Policy implementation immediately follows the enactment of legislation. Because legislation seldom contains explicit language on how it is to be implemented, details are left to the process of rule making. A formal part of the implementation phase, the dissemination of rules is accomplished by specific implementing organizations. For example, the provincial governments, while involved in passing legislation related to the regulation of nurses, leave the implementation, promulgation, and enforcement of specific legislation related to the licensing and regulation of nurses to the provincial and territorial colleges and Associations of Nursing. Thompson and Fossett (2009) categorize the interaction between some implementing organizations and affected interest groups as highly strategic. Interest groups routinely seek to influence rule making, because they are so often affected by rules established to implement health policies. Lobbying is one of the major means by which interest groups attempt to influence policy makers. Lobbying is especially intense when various interest groups disagree over the formulation of a particular policy.

Policy Modification

As the third phase of the policy-making process, policy modification occurs when the outcomes, perceptions, and consequences of existing policies indicate that either the original problems still exist, or new problems have arisen from unforeseen circumstances or from the policy itself. The policy modification phase is intended to be a kind of feedback loop into the agenda-setting and legislation-development stages of the formulation phase—potentially creating new legislation—and into the rule-making and policy operation stages of the implementation phase, stimulating changes in rules or operations. Many programs are routinely amended, some of them repeatedly, over a period of many years. These modifications may reflect, among other things, the development of new technologies, changing economic conditions, and public demand (Longest, 1995).

Nursing as a Political Force

Knowing all that goes into passing bills and enacting legislation from chapter 7 and earlier in this chapter, you might be asking yourself how these processes are relevant to individual nurses. Certainly, nurses can and should be involved in the passing of both public and private bills by helping to elect members of Parliament through their individual votes, lobbying for bills to be proposed or passed, and acting as expert witnesses during the process of parliamentary debate and discussion of bills as they are moved through the House of Commons and Senate on their way to becoming laws.

Nurses can lobby for bills to be proposed or introduced through Parliament. For example, nurses in Canada were an active part of proposing mandatory bicycle helmet laws for children. In everyday practice, nurses see the individual effects of many kinds of public and social issues (e.g., second-hand smoke, riding all-terrain vehicles [ATVs] without helmets, lack of access to healthy options, lack of clean water) and they often have good ideas about strategies to reduce both morbidity and mortality that can be translated into legislation protecting public interests. Nurses also have strong opinions about professional issues that have legal implications and are usually governed by provincial acts, issues such as scope of practice and entry to practice. As knowledgeable consumers of health care, professionals whose practice is regulated by the government, and morally and ethically sensitive advocates for patients, nurses *should* be highly politically involved. Furthermore, as the largest group of health care professionals in Canada, made up of women and men from diverse backgrounds and experiences and espousing varying values, beliefs, and opinions, nurses are highly representative of the Canadian public as a whole.

There are many kinds of political issues that should be, and are, of interest to nurses. We have identified four categories of political issues in Figure 14-2, including political–ethical issues, political–social issues, professional issues with professional implications, and those involving public health. Nurses' opinions on these issues may be based on both personal and professional experiences, ethical orientation, religious or spiritual beliefs, cultural norms, and other factors that have an impact on how persons develop their own sets of values, norms, and beliefs. Naturally, there is much debate and discussion arising from a healthy diversity of opinions about many of the issues identified in Figure 14-2.

FIGURE 14–2 **SELECTED EXAMPLES OF POLITICAL ISSUES**

Many of the political issues listed below are not exclusively "social" issues or "ethical" issues. In fact, many fall into more than one category. For example, issues around genetic testing certainly have ethical implications, but they are also considered to be social issues, as they have implications for the health of groups of persons. As another example, the mandated use of child seats or motorcycle helmets is a social issue (because it represents a limit on personal freedom) with public health implications.

The following are examples of some political issues in Canadian health care.

Political–ethical issues

- Abortion
- Genetic testing and research
- Reproductive technologies

(Continued)

- Contraception
- Organ procurement and transplantation
- Informed consent
- Age of consent
- Euthanasia and assisted suicide
- Access to care

Political–social issues

- Privacy of health records
- Tobacco legislation
- Accessibility for persons with disabilities
- Health of Aboriginal persons
- Urban and rural health priority setting
- Health care reform initiatives
- Listing and delisting of provincially covered health services

Political issues with professional implications

- Entry to practice
- Scope of practice
- Use of advanced practice nurses and prescriptive authority
- Use of non-regulated health care professionals
- Research funding
- Safety and workplace legislation

Political issues involving public health

- Bicycle helmet laws
- Seatbelt and child safety-seat laws
- Clean air legislation
- Water quality
- Disaster readiness and pandemic flu planning
- Pollution control
- Treatment and reporting of STIs
- Mandatory reporting of child abuse and neglect
- Mandatory gunshot wound reporting
- Mandating and/or availability of flu shots
- Food safety and labelling
- Substance abuse and "clean needle" or harm reduction programs

Ethics in Policy Making

Because policy affects people's lives and relationships and is often part of the distributive justice process, policymaking is an inherently ethical endeavour. The outcomes and consequences of most health policies affect large groups of people. There are two equally important functions of ethics in public policy making. In the *policy formulation* phase, ethics can guide the original development of new policies. Ethics is also useful in the *policy modification* phase, as a means to legitimately criticize policies that have already been implemented (Thompson, 1985). There is, however, some practical difficulty in adhering strictly to specific ethical principles during the policymaking process. Discussing the complexity of policymaking and ethics, Beauchamp and Childress (2009) write:

> Policy formation and criticism involve more complex forms of judgment than ethical theories, principles and rules can handle on their own. Public policy is often formulated in contexts that are marked by profound social disagreements, uncertainties, and differing interpretations of history. No body of abstract moral principles and rules can determine policy in such circumstances, because abstract norms do not contain specific information to provide direct and discerning guidance. The implementation of moral principles and rules must take account factors such as feasibility, efficiency, cultural pluralism, political procedures, pertinent legal requirements, uncertainty about risk, and noncompliance by patients. Principles and rules provide the moral background for policy formation and evaluation, but a policy must also be shaped by empirical data and by information available in fields such as medicine, nursing, public health, economics, law, biotechnology and psychology. When using moral principles or rules to formulate or criticize public policies, we cannot move with assurance from a judgment that an *act* is morally right (or wrong) to a judgment that a corresponding *law* or *policy* is morally right (or wrong). The judgment that an act is morally wrong does not necessarily lead to the judgment that the government should prohibit it or refuse to allocate funds to support it. (p. 9)

Beauchamp and Childress are not suggesting that health policy is so complex as to prohibit the strict and exclusive use of specific rules or principles in guiding policy formulation; rather, the authors suggest that ethical considerations must be accompanied by the rational use of empirical data.

Research and Policy

In order to prevent the formulation and implementation of policies based upon unsubstantiated beliefs or personal values, when we are interested in an issue, we must furnish officials with important and reliable information. If they have reliable facts and research findings, policy makers are able to identify problems, make comparisons, confirm trends, and establish policy based on evidence (Donley, 1996). Because time is a precious commodity, officials are often more interested in empirical research findings than in unsubstantiated personal opinion. Pender (1992) suggests that nurses who plan to discuss policy with officials carefully review research findings that pertain to the issue and be ready to quote a few particularly compelling or attention-getting statistics. Cost savings will often get attention when other facts elicit little response.

The federal government recognizes the importance of health care research in the development of policy. Here are three examples of how research and policy interact in Canada. First, the Policy Research Initiative (PRI) is a neutral research organization within the federal government responsive to emerging issues in Canadian society. The broad aims of this initiative are twofold: To connect those involved in policy research, both within the government and external to it, with those in the policy-setting areas in government, and to advance research on emerging and pressing issues. Furthermore, the PRI helps to ensure that effective knowledge transfer takes place between policy makers and researchers.

Second, the Canadian Policy Research Network (CPRN) is an independent, not-for-profit organization funded by a variety of sources, including federal and provincial governments. This organization conducts research and public consultatory processes to find out what kinds of socioeconomic issues are important to the public, e.g., health care, education, sustainable environments and communities, family supports. The network makes its research and data available to federal, provincial, and local governments to assist in policy-making processes.

Finally, organizations at a provincial level, such as the Institute for Clinical Evaluative Sciences (ICES) in Ontario, function independently to provide scientific research data to assist policy makers in health care delivery. ICES profiles its research work through publications such as atlases and investigative reports, as well as peer-reviewed journals in health care. Organizations at the provincial level, such as ICES, can also be mandated by the government to conduct research in specific areas of interest, or in areas that require more urgent data in order to make effective policy decisions on an urgent or emergent basis (e.g., SARS).

There are many research policy centres in universities across Canada that provide training and conduct research on health policy issues. Some examples are the Centre for Health Services and Policy Research at the University of British Columbia, the Canadian Research Institute for Social Policy at the University of New Brunswick, the Children's Health Policy Centre at Simon Fraser University, and the Health, Law and Policy Group at the Faculty of Law in the University of Toronto.

NURSING, POLICY, AND POLITICS

Not since the days of Lavinia Lloyd Dock have nurses been so actively involved with policy making and politics. It is through the perspective of knowledge, experience, and intimacy with the health care needs of the population that nursing is in a unique position to bring balance to the policy making process (Murphy, 1992). Moreover, professional codes of ethics identify the goals and values of the profession, and explicitly call for nurses to be involved in policy formulation. For example, the ICN *Code of Ethics for Nurses* (2000) calls for nurses to share with society the "responsibility for initiating and supporting action to meet the health and social needs of the public, in particular those of vulnerable populations." The Canadian Nurses Association notes that, "If we think of health as something broadly defined and influenced, we begin to arrive at the inescapable conclusion that to be concerned with health is to be concerned with the social context, and that nursing is, indeed, a political act." (Canadian Nurses Association, 2000).

The formulation of health policy requires strong nursing leadership and an understanding of the nature of local and national policymaking and priority setting. Calling for the political empowerment of nurses, Batra (1992) charges that if we are serious in our efforts to promote health, we must understand the crucial role of public policy. To do this, we must develop the ability to think, teach, research, and act in ways that are relative to policy; we must be aware of the impact that policies have on health and on our clinical practice; we must conduct research on health policy issues; and we must find strategic ways to influence federal and provincial policy agendas. Recognizing health problems as policy issues naturally leads nurses to move into the realm of policy formulation.

Why Should Nurses Be Involved in Politics?

From the bedside to the arenas of health policy, nurses can make a difference. According to many nurse scholars, professional practice involves political action, including influencing others, advocating for and empowering persons and groups, and challenging unfair or oppressive politico-social structures (Des Jardin, 2001; Thomas, Billington & Getliffe, 2004). The benefits of being politically active are clear. Nurses' values are brought to the policymaking table, and through political activism nurses can lobby for redress of the social injustice and health inequities that they encounter in their day-to-day practice. Through not only direct care, but political activism, nurses can make a difference in the lives of others, improving quality of care and having an influence upon determinants of health. Political lobbying and activism can also be on behalf of the profession as well—speaking out for the needs and policies of nurses, as a unique group. In Canada, nursing professional associations (e.g., the Association of Registered Nurses of BC (ARNBC) and the Registered Nurses Association of Ontario (RNAO)) are much more politically active than their respective regulatory bodies, taking clear political stances on important and timely health care and nursing issues. Nurses may align with their professional associations' views or stances, or may find these organizations a good place to engage in debate or learn about how to be more politically active. A clear part of nurses' professional role is being politically active, and becoming involved in some way is an important step to being more influential as a profession.

Nursing's Political Strengths

Nursing enters the political arena with some notable strengths. First, as the most sizable group of health care providers, the nursing profession boasts an extremely large number of political constituents. Acting together, the nation's nurses have the potential to be a formidable political force. Second, nurses have traditionally been perceived in a favourable light. Nurses are viewed as being much less self-interested than any of the other major health-related interest groups (Hadley, 1996). Third, once nurses become involved in health policy, they usually continue to be active (Gebbe, Wakefield & Kerfoot, 2000).

Nursing's Political Weaknesses

The profession, as a political whole, also has a number of weaknesses in the ability of the profession to be politically strong. First, because of being relatively new to the political arena, many nurses are not astute or comfortable in policy making or lobbyist roles. Second, there has historically been a lack of ideological and political unity within the profession, a weakness Hadley (1996) believes stems from the lack of uniform educational requirements and titles. Third, nurses may shy away from being involved in political activism due to a perceived conflict between professional values and political involvement (Des Jardin, 2001). Fourth, though nurses comprise the largest number of professionals, there are fewer dollars in nursing funding specifically earmarked for intense lobbying than are available in many other special-interest groups. Finally, in nursing education, we have typically provided little or no education regarding how to be politically active. While programs now include courses on current trends and issues, even today very little attention is given to teaching nursing students how to engage in political activism. We do equip nursing students with skills and knowledge in advocacy; however, these skills are often related to advocacy for individual patients and not groups or communities. Fortunately, some programs now include more emphasis on political activism, recognizing the evolving roles of nurses in a variety of communities.

Policy Goals for Nursing

How do nurses become aware of the issues that are important and require energy and focus? Each one of us has a responsibility to reflect on problems and potential solutions. In addition, one of the major functions of professional organizations is to provide leadership and assistance to members in political and other matters. In the Canadian Nurses Association's most recent revision of its *Code of Ethics for Registered Nurses* (2008), nursing practice is defined as "direct care (which includes community and public health), education, administration, research and policy development." (p. 1)

THINK ABOUT IT

Nurses Take Positions on Political Issues

The Canadian Nurses Association has been a powerful lobbying force for many years. Issues of interest to members of the organization are freely accessible through the CNA's Web site at http://www.cna.aiic.ca. The site includes a section titled "Nursing and the Political Agenda," with links to public opinion polls on current political health care issues. The CNA has also produced a number of position statements, fact sheets, research summaries, presentations and briefs, and open letters to governments. The CNA has been actively involved in political activism and advocating for policy in a number of areas, including environmentally responsible activity in the health care sector, screening for alcohol and drugs in the workplace, promoting culturally competent care, ensuring patient safety, monitoring entry to practice, and providing care at the end of life. The CNA has also been actively involved in presenting briefs to the government on current issues. These briefs, which can be found on the Web site, address many diverse interests, such as the *Brief to the House of Commons Standing Committee and Human Resources, Social Development and the status of Persons with Disabilities;* and the *Brief to the National Advisory Committee on SARS and Public Health: Lessons Learned and Recommendations.* Through these and other briefs and their presentations, the CNA demonstrates political activism, solidarity, and leadership. These are only a few examples of the kinds of issues the CNA has been involved in over the past decade.

- What are the reasons for the CNA to publish position statements and fact sheets? Who benefits and why?

- Should nurses be concerned with issues such as mandatory gunshot wound reporting or screening for drugs and alcohol in the workplace? Why or why not?

- What are the socio-political issues that you feel are most important in health care today, nationally, in your province or territory, and in your city or community?

- Think of one socio-political issue that is important to you today. How would you begin to think about being politically active and advocating for health policy for this issue?

LOBBYING

Sometimes nurses are legitimate members of governmental or institutional policy-making bodies. More often, the nurse's role in policy formulation, implementation, and modification is that of lobbyist. "**Lobbying** is the art of persuasion—attempting to convince a legislator, a government official, the head of an agency, or a state official to comply with a request—whether it is convincing them to support your position on an issue or to follow a particular course of action" (deVries & Vanderbilt, 1992, p. 1). Though many special-interest groups employ lobbyists, every nurse can be a lobbyist and should lobby on issues of concern. Lobbyists have a powerful voice in determining the policy-making process, from agenda setting to policy modification. In fact, some nurses believe it is a nurse's duty to participate in political **activism**. Hagerdorn defines activism as "a passionate approach to everyday activities that is committed to seeking a more just social order through critical analysis, provocation, transformation, and rebalancing of power" (1995, p. 2). Activism promotes "exposing, provoking, and unbalancing the social power that maintains people in a state of disease, while simultaneously nurturing caring" (1995, p. 2). Others believe that constrained, subtle, and persistent political activity is more effective in the long term than overt activism.

To be effective in the political domain, nurses are charged to become politically astute. According to Jennings, "One can have the best policy proposal on the table but if he or she doesn't know how to play the political game, all will be lost. Nurses must be very adept at discerning who has the power in the policy arena and how to link to that source" (1996, p. 4). Knowing the "power players" and understanding the processes in the political arena is one of the most important steps in the lobbying process.

Methods of Lobbying

The most familiar type of lobbying is the face-to-face approach. This process involves either meeting directly with a policy maker to request a desired action, or testifying at a hearing. When possible, both paid and volunteer lobbyists should utilize the face-to-face method of lobbying. A second form of lobbying is **grassroots lobbying**. Grassroots lobbying involves mobilizing a committed constituency to influence the opinions of policy makers. Different types of grassroots lobbying include organized letter writing, and implementing campaigns designed to mobilize public opinion.

One of the most important facets of lobbying is knowing whom to lobby. In seeking help to promote a particular legislative agenda, nurses want to begin by enlisting policy makers who have the following characteristics: (1) legitimate power, (2) an interest in the problem, (3) an affinity for nursing or for health care issues in general, (4) time and energy to invest in the process, (5) the respect of colleagues, and (6) committee or other positions that are appropriate to the particular legislation. Finding an official with all of these characteristics will greatly improve the probability of legislative success. New lobbyists waste time and energy lobbying officials who are not interested, have conflicting loyalty, are powerless, or are not respected by their colleagues. The first step in lobbying is to connect with the appropriate policy makers.

The Lobbying Campaign

Once nurses have identified the appropriate policy-making officials and are familiar with the issues and the legislative and regulatory process, the lobbying campaign can begin. There are two basic types of lobbying: direct and indirect. Indirect lobbying strategies are geared toward influencing public opinion, which in turn will influence policy makers. Methods of indirect lobbying include media broadcasts; newspapers and other written materials; dissemination of the results of opinion polls; paid advertisements; educational campaigns; and organizations' agendas. Direct methods include party platforms, political elections, influence of committees, agency regulations, face-to-face lobbying, letter writing, and contact with policy makers during social events (deVries & Vanderbilt, 1992).

Preparing for Political Action of Any Kind

There are three steps in preparing to engage in political action of any kind, including lobbying, for a specific cause (Canadian Nurses Association, 2000). These steps involve thoughtful assessment of the situation and context in which policy making occurs related to the specific issue you are concerned about.

- Conduct research and educate yourself in order to speak in a knowledgeable and informed way. You also need to have a good understanding of the processes and levels of government in order to aim your lobbying actions most effectively.

- Enlist interested and informed allies to your lobbying cause. There is strength in numbers, and governments will pay attention to large interest groups and groups that have persons with particular expertise.

- Make sure you have identified the "right" group of decision makers before you begin lobbying. Is this really the group that can help enact the change you want? Is there more than one decision-making group you should be targeting? Should you be involving private industry or corporations as well?

Letter Writing

Handwritten, personal, mass letter writing is a powerful grassroots lobbying technique. Certain letter writing techniques have been found to be more effective; here are some practical tips for letter writing:

- Whenever possible, individualize and legibly handwrite or type letters on personal stationery. Though more effective than no letters at all, form letters are much less likely to be read by officials than individualized letters.

- Write the letter in your own words, using your own thoughts and logic and drawing pertinent inferences.

- Identify yourself as a nurse and state your reason for writing in the first paragraph, including the title and number of the legislation in which you are interested.

- Be specific and include key information and examples supporting your position.

- Be explicit. Tell the official exactly what you want.

- Be brief but informative. Keep your letter to a maximum of one to two pages.
- Include only one topic in each letter.
- Never threaten or use hostility. This immediately destroys your chances of developing a co-operative relationship.
- Offer your assistance as a resource.
- Promptly thank the official for favourable votes.
- Using technology to communicate with large groups of people is highly effective. Legitimate Web sites, blogs, wikis, and discussion boards can get messages out or enlist allies.
- Carefully choosing the places you want to send your message and how it is communicated is key to maintaining credibility.
- It helps to have a strong and dependable media outlet through which to communicate your message. Garnering media attention for your issue can be an essential way of reaching larger groups of people. Of course, newspapers, television, or radio news programs can have specific political agendas and perspectives, so research these and develop trusting and sustainable relationships with media personnel who you feel may be able to present your issue effectively (Canadian Nurses Association, 2000).

Personal Visits

A personal visit is usually a more powerful lobbying tool than letter writing. Whenever possible, nurses should seize the opportunity to meet with policy makers face to face. Following are a few suggestions for personal visits with policy-making officials:

- Be prepared. Develop your plan of action and know what you intend to say.
- Be on time for your appointment, and be patient if the official is late.
- Be courteous, greet the official with a firm handshake, introduce yourself, and present your business card.
- Identify the subject of the meeting and present your facts in an orderly, succinct, and direct fashion.
- Support your position with personal experiences and anecdotes; use valid research and statistics when appropriate.
- Keep your presentation simple. Avoid technical language and professional jargon. Your goal is to inform and influence, not to impress.
- Close the meeting strongly and effectively, asking for the official's support.
- Leave a short fact sheet summarizing the issue and your position. Include the names and telephone numbers of contact people.
- Send a letter within a few days thanking the official for the meeting, restating your position, and including any information requested during the meeting.

THINK ABOUT IT

Be Careful of Your Wording

Nurses must choose their words carefully when lobbying. One nurse relates a story of her first experience testifying before a government committee. Feeling her presentation was well prepared and would be effective, the nurse decided at the last minute to substitute the words *nurse voters* for the word *nurses*. There were many people giving testimony that day. Following the completion of the testimony phase, the legislators were given an opportunity to make comments or ask questions. There were no questions. Every comment was directed toward the nurse, who was surprised to learn that the legislators perceived the term *nurse voters* to indicate a veiled threat. They did not hear the substance of the presentation, but rather the perceived threat, "If you do not support our position, we will vote you out of office." By unintentionally giving this impression, the nurse may have damaged a productive relationship with these legislators. The legislation that the nurses were supporting failed.

- Why do you think the nurse changed the wording of her presentation in the first place?
- What words would you have used?
- Describe similar circumstances when you were speaking and the reaction of the listeners was based upon their inferences from your choice of words rather than their intended meaning.
- How can nurses avoid mistakes of this sort?

Political Campaigns

One very effective direct lobbying technique is for nurses to become involved in either supporting candidates or running for elective office themselves. According to Wakefield (1990), nurses are encouraged to get involved in lobbying for specific legislation, not realizing that the ability to influence decisions occurs long before the issues are revealed to the public. Wakefield suggests that nurses become involved in campaigns and elections. This can be done in any number of ways. First, nurses should become involved in political-party organizations. Political-party activity serves as a vehicle for developing important relationships with elected officials, and involvement in a political party is essential to building a political network. Second, nurses can become involved through provincial nurses' associations. These organizations provide an opportunity to meet candidates, form relationships, and offer candidates forums. Forums remind a candidate that nurses are an organized group interested in politics and public policy and acquaint nurses with the candidate's positions on important issues. Third, nurses can become actively involved in campaigning for candidates who support their positions on various health care issues. This may take the form of campaigning door to door, stuffing envelopes, or publicly endorsing candidates. Actively supporting candidates for public office helps to forge relationships with officials and elect candidates to public office who will sympathize with issues important to nurses. Involvement with political parties and the consequent relationships with public officials can also lead to either nurses' candidacy and election to public office, or nurses' appointments to important policy-making positions.

SUMMARY

Many political issues are important to nurses. Most issues that nurses are actively concerned about are related to health policy: issues of a moral nature; issues related to professional regulation; issues related to public health; and issues related to distributive justice. Fulfilling the role of advocate, nurses are challenged to become politically active: to know about and become involved with important issues; to learn the political process; to form relationships with public officials; and to become astute in methods of influencing health policy.

CHAPTER HIGHLIGHTS

- The term *political* relates to the policy-making process within the government.
- Political issues are those that are created, affected, or regulated by any of the government branches.
- Political parties are organized groups with distinct ideologies that seek to form the government.
- Health policies influence the actions, decisions, and behaviours of people in the domain of health.
- Society's definition of health reflects how far society is willing to go toward maximizing the health of citizens.
- Allocative health policies are designed to provide benefits to a distinct group.
- Regulatory policies are designed to influence others through directive techniques.
- The health policy process includes the phases of policy formulation, policy implementation, and policy modification.
- There are two important functions of ethics in public policy making—guiding the original development of policies and criticizing previously implemented policies.
- Nurses are able to affect health policies through various political means.

DISCUSSION QUESTIONS AND ACTIVITIES

1. Explore the CNA's Web site at http://www.cna-aiic.ca. Review some of the presentations and briefs. How do some of these issue relate to current issues in nursing ethics?

2. Discuss the issues listed in Figure 14–2 in class. How do your classmates' positions compare to those of the major political parties? Are each student's opinions politically consistent from one issue to another?

3. Discuss the following question in class: What purpose do political parties serve?

4. Compile a list of political issues and classify them as to which branch of government the issue is most closely aligned with—administrative, judicial, or legislative.

5. Discuss methods for influencing health policy in the administrative and judicial domains.

6. Compile a list of at least five political issues related to health that have been decided within the judicial domain. How have the judicial decisions affected health care delivery?

7. Compile a list of political issues related to moral values. Discuss the role of the professional organization in guiding members' actions related to these moral issues.

8. Discuss popular definitions of health and determine how each definition, if adopted by government, would affect health care delivery.

9. Discuss the role of ethics in policy making.

REFERENCES

Batra, C. (1992). Empowering for professional, political, and health policy involvement. *Nursing Outlook, 40*(4), 170–176.

Beauchamp, T. L., & J. F. Childress (2009). *Principles of biomedical ethics* (6th ed.). New York: Oxford University Press.

Canadian Nurses Association. (2000). Nursing as a political act. *Nursing Now.* May 2000. Ottawa: Canadian Nurses Association.

Canadian Nurses Association. (2008). *Code of ethics for Registered Nurses.* Ottawa: Canadian Nurses Association.

Des Jardin, K. (2001). Political Involvement in Nursing — Politics, Ethics, and Strategic Action. *AORN Journal 74*(5), 614–622.

deVries, C. M., & M. W. Vanderbilt (1992). *The grassroots lobbying handbook: Empowering nurses through legislative and political action.* Washington, DC: American Nurses Association.

Donley, R. (1996). Shaping health policy. *Nursing Policy Forum, 2*(1), 12–19.

Gebbe, K. M., M. Wakefield & K. Kerfoot (2000). Nursing and health policy. *Journal of Nursing Scholarship, 32*(3), 307–315.

Hadley, E. (1996). Nursing in the political and economic marketplace: Challenges for the 21st century. Nursing Outlook, *44*(1), 6–10.

Hagerdorn, S. (1995). The politics of caring: The role of activism in primary care. *Advances in Nursing Science, 17*(4), 1–11.

International Council of Nurses. (2000). *The ICN code of ethics for nurses*. Geneva, Switzerland: International Council of Nurses.

Jennings, C. (1996). Politics and nursing do mix! *Nursing Policy Forum, 2*(3), 4.

Longest, B. B., Jr. (1995). *Health policymaking in the United States*. Ann Arbor, MI: AUPHA Press/ Health Administration Press.

Murphy, N. (1992). Nursing leadership in health policy decision making. *Nursing Outlook, 10*(4), 158–161.

Pender, N. (1992). Making a difference in health policy. *Nursing Outlook, 40*(3), 104–105.

Romanow, R. (Commissioner). (2002). *Building on values: The future of health care in Canada*. Ottawa: The Romanow Commission.

Thomas, S., A. Billington & K. Getliffe (2004). Improving continence services — a case study in policy influence. *Journal of Nursing Management,* 12, 252–257.

Thompson, D. (1985). Philosophy and policy. *Philosophy and Public Affairs, 14*(2), 205–218.

Thompson, F. J., & J. Fossett (2009). The enduring challenge of health policy implementation. In J. A. Morone, T. J. Litman & L. S. Robins, eds., *Health politics and policy* (4th ed.). Albany, NY: Delmar.

Wakefield, M. (1990). Political involvement: A nursing necessity. *Nursing Economics, 8*(5), 352–353.

WEBSITES

Institute for Clinical Evaluative Studies (ICES)

   http://www.ices.on.ca

Canadian Policy Research Networks (CPRN)

   http://www.cprn.ca

Policy Research Initiative (PRI)

   http://www.policyresearch.gc.ca

Centre for Health Services and Policy Research at the University of British Columbia

   http://www.chspr.ubc.ca

Canadian Research Institute for Social Policy at the University of New Brunswick

   http://www.unb.ca/crisp/index.php

The Children's Health Policy Centre at Simon Fraser University

   http://www.childhealthpolicy.sfu.ca

Health Law and Policy Group at the University of Toronto Faculty of Law

   http://www.law.utoronto.ca/healthlaw

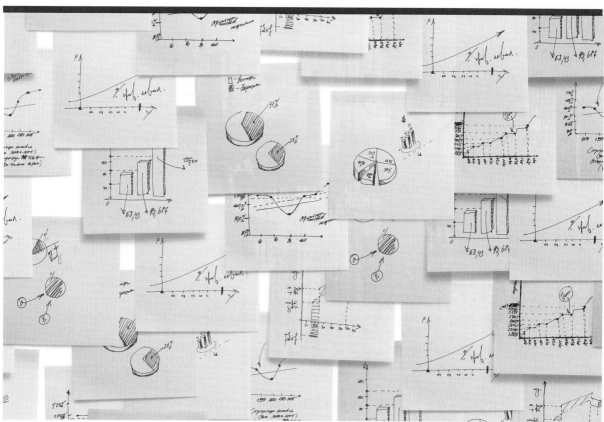

iStockphoto/Thinkstock.com

CHAPTER **15**
ECONOMIC ISSUES

OBJECTIVES

After completing this chapter, the reader should be able to:

1. Describe the role of economics in health care.
2. Explain the concept of distributive justice.
3. Discuss utilitarian, libertarian, communitarian, and egalitarian theories.
4. Discuss basic questions related to the distribution of health care resources.
5. Describe recent trends in health care economics and the relationship of economic trends to the delivery of health care.
6. Discuss ideas around Canadian health care reform.

INTRODUCTION

Nursing, other health care professions, and the overall health care delivery system exist to deliver health care to society. Over the past several decades, dynamic forces have worked together to create a complex system that has been called one of the best in the world. From advances in knowledge and technology to changes in health care financing, the system has experienced rapid and drastic changes. It is not unusual, today, to hear the term "crisis" used to describe the state of the current health care system. The crisis in health care refers to grave concerns over our ability to sustain a system that is incredibly costly, while assuring high quality and access to health services. With rising costs, changing demographics, and evolving needs, the system requires significant reform. The health care system in Canada is one with an ever-increasing demand for a finite amount of services; alongside cuts from the federal government to support health care, the system is strained at best, ailing at worst. The extremely high costs of new technologies and the push to use them in managing illness and disease is driving the cost of health care up significantly. The high cost of technology-heavy acute care means that resources for areas like public health, population health, and health promotion—all areas integral to the prevention of illness and disease—are few. Thoughtful, systematic, ethical priority setting at all levels of care—the bedside, institutions, and agencies, as well as governments—is needed to try to devise solutions to the current problems in health care.

OVERVIEW OF TODAY'S HEALTH CARE ECONOMICS

The history of economic thought is closely associated with the utilitarian movement in the last century (Honderich, 1995). One of the main assumptions in traditional economics is that we should judge the institutions of a society by the preferences of the people that those institutions affect. There are different ways to judge the overall preferences of society. One method claims that one arrangement is better than another only if it satisfies the preferences of some people and does not frustrate the preferences of any others. This idea is at the centre of what is known as welfare economics. Another method suggests that institutions are properly judged only according to the preferences of the people they affect; therefore, the institution of health care should be judged by the people it serves. Discussion and debate about the current state of health care economics is integral to the process of evaluating the present system and formulating one that is more just.

Today's problems in the health care system have a long history, with many intervening factors. We have produced a system with progressively higher standards that require the most and the best care for most of the population, regardless of cost. This spiralling pattern is combined with a lack of accountability caused by a third-party reimbursement system that (in the past, at least) did not require providers or patients to be careful of cost. This has led to a skewed model that focuses heavily on technology and personal autonomy, while ignoring basic principles of social responsibility and distributive justice. This system features an odd split between those who help make the spending decisions (patients, physicians, and allied health care professionals) and those who must actually pay for the costs of those decisions (provincial governments and private insurance companies). (Morreim, 1995; Starfield, 2010). Moreover, there are staggering contrasts within this system. In some instances, hundreds of thousands of dollars are spent on what is recognized by many as futile care yet many others wait for urgent care in long queues. Patients often complain about long waits in emergency rooms, for consultations with specialists, or for imaging (CT, MRI), and for urgent surgeries such as hip or knee replacements. This is felt to be at odds with a system that, in some cases, will allow extensive diagnostic testing or intensive care for patients at the end of life with no hope of active recovery or remission. While these are very different situations, for many, they represent a lack of fairness and consistency and instead reflect inconsistent values and decision-making processes across different contexts in health care.

Within the traditional fee-for-service system, medicine is predominantly driven by codes of ethical behaviour and patients' rights statements, with a strong focus on the principle of autonomy. This model focuses on the individual patient, protects physician autonomy, promotes treatment that offers potential benefit or prolonged life, and appears to assume unlimited resources. Clearly, there are ethical problems associated with this model, including overutilization, priority setting based only on a narrow set of values and rationing on the basis of financial means primarily (Biblo, Christopher, Johnson & Potter, 1996).

ASK YOURSELF

Paying for Futile Care

One often hears stories about elderly patients with terminal illness, and even "do not resuscitate" status, who remain in intensive care settings for extended periods of time, often because of family members who insist that everything be done for their loved one.

- Is the expenditure of expensive health care resources appropriate for these types of situations? Explain your position.
- Who should bear the financial burden for futile care?
- What are the ethical principles that conflict in situations of this sort?

In many other countries, health care is also a priority from an economic perspective. Around the world, costs are increasing with the use of more advanced technology.

Three basic types of health care systems exist. First there is the national health systems model, in which health care priorities are set and services are organized and delivered by a national system, either in a centralized way, as in Cuba and Russia, or in a decentralized, more local way, as in Sweden and Finland. In the second model, the public insurance model, such as Canada has, health care services are publicly financed but delivered by others; in this case, provincial and territorial governments and institutions. In the third model, the entrepreneurial model, patients must be able to pay for health services, which are provided by private providers in a relatively free or open market. The United States is a prime example of such a model of health care.

The health care systems model in the United States is a source of constant debate. In an essay on reforming American health care, DeBlois, Norris, and O'Rourke (1994) discuss the problems with the U.S. health care financing system. While some of the problems are unique to the American system, others are shared by all types of health care systems. Though most people agree that modern health care in the United States is highly sophisticated and technologically advanced, they also recognize that there are many deficiencies in the system. One key problem is the lack of primary care in the U.S. Strong primary care infrastructure has been demonstrated to contribute to better health of populations, and improved health for those who are more vulnerable or marginalized (Starfield, 2008; 2010; Starfield & Shi, 2002). First, nearly 20 percent of the U.S. population has no access to health care services and resources. Second, health care costs are accelerating at an unsustainable annual rate, consuming a huge portion of the gross domestic product. Third, the high cost of health care threatens the competitiveness and profitability of business and industry. Fourth, the benefits to the individual and corporate providers within the system are often pursued at the expense (and sometimes harm) of persons who are in need of health care. DeBlois *et al.* (1994) propose that the real problems with the American system continue to be related to its priorities, and the values and commitments that support them, the most significant of which are:

1. an extreme form of individualism that routinely and consistently places individual interests above concerns about the community of persons;

2. an endorsement of profit-making as a primary motive for providing health care services; and

3. an uncritical acceptance of technology as morally neutral and as unambiguous in the service of human goods and goals. (1994, p. 55)*

DeBlois *et al.* (1994) also charge that the health and well-being of people subjected to a system under the influence of these values are often threatened by the kinds of services offered, the manner in which they are provided, and the priorities that determine both. Further, if improvements in the system are intended to promote the health and well-being of people, those efforts need to be ethically grounded and to challenge the values that drive this type of system.

Challenging the status quo and the overarching values is an important part of examining a health care system, critically and ethically. While the U.S. system values individualism, the Canadian system espouses a more communitarian-based value system, in which the health of individuals, groups, and communities are valued above individual freedom and liberty. In the U.S. system, despite the emphasis on liberty and freedom of individual choice, many people are left without any freedom of choice and without the funds to afford basic health care. Still others, who can afford

---

* "*A primer for health care ethics: Essays for a pluralist society,*" de Blois, J., Norris, P., & O'Rourke K., © 1994 Georgetown University Press.

a minimum of care, find that they are plunged into debt or financial collapse when faced with a catastrophic illness. These are not choices, but severe consequences of such a system.

DISTRIBUTIVE JUSTICE

The ethics of **justice** relates to fair, equitable, and appropriate treatment in light of what is due or owed to persons (Beauchamp & Childress, 2008). As mentioned in Chapter 3, the relevant application of the ethical principle of justice within the health care system focuses on the fair distribution of goods and services. This application is called **distributive justice**. Beauchamp and Childress (2008) define distributive justice as the fair, equitable, and appropriate distribution of diverse benefits and burdens such as property, resources, taxation, privileges, and opportunities. Because there is always a scarcity of resources and competition for resources and services, it is impossible for all people to have everything they might want or need. It is important to remember that, in Canada, while health care is of paramount importance, other social programs such as welfare, education, and the public retirement income system are also important to maintaining the health and security of persons. Each time we claim that more funds must be provided for health care, we need to reflect upon the fact that this will necessarily mean funds will be taken away from another type of social program. With the way that health care funds are provided by the federal government to the provinces and territories, each individual province or territory is responsible for deciding how resources should be divided between various social programs. Is education more important than health care? We know, for example, that literacy and education are determinants of health, and neglecting them will have negative effects on the health and well-being of citizens. We also know that if we neglect to provide adequate health care and disease prevention, children may be prevented from being able to go to school. Thus it is difficult to say that one kind of social program should have higher priority than another without the result being devastating effects on groups of persons and individuals.

One of the primary purposes of government is to formulate and enforce policies that deal with the distribution of scarce resources. To put it simply, distributive justice deals with how the "pie" of health care will be divided among many hungry persons. One can choose to divide the pie equally in similar-sized pieces or to give more to those who are younger, sicker, or more vulnerable. There is no easy solution, nor is there a solution that will please everyone. Many people have divergent opinions on what constitutes "fair" distribution of a scarce resource like health care. Some say that funds should be focused on acute care, while others propose that disease prevention should get more resources. Many argue that we should spend more money on children's care and cancer, while others say that more resources should be diverted to care of the elderly and frail persons. If we return to our analogy of a pie being divided up between a number of hungry people, we can easily see how we might find markedly different approaches to dividing up the pie, depending on who is responsible for making the decisions. Some may feel that those who are most hungry should have the most, while others might feel that the children, by virtue of being at a stage of high growth and development, need the largest pieces of the pie. Others may choose to give everyone an equal piece simply to avoid making judgments about what attribute (hunger, age, health) is most important when rationing out the pie, or, for that matter, health care resources. Daniels (1994, p. 27) states

> Rationing decisions, both at the micro and macro levels, share three key features. First, the goods we often must provide — legal services, health care, educational benefits — are not sufficiently divisible (unlike money) to avoid unequal or "lumpy" distributions. Meeting the educational, health care, or legal needs of some people, for example, will mean that the requirements of others will go unsatisfied. Second, when we ration, we deny benefits to some individuals who can plausibly claim they are owed them in principle; losers as well as winners have plausible claims to have their needs met. Third, the general distributive principles appealed to by claimants as well as by rationers do not by themselves provide adequate reasons for choosing among claimants. They are too schematic; like my "fair equality of opportunity" account of just health care, they fail to yield specific solutions to these rationing problems. Solving these problems thus bridges the gap between principles of distributive justice and problems of institutional design.*

Many areas of health care are affected by the issue of distributive justice: Which population groups should be the recipients of health care resources? What percentage of society's resources is it reasonable to spend on health care? Recognizing that health care resources are limited, which aspects of health care should receive the most resources? These are important questions, and they are both practical and ethical in nature.

Many people may think that in Canada everyone gets an "equal" share, so why should we be concerned with how resources are allocated? However, history has demonstrated that, even in a system based on universality and reasonable access—two key guiding principles of the *Canada Health Act* (1984)—there are still some who get more or less benefit from the health care system. People living in remote areas in the north, or rural areas, even in densely populated provinces such as Ontario or Quebec, have difficult accessing specialists and even family doctors for routine care. Those living in small provinces such as Prince Edward Island have no access to a number of important specialties and are forced to travel long distances to access care that someone living in downtown Edmonton or Vancouver could access quite easily. Keep in mind, as well, that the *Canada Health Act* and the universal health care system covers only hospital and physician care. Allied health services, such as psychological services, occupational or physical therapy, vision care, prescriptions, and dental care are not covered by the *Canada Health Act* and are considered out-of-pocket expenses, unless you are fortunate enough to be covered for these kinds of health expenditures through your employer (or your spouse's or parents' employer).

---

* "Four Unsolved Rationing Problems A Challenge" by Norman Daniels. © 1994 *The Hastings Center Report* Vol 24 No 4 pp 27–29.

Many people have jobs that do not provide benefits and may therefore have difficulty paying for dental care, glasses, psychological treatment, or physiotherapy if they require it. Many people need these types of allied services; however, the requirement to pay for them means that often those who need them will not get them. Furthermore, some provinces still require a type of out-of-pocket payment, called a premium, on a monthly basis to subsidize health care. Alberta is one province that, up until 2009, still required citizens to pay monthly premiums. In some areas in Canada, there are many people who do not have legal status, that is, they have come to Canada and have not been able to achieve legal status. In some urban areas, there are large numbers of people without legal status, and although they are living here in Canada, and many times have complex health needs related to difficult situations from which they have fled, they cannot access health care, as our system is set up for Canadian citizens, and not visitors or foreigners, to access without cost.

So, even in what many consider to be a "fair" and "equitable" system, there are still inequities and problems with how health care is distributed; we must examine these inequities and problems through an ethical lens.

Entitlement

In deciding questions of distributive justice, we must ask, "Who is entitled to these services?" As with all of ethics, there is no universally accepted answer. Distribution of limited resources is the function of various levels of governing bodies. In attempting to distribute limited resources fairly, leaders will seek systematic means of deciding. Historically, these questions have been answered by such **material rules** as: to each person an equal share, to each person according to need, to each person according to merit, to each person according to social contribution, to each according to the person's rights, to each person according to effort, to each person according to ability to pay, or to each person according to the greatest good to the greatest number. Most societies will utilize several of these principles in establishing public policies.

ASK YOURSELF

Is Health Care a Right or a Privilege?

- Picking up on our discussions from Chapter 13, remember whether you decided that health care is a right or a privilege. Reflect for a moment on the reasons that underpin your decision.

- Should all people have access to the same health care services? Should ability to pay ever influence access to health care services?

- If you believe health care is a right, how much health care is each person entitled to?

(Continued)

- What about the fact that many people are born into situations of destitution, war, and poverty and cannot afford or access quality health care? As citizens of a country with highly developed health care, what do we owe others?

- In Canada, some health care services are not universally covered, such as dental care and reproductive technologies like in vitro fertilization. Do you think that either of these two services should be covered by the health care system? If so, why? Did you feel that one should be covered and not the other? Again, ask yourself why.

- Cosmetic surgery procedures are, for the most part, not covered by our public health care system. However, some procedures that are cosmetic in nature, but done for reasons of repair after a trauma or accident, are covered by public insurance. Do you agree with this? Why or why not?

Right to Health Care

In examining who should receive care, we ask questions about the basic right to health care. Is health care a right or a privilege? This is a question that is debated fiercely in the media, in the professional and political arenas, and around the dinner table. Is society responsible for providing health care for all citizens, and, if so, to what degree? Should each person be eligible for minimum basic health care, or should everyone be allowed to have everything there is to offer, from organ transplants to tummy tucks to in vitro fertilization, if they wish? Which is preferable—a strict free-market system that would provide health care services only to those who can pay, or a system responsible for the health care needs of all citizens? If health care is a right and health care resources are scarce, what resources should be allocated to which group of people? These and other questions fuel the debate about the right to health care, even in Canada.

Discussion of health care as a right is not new. On December 10, 1948, the General Assembly of the United Nations adopted the Universal Declaration of Human Rights, which identifies medical care as a necessary social service, ensuring the right to a standard of living adequate for health and well-being (Giesen, 1994).

The issue of health care as a right has some basis in constitutional law. In Canada, our most important constitutional document is the *Charter of Rights and Freedoms*. While many Canadians consider health care to be a right, there is nothing in the *Charter* that describes such a right (Kirby, 2002). As Kirby explains, the *Canada Health Act* notes that the goal of an intact and strong Canadian health care policy is "to protect, promote and restore the physical and mental well-being of residents of Canada and to facilitate reasonable access to health services without financial or other barriers" (Kirby, 2002, p. 100). While this language notes the importance of health care, and access to care without the ability to pay being a factor, it does not confer a right to health care. Yet, as Canadians, we use that language frequently to describe our feelings about health care and health policy. There is no legal document actually describing a right to health care in Canada. Although policies and government agencies exist to provide health care and ensure access to some health services, this does not mean that health care is a right, backed up by the legal or constitutional systems. However, Kirby also notes that some people who have been denied access to particular services or who have been forced to seek services in other jurisdictions as a result of local cuts or services not locally provided, have turned to the *Charter of Rights and Freedoms* to try to stake their claim to a right to health care.

THINK ABOUT IT

A Constitutional Right to Health Care?

One commonly cited case in Canada is *Auton (Guardian ad litem of) v. British Columbia (Attorney General).* In this case, Connor Auton, a preschooler diagnosed with autism spectrum disorder, was denied access to intensive behavioural intervention therapy (IBI) in his home province of British Columbia. Connor's parents, believing that they had a constitutional right to health care for Connor, which they felt should include IBI therapy, cited section 15(1) of the *Charter of Rights and Freedoms,* citing that failure to provide this therapy to their son violated this section of the *Charter,* which states that individuals should have equal treatment without being discriminated against for reasons of race, birthplace, skin colour, religion, gender, age, or disability. As a person with a diagnosed disability, for which there was documented treatment, along with documentation demonstrating the importance of early preschool intervention, Connor, his parents claimed, was being discriminated against by not being able to access appropriate care that should have been made available to him. While the provincial courts concluded that Connor did have a right to IBI therapy and that it should be provided, the Supreme Court of Canada overturned the decisions of the lower courts to conclude that there is no constitutional right to receive therapy for children such as Connor.

- When you read cases like this one, do you think that Canadians have a "right" to health care? If so, what does that mean to you?

- How far would you go to fight for access to health care services?

- Do you think that the lower or higher courts were right in this case? Why?

In the United States, the President's Commission for the study of Ethical Problems in Medicine and Biomedical and Behavioral Research reported that neither the Supreme Court nor any appellate court had found a constitutional right to health care (President's Commission for the Study of Ethical Problems in Biomedical and Behavioral Research, 1983) . Despite the statement by the Commission, federal and state statutes have been interpreted to provide statutory rights in the form of entitlements to some vulnerable groups. As a consequence, some vulnerable groups have benefited from many legal decisions. In the U.S., vulnerable groups have typically included any uninsured individuals, especially those who are older adults, children or persons, and those who are very poor (Jones & Sheppard, 2012). Bandman and Bandman (1978) argue that the common welfare clause of the U.S. Constitution implies the protection of basic needs, including a right to the protection of health.

Health care as a right is not a universal belief. There are those who believe that health care is a privilege to be enjoyed by some, but beyond the common advantage of all citizens. The entrepreneurial model of libertarianism declares that health care is not a right, but a commodity that must be purchased on the open market like any other service. This model equates the health care professional's right to conduct a practice and charge fees with the right of other businesses to do so. It can be argued that this model provides health care only for those who can pay, or for those who are given health care services as a gift. It is hypothesized that, as a result of a free market system of health care delivery, supply-and-demand and pricing competition would result in lower health care costs. This in turn would result in health care services becoming more accessible to a larger portion of the population. Except for the fact that professionals can choose to provide services free of charge, this model makes little allowance for children and the very poor (Bandman & Bandman, 1978; Beauchamp & Childress, 2008).

The working poor (i.e., those who have full-time jobs but may just barely be able to afford the necessities of living, remain in debt, and cannot see relief) make up a significant percentage of the population. For individuals and families in that situation, having to pay for health care is devastating and unrealistic. In Canada today, families like this have access to physician, hospital, and allied health care services, but may not be able to afford dental care, prescription drugs or eye glasses. So there are inequities in all systems, even ones that "seem" to be more fair.

How Much and to Whom?

If one accepts that health care is a right or that society has an ethical obligation to provide health care services to vulnerable populations, then one is required to examine the question of *how much* health care is to be provided, and *to whom*. There are two broad views about the right to access to health care: some believe all should have equal access to health care, while others believe the right extends only to a decent minimum of health care with an understanding that priority setting may mean queues or marked differences in access to care. Consider the following case.

 CASE PRESENTATION

Lucy is a twenty-three-year-old woman with a history of depression who has been hospitalized with episodes of severe depression, suicide attempts, and incidents of "cutting" herself. She had to drop out of university and spent a great deal of time in an inpatient unit getting treatment for her depressive episodes. She is now on antidepressants, feeling well, and able to live independently in the community. She would like to return to school to become a physiotherapist, but is concerned about a number of significant scars on her arm from cutting herself. She is worried about the stigma of having them seen by her fellow students or friends and feels that she may not be able to cope with this. When she sees a plastic surgeon about surgery to repair and cover the scars, she says, "I think I can finally move forward in my life, if only we can make these scars less visible."

Tenille is a thirty-five-year-old woman, who, along with her partner, Carlos, has been trying to conceive a child for a number of years. Tenille has had a barrage of tests that demonstrate she is capable of conceiving and Carlos also has had tests to confirm his fertility. Tenille and Carlos both work at a factory, in the shipping office. While they make a good living, they cannot afford the costs of monthly in vitro fertilization, which, their doctor has told them, is their only chance to have a child.

George is 78 years old and a retired mechanic. He and his wife, Jacqui, have saved for many years in order to be able to retire somewhere warm and sunny. They spend ten months of the year in Florida, in Fort Lauderdale, where they purchased a small condominium. They return home to Canada for one month at Christmas, to see their children and grandchildren, and one month in the summer, when it is too hot in Florida for Jacqui, who has asthma. They still maintain a small apartment in Winnipeg, but only spend two months a year there. While they are in Florida, George sustains a heart attack. The cardiologist tells him that he has serious triple vessel disease and requires bypass surgery. George insists that the doctor make arrangements to fly him home to Winnipeg, where he can have his surgery and "be at home."

- Should all of these treatments and interventions be provided without charge to the individuals? Why or why not?

- Are these "medically necessary" treatments? If so, what makes a treatment "necessary," in your opinion?

- If you were a decision-maker, what would be your reasons for not covering any of the three treatments described above? How would you justify your decision?

Fair Distribution

Few people would argue that there are enough resources to pay for all services. Think about your household budget. If you have only $300 to spend on Christmas gifts for your three sisters and you also need to purchase groceries for the week and antibiotics for yourself, it would be foolish to spend $150 on one gift. By doing that, you would ensure that your sisters would not be treated equitably, that you probably would not be eating very well for the next week, and that you would not feel well anyway, since you could not afford your prescription medication. The same principle applies to health care dollars. The limited public budget must be divided among many competing interests. In order to maintain a functioning infrastructure, the government must ensure that public schools, highways, police, education, social assistance, and other services in the public domain have a proportionate share of the total budget. Policy makers are charged with the difficult task of making equitable decisions about distribution of resources. These decisions must balance health care spending with other programs, and must carefully avoid both extravagant excess spending and frugality that would threaten the health of citizens.

Distribution of Resources

Limited health care dollars must be spent wisely. There are several different criteria that have been proposed to make distributive justice decisions. One method involves making judgments about cost in relation to predicted benefit. For example, we could question the practice of allowing patients in the last stages of terminal illness to monopolize limited and expensive intensive care beds, thus utilizing the most expensive kind of health care for the least benefit. Some propose that the best way to avoid making arbitrary decisions in these kinds of situations is to set mandatory guidelines. For example, some suggest that expensive therapies, such as dialysis or organ transplant, be reserved only for those below a certain age. A second method involves making judgments about the usefulness of given therapies. Immunizations, for example, are cost effective and benefit a large percentage of the population. Some would suggest that the most utile therapies (the ones that are less costly and nearly guaranteed to help a large number of people) are the ones that should have priority.

Theories of Justice

Distributive justice is based upon common morals and ethics. Several theories have been proposed to determine how resources and services should be distributed. Utilitarian, libertarian, communitarian, and egalitarian theories are examples of popular theories of justice. Because of society's fragmented beliefs about social justice, no single theory can be expected to bring coherence to the situation.

Recognizing that no single theory will satisfy society by fulfilling all principles, we suggest that several theories of justice be used to understand competing social goals.

Egalitarian Theories

Egalitarian theories are related to the concept of equality, in which people who are similarly situated should be treated similarly, though much depends on what kinds of similarity count as relevant and what constitutes similar treatment (Honderich, 1995). Promoting ideals of equal distribution of social benefits and burdens, egalitarian theories recognize the social obligation to eliminate or reduce barriers that prevent fair equality of opportunity. These theories are cautiously formulated to avoid requiring equal sharing of all possible social benefits. A leading proponent of egalitarianism,

John Rawls, suggests that in making decisions of justice, one should examine the situation behind a veil of ignorance. In this hypothetical situation, "no one knows his place in society, his class position or social status, nor does anyone know his fortune in the distribution of natural assets and abilities, his intelligence, strength, and the like" (1996, p. 567). This veil of ignorance ensures that no one is able to design principles to favour his or her own particular condition. Supporters of Rawls's theory recognize a positive social obligation to eliminate or reduce barriers that prevent fair equality of opportunity, and suggest that health policy formulated according to egalitarian principles would guarantee a safety net or minimum floor that citizens would not be allowed to fall below (Beauchamp & Childress, 2008).

Utilitarian Theories

Based, in general, upon the rule that it is good to maximize the "greatest good for the greatest number," **utilitarian theories** favour social programs that protect public health and distribute basic health care equally to all citizens. This is based on the belief that the outcome of these programs maximizes utility. Although these theories are the basis of many social programs, there are problems in their application. For example, because utilitarianism places aggregate social good before individual rights, a utilitarian model may support maximizing utility while limiting resources directed toward some of society's sickest and most vulnerable populations (Beauchamp & Childress, 2008).

Libertarian Theories

Libertarian theories propose that the just society protects the rights of property and liberty of each person, allowing citizens to improve their circumstances by their own effort. Libertarian theories support a private citizen's or group's right to own and manage a health care business. Libertarian theory does not classify health care as a right, but rather as a commodity that operates on the material principle of ability to pay either directly or indirectly through insurance. Strict libertarians view taxation as an unjust redistribution of private property, but do not oppose other methods of distribution if they are freely chosen (Beauchamp & Childress, 2008).

Communitarian Theories

Communitarian theories place the community, rather than the individual, the state, the nation, or any other entity, at the centre of the value system. Less fully developed than utilitarianism or libertarianism, communitarianism emphasizes the value of the public good and maintains that values are rooted in communal practices. Communitarians believe that human life will go better if collective and public values guide peoples' lives. They have a commitment to facilities and practices designed to help members of the community develop their common goals and interests and hence their personal lives (Honderich, 1995). Modern communitarian writers disagree about how to apply these theories to health care access. Some propose a federation of interlinking community health programs that are democratically administered by citizen-members. In this model, each individual program would determine which benefits to provide, which care is most important, and whether expensive services will be included or excluded. Another communitarian theory holds that community tradition includes commitments of equal access to health care, and suggests that as long as communal funds are spent, services must be equally available (Beauchamp & Childress, 2008).

ASK YOURSELF

Making Fair Decisions

- Which theory of distribution appeals to you as the most fair and equitable? Why?
- Do you think the theory you chose would be fair to all people in all circumstances? Discuss your thinking.
- Could you combine two or more theories to make a system that is fair and equitable?

RECENT TRENDS AND HEALTH ECONOMIC ISSUES

Questions of ethics and distributive justice began to be discussed well before the mid-1990s. Claims that Canada was experiencing a crisis in health care economics have escalated over the last two decades, with increasing demands for covered services and long waiting lists for procedures such as hip and knee replacements and cardiac surgery. Skyrocketing expenditures and a general tightening of health care dollars resulted in fiscal scarcity. The federal government has responded by attempting to gain control over expenditures. The tightening of health care budgets, while consistent across a number of sectors (public health, health prevention), is most noticeable in acute care. Shifting the traditional focus away from the welfare of patients, many hospitals devised ways to cut costs, improve their bottom line, and increase efficiency by contracting out services such as laundry, catering, and cleaning.

With excessive health care costs, long queues for care, and demands by the public for more accountability and transparency in the 1980s, the broad concern was that the system, in its form at that time, was unsustainable. While the Canadian system still costs less than other kinds of systems—such as an entrepreneurial model based in the private market, as exists in the United States—rising costs in a country like Canada, where funds are shared among several social programs, meant that there was also a significant threat to other public sectors that make up part of our social safety net, such as education, old age benefits, and welfare. The public felt at that time that there was not enough accountability on behalf of the government, that misspending or overspending might be occurring, and that there was not enough public consultation on how priorities in health care should be set.

The 1990s

In the early 1990s, the federal government reduced transfer payments to the provinces and territories in an attempt to control spending and reduce a large deficit. Over the next few years, these transfer payments for health care, education, and other social services were further reduced. In turn, the provinces and territories were forced to cut spending in these sectors to accommodate the decreased federal funding. Sharp cutback strategies included hospital amalgamations, reductions in beds on units, pressure to reduce the length of stay for patients, and longer waiting lists for non-urgent or non-emergent surgeries, as well as moving care from the hospital to outside the hospital system, where it is not covered by the *Canada Health Act* and therefore must be paid for by private insurance coverage or by individual patients. The system truly was in crisis. These cutbacks resulted in decreased satisfaction and worrying concerns on behalf of the public. With the public concerned by an aging population; the costs of increasing technologies; an evolving shortage of qualified health care providers, including family physicians and hospital-based nurses; and long waits and lack of access to care, it was clear that some kind of reform was needed (Hughes Tuohy, 2002).

Some of the broader problems in the system included things like fragmentation of care, lack of co-ordination of care, and episodic and illness-based care with a lack of focus on preventative care. All these problems, some of which persist today, result in higher costs and a system that is, therefore, difficult to sustain.

At the level of health policy at that time, there were three important issues in the area of reform. First, there was a feeling that there was an ongoing, growing political assault on the Canadian health care system. Noted erosion in other publicly held value-based programs, such as education, social programs, and care of the environment, meant that the perception, at a policy level, was that social programs that reflected Canadian values and beliefs were no longer a governmental priority. Second, with changing values, stronger trade relationships with the United States, and demands for choice, came the rise of a greater emphasis on providing health care through a "free market" approach; to provide people with choices if they wanted them, and possibly consider the creation of a two-tiered system. Alongside these kinds of pressures, the force of globalization added demands for greater harmonization between different, interacting markets. Much of the force of globalization is of course driven by the strongest players, so the call for harmonization was, and often remains, to adhere primarily to U.S. norms (Spalding, 2000).

Today

From a policy perspective, the concern with how health care is provided is an important one, but the issues are greater than simply the "site" of care. The issues were, and continue to be, much larger. Concerns with efficiency are reflected in the broader discussion of the possibilities of a two-tiered system. Concerns over site of care (i.e., hospital versus the community), are in turn reflected in discussions about considerations of other types of health care systems and markets. Policy makers ask themselves serious and difficult questions about the implications of introducing other kinds of delivery methods in order to save the system money. Should we make health care an industry? Should we inject it with additional funds from the private sector? Should the patient now be a client or consumer of health care?

The discussion of the privatization of health care is an ongoing debate with markedly different views as to just how much of the provision of health care should be privatized. Clearly, elements of privatization exist already in our system. First, the provision of care by practitioners other than medical doctors is often provided on a private basis, where patients pay out-of-pocket or through coverage by private health insurance companies. Second, as only services and therapies deemed to be in the category of "medically necessary" are covered by our health insurance model, many services, treatments, and therapies must be paid for by patients. Third, many services in hospitals and acute-care centres other than the provision of health care are privatized. Cafeterias, cafés, gift shops, cleaning, and laundry services are outsourced to private companies, with the goal of saving hospitals money and increasing efficiency. Finally, many hospitals and health care institutions accept private donations from philanthropic individuals, naming wings, centres, and atriums after private donors. So we see that our health care system has elements of privatization throughout. To claim that there is no privatization in our system is false. The debate over privatization, however, concerns just *how much* privatization we should allow, and what the limits should be for privatizing health care services.

 CASE PRESENTATION

Chaoulli v. Quebec is a landmark court case that has helped to shape the debate over the privatization of health care. Jacques Chaoulli, a physician in Montreal, observed that there were excessively long wait times for patients who required care, including one 73-year-old patient, George Zeliotis, who was in need of a hip replacement but was waiting in a year-long queue for his surgery. Dr. Chaoulli and his patient claimed that the ban on private medical care in the face of these kinds of excessively long waits violated patients' rights to life, liberty, and security as described in the *Canadian Charter of Rights and Freedoms* and the *Quebec Charter of Human Rights and Freedoms*. Their fight took them to the Supreme Court of Canada, which found in favour of their claim. The key argument articulated throughout the case was whether or not the ban on privatized health care was a protection of the health care system or rather a violation of human rights. The

Supreme Court judgment resulted directly in the establishment of wait-time guarantees in Quebec, and has opened up the discussion of private health care, especially in provinces with explicit bans on privately-funded and provided medical care: Ontario, B.C., Quebec, Nova Scotia, Alberta and Manitoba. (Kondro, 2006).

THINK ABOUT IT

- Think about the key argument in the case, as outlined above. Do you agree that a legal ban on private health care protects patients or deprives them of a basic right?

- The aftermath of the Chaoulli case has resulted in a more open discussion of private *versus* public health care. It has also resulted in various organizations, regulatory bodies, and professional associations making public statements about their views on the debate. Think about your professional association or regulatory body—do you know their stance on the issue? Do you agree with their view?

As a result of the pressures to reform the health care system, two important reform documents were produced in Canada. Both released in 2002, the *Romanow Report* and the *Kirby Report* called for significant changes in the way that health care is delivered in the country. While these reports are now a decade old, the principles for reform that they call for are still highly relevant and not yet actualized. Both are available on line, in French and English.

Challenges to the Health Care System, According to the Romanow Commission Report

- An overall lack of accountability in the health care system
- Lack of transparency over spending, priority setting, and decision making
- Lack of seamlessness between services, sectors, disciplines
- Increased pressure to privatize services
- Focus on illness-based, acute, and episodic treatment
- Accessibility is not consistent, as those in rural and remote areas have less access to services than those in urban areas
- Resources are not being used optimally or appropriately

(Continued)

- The *Canada Health Act,* while perhaps somewhat outdated and restrictive, has values that need to be reaffirmed, but the act must also be modernized, reflecting current contexts (e.g., more appropriate definition for "medically necessary" health care in light of ongoing debates and divergent opinions as to what this term means)
- Poor information dissemination and poor management of health information, leading to lack of continuity of care
- A need for more emphasis on primary health care/health promotion and shift away from hospital care and disease treatment
- Not enough focus on long-term strategies for increasing the sustainability of the system and better health for all Canadians
- Waiting lists need to be better and more consistently managed
- Need for increased acknowledgment of diversity of needs across cultures, ages, areas, abilities, etc.
- National platform needed for home care
- Coverage of home care services through the *Canada Health Act*
- Need for improved and better covered community mental health care and palliative care services
- Need more integration between "pharmacare" (i.e., the provision of drugs) and medicare
- Lack of a national "drug agency" to oversee and monitor pharmaceutical activity/ quality/delivery
- Poor Aboriginal health.

(Romanow, 2002)

While it is clear that there are problems in our system, as with any high-cost, high-demand system, there are different kinds of problems in all sorts of health care systems. Evaluation and reform of health care systems is an ongoing activity all over the world. If we look at the United States, for example, with each presidential election, candidates bring forth their ideas for new and innovative ways to provide health care. Often there is acknowledgment that a "Canadian-style" system may be a direction to aim toward; however, it would require significant overhauling of the managed-care system.

Interestingly, when we look at other systems of providing health care, we note that different kinds of inequities and challenges prevail. The American managed-care system is defined by Chang, Price, and Pfoutz as a "health care system willing to be held accountable both clinically and financially for the health outcomes of an enrolled population for a capitated (fixed) payment" (2001, p. 299). It is further described as an integrated form of health care delivery and financing that represents attempts to control costs by modifying the behaviour of providers and patients. Managed care moves away from a system focused on patient and provider autonomy and instead aims to focus on cost-based analysis of effectiveness of care and quality of priority setting and decision making. While there are many claims that managed care helps cut costs, in fact, it costs significantly more than the Canadian system, by virtue of skyrocketing administration costs. Compared to Canada, in which approximately 9 percent of our GDP is spent on health care, the American system costs roughly 14 percent of the GDP (and leaves a fifth of the population without medical care). Furthermore, administrative costs, as noted, are markedly lower—10 percent in Canada, compared to 24 percent in the United States (Spalding, 2000) and the gap between the two countries, in terms of amount spent on administration costs, is consistently increasing (Starfield, 2010; Woolhandler, Campbell & Himmelstein, 2003). Many Canadians view the American system as being driven by the patients' ability to pay, as opposed to the Canadian system, which guarantees reasonable access to care, regardless of income or ability to pay.

Managed care has profound ethical implications. Based on the assumption that the basic ethical criterion for the planned organization of the system and allocation of resources in any health care setting at the policy level is the well-being of the group of individuals for whom the decisions are being made, scholars at the Center for Practical Bioethics in Kansas City, Missouri, have commented on the relationship between this ethical criterion and a managed-care system and have developed a list of considerations to be used by managed-care organizations for guidelines on how to ethically ration care. These considerations include: valuing caring as an ethical obligation and an inherent benefit, and ensuring that health care professionals understand that their primary duty is to benefit patients through the provision of care. Care that is deemed to be futile or of no potential benefit should be avoided, with careful consideration of the patient's and family's view of futility, as well as the health care professional's view. Care that is neither clearly beneficial nor clearly futile, but rather of questionable benefit, should not be allocated based on cost constraints but rather on assessment of therapeutic value. The authors also state adamantly that some types of care should never be subject to rationing, such as palliative care, and that care should never be denied based on lifestyle choices. In terms of considerations for how rationing should occur, Biblo and colleagues recommend that persons who are particularly vulnerable or marginalized should be given special consideration, and that discrimination should not occur. Finally, in what is a very interesting recommendation, the authors note that those who are making difficult decisions about allocation of resources should reflect upon what they would want for themselves to guide them in their decision-making processes (Biblo *et al.*, 1996).

CASE PRESENTATION

Challenges in Our Health Care System

Many rural hospitals have centralized services for dialysis, where patients from a large geographical area come to be dialyzed. As the patient population and the acuity changes, the nurses on these units have to set priorities as there are a limited number of dialysis machines and, therefore, a finite number of dialysis spots each week.

(Continued)

In this case, the weekly schedule for this particular dialysis unit at a rural hospital is very full and the nurse manager has to make some difficult decisions about how dialysis can be provided to a larger number of patients than there are available spots. So he decides that the unit will make some patients wait until they are demonstrating signs of fluid overload (i.e., difficulty breathing) to be dialyzed.

Mr. M is a dialysis patient who has been on the unit for a number of years. He is a retired principal of a local high school and many of the nurses know him well. Mr. M has a history of not managing his disease well and, despite getting lots of good advice from the nurses, has been quite negligent at managing aspects of his own health. He has been bumped off of the dialysis schedule this week to make room for a very ill young woman, Miss S, who has just arrived in Canada from Ghana, where she was unable to access adequate medical care for her congenital kidney disease, which has worsened suddenly. She is not a Canadian citizen, and is now staying in the county with refugee status, with her sister, to access dialysis. She has a young son at home being cared for by her aunt, and she is a single mother. She is quiet and scared when she comes to the unit with her sister.

Some of the nurses on the unit go for their coffee break and they discuss that they are upset that Mr. M, a likeable and familiar patient, will have to wait to be dialyzed. He has required more frequent dialysis lately and they know that he will be uncomfortable and in some degree of distress at home while he waits. One nurse says, "He's been paying taxes all his life! Why should he wait?" Another nurse adds, "But he's contributed to his disease. Hers isn't her fault!" Everyone seems to have a different opinion about who should have been a priority for dialysis.

 THINK ABOUT IT

- Do you think that the right decision was made to make Mr. M wait for dialysis to make room for the acutely ill Miss S? Why or why not?

- If paying taxes is a justification for receiving better health care, then what about children? Should we deny them care because they haven't yet paid taxes?

- One nurse states that Mr. M has contributed a great deal to the local community, whereas Miss. S has not. Do you think that this should be a consideration in deciding who gets dialyzed first?

- What criteria would you use if you were the nurse manager and had to make this difficult decision?

SUMMARY

Because health care is a scarce resource, citizens rely upon social institutions to make fair and equitable distributive justice decisions. There is little consensus on basic ethical questions such as *How should people receive health care resources? Is there a right to basic health care? How much should be spent on particular health care services? What percentage of the society's overall resources should be invested in health care?* Egalitarianism, utilitarianism, libertarianism, and communitarianism are theories that attempt to describe fair means of distributing resources. Recent focus on problems related to the sustainability of Canada's health care delivery system has prompted debate on practical issues of distributive justice and accountability. In any health care system, when setting priorities or making decisions around reform, close attention must be paid to overarching values and ethical standards in health care.

CHAPTER HIGHLIGHTS

- The history of economic thought is closely associated with the utilitarian movement in the last century.
- The traditional health care system in Canada is a public insurance model.
- Justice relates to fair, equitable, and appropriate treatment in light of what is due or owed to persons, and recognizes that giving to some will deny receipt to others who might otherwise have received these things.
- Distributive justice is the fair, equitable, and appropriate distribution of benefits and burdens. Theories of distributive justice seek to render diverse principles coherent.
- Egalitarian theories are related to the concept of equality in which people who are similarly situated should be treated similarly.
- Utilitarian theories are based upon the rule that it is good to maximize the greatest good for the greatest number.
- Libertarian theories propose that the just society protects the rights of property and liberty of each person, allowing citizens to improve their circumstances by their own effort.
- Communitarian theories place the community, rather than the individual, the state, the nation, or any other entity, at the centre of the value system.
- Scarcity of health care resources has led to a rethinking of the structure of health care economics.
- Managed care gives rise to ethical problems associated with balancing utilitarian views of cost-effective care with a respect for persons and the traditional view of a duty to care.
- Health care evaluation and reform is an ongoing activity in Canada, in order to ensure high quality and ethical care.

DISCUSSION QUESTIONS AND ACTIVITIES

1. Discuss current problems in health care economics with classmates. Is there a consensus regarding root causes, right to health care, or the role of the government as a payer for health care services?

2. Go to the library and find a basic economics textbook. How does the health care system differ from other publicly-funded systems? Should it? Why or why not?

3. Discuss the influence of utilitarian theory on the economics of the current health care system.

4. How do patient and provider autonomy affect health care delivery and financing?

5. Define distributive justice. In class, discuss the material rules of distributive justice. Which material rule is most popular among classmates?

6. What method of distributing goods and services do you think is fair and equitable? Do your classmates agree with your theories?

REFERENCES

Bandman, E. L., & B. Bandman (1978). *Bioethics and human rights: A reader for health professionals.* Boston: Little, Brown.

Beauchamp, T., & J. Childress (2008). *Principles of biomedical ethics* (6th ed.). New York: Oxford University Press.

Biblo, J. C., L. J. Christopher, L. Johnson & R. L. Potter (1996). *Ethical issues in managed care: Guidelines for clinicians and recommendations to accrediting organizations.* Bioethics Forum, 12(1), MC/1-24.

Chang, C. F., S. A. Price & S. K. Pfoutz (2001). *Economics and nursing: Critical professional issues.* Philadelphia: Davis.

Daniels, N. (1994). Four unsolved rationing problems: A challenge. *Hastings Center Report, 24*(4), 27–9.

DeBlois, J., P. Norris & K. O'Rourke (1994). *A primer for health care ethics: Essays for a pluralistic society.* Washington, DC: Georgetown University Press.

Giesen, D. (1994). A right to health care?: A comparative perspective. *Health Matrix, 4*(2), 277–295.

Honderich, T., ed. (1995). *The Oxford companion to philosophy.* New York: Oxford University Press.

Hughes Tuohy, C. (2002). The cost of constraint and prospect for health care reform in Canada. *Health Affairs, 21*(3), 32–46.

Jones, D.J. & Sheppard, C. (2012). *Advancing Americans' right to health. The Globe and Mail,* June 28, 2012. Retrieved August 20, from http://m.theglobeandmail.com/commentary/advancing-americans-right-to-health/article4378240/?service=mobile

Kirby, M. J. L. (2002). The health of Canadians: The federal role. *Final Report.*

Kondro, W. (2006). Chaoulli decision resonates one year later. *Canadian Medical Association Journal, 175*(1), 17–18.

Morreim, E. H. (1995). *Balancing act: The new medical ethics of medicine's new economics.* Washington, DC: Georgetown University Press.

Rawls, J. (1996). A theory of justice. In J. Feinberg, ed., *Reason and responsibility: Some readings in basic problems of philosophy* (pp. 567–572). Belmont, CA: Wadsworth. (Reprinted from J. Rawls, *A theory of justice,* 1971, Cambridge, MA: Harvard University Press)

Romanow, R. (Commissioner). (2002). *Building on values: The future of health care in Canada.* Ottawa: Romanow Health Care Commission.

Spalding, K. (2000). Introduction to politics and health policy. Lecture in course entitled "Nursing and the health care system: Policy ethics and politics." Faculty of Nursing, University of Toronto.

Starfield, B. (2008). Access, primary care and the medical home: Rites of passage. *Medical Care, 46*(10), 1015–1016.

Starfield, B. (2010). Reinventing primary care: Lessons from Canada for the United States. *Health Affairs, 29*(5), 1030–1036.

Starfield, B., & L. Shi (2002). Policy relevant determinants of health: an international perspective. *Health Policy, 63,* 201–218.

Woolhandler, S., T. Campbell & D. U. Himmelstein (2003). Costs of health care administration in the United States and Canada. *New England Journal of Medicine, 349,* 8, 768–775.

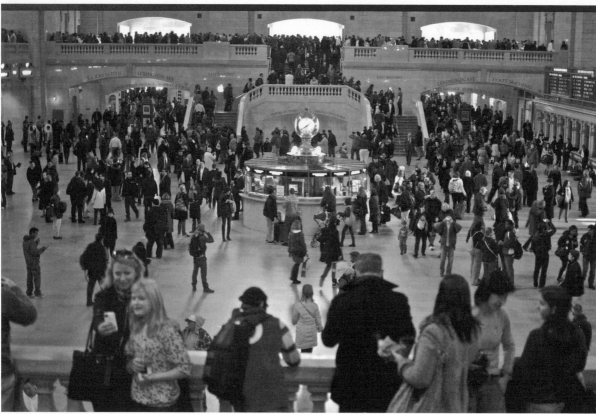

Jay Lazarin/iStockphotos.com

CHAPTER **16**

SOCIAL ISSUES

Based on a previous version of this chapter written by
Mary Jo Butler.

OBJECTIVES

After completing this chapter, the reader should be able to:

1. Review and discuss the social determinants of health and why these are imperative to consider in the provision of nursing care.

2. Explain how social conditions such as poverty, homelessness, intimate-partner violence, an increasing elder population, and racism affect health.

3. Apply the concept of justice to vulnerable populations, elaborating on the implications for society and the health care system.

4. Discuss the application of beneficence and non-maleficence to vulnerable groups in light of today's health care system.

5. Identify the pros and cons of promoting autonomy for health care decision making among vulnerable populations.

6. Analyze evidence of victim blaming within the health care system.

7. Illustrate application of the concepts of advocacy and nonviolence to care of vulnerable populations.

8. Examine current research for application to culturally diverse groups.

INTRODUCTION

Health is unquestionably a product of people and their environment. Thus, social conditions that alter the person and the environment interchange process are critical concerns for nurses and nursing students. Nurses confront social issues that shape the health and health care management of individuals on a daily basis. These social issues may create conflicts in values and ethical dilemmas that must be addressed in order to determine the appropriate health care interventions for the individuals involved. The purpose of this chapter is to help clarify the principles inherent in decision making when social issues create ethical dilemmas for the nurse.

SOCIAL ISSUES

As we know, health is determined by the complex interplay between many factors, including social and economic factors, our decisions and behaviours and the actual environment we live in. These factors are referred to as the social determinants of health and are extremely important for nurses to consider in the holistic care of any patient. Think about a patient recovering from surgery at home and just how important that home environment is. A person without access to running water or nutrient-rich foods, living in an unclean, noisy, or unsafe environment, or exposed to violence in the home, will have a much more difficult time recovering. Even simple nursing instructions for discharge that might include a sitz bath or a clean dressing may be impossible to follow for a person living in a shelter or on the street. To fail to consider the social determinants of health when providing care is to fail to acknowledge the many factors that have an impact upon a person's ability to maintain a particular level of health.

The Public Health Agency of Canada includes the following as social determinants of health: poverty and social status, employment status and working conditions, level of education and literacy, the presence of social supports and networks, social environments, physical environments, healthy child development, the kinds of health services that are available and accessible, culture, gender, biological personal health practices, and ability to cope (Public Health Agency of Canada, 2011). The World Health Organization identifies similar social determinants, with the addition of stress, social exclusion, and food security (Wilkinson & Marmot, 2003). When we look carefully at these determinants, we can see how social issues can have a direct and an indirect impact on the health of individuals and communities. Many pervasive social issues that are relevant to the social determinants of health are of special concern to health care providers today.

What are nurses' responsibilities in relation to the social determinants of health? As a starting point, nurses must understand the impact that the social determinants of health have on individuals and groups. Incorporating these factors into any assessment of individuals or groups is imperative. These factors must be considered in decisions about treatments, interventions, or resources. Nurses must advocate for appropriate resources and policies that address the impact of the social determinants of health. Furthermore, nurses should be advocating for additional research into the impact of these social and structural issues on health; in other words, going beyond a fairly exclusive focus on individual responsibility for health and wellness (CNA, 2005; Ling Yu & Raphael, 2004).

Poverty, homelessness, intimate-partner violence, an increasing elder population, and racism are examples of some of these very important concerns. We address these selected issues briefly in this chapter, along with guiding principles for related ethical decision making.

Poverty

Poverty is growing worldwide, and it is known to have a negative impact on both the health of individuals and the receipt of health care services—and it is prevalent in North America (Catley, 1992). People living in poverty are often sicker than people with adequate financial resources. Not only is poverty detrimental to the health of all individuals living with inadequate resources, it produces a next generation of citizens with more health problems than usual. Poverty can affect health in many serious and profound ways, not just physically (Wilkinson & Marmot, 2003). The psychological effects of poverty include helplessness and lack of control over one's daily life, both of which correlate strongly with poor health outcomes (Wallerstein, 1992). Children living in poverty have a higher incidence of conditions associated with trauma, drugs, burns, and mental illness (Wessell, 1992).

Children living in poverty are more likely to experience poor nutrition, inadequate exercise, and illnesses from environmental factors. They are also more likely to sustain physical injuries, be harmed in a fire, or be victims of homicide, compared to children not living in poverty (Canadian Institute of Child Health, 2001). They are more likely to grow up with chronic illnesses that require extensive health care resources. In Canada, the rate of children living in poverty is rising, with an estimated 15 percent of children living in after-taxes poverty, which translates to about one in six children. (CICH, 2000; Curry-Stevens, 2004). While the rate is lower than in the United States (22 percent), it is still higher than in countries such as France (7 percent), Sweden (3 percent) and the United Kingdom (10 percent). Children of lone-mother families, Aboriginal children, and children from visible minorities are all at a significantly higher risk for living in poverty, according to the most recent edition of *Health of Canada's Children*. According to CICH, "Children who live in poverty encounter more hurdles to healthy development and are, consequently, at an elevated risk for a wide range of negative health outcomes" (CICH, 2001, p. 2).

In a discussion of poverty in Canada, Raphael notes that while there are many discourses about poverty, or ways to think and talk about poverty, many of these discussions are at the level of the individual living in poverty (Raphael, 2001). While he acknowledges that, in fact, poverty does have a marked effect on the health and well-being of individuals, he instead suggests that we think about the kinds of community, social, economic, and environmental structures that can "support or limit the health status of those living in poverty." (p. 224).

According to Raphael (2001), there are three main reasons Canadians should be concerned with economic inequality and poverty: (1) it contravenes international notions of basic human rights; (2) it may also strain the health care system and social safety net of the country through the increased health care needs and problems of those living in poverty; and (3) the connection between the degree of economic inequality and both higher mortality rates (at all ages) and lower life expectancy is clear, thus posing a threat to all Canadians living in situations of economic disadvantage.

CASE PRESENTATION

Socioeconomic Influences on Health

Martha is a sixty-nine-year-old woman who lives in a substandard third-floor apartment in social housing in a relatively unsafe neighborhood. She gets by each month on money from Old Age Security along with some additional money in the form of a Guaranteed Income Supplement. She supplements this by working as a cleaning lady for three families, and is paid in cash. She uses public transportation to go to and from her job, spending $5.00 each working day on bus fare.

Martha helps her alcoholic single daughter, age forty-seven, with two teenage children, especially when her daughter is experiencing a drinking binge. The children frequently stay with Martha and rely on her for food, shelter, and love. Martha's husband is also an alcoholic and has not been home for two years; however, he does occasionally call from a homeless shelter or treatment facility. Neither her daughter nor her husband contribute to household expenses, but Martha remains devoted to her family, especially her two grandchildren.

Martha is 5'8" tall and weighs 285 pounds. She has hypertension, with her blood pressure ranging from 200/90 to 250/110. She is on medication for her blood pressure, and the physician has linked her with a home health nurse to encourage a diet and simple exercise regime for her obesity and hypertension. She is beginning to show signs of Type II diabetes and has been encouraged to lose weight and adhere to a diabetic diet. In addition, she has some small ulcerations on her left ankle.

The home health nurse visits Martha and instructs her in the care of her ulcers, advising her to keep her left foot elevated as much as possible. The nurse spends considerable time explaining a 1200-calorie diabetic diet with moderate sodium restriction, and talks with Martha about the need to begin walking as soon

(Continued)

as the ulcers on her foot heal. Martha lets the nurse know she used to attend a weight control group and understands low-fat and diabetic diets. However, she says coming home to her usual dinner of high-fat, prepared foods is her only daily pleasure. "I've lived sixty-nine years on this diet, don't wish to change, and have nothing to lose if I remain on it the rest of my life." She also points out that the sidewalks in her neighborhood need significant repair in order to be safe for taking walks. In addition, she indicates that she is too tired to exercise after working all day.

THINK ABOUT IT

Who Decides What Is Best for a Patient?

- Consider Martha's decision to ignore recommendations regarding diet, exercise, and, perhaps, care of her ankle ulcerations, in relation to autonomy, beneficence, and non-maleficence.
- What two principles are "at odds" here?
- Since the principle of beneficence requires actively doing good for Martha, who decides what is good?
- How would the home care nurse decide how to best help Martha?

Homelessness

Homelessness is a difficult social phenomenon to capture, characterize, or assume we can understand. There are many assumptions about people who are homeless—that they all have issues with drug addictions or that they chose to reject other lifestyles. Many of these assumptions are simply not true and instead represent a lack of insight into the growing phenomenon of homelessness in Canada. While acknowledging how difficult it is to capture an accurate number of homeless persons, Murphy (2000) estimated that, in 2000, there were between 15 000 and 20 000 homeless persons in urban centres across Canada. This number is increasing and today, the numbers of homeless people in Canada may be closer to ten times Murphy's original estimate. Additionally, Murphy notes that while these numbers represent those who do not have a permanent address, there are many more people living in what most of us would classify as barely acceptable housing with substandard amenities, poor construction, health hazards, and hygiene risks. The numbers of those living in inadequate housing may be even more difficult to capture accurately than the numbers of homeless people.

In Canada, homelessness can be thought of in three different ways that exist, to some degree, on a spectrum. First, there is *relative homelessness*, in which people may live in sub-standard housing, or be at serious risk of losing the home that they have. The second category is *hidden or concealed homelessness,* in which persons may live in a car, or with friends or family, and may move frequently between various options. Finally, *absolute homelessness* refers to those who live on the street or in temporary shelters (Echenberg & Jensen, 2008). An estimated 150,000 persons live with some form of homelessness in Canada (Pye, c. 2007), although other sources claim that this number markedly underestimates the true number of homeless Canadians, thought to be 300,000 in total (Echenberg & Jensen, 2008). The lack of dependable and accurate statistics on homelessness in Canada has been widely criticized, both from within our country and internationally (Echenberg & Jensen, 2008; UN Committee on Economic, Social and Cultural Rights, 2005).

There are many complex causes of homelessness and to characterize all those living on the street or in shelters as having similar issues and personal histories would be markedly inaccurate. Men, women, children, and families are affected by homelessness, and the causes of their homelessness relate to multiple factors. Some hypotheses concerning the increasing rates of homelessness in urban centres across Canada include the lack of affordable housing for those living on lower incomes, the gentrification of downtown areas with the resulting displacement of poor people, and the trend toward community living and the de-institutionalization of those with mental illnesses.

Like others living in poverty, homeless people suffer from acute and chronic health problems. Burg (1994) categorizes their health problems as those resulting from limited access to care, those coincident with homelessness, and those associated with the psychosocial burden of homelessness. Health problems resulting from limited access to care include exacerbated or advanced conditions that would have responded to early and thorough intervention. Health problems coincident with homelessness include illnesses resulting from living with inadequate nutrition, warmth, hygiene, safety, and other basic needs. Health problems associated with the psychosocial burden of homelessness are primarily mental illnesses, suicide, assault, and substance abuse, which can dull the anxiety of homelessness.

Mondragon (1993) describes the pervasive assumptions that underpin some models of health promotion. These assumptions view health as the absence of disease and associate common diseases with controllable risk factors. Thus, the key to improved health is deemed to be the provision of knowledge and skills to individuals. It is assumed that people will use self-determination, individualism, and responsibility to secure adequate housing, employment, and proper nutrition. While this model may benefit people with good education, a continuum of options, and resources to elicit change, it is less relevant to those who face limited choices by virtue of their socio-economic status.

CASE PRESENTATION

Few Choices

Diane is a forty-two-year-old woman with a history of mental illness, asthma, and former drug dependency, who has been living, sporadically, for the past three years, on the streets. She occasionally has been admitted to hospital for acute exacerbations of her illnesses and for problems with her medications. For the most part, however, she is able to survive and look after herself with the resources available to her, including street health nurses, shelters, and soup kitchens. She is able to work occasionally cleaning a local church and is paid in cash, which she carefully carries with her and spends judiciously.

Christopher is her primary outreach nurse from the local clinic. He meets with Diane, usually in a local coffee shop, once a week. This week, when they meet, it is apparent that Diane is upset. She tells Christopher that the women's shelter has closed temporarily and the women who depend on this shelter are now sleeping in the men's shelter down the street. She tells Christopher that "the neighbourhood is changing" and she doesn't feel safe any longer. Christopher knows that there have been issues with violence in the men's shelter and the supervision is less than ideal. However, it is now November and the weather has become cold and rainy.

Diane tells Christopher that she feels she cannot sleep in the men's shelter. She was a victim of intimate-partner violence a number of years ago and cannot expose herself to that potential risk again. She informs Christopher that she will sleep in the park across town because she feels safer and knows of hidden spots in which she can make a place to sleep. She tells Christopher that she has a male friend who has told her he will be with her at night to help and protect her. Christopher knows that Diane's friend is a drug dealer with a history of violence and feels that will put Diane at risk for returning to taking street drugs. Additionally, sleeping in the park across town means that she cannot meet Christopher regularly anymore, as it will be difficult for her to get to the park and back again for their weekly meetings.

Christopher asks Diane to reconsider. Given the challenges of managing her medications, her risk for entering into drug use again, the obvious health and personal safety risks of sleeping in the park, and the loss of the regular contact with her primary nurse, Diane's plan hardly seems like a good idea, and Christopher tells her so. He tells her that he is concerned about her and that he feels she would be exposing herself to a number of serious risks with her plan. He also tells her that he is worried that her male friend is coercing her into moving across town. Christopher tells Diane that he would be willing to speak and work with the shelter managers to make sure that improved safety measures are taken, especially with the influx of women clients. He also recommends a fairly close "Out of the Cold" program that provides safe shelter, bus tickets, and a hot meal, but only two nights a week.

Diane listens to Christopher but insists that this is the plan she must follow, despite the risks.

? THINK ABOUT IT

- How would a deontologist analyze this case and reflect on what action, if any, Christopher should take?
- How should we decide what is in Diane's best interests?
- Given that Christopher feels Diane is not making rational or sensible choices, what might he do, if anything? What would he be justified in doing? What would be ethically problematic and why?
- Would restricting Diane's autonomy, at this time, be either reasonable or in her best interests?

Intimate-Partner Violence

A third common social condition affecting health and health care delivery is intimate-partner violence, the most common but least reported crime in North America. Estimated numbers of abused women range from two to twelve million per year, but it is now accepted that both men and women can be victims of intimate-partner violence (IPV). Statistics indicate that, in 2010, there were 363 reported cases of IPV per 10,000 persons, which translates to a total of approximately 102,000 Canadians who reporting being abused by their partner or spouse (Sinha, 2012). Of course, these numbers must be considered carefully, keeping in mind the fact that many cases of IPV will not be reported to police or any other authority.

Definitions of IPV have evolved over the past ten to twenty years from only including spousal abuse involving female victims to now including instances of abuse against men, abuse in common-law marriages, and other kinds of intimate relationships that could potentially involve violence, including dating relationships (Sinha, 2012). Since this inclusion, it has been noted that, contrary to what we might expect, younger people (aged 15 to 24) are more at risk of spousal abuse or being killed by a spouse, while those in their late 20s to early 30s are more at risk of dating violence (Sinha, 2012).

Intimate-partner violence against women flows from a historical position of sexism. Eisler (1987) describes how select tenets of Judaism, Christianity, and Islam support patriarchy, the perceived inferiority of women, and the concept of women as the property of men. Remnants of these beliefs are still threaded through society, affecting the way families socialize their children and the way communities tolerate gender inequity. Butler and Weatherley (1992) and Roberts (2000) indicate that women have long been defined by the mothering role and dependence on men in North American society. While these role definitions are changing, events in society continue to perpetuate gender inequity. As long as gender inequity exists, intimate-partner violence against women will remain a social problem.

Women are not the only victims of intimate-partner violence. Men can also be victims of violence in their homes; however, women remain at greater risk in terms of frequency and severity of violence, about four times more at risk than men for being victimized, sexually assaulted, or killed by an intimate partner (Canadian Centre for Justice Statistics, 2011; Sinha, 2012). Fewer than one-third of all victims of intimate-partner violence ever report their problem or seek help. This may be due to any number of reasons, including embarrassment, fear for their own safety or the safety of children involved, or a suspicion that the judicial system will not be able to protect them from violence.

The vast majority of abused women eventually leave their abusive partners. However, leaving is a process that takes time, energy, and resources. Many abused women will leave and return to their abusive partners several times before permanently terminating the relationship. Esposito (1993) attributes this to several factors: the inability to find housing or suitable jobs; the fear, loneliness, or poverty that results from being out on their own; concern for children who are experiencing relocation and other difficulties; relentless pressure from family and friends to try harder to make the relationship work; and poor support from the criminal justice system. It is sometimes easier to return to a familiar though unpleasant situation than to start over and deal with numerous unknowns.

Intimate-partner violence affects women of all socio-economic, racial, and ethnic groups (Esposito, 1993; Morbidity and Mortality Weekly Report, 2000). Many women living in violent relationships will experience poor health. Women living in abusive situations experience acute traumatic injuries and chronic physical and emotional problems (Butler & Weatherley, 1992; Kernic, Wolf, & Holt, 2000). They are especially vulnerable to battery during pregnancy, and at a higher risk than women not exposed to violence for poor pregnancy and birth outcomes, including low birth weight, fetal distress, and fetal death (Bohn, 1990; Sinha, 2012). The health care system may, in part, add insult to abused women's' injuries. Women can feel humiliated, neglected, and blamed for the abuse by a health care system that minimizes the abuse, makes insufficient referrals, and fails to acknowledge abuse as the culprit of serious presenting injuries (Bradbury-Jones *et al.*, 2011; Campbell, Pliska, Taylor & Sheridan, 1994; Gutmanis *et al.*, 2007). Even today, in many health care settings women's' injuries resulting from intimate partner violence go unrecognized or unexplored and victims continue to feel that their complex health care needs are not addressed or met (Bradbury-Jones *et al.*, 2011; Humphreys & Thiara, 2003). Furthermore, as noted in a systematic review, victims found that responses of health care professionals to IPV ranged from unhelpful to inappropriate (Robinson & Spilsbury, 2008; Sundborg *et al.*, 2012) As a result, many women leave health care settings without having intimate-partner violence addressed, remaining isolated and uninformed about their options (Fishwick, 1995; Robinson & Spilsbury, 2008).

CASE PRESENTATION

Suspicions of Abuse

Maria is a twenty-five-year-old woman who made an initial visit to the clinic for prenatal care when she was eighteen weeks pregnant. She has returned for a second prenatal visit at twenty-two weeks gestation. Maria has a four-year-old son and a two-year-old daughter. Her record indicates she had several bruises, lacerations, and a black eye during her last pregnancy that she attributed to clumsiness. Her two-year-old weighed four pounds, eight ounces at birth and was seventeen inches long.

As part of routine prenatal care for the most recent pregnancy, Maria was tested for HIV antibodies. The test was positive, and the physician and nurse conveyed this information to Maria during her second prenatal visit. Maria, of course, was upset. She admitted that her spouse has been physically abusing her for some time and that both have used intravenous drugs in the past. She has had no sexual partners other than her spouse.

The nurse encourages Maria to tell her spouse that she is HIV positive so that he can be tested for antibodies. She also encourages use of condoms during sexual intercourse to help avoid transmission to her spouse should he not be infected. Maria insists that her husband refuses to use condoms. In addition, she says he would "kill" her if he knew she was HIV positive.

The nurse encourages Maria to go to a temporary shelter for abused women and links her to both a counselor and a social worker from the public health department who help her devise a safety plan. However, Maria ultimately decides to go home because she cannot abandon her children, and she does not want them in a shelter. She knows she cannot make it on her own, as she has neither income nor job skills. She requests that the clinic not interfere and that they allow her to decide if, when, and how she will notify her spouse about her HIV status.

THINK ABOUT IT

When Patient Choices Place Them at Risk for Harm

- Consider the principle of autonomy when determining the appropriate decision in this situation. Remember that confidentiality is an inherent part of autonomy.

- What do you think is in Maria's best interest, at this point? How best can the clinic nurse support her?

(Continued)

- If it is revealed that Maria's children have witnessed her being abused by her spouse, is this a situation which a registered nurse is mandated to report?

- Can the nurse force Maria to seek help or go to a shelter? If not, how can she best support Maria and help to ensure her safety?

Increasing Elder Population

In addition to poverty, homelessness, and intimate-partner violence, the elderly are a growing population worldwide (Catley, 1992). In Canada, our elderly population is rapidly growing, as baby boomers age. People are living longer due to healthier diets, vaccines, and better living conditions (Windom, 1988). Certainly, advances in health care knowledge have contributed to greater longevity. However, many elderly, especially from minority populations, live on inadequate incomes, even with social safety nets such as the Guaranteed Income Supplement program (Hall, 1993; Service Canada, 2012). The elderly have much higher rates of poverty; notably, those who are elderly and living alone, unattached to families, have a significantly higher rate of poverty than any other age group. In 2004, elderly women living alone had the highest rates of poverty for any elderly persons (17%), while eleven percent of elderly men living alone were reported to be living in poverty. (Canadian Council on Social Development, 2007). Vast numbers of the elderly are socially isolated, in need of work to survive, and susceptible to economic hardship. Chronic illnesses; pain, especially from arthritic processes; frailties; and disabilities occur with increasing frequency as people age (Tebb, 1995). Health problems contribute significantly to the social isolation and financial burdens that may accompany aging.

The assumption in current prevailing health care models is that the frail elderly will be cared for at home by friends and family to alleviate strain on the health care system. In reality, family members may be unable to provide needed support due to geographical distance from the frail elderly family member or other personal responsibilities. Skaff and Pearlin (1992) describe how caregivers of the elderly experience emotional and financial strain. The caregivers often have to help with finances of the elderly, since their fixed incomes cannot cover the basic cost of living as well as health care expenses. Reliance on friends and family for health care of the frail elderly is especially problematic for elderly people who do not have the necessary social or financial resources. The shift to caring in the home and the emphasis away from institutionalized care has two distinct effects. While many elderly people would prefer to live in their own homes, they may require either intensive or specialized care if they are frail or ill. Lay family members may not be able to provide the level or intensity of care required. More emphasis and resources need to be directed toward strengthening and supporting home care initiatives (Romanow, 2002).

CASE PRESENTATION

Aging, Poverty, and Illness

Mr. Chang is a sixty-five-year-old widower with chronic kidney disease. He is supposed to receive dialysis three times a week, but frequently misses his appointments due to not having transportation or not feeling well. His only hope for a cure is a kidney transplant, which Mr. Chang really wants. Mr. Chang is very frail with many health problems. He lives alone in a small garage apartment and the landlord is threatening to evict him because he is behind in his rent payments. Mr. Chang lives on a small pension. As Mr. Chang lives in Ontario, most of his prescription costs are covered by the Ontario Drug Benefit Program. However, some costs and health products are not, and Mr. Chang has to pay for these expenses out of his pensions.

A home health nurse used to transport Mr. Chang to dialysis occasionally, as Mr. Chang lives outside the city limits and is unable to access public transportation services. The nurse also helps Mr. Chang with his activities of daily living and showers. Additionally she provides strong support to him and assists him with his medications. Finally, she has helped advocate for Mr. Chang with his landlord. The clinic does not believe Mr. Chang is a candidate for a transplant, due to his frailty. Due to cuts in home care, the nurse is no longer able to visit Mr. Chang unless he has a specific need such as a dressing change or intravenous medication. No volunteer organizations for transport to hospital exist in Mr. Chang's area.

THINK ABOUT IT

What Health Care Should Society Provide for Its Citizens?

- Consider the principle of justice in deciding if health care is a right or a privilege. If health care must be rationed, who decides what services an individual will receive?

- Should we, as a Canadian society, be willing to provide health care for all?

- Is there a level of care that society should provide to all citizens? Explain.

- What is fair for Mr. Chang?

Racism

Racism is another social concern that affects health. The term "race" generally refers to an attribute that allows classifications of human beings on the basis of certain biological characteristics (Melville, 1988). Although no racial group of people ascribes to the same cultural beliefs and practices, it is often race that stereotypes a group of people or engenders ethnocentric beliefs and moral conflicts in values. Brown (1991) believes racism is an ethical problem based on inadequate respect, violation of personal boundaries, and an imbalance of power.

Racism exists today despite strong legal frameworks, policies, and laws opposing racism and racially based discrimination in Canada and in countries around the world (Minister of Public Works and Government Services, Canada, 2005). The International Convention on the Elimination of All Forms of Racial Discrimination, ratified by Canada in 1970, calls upon governments to eliminate racial discrimination and ensure equality for all in terms of human rights and freedoms. The *Canadian Charter of Rights and Freedoms* outlines the fundamental rights of all those living in Canada and it is entrenched within the constitution. Specifically, Section 15(1) states "every individual is equal before and under the law and has the right to equal protection and equal benefit of the law without discrimination" (1982). Furthermore, Section 35 confirms the historical and treaty rights of Aboriginal persons. Other relevant legislation includes the *Canadian Human Rights Act;* the *Canadian Bill of Rights;* the *Employment Equity Act;* the *Official Languages Act;* the *Canadian Multiculturalism Act;* the *Immigration and Refugee Protection Act;* and the *Citizenship Act.* A link to each of these is provided at the end of this chapter.

Racism in Canada persists. In a 2003 Ipsos-Reid survey sponsored by the Centre for Research and Information on Canada and *The Globe and Mail,* over 70 percent of respondents felt that racism persists in Canada. In other research, almost forty percent of visible minorities reported that they felt they had been discriminated against because of ethnicity or culture. This included 50 percent of blacks and over 30 percent of South Asian and Chinese persons (Statistics Canada, 2002). Almost half of all Aboriginal persons not living on reserves reported being a victim of racial discrimination in a 2003 report (Minister of Public Works and Government Services, Canada, 2005). Furthermore, in a separate survey one year earlier, more than half of all the Canadians surveyed felt that racism separates Aboriginal persons from the rest of Canadian society (Minister of Public Works and Government Services, Canada, 2005). The reality is that the stereotypical "face" of Canada has changed and nearly half of all Canadians are from an ethnic origin other than British, French, or native-born Canadian. We are a multicultural society and enjoy the advantages of this. However, not all persons are able to enjoy the advantages of a rich multicultural society, as they experience racial and ethnic discrimination in various contexts and situations in their daily lives.

Poverty and racial discrimination can be linked as barriers to opportunities and advantages. The 2001 Census report notes that over 20 percent of all immigrant families in Canadian cities are low-income families. The rate for non-immigrant families in the same geographic areas is almost ten percent lower (Census of Canada, 2001).

There is significant interface of poverty, homelessness, intimate-partner violence, an increasing elderly population, and racism. Poverty underpins homelessness. Women experiencing intimate-partner violence move frequently and often deal with homelessness and poverty as they try to improve their situations (Bassuk, Dawson & Huntington, 2006; Kanna, Singh, Nemil, & Best, 1992). Goodman (1991), Campbell (1993) and Jewkes (2002) provide data that poverty and homelessness are linked to a higher rate of intimate partner violence and other kinds of abuse. The elderly are often made homeless as they face mounting health care and medication costs and living costs on a fixed income. People who are experiencing poverty, homelessness, aging, intimate-partner violence, and racism are vulnerable to poor health and inadequate health care delivery. Often these vulnerable groups are the least powerful and vocal persons in society, yet they are the groups most affected by ethical decisions regarding health and health care (CNA, 2005; Raphael, 2004; Wessell, 1992).

These social situations represent examples of classism, sexism, ageism, and racism. Each indicates prejudice or discrimination against a particular class, gender, age group, or racial group. The implication is that one group of people is held to standards espoused by another group. Statistical data on these social situations, and the health of persons experiencing the social situations, explain why a feeling of helplessness may emerge when social situations are so intrinsically intertwined with health. Yet treating a person's symptoms without attending to the root causes of the problem may be viewed as inadequate health care.

ETHICAL PRINCIPLES APPLIED TO SOCIAL ISSUES

The common principles most essential in unravelling ethical dilemmas encompassing social issues include justice, non-maleficence, beneficence, and autonomy. A brief discussion of each principle follows.

Justice

Justice is the duty to treat all people fairly without regard to age, socioeconomic status, race, or gender. This implies a fair distribution of the benefits and burdens among members of a society, with equal treatment to all or to those most in need. A frail elderly man, beloved by his family, might receive an expensive but desired transplant procedure based on justice, even though there is only a moderate chance that the extensive surgery will prolong life or improve the quality of life.

Non-maleficence

Non-maleficence is the duty to prevent or avoid doing harm, whether intentional or unintentional. This could mean making sure a seriously ill research participant has full information on the risks of entering a clinical trial. It might also entail ensuring a safe, hygienic environment before the release from hospital of a newborn infant and mother suffering from poverty or homelessness.

ASK YOURSELF

Who Should Receive Limited Health Care Resources?

- In this day of declining health care resources, should those with the greatest need or those who have contributed to society receive expensive restorative procedures? Or should these procedures be available to all? Support your position.

- When thinking about this question, also consider how you think all health care resources should be allocated, if not by need?

Beneficence

Beneficence is the duty to actively do good for patients. It requires careful consideration of the best interests of others, and the ability to see issues and challenges from the perspective of another person. Thus, the homeless woman with leg ulcers and diabetes who walks all day and stands in lines in poor shoes and in all types of weather to secure free meals and safe sleeping quarters must receive treatment for the leg ulcers that will ensure adequate diet and rest, elevation of the legs, and proper hygiene. Treatment would have to go beyond the usual prescriptions for drugs, and address the social conditions contributing to the physical problems.

Autonomy

Autonomy is the patient's right to self-determination without outside control. Related to this principle are the principles of veracity, privacy, confidentiality, and respect for all persons. Little (2000) reminds us that we must develop our sense of autonomy. She suggests that autonomy involves a set of skills that various people possess to greater or lesser degrees. In order to have these skills, we often need someone to help us cultivate them, a context that sustains them, and help in exercising them when we are in a vulnerable position. One of the skills involved is the capacity to think through different options and imagine possibilities. Autonomy would direct us to work with an abused woman to develop a stronger sense of herself and to help her to see various options and available support. Autonomy would also honour her choice to return home, even if her safety is a concern, continuing to offer support as she struggles with difficult decisions. We must always consider as well how factors such as the chronic stress of living with abuse affect a person's ability to act autonomously (Limandri & Tilden, 1993).

THINK ABOUT IT

The Impact of Social Conditions on Vulnerable Groups

Consider how social conditions affect vulnerable groups such as children, people with mental health challenges or physical disabilities, and people who are institutionalized or incarcerated.

- Discuss the factors that make these populations vulnerable.
- Describe the issues related to these populations that give you concern as a nurse.
- Discuss the ethical concerns related to the needs and care of people in these groups.
- How would you apply principles of justice, non-maleficence, beneficence, and autonomy to health care concerns with people in each of these groups?

PERSONAL IMPEDIMENTS TO INTERVENING WITH VULNERABLE GROUPS

Working with persons who are poor, homeless, experiencing intimate-partner violence, or are otherwise vulnerable requires the exploration of one's own personal values to ensure that one's own attitudes, values, and beliefs do not interfere with health care. Price, Desmond, and Eoff (1989) caution that victim blaming is a real phenomenon that can colour attitudes and interactions.

Victim Blaming

Victim blaming tends to hold the people burdened by social conditions accountable for their own situations and responsible for needed solutions. Victim blaming is often evident in language. If there is evidence of personal or system wide victim blaming, a new world view may be needed. However, it is important to note that when we hear a nurse voicing notions of victim blaming, this is likely a direct result of his or her own experiences and challenges, so a sensitive exploration of attitudes is required. A desirable world view would see all persons as autonomous beings who deserve to be treated with dignity and fairness. Unfortunately, the health care system may not be designed to extend the needed degree of autonomy to all persons. Nurses and other health care providers are generally educated to make decisions, considering the best interests of others. Sines (1994) describes how prominent power relationships interfere with therapeutic practice and desirable client outcomes. To respect others by allowing them to make choices and decisions, when they are capable of doing so, requires an attitude of caring with a focus on advocacy. This implies guarding patient rights, preserving patient values, championing social justice in health care, and serving as the conservator of the patient's best interests (Sines, 1994). Re-educating nurses and other providers to enhance the advocate role may lead to improved care within a health care agency and empower individuals.

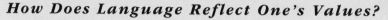

ASK YOURSELF

How Does Language Reflect One's Values?

How do the values reflected in the language of the following statements imply victim blaming?

- Most young, single, poor women get pregnant to increase their social assistance benefits.
- If poor, homeless people would take more responsibility for themselves, they could improve their situation. There are jobs out there for people who want to work.
- The highest calling for a woman is to be the family nurturer.
- If an abused woman wanted help, she would just leave the abusive relationship.
- An important part of assessing for intimate-partner violence is to ask what the woman was doing or if she was drinking right before she was victimized.
- Resistance to change is a normal part of aging.
- Loss is a normal part of aging.
- All five senses tend to decline as a person ages.
- How did they get HIV? Are they innocent victims who acquired it through a blood transfusion?
- She should have known better. If you don't use condoms, you'll be at risk for STIs.
- Since most low-income persons do not comply with therapies, it is not cost-effective to spend too much time with them on health education.
- What did you expect? Look at how her mother behaved.
- People can get ahead if they take advantage of life's opportunities.

Language of Violence

Another possible impediment to intervention, specifically connected with the social situation of violence, is the mode of violence that colours speech and actions. Ewing (1987) describes how the health care system uses metaphors of violence such as "attacking" germs, "battling" disease, "plotting strategies" against or "defeating" invasive cells and unwanted organisms, and, ultimately, "suffering defeat" or "achieving victory." The prevailing mindset behind this strategy of confrontation is the antithesis of a needed compassionate approach that values nonviolence. This is especially true for persons experiencing intimate-partner violence. Language that supports violence can inadvertently lead to victim blaming, or covertly encourage futile and dangerous retaliation. Additionally, use of such language may prevent the creation of a safe environment for women or victims of abuse in the health care setting. Indeed, a first step in effective intervention with those experiencing violence is to create a milieu that emphasizes nonviolence. The message has to be clear that violence of any form is wrong and, generally, illegal. This may necessitate a change in how health care providers approach and work therapeutically with people experiencing violence.

SOCIAL ISSUES AND SCHOLARSHIP

Many health care interventions are, quite properly, based on research; however, nurses need to ask if the underlying research may create problems based on classism, sexism, or racism. For example, growth and development knowledge has traditionally been based largely on studies of the experiences of white heterosexual men (Gilligan, 1982). Thus, the application of growth and development theory to both genders and to other races requires prudence. Campbell (1993) provides excellent data that assumptions about the abuser in intimate-partner violence situations are often based on the sex-role socialization in many families, and therefore does not explain the violence in families of other cultures, for example. Demi and Warren (1995) and Vasquez and Eldridge (1994) explore the issues of valid research for vulnerable populations, pointing out that the way family is defined and the systems for recruiting and retaining families contribute to the inability to generalize research findings. In addition, many of the research instruments in use are not designed for diverse and vulnerable populations.

Some research has viewed women as inferior to men and non-white groups as inferior to whites (Vasquez & Eldridge, 1994). These historical roots have contributed to a dearth of scholarly studies on women and visible minorities. This means that classroom teachings and clinical knowledge may be based on inadequate research for minority populations.

There is an ethical responsibility to teach nurses how to provide care to diverse cultural groups. Thus, faculty and students must be cognizant of the benefits of selected interventions for all population groups. In addition, they must be vigilant in avoiding generalizations of research findings to diverse population groups. Research on vulnerable populations needs to be done to make sure there is an adequate data base for working with those growing populations that are experiencing social issues such as poverty, homelessness, intimate-partner violence, unhealthy aging, and racism.

SUMMARY

This chapter focused on ethical dilemmas that emerge when health care is considered for vulnerable population groups. Ethical decisions related to health care for vulnerable populations confront nurses who work with those experiencing the social conditions of poverty, homelessness, domestic violence, unhealthy aging, and racism on a daily basis. Since values affect professional behaviour, nurses must analyze their personally held values as well as those of the health care agency where they are employed for appropriate consideration of justice, beneficence, non-maleficence, and autonomy. Nurses who work with vulnerable groups need to utilize these principles in ethical decision making. Nurses must consider the impact and validity of health care interventions and research on vulnerable populations, and ensure that what nurses teach both in the classroom and to patients is based on research applicable to the populations being served and studied.

CHAPTER HIGHLIGHTS

- Poverty, homelessness, intimate-partner, being elderly, and racism can have a direct impact upon health states of persons. Limited choices and lack of appropriate treatment options often interfere with the best health care for these vulnerable populations.

- Applying the concept of justice to vulnerable populations can change the way society and the health care system provide health care. Addressing the social conditions of the individual with an illness or disease is basic to health care.

- Non-maleficence and beneficence may clash with autonomy when providing care for vulnerable populations.

- Victim blaming, evident in covert or overt beliefs that all people are accountable for their own situations and responsible for solutions, interferes with health care delivery for vulnerable populations and is evidence of sexism, classism, or racism.

- Advocacy and caring—which are ways to go beyond delivering health care that is grounded in sexism, classism, and racism—require letting go of the power relationships that often dominate health care delivery.

- Clearing speech patterns and other behaviours of words and actions that are based on violence is a step toward therapeutic interventions with those who experience violence in their lives.

- Findings from research studies may not be applicable to vulnerable populations if the vulnerable people themselves are not part of the study population.

DISCUSSION QUESTIONS AND ACTIVITIES

1. Visit a homeless shelter or shelter for abused women. Interview residents about their health and ability to access health care.

2. Spend a few afternoons volunteering in a soup kitchen. Talk with people who come in for free meals about their health problems and ability to access health care.

3. Spend some time with a home health nurse or Meals on Wheels, making contact with the elderly who live at home alone. Explore with them their perceptions of quality of life, health dilemmas, and needs.

4. Work with classmates to develop a "health fair" for the homeless, discussing the value of typical activities and materials made available at traditional fairs, while designing a more relevant approach.

5. How many examples of toys, advertisements, acting roles, literature, child-rearing practices, and the like can you identify that continue to perpetuate the woman's role as one of caregiver or sexual object? Discuss how the examples contribute to gender inequity for women.

6. Look at the community where you live. What are the important social issues in this community? How are vulnerable people supported?

7. In Canada today, despite our universal health care system, many people still experience barriers to accessing care. What are the reasons for this? Is health care a right or a privilege? What can nurses do to help remove barriers to care?

REFERENCES

Bassuk, E., R. Dawson & N. Huntington (2006). Intimate partner violence in extremely poor women: Longitudinal patterns and risk markers. *Journal of Family Violence, 12,* 387–399.

Bohn, D. K. (1990). Domestic violence and pregnancy: Implications for practice. *Journal of Nurse Midwifery, 35,* 86–98.

Bradbury-Jones, C., Duncan, F., Kroll, T., Moy, M., & Taylor, J. (2011). Improving the health of women living with domestic abuse. Nursing Standard 25, 43, 35–40.

Brown, L. S. (1991). Antiracism as an ethical imperative: An example from feminist therapy. *Ethics and Behavior, 1,* 113–127.

Burg, M. A. (1994). Health problems of sheltered homeless women and their dependent children. *Health and Social Work, 19,* 125–131.

Butler, S. S., & R. A. Weatherley (1992). Poor women at midlife and categories of neglect. *Social Work, 37,* 510–515.

Campbell, D. W. (1993). Nursing care of African-American battered women: Afrocentric perspectives. *AWHONNS Clinical Issues in Perinatal and Women's Health Nursing, 4,* 407–415.

Campbell, J. C., M. J. Pliska, W. Taylor & D. Sheridan (1994). Battered women's experiences in the emergency department. *Journal of Emergency Nursing, 20,* 280–288.

Canadian Centre for Justice Statistics [Statistics Canada] (2011). *Family violence in Canada: A statistical profile.* Retrieved June 11, 2012 from http://www.statcan.gc.ca/pub/85-224-x/85-224-x2010000-eng.pdf

Canadian Charter of Rights and Freedoms. (1982). Retrieved June 10, 2012, from http://laws-lois.justice.gc.ca/eng/charter/

Canadian Council on Social Development. (2007). *Economic security: Poverty.* Retrieved June 10, 2012, from http://www.ccsd.ca/factsheets/economic_security/poverty/index.htm

Canadian Institute of Child Health. (2000). *The health of Canada's children: A Canadian Institute of Child Health profile* (3rd ed.). Ottawa: Author.

Canadian Institute of Child Health. (2001). *Income inequity: A Canadian Institute of Child Health fact sheet.* Ottawa: Author.

Canadian Nurses Association (2005). *Social determinants of health and nursing. A summary of the issues.* Retrieved June 10, 2012 from http://www2.cna-aiic.ca/CNA/documents/pdf/publications/BG8_Social_Determinants_e.pdf

Catley, C. M. (1992). Global considerations affecting the health agenda of the 1990s. *Academic Medicine, 67,* 419–424.

Census of Canada. (2001). Retrieved January 20, 2009, from http://www12.statcan.ca/english/census01/home/index.cfm.

Commission on the Future of Health Care in Canada. (2002). *Building on values: The future of health care in Canada — Final Report.* Retrieved January 20, 2009, from http://www.hc-sc.gc.ca/hcs-sss/hhr-rhs/strateg/romanow-eng.php.

Curry-Stevens, A. (2004). Income and income distribution. In D. Raphael (Ed.) *Social determinants of health – Canadian perspectives.* Toronto: Canadian Scholars' Press Inc.

Demi, A. S., & N. A. Warren (1995). Issues in conducting research with vulnerable families. *Western Journal of Nursing Research, 17,* 188–202.

Echenberg, H. & H. Jensen (2008). *Defining and enumerating homelessness in Canada.* Parliamentary Information and Research Service. Retrieved June 11, 2012 from http://www.parl.gc.ca/Content/LOP/ResearchPublications/prb0830-e.pdf

Eisler, R. (1987). *The chalice and the blade.* San Francisco: Harper & Row.

Esposito, C. N. (1993). Abuse: Breaking the cycle of violence: The victim's perspective. *Trends in Health Care, Law, and Ethics, 8,* 7–11.

Ewing, W. A. (1987). Domestic violence and community health care ethics: Reflections on systemic intervention. *Family and Community Health, 10,* 54–62.

Fishwick, N. (1995). Getting to the heart of the matter: Nursing assessment and intervention with battered women in psychiatric mental health settings. *Journal of the American Psychiatric Nurses Association, 1,* 48–54.

Gilligan, C. (1982). *In a different voice.* Cambridge, MA: Harvard University Press.

Goodman, L. A. (1991). The prevalence of abuse among homeless and housed poor mothers: A comparison study. *American Journal of Ortho Psychiatry, 61,* 489–500.

Gutmanis, I., C. Beynon, L. Tutty, C. N. Wathen & H. L. MacMillan (2007). Factors influencing identification of and response to intimate partner violence: a survey of physicians and nurses. *BMC Public Health, 7,* 12.

Hall, C. (1993). Long term care and the minority elderly. *Pride Institute Journal of Long Term Health Care, 12,* 3–8.

Jewkes, R. (2002). Intimate partner violence: Causes and prevention. *The Lancet, 359,* 9315, pp. 1523–1429.

Kanna, M., N. Singh, M. Nemil & A. Best (1992). Homeless women and their families: Characteristics, life circumstances, and needs. *Journal of Child and Family Studies, 1,* 155–165.

Kernic, M. A., M. E. Wolf & V. L. Holt (2000). Rates and relative risk of hospital admission among women in violent intimate partner relationships. *American Journal of Public Health, 90*(9), 1416–1420.

Limandri, B. J., & V. P. Tilden (1993). Domestic violence: Ethical issues in the health care system. *AWHONNS Clinical Issues in Perinatal and Women's Health Nursing, 4,* 493–502.

Ling Yu, V. & D. Raphael (2004). Identifying and addressing the social determinants of the incidence and successful management of type 2 diabetes mellitus in Canada. *Canadian Journal of Public Health, 95*(5), 366–368.

Little, M. (2000). Introduction to the ethics of care. Presentation at *New century, new challenges: Intensive bioethics course XXVI,* Kennedy Institute of Ethics, Georgetown University, Washington, DC, June 10, 2000.

Melville, M. B. (1988). Hispanics: Race, class, or ethnicity? *The Journal of Ethnic Studies, 16*(1), 67–83.

Minister of Public Works and Government Services, Canada. (2005). *A Canada for all: Canada's action plan against racism—An overview.* Ottawa: Government of Canada. Retrieved January 20, 2009, from http://www.cic.gc.ca/multi/pln/pdf/action-eng.pdf.

Mondragon, D. (1993). No more "Let them eat admonitions": The Clinton administration's emerging approach to minority health. *Journal of Health Care for the Poor and Underserved, 4,* 77–82.

Morbidity and Mortality Weekly Report (2000). Prevalence of intimate partner violence and injuries—Washington, 1998. (July 7, 2000), 49 (26), 589–592.

Murphy, B. (2000). *On the street: How we created the homeless.* Winnipeg: Shillingford Publishing.

Price, J. H., S. M. Desmond & T. A. Eoff (1989). Nurses' perceptions regarding health care and the poor. *Psychological Reports, 65,* 1043–1052.

Public Health Agency of Canada (2011). *What determines health?* Retrieved June 10, 2012 from http://www.phac-aspc.gc.ca/ph-sp/determinants/index-eng.php

Pye, S. (c. 2007). *The homeless individuals and families information system (HIFIS) initiative. Using information and communication technologies to build knowledge and understanding on homelessness.* National Secretariat on Homelessness. Retrieved on June 10, 2012 from http://www.homelesshub.ca/ResourceFiles/usinginfotech_e.pdf?AspxAutoDetectCookieSupport=1

Raphael, D. (2001). From increasing poverty to societal disintegration: How economic inequality affects the health of individuals and communities. In P. Armstrong (Ed.), *Unhealthy Times* (pp. 223–246). Don Mills: Oxford University Press.

Raphael, D. (2004). An Introduction to the social determinants of health. In Raphael, D. (Ed.) *Social determinants of health: Canadian perspectives.* Toronto: Canadian Scholars Press.

Roberts, D. (2000). Race, gender, justice, and reproductive health policy. Presentation at *New century, new challenges: intensive bioethics course XXVI,* Kennedy Institute of Ethics, Georgetown University, Washington, DC, June 9, 2000.

Robinson, L., & Spilsbury, K. (2008). Systematic review of the perceptions and experiences of accessing health care by adult victims of domestic violence. *Health and Social Care in the Community. 16, 1,* 16–30.

Service Canada (2012). *The Guaranteed Income Supplement.* Ottawa: Service Canada. Retrieved August 22, 2012 from http://www.servicecanada.gc.ca/eng/sc/oas/gis/guaranteeddincomesupplement.shtml.

Sines, D. (1994). The arrogance of power. A reflection on contemporary mental health nursing practice. *Journal of Advanced Nursing, 20*, 894–903.

Sinha, M. (2012). *Violence against intimate partners.* A publication of Statistics Canada. Retrieved on June 11, 2012 from http://www.statcan.gc.ca/pub/85-002-x/2012001/article/11643/11643-2-eng.htm#tphp

Skaff, M. M., & L. J. Pearlin (1992). Caregiving: Role engulfment and the loss of self. *Gerontologist, 32*, 656–664.

Statistics Canada. (2002). *Ethnic diversity survey: Portrait of a multicultural society.* Retrieved January 20, 2009, from http://dsp-psd.communication.gc.ca/collection/statcan/89-593-X/89-593-XIE.html.

Sundborg, E.M., N. Saleh-Stattin, P. Wändell & L. Törnkvist (2012). Nurses preparedness to care for women exposed to Intimate Partner Violence: a quantitative study in primary health care. *BMC Nursing, 11*, 1.

Tebb, S. (1995). An aid to empowerment: A caregiver well-being scale. *Health and Social Work, 20*, 87–92.

UN Committee on Economic, Social and Cultural Rights (2005). *UN Committee on Economic, Social and Cultural Rights: Concluding observations, Canada.* Retrieved June 10, 2012 from http://www.unhcr.org/refworld/docid/45377fa30.html

Vasquez, M. J. T., & N. S. Eldridge (1994). Bringing ethics alive: Training practitioners about gender, ethnicity, and sexual orientation issues. *Women & Therapy, 15*, 1–6.

Wallerstein, N. (1992). Powerlessness, empowerment, and health: Implications for health promotion programs. *American Journal of Health Promotion, 6*(3), 197–205.

Wessell, M. L. (1992). Said another way: An ethical issue for a profession for all seasons. *Nursing Forum, 27*, 29–33.

Wilkinson, R. & M. Marmot (Eds.) (2003). *Social determinants of health: The solid facts.* Second edition. Copenhagen: World Health Organization. Retrieved on June 10, 2012 from http://www.euro.who.int/__data/assets/pdf_file/0005/98438/e81384.pdf

Windom, E. (1988). An aging nation presents new challenges to the health care system. *Public Health Reports, 103*, 1–2.

WEBSITES

The Canadian Charter of Rights and Freedoms

   http://laws.justice.gc.ca/en/charter/

A Canada for All: Canada's Action Plan Against Racism

   http://www.pch.gc.ca/multi/plan_action_plan/index_e.cfm

The Canadian Human Rights Act

   http://laws.justice.gc.ca/en/H-6/index.html

The Canadian Bill of Rights

   http://laws.justice.gc.ca/en/C-12.3/index.html

The Employment Equity Act

   http://laws.justice.gc.ca/en/E-5.401/

The Official Languages Act

http://laws.justice.gc.ca/en/O-3.01

The Canadian Multiculturalism Act

http://www.canadianheritage.gc.ca/progs/multi/policy/act_e.cfm

The Immigration and Refugee Protection Act

http://www.irb-cisr.gc.ca/en/about/publications/irpa/index_e.htm

The Citizenship Act

http://laws.justice.gc.ca/en/C-29/index.html

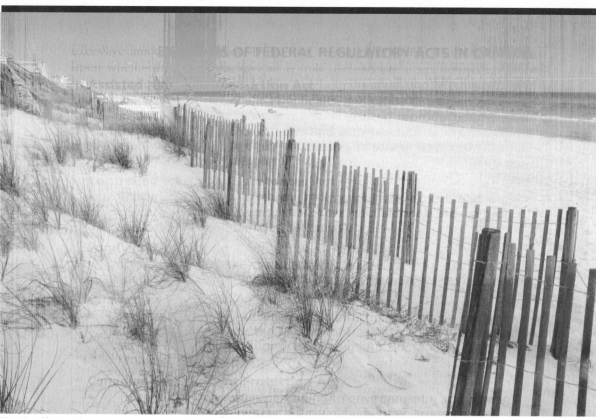

Vivian Fung/Shutterstock.com

CHAPTER 17
ISSUES OF GENDER AND CULTURE

Based on a chapter written by Sandra L. Cotton and a chapter written with the collaboration of Mary Gail Nagai-Jacobson.

OBJECTIVES

After completing this chapter, the reader should be able to:

1. Describe historical bases of gender issues in nursing.
2. Describe factors associated with and the impact of sex discrimination in nursing.
3. Discuss sexual harassment within a nursing context.
4. Discuss communication issues related to gender.

5. Describe nursing issues related to modern sexism.

6. Describe factors associated with cultural sensitivity within nursing.

7. Discuss the influence of culture on health and health care decisions.

8. Identify approaches for dealing with transcultural issues in nursing.

9. Discuss issues related to the use of complementary therapies by patients.

10. Identify legal considerations related to transcultural issues.

INTRODUCTION

In a perfect world, people would consistently relate to each other with mutual respect and empathy. Unfortunately, the reality of our lives is that our interactions are sometimes clouded by prejudice, incorrect assumptions, or lack of understanding. The diverse workplace is a common arena for many societal issues to manifest that may be grounded in issues related to gender or culture. Issues such as employment equity, employment opportunities, sexual harassment, and role strain are but a few examples of the kinds of conflicts that may be encountered in professional relationships. Our culture and gender may mean that we embrace different personal values, but as health care professionals, we must be aware of our personal values, while also being attuned to those of others around us, and able to reflect on the ways that factors such as our culture and our gender influence our values development. Furthermore, the social construction of gender and culture can have an impact on how we think of ourselves in relation to other diverse colleagues and patients, and how we evaluate or think about their choices, which may well be different from our own.

There are two basic approaches to dealing with these kinds of issues. We can simply pretend that they do not exist. This approach may result in increased frustration as unresolved feelings and issues play out on the job. Alternatively, we can become aware of the issues and define ways to deal with the realities of our diverse, multicultural society in a straightforward, genuine and thoughtful way. This chapter focuses on the latter approach and explores issues concerning both gender and culture in the nursing workplace.

HISTORICAL PERSPECTIVES AND OVERVIEW OF GENDER-BASED ISSUES

The legalization of same-sex marriage in Canada in 2005 through the passing of the *Civil Marriage Act* was met with both jubilation and vocal opposition, mostly from various church and conservative groups. Some, like the Catholic Church, organized formal protests against the Chrétien government. With over 40 percent of the Canadian population noting an affiliation with the Catholic Church (Statistics Canada, 2005), it was important for two things to happen. First, it was critical to hear both sides of the argument and differentiate between deep-seated religious beliefs and homophobia. Second, it was, and remains, important to not assume that all those who list themselves as having an affiliation with the Catholic Church share the same views as those in the Church with the most power, who are also highly vocal in the public sphere.

In the United States, the passing of the California ballot proposition known as Proposition 8 restricted the state's Constitution so that it limited the definition of marriage to being between only a man and a women. Campaigns against the passing of Proposition 8 were widespread and continuing as the state put the Proposition into immediate effect the day after the 2008 election. In early 2012, a U.S. federal court declared that California's ban on same sex marriage, found in Proposition 8, was unconstitutional. Since then, activists have stated that they are willing to take their opposition to the ban forward to a higher court, and possibly all the way to the U.S. Supreme Court.

These two events demonstrate that there is still significant discrimination against lesbians and gay men, whether in the workplace or in their efforts to seek, ensure, and enjoy the same kinds of rights that everyone in society is due. Discrimination and marginalization of persons for reasons related to gender persist and the example of the legalization of same-sex marriage helps to highlight these inequities.

Gender in nursing has been a topic of much discussion and reflection. While some authors contend that most have come to accept the term *"nurse"* as "a person who tends to the needs of the sick" (Ellis and Hartley, 2003, p. 150), discussion persists concerning exactly what a person who provides nursing care should be called, and how, if at all, this relates to the gender of the person providing the care (Bernardi, 1996).

In her comprehensive work, *Woman as Healer,* Achterberg chronicles the journey of women in healing professions. Citing the masculinisation of medicine as one of many issues that challenge nurses, Achterberg states that, although nursing has gained professional status, it suffers in some contexts because of issues of "nurses' functioning subordinate to multiple layers of authority" (1990, p. 177). The feminization of nursing and women's work, alongside the social construction of gender, has contributed to the real and perceived lack of power of nurses, relative to physicians (Porter, 1992). In discussing the position of nurses relative to other health care professionals, in particular physicians, gender is thought to be of great importance. While many would eschew these differences, citing evidence of the increasing numbers of females in medical school and males in nursing school, societal views of these two professions remain entrenched in images of the nurse as female and the physician as male.

Societal Expectations

As nursing continues to be a predominantly female profession, societal issues that have affected women have also been reflected in nursing. Women have been socialized to achieve or be less than they are capable of becoming. This reluctance to achieve is evident in the lack of women in positions of power, especially in the political arena (Hamilton, 1996). Although more recent societal influences have had a positive impact in this regard, nursing is still a female-dominated profession, which unfortunately has a history of oppression that many believe it has yet to overcome.

ASK YOURSELF

Is There Gender Stereotyping in Nursing?

- In what ways do you think nurses can help dispel this declining but continuing stereotype?
- How would you respond if your son or daughter chose nursing as a profession? Would you encourage him or her? Why or why not?

Authors such as Achterberg (1990), Kane & Thomas (2000), Kavanagh (1996), and Lewenson (1996) believe that nurses have been forced to work within a framework that focuses on societal expectations of women and what is considered women's work. In what has been termed the medicalization of North American society, nursing has been forced to overcome the prejudices of a society that has historically embraced the bio-medical curative model of health care. As diversified users of our health care system are demanding more sophisticated and culturally congruent care, nurses are in a prime position to provide high-quality, relevant, individualized care. If nursing is to be successful in this and other arenas, it must concomitantly address issues of territoriality, power, and authority within its own ranks as well as with other health care professionals.

GENDER DISCRIMINATION IN NURSING

Historically, women have worked for lower pay than their male counterparts. Employment equity is generally protected by federal and provincial legislation. Over the past thirty years, many initiatives have been undertaken to address pay inequity on the basis of gender. The United Nations Convention on the Elimination of All Forms of Discrimination Against Women, adopted in 1979 and now under the auspices of the Office of the High Commissioner for Human Rights in Geneva, attempted to define discrimination and to facilitate the elimination of discrimination at national levels in all UN countries (Office of the United Nations High Commissioner for Human Rights, 1979). There are laws governing employment equity in provinces across Canada, and equal pay for equal work is a right protected by the *Canadian Human Rights Act*, specifically the Equal Wages Guidelines (1986). Additionally, in 2001, a pay equity task force was formed by the federal government to find ways to address employment equity and implement the changes necessary to ensure pay equity and to keep pace with the changes of a modern society and the dynamic nature of the workplace (Department of Justice Canada, 2001).

Despite these laws and more legislation and activism, women still earn less than men, on average, for the same work. In fact, one source notes that, as of 2005, a woman gets paid, on average, 70 percent of what a man earns in a similar position (Canadian Labour Congress, 2005). Salaries in nursing remain low compared with other professions that require comparably high levels of skill, education, and responsibility. Some suspect that the increasing presence of men in nursing is helping to raise salaries; however, other economic considerations, such as nursing shortages, fair-labour-related legislation, and collective bargaining, may be responsible (Ellis & Hartley, 2003). Although a disparity in earnings, known as a *pay gap*, exists between men and women of many occupations, the gap is considerably narrower for nurses (Reskin & Padavic, 1994). The fact that a gap exists at all is striking, in that men comprise only a small percentage of the nursing profession (Benokraitis & Feagin, 1995). As Gilloran (1995) notes, the development of a patriarchal structure within nursing, with fewer women in senior management positions, may account for this gap. However, this trend is also changing.

According to sociologist Christine Williams (1995), issues of comparable worth are a real concern for nurses. Williams identifies several hidden advantages to being a man in nursing, particularly related to hiring and promotion. Williams' work supports Gilloran's (1995) assertions of gender disequity, as men are typically tracked into higher paying and more prestigious positions. Even in a predominantly female profession, women may be experiencing a form of economic gender discrimination.

Expanding Numbers of Men in the Profession

Although the number of men in nursing has increased steadily, men still comprise a relatively small percentage of all practising RNs in Canada (Canadian Nurses Association, 2011). Sullivan (2000) stresses the value of gender diversity in nursing, noting that men play an important role in the profession. Citing societal stereotyping as one of the major limiting factors for men in nursing, Squires (1995) may be categorizing men further when he asserts that health care reform that increases responsibility and autonomy will attract more men to the nursing profession. Perhaps what Williams (1995) perceives as hidden advantages for men in nursing adds some credence to Squires's assertions. Despite these and other stereotypes, Squires considers the lure of nursing to be universal regardless of gender. Noting the challenge, variety, and excitement of nursing, Squires is quick to acknowledge that the road men in nursing have travelled thus far has not been without controversy.

Gender and Caring

In 2009, the total number of nurses in Canada was 284,690 (including NPs), with only 6.2 percent or approximately 16,475 of those nurses male (Canadian Nurses Association, 2011). Canada is lagging behind other countries, such as the United Kingdom, where over 25 percent of all nurses are male. This number, according to a 2007 *Canadian Nurse* article, is rapidly increasing in the United Kingdom (Tosh-Kennedy, 2007). In the United States, the percentage of male nurses in the total nursing population is also increasing, but remains closer to Canada at approximately 9 percent (U.S. Department of Health and Human Services Health Resources and Services Administration, 2010).

Canadian research shows that rates of attrition from nursing programs are higher for male students than female, with rates of almost 50 percent, compared to an average attrition rate of 20 percent for their female colleagues (Tosh-Kennedy, 2007). As the number of men in nursing increases, research directed toward gender-related issues in the profession has begun to emerge (Ekstrom, 1999; Gilloran, 1995). For example, many authors have focused nursing research on caring as it relates to gender. Although much of this work is in its infancy, research questions related to possible differences in the learning or expression of caring as it relates to the gender of the student, educator, or recipient of care demonstrate the attention these and other issues in nursing have commanded. Recognition of the need to explore gender became evident for Peter and Gallop (1994) in their comparative study designed to examine whether caring uniquely reflected the moral orientation of nursing students. They discovered that differences in caring noted between medical and nursing students appeared to be related to gender differences. A study exploring the relationship between nurse gender and both nurse and patient perceptions of caring found no significant difference in actual caring according to nurse gender (Ekstrom, 1999). However, from both nurse and patient perspectives, expectations of certain nurse caring behaviours were lower for male nurses.

Ironically, a gender bias may already exist in the literature that focuses on caring. Chinn (1991) devoted an entire anthology to caring, but did not explore gender in relation to caring, except as it related to economic gains (or lack thereof) for male faculty members in male-dominated academic centres. The exclusion of men by Grigsby and Megel (1995) as they explored the caring experiences of nursing faculty is another example of current nursing research that does not include men.

Despite an increased interest in the caring aspect of nursing, Begany (1994) perpetuates a nursing stereotype by equating the positive attribute of caring to images of nurturer or handmaiden. Some men in nursing may already experience a form of gender discrimination with regard to the stereotypical belief that all men in nursing are homosexuals. This stereotype is rooted in gender-based role assumptions, such as Begany's, related to the caring attributes that many perceive as feminine. Because nursing has historically been viewed as "women's work," men in nursing have been stereotyped as feminine. Often, assumptions are made that male nurses must be homosexual. Even though Williams (1995) found there were hidden advantages in nursing for men, she also discovered that, ironically, these "opportunities . . . may extend only to those who exhibit conventional masculine characteristics, including a heterosexual orientation" (p. 65).

THINK ABOUT IT

Do Men and Women Express Caring in Different Ways?

- What do you think of Begany's (1994) images of caring? What does caring mean to you?

- Williams (1995) believes that organizations are gender-biased in how they regard masculine behaviours versus feminine ones. She suggests

(Continued)

the development of gender-sensitive evaluation tools that would acknowledge women's contributions to the profession. If you were appointed to develop such an evaluation tool, what attributes would your tool reward and recognize as unique to women? What justice issues may be involved in using gender-sensitive evaluation processes?

- Do you think that there are specific benefits to having nurses who are men? If so, how do these differ from the benefits of nurses who are women?

As more men enter the profession, additional gender issues may be identified. According to one author, some areas of nursing have more male nurses than others, including mental health, intensive care, and the operating and emergency rooms (Vere-Jones, 2008). Why some areas attract and retain male nurses more than others is an area for further research and discussion. For example, once in the workforce, men in nursing may experience difficulty when cross-gender mentoring relationships exist (Feist-Price, 1994). Feist-Price notes several potential adversities in cross-gender mentoring relationships, mainly related to communication differences between men and women (Tannen, 1990). Feist-Price further notes that cross-gender mentoring relationships have successful outcomes, especially when formal mechanisms are in place to deal with issues as they arise. One final implication for nursing may be in the area of caring. If differences in the development or expression of caring in male nurses actually exist, these and other differences need to be explored and further utilized to improve the practice of nursing and optimize gender differences. However, there is a persistent lack of strong male role models in nursing, along with few positive or realistic media representations of male nurses (Anonymous, 2007; Meadus & Creina Twomey, 2007). Add to that almost no targeted recruitment strategies for young males seeking career counselling in high school or university to even suggest nursing as a viable, fulfilling, and challenging career. One small grass-roots group is hoping to work to attract more young men into nursing. The Men in Nursing Interest Group (MINIG), a group established through the Registered Nurses Association of Ontario, is working hard on outreach and media activities, to dispel myths about male nurses and promote a professional career with so many options, to young men who, up until now, rarely considered nursing as a viable career choice (Anonymous, 2007). These issues imply that, certainly, unless more strategies are put in place to recruit, attract, and retain more men in the profession, we will continue to have small numbers of male nurses in Canada.

SEXUAL HARASSMENT IN NURSING

Bullough (1990) describes Florence Nightingale's encounters with harassment and the prevailing strategy of the day "to gain respect" through being a lady (Nightingale, 1859). Bullough contends that sexual harassment has been a recurring theme in Western nursing. The Supreme Court of Canada defines sexual harassment as "unwelcome conduct of a sexual nature that detrimentally affects the work environment or leads to adverse job-related consequences for the victims." (*Marinaki v. Human Resources Development*

Canada, 2000). The Ontario Human Rights Commission notes that sexual harassment is unwanted words or actions that are related to gender or of a sexual nature. Often referred to under the umbrella of workplace harassment, sexual harassment may include touching in a way that is inappropriate or uninvited; staring or making comments in a sexual way; being verbally abusive because of gender; making sexual requests, jokes, or remarks about a person or about a specific gender; or displaying sexually offensive images of any kind to others (Ontario Human Rights Commission, 2008). There are two important things to note about sexual harassment. First, it may not be overtly sexual in nature, despite its label. It may refer to being bothered or harassed simply because of gender. Second, sexual harassment doesn't only happen to women; it can happen to anyone, in any situation (Ontario Human Rights Commission, 2008). Nurses may not immediately recognize or label the behaviours as sexual harassment, and, according to Madison and Minichiello (2000), often have difficulty finding appropriate words to describe the experience concisely. Madison and Minichiello (2000) go on to identify some key indicators of sexual harassment by individuals:

- A feeling of having your space invaded or being cornered;
- A feeling of being disrespected;
- Noting behaviour that feels forced or too friendly.

According to the same authors, indicators of an environment or workplace in which sexual harassment might happen more readily may include:

- Other persons confirming that they have been harassed;
- Power or administrative structures that support or protect the harasser while providing limited options for the harassed;
- A workplace where sexual innuendo, images, or humour is common or tolerated.

Bullough (1990) suggests that nurses need to employ specific strategies to combat sexual harassment.

ASK YOURSELF

Discrimination and Inequality in Nursing

When we talk about issues of women's rights or sexual discrimination (which can affect both genders), we need to be pay attention to the fact that many forms of discrimination can occur. Section 15 of Canada's *Charter of Rights and Freedoms* (1982) clearly precludes any form of discrimination or practised inequality, with the exception of affirmative action for the purpose of ameliorating the situation of marginalized individuals or groups.

(Continued)

15. (1) Every individual is equal before and under the law and has the right to the equal protection and equal benefit of the law without discrimination and, in particular, without discrimination based on race, national or ethnic origin, colour, religion, sex, age or mental or physical disability.

(2) Subsection (1) does not preclude any law, program or activity that has as its object the amelioration of conditions of disadvantaged individuals or groups including those that are disadvantaged because of race, national or ethnic origin, colour, religion, sex, age or mental or physical disability.

- Do issues of discrimination affect nurses in a unique way?
- As advocates for others, discuss what responsibility you think nurses have in relation to marginalized or vulnerable populations, such as the homeless or persons without legalized status.
- Reflect on experiences you have had, in which you might have felt discriminated against, by virtue of your gender, abilities, religion, age, or ethnic origin. How did you feel? What did you do? How would you approach a situation like this again, if you encountered it?

We do not need to venture far to find images that reinforce the view that nurses are sexual objects. A quick Google image search, tour of the humorous *Get Well* section at your local greeting card shop, or costume rental store at Hallowe'en will graphically illustrate this point. Although sexual harassment does not recognize gender boundaries, clearly sexual harassment has historically been the bane of women. As more men enter the nursing profession, issues concerning sexual harassment directed toward them or from them may emerge. Research is needed that is directed toward understanding issues concerning sexual harassment in nursing, how best to address the needs of men in nursing, and the implications for the women with whom they work.

COMMUNICATION ISSUES RELATED TO GENDER

How nurses communicate with each other, their patients, and their colleagues has long been discussed in the nursing literature (Campbell-Heider & Hart, 1993; Corser, 1998). Nurses need to address how changing societal roles and expectations relate to the practice of nursing, and what research is needed to promote and bring about positive change.

"The Doctor–Nurse Game"

A gender division of labour has been a significant factor in how nurses, who are primarily women, and physicians, a traditionally male-dominated profession, relate to each other in health care settings. Initially described as the *doctor–nurse game* (Stein, 1967), issues regarding communication with physicians remain an area of primary concern for many nurses (Anderson, Maloney, Oliver, Brown & Hardy, 1996). Favourable patient outcomes have been positively associated with successful nurse–physician communication (Shortell, Zimmerman, Rousseau, Gillies, Wagner, Draper, Knaus & Duffy, 1994).

Many nurses still use less-than-straightforward methods to manage conflict among themselves or between nurses and physician colleagues (Valentine, 1995, 2010). Valentine indicates that staff nurses and nurse managers are most comfortable using avoidance or compromise as their primary method of conflict management. These methods may be reinforced by nursing educators, whom Valentine found also employed avoidance as their most frequent conflict management tool (1995, 2010). According to Tannen (1990), the primary reason for these and other communication conflicts relates to identifying and understanding gender differences in communication. Previously linked to societal roles and expectations of women, the "doctor–nurse game" was re-examined by Stein, Watts, and Howell (1990). The authors found that a more humanistic public image of physicians and the increasing numbers of female physicians and male nurses have generally improved physician–nurse relations.

THINK ABOUT IT

Do Men and Women Communicate Differently?

Tannen (1990) asserts that men and women communicate from such differing frames of reference that their communication could be considered a cultural clash of sorts.

- What has your experience been in this area?
- What communication concerns with fellow students, faculty, patients, or physicians have you experienced in your program of study?
- How would you rate the nurse–physician communication in your clinical agencies? Describe why.
- Describe potential gender-based differences in communication.

With females comprising nearly 50 percent of students entering medicine, and a slowly increasing percentage of males entering nursing school, perhaps the patriarchal system of health care will shift. The implications this may have for nursing remain unknown.

Communicating with Patients

Today, one trend that has seeped into health care from the street is the casual nature of attire and approach to work (Twenge, 2006). In nursing, uniform policies and requirements have changed to reflect a more casual society, with a concern for comfort over formality. Starched white dresses, hats, and polished shoes have been replaced by scrubs, T-shirts, and casual wear. While this has advantages—making nurses appear to be more friendly and accessible—it also has a downside. Many people find that it is difficult to tell what roles people play in health care environments, because their dress does not help to identify them as uniquely-skilled professionals. Furthermore, the casual comfortable nature of nursing dress is seen by many as unprofessional and indicative of a casual approach to work as well as appearance. While it would be foolhardy and impractical to return to the formal traditional dress of nurses as noted above, it is worth giving thought to what you look like when you approach patients—remembering that you are there as a trusted, capable, and highly skilled professional. To some degree, your appearance should reflect that. For example, scrubs with teddy bears on them may be appropriate for a pediatric unit, but would not be appropriate for an adult setting and might inadvertently suggest to patients a message of incompetence or immaturity.

Through the informal dress and communications, nurses may in fact be sending powerful negative messages to their patients and medical colleagues. The bedside manner of nurses is discussed by Campbell-Heider and Hart (1993), who note that the tone of familiarity expressed by nurses who use their first names with patients may translate sociologically into persistent stereotypic themes and become a mechanism of social control. While superior nursing care may reduce these stereotypes, Campbell-Heider and Hart discuss the role of deliberative communication strategies, both verbal and nonverbal, in accelerating professional recognition.

Successful interpersonal communication with patients is central to the practice of nursing. In relation to sensitive issues and sexuality, Propst (1996) found that registered nurses' communication practices are lacking. Only half of the respondents in her sample of women's health nurses discussed issues concerning sexuality with their patients. Even in a specialty practice area, such as women's health, nurses are not immune to communication issues when sensitive topics are involved.

MODERN SEXISM

Even though women have made tremendous inroads in the workplace, Benokraitis and Feagin reported in 1995 that sex inequality was a major problem, and it continues today. **Sexism** is "the assumption that members of one sex are superior to those of the other" (Kavanagh, 1996, p. 296). In our predominantly male-oriented health care system, issues concerning sexism may manifest themselves in power struggles for reimbursement, as nurses take on advanced practice roles. Unfortunately, even within the nursing profession, issues of sexism related to men in nursing are present. An example of this is the male colleague who feels he has a hiring edge over women in nursing, because he never needs to be off for maternity leave or stay home from work to care for sick children.

ASK YOURSELF

Are Male Nurses Perceived as More Competent?

Benokraitis and Feagin (1995) interviewed male nurses. The authors report that physicians view male nurses as being more competent than their female counterparts. They also found that female nurses were often ignored, whereas male nurses' opinions were valued.

- Have you observed this behaviour in your clinical or classroom settings?
- How could you best deal with this form of modern sexism?

SEXUAL ORIENTATION

Heterosexism is "the assumption that everyone is or should be heterosexual, and that heterosexuality is superior and expectable" (Kavanagh, 1996, p. 296). We must be alert for this form of sexism directed toward patients and some nurses (Stevens, 1995; Williams, 1995). Van Ooijen and Charnock (1995) note that very little attention is given to addressing this and other gender issues within the nursing curriculum, despite the belief that developing an understanding of these issues may have a tremendous effect upon nursing care.

Lesbians and gay men may be the largest minority group in nursing. These nurses are practising in every province and working in every hospital. Fearing sexual harassment or discrimination from co-workers, superiors, and bureaucratic systems, many remain reluctant to have their sexual orientation known.

Sexual harassment and bigotry is a fact of life for many lesbians and gay men. These kinds of attitudes can range from prejudice to homophobia. Prejudice that operates on the institutional level leads to discrimination. More extreme forms of bigotry include harassment and physical violence. Zurlinden (1997) writes, "Unmasked, homophobia is really hatred, willful ignorance, mean-spiritedness, and narrow-mindedness. People suffering from homophobia do not run screaming in terror when they encounter a lesbian or gay man. Instead, they assume they are justified to be cruel; to discriminate in housing, employment, and education; and to pass laws to prevent gay men and lesbians from enjoying the civil liberties that other Americans take for granted" (p. 11).

Within institutions, hidden *bigotry* can be insidious, damaging, and difficult to change, or even prove. Some employers systematically discriminate against lesbians and gay men through hiring, promotion, and disciplinary practices. This may be the result of institutional policy, discriminatory administrative practices, punitive supervisors, or discrimination by co-workers (Zurlinden, 1997). Discrimination may also take the form of not offering employment benefits that are available to heterosexuals. Though many employers extend spousal benefits such as health insurance, life insurance, and maternity leave to same-gender couples, these may not be available everywhere. The International Council of Nurses *Position Statement on Ethical Nurse Recruitment* cites freedom from discrimination as a guiding principle, stating that "Nurses have the right to expect fair treatment such as working conditions, promotion and continuing education" (ICN, 2007).

While there has been progress in recognizing and dealing with issues of discrimination against persons for their sexual orientation, much remains to be done. Tolerance for behaviours, language, or practice that discriminates against persons for their gender or sexual orientation, in any context or institution, is difficult to understand or endorse in any way. Federal and provincial position statements and legislation exist for supporting non-discriminatory practices and having zero tolerance for anything otherwise. However, leading organizations such as the Canadian Nurses Association and provincial nursing regulatory bodies should take stronger stances on this issue in a public way.

TRANSCULTURAL ISSUES

We live in a multicultural society, alive with diversity. Such diversity of people and backgrounds provides a richness to our lives, yet challenges our abilities to appreciate, rather than judge or fear, differences. **Culture** is a complex phenomenon that can be defined as the worldview, lifestyle, shared knowledge, symbols, and rules for guiding behaviour and creating some degree of shared meaning within a group of persons (Aboriginal Nurses Association of Canada, 2009; Racher & Annis, 2007). **Diversity** is encountered wherever there are differences, whether these be gender, age, socioeconomic position, sexual orientation, health status, ethnicity, race, or culture (Kavanagh, 1993). Dealing with diversity is an essential component of nursing care. Nurses need competence in providing culturally appropriate care. **Cultural competence** (Engebretson & Headley, 2000; Waters, 1996) includes **cultural awareness**—knowledge about values, beliefs, behaviours, and the like of cultures other than one's own—and **cultural sensitivity**—the ability to incorporate the patient's cultural perspective into nursing assessments and to modify nursing care in order to be as congruent as possible with the patient's cultural perspective.

The same phenomenon may be viewed differently by people from different cultures, because culture teaches us to understand a perception of reality. A good example is the experience of death and dying, and how different cultural beliefs result in very divergent perspectives on this universal and real experience. Another way of appreciating different perspectives is to consider what we see when we are in the valley, compared with what we see from halfway up the mountain or the view from the top of the mountain. Different perceptions of the same reality derive from the perspectives from which it is viewed. One view of reality is not more correct than the other; the different views merely come from different perspectives.

The most recent Canadian census data, available post-analysis, notes that one-fifth of the total population of Canada comprises persons who identify themselves as immigrants, i.e., persons who are, or have ever been, landed immigrants (Statistics Canada, 2006). Of the over six million persons who identify as immigrants in Canada, over 1.1 million immigrated between 2001 and 2006. What is not captured in the census, of course, are those persons who may be in Canada as refugees, or with no legal status. Undocumented evidence supports that these numbers may be increasing and that the needs of persons in such groups to maintain health and well-being is of the utmost importance to bring to the attention of the public. Many of the lives of persons without legal status are precarious, invisible to others, and highly dangerous, both in their place of origin and here in Canada. Persons living without legal status may not have access to health care, child care, social services, or other important supports. In cities and communities across Canada, attention must be given to the plight of such persons and how best to accommodate and meet their needs, in a holistic and compassionate manner, given the diverse contexts of each story and situation.

The Canadian Nurses Association (2000) notes that cultural diversity is not merely an issue for large urban areas, as trends demonstrate that increasing numbers of immigrants are moving from major cities out into smaller communities and rural areas.

The census also notes that of the total population of Canada, only half of all persons identify English as the first language used at home in childhood and still understood (Statistics Canada, 2006). This has a tremendous impact on communication and education within the therapeutic nursing relationship.

Other changes in the demographics of Canadians have an effect on how health care should be provided in a holistic and relevant manner. Approximately 45 000 persons identified as being in a same-sex relationship, living in the same household. This is likely to be not only an underestimation of reality, but additionally, not reflective of many same-sex relationships in which persons do not cohabit. Of the 45 000 persons, 7000 identify as married. Again, while these are underestimations and mere glimpses of Canadian demographics, it is clear that the faces of Canadian identity and the notion of family in Canada have been, and are, rapidly changing. In turn, nursing as a profession must not only reflect these kinds of changes by ensuring access to the profession for persons of diverse cultures, races, genders, abilities, and sexual orientation, but also openly discuss, reflect upon, and educate nurses about diversity and the notion of comprehensive cultural competence (Leininger, 2002).

ASK YOURSELF

How Do You Deal with Diversity?

Consider a situation in which you judged someone you did not know because she or he was different from you.

- What about the person or situation triggered your judgment?
- Why do you think you reacted to the person or situation the way you did?
- How and from whom did you learn to react in this way?
- What has helped you to understand diversity?
- How can nurses learn to appreciate rather than fear diversity among colleagues and patients?

Understanding Culture

Self-awareness is a key factor in dealing with transcultural issues. The best starting point for becoming sensitive to the culture of another is to understand our own culture and its influence on our perceptions and behaviours. As we have noted, **culture** is a complex phenomenon that can be defined as the worldview, lifestyle, shared knowledge, symbols, and rules for guiding behaviour and creating shared meaning within a group of persons (Aboriginal Nurses Association of Canada, 2009; Racher & Annis, 2007). These *learned rules and meanings* are passed from one generation to the next in formal ways, such as through educational settings, and in informal ways, such as through role modelling. Unique cultural expressions can be observed within many groups of interacting individuals—for example, the culture of the deaf community, prison culture, or the culture of health care. We need to recognize that each of us is part of a culture and to identify values, beliefs, and behaviours that we hold dear, as these reflect our own cultural perspective. In this process we each must be alert to our own, **culture** is a complex phenomenon that can be defined as the worldview, lifestyle, shared knowledge, symbols, and rules for guiding behaviour and creating shared meaning within a group of persons **ethnocentrism**, reflected in the tendency to judge behaviours of someone from another culture by the standards of our own culture.

Nurses must develop cultural sensitivity, which implies understanding the behaviours and values of another culture within the context of that culture, without imposing our own cultural values on others. In this process we must avoid **stereotyping**, which is expecting all persons from a particular group to behave, think, or respond in a certain way based on preconceived ideas. Every culture contains variation, and some people within the group may not subscribe to all beliefs and values attributed to that culture.

Understanding Diversity

Culturally competent nurses, writes Maier-Lorentz (2008), are those who are not only sensitive to issues and differences "related to culture, race, ethnicity, gender and sexual orientation" (p. 37), but are also willing and eager to engage, on a continual basis, in achieving a seamless ability to work with persons without having cultural differences constrain or confine the therapeutic relationship.

Leininger (2002) notes that cultural competence, at its best, implies a strong awareness of diversity, skills in transcultural knowledge developed over time, and a strong personal and professional respect for those from varying cultures or contexts.

For many, the notion of cultural competence means having an awareness of the varying values and beliefs others may hold, as a result of their culture, race, birthplace, or ethnicity. However, in today's world, cultural competence implies that we also understand that the values and beliefs of others are due to factors related to gender, sexual orientation, family structure, political stance, and socioeconomic status. Differences in approaches to health and illness may arise from sources other than one's culture. As care providers to a wide variety of diverse persons, in terms of factors other than simply culture, nurses need to be aware that, for all of us, our worldview and value system are developed out of other kinds of experiences and personal characteristics. Developing cultural competence, as Leininger and others characterize it, means exploring more than just culture in order to provide holistic care.

Furthermore, in today's multicultural societies, especially in urban centres such as Toronto, Montreal, and Vancouver, many cultures and ethnicities overlap and have far less defined boundaries than in the past. Many persons are born in other countries but identify as Canadian, having immigrated to this country. Identifying persons or assuming values and beliefs based on a person's accent or skin colour is highly problematic. Naively, nurses may not expect that someone who is originally from the Indian subcontinent would not embrace the practices of Ayurvedic medicine to treat and heal illness. Or they may be surprised that a person who is not Chinese adopts practices from Chinese medicine to maintain health or manage chronic illness. Certainly, nurses must deal with their own stereotypes and programmed expectations in order to achieve true cultural competence.

Cultural Safety

The notion of cultural safety (Aboriginal Nurses Association of Canada, 2009; University of Victoria, 2008) goes beyond the three concepts of cultural awareness, cultural sensitivity, and cultural competence, while acknowledging their importance. **Cultural safety** "involves the recognition that we are all bearers of culture and we need to be aware of and challenge unequal power relations at the individual, family, community, and societal level" (University of Victoria, 2008, p. 1). This concept challenges us, in discussions of culture and diversity, to be more open about issues of oppression, unequal power, and social and political contexts that underlie beliefs, practices, and language. The Aboriginal Nurses Association of Canada and the Canadian Association of Schools of Nursing have jointly published a document that is now widely used in nursing education across Canada, titled *Cultural Competence and Cultural Safety in Nursing Education* (2009). In addition to presenting a more contemporary and Canadian perspective on culture in nursing, this document specifically addresses the need to recruit and retain more First Nations, Métis, and Inuit nurses, to better prepare nursing students to work in Aboriginal and First Nations communities, and to more thoroughly present the historical and contextual legacies of Aboriginal persons, along with an emphasis on cultural safety in caring for clients across cultures, and specifically clients from First Nations, Inuit, and Métis populations. The document provides a curriculum framework alongside core competencies that should be incorporated into contemporary nursing education programs across Canada (Aboriginal Nurses Association of Canada, 2009).

ASK YOURSELF

How Might Ethnocentrism Affect Nursing Care?

Consider the varied meanings the following behaviours may have, depending upon the cultural context in which they occur: direct eye contact may

(Continued)

connote honesty or intrusion; a firm handshake may be viewed as confident
or hostile.

- How might behaviours such as these be judged by people within the
  dominant culture in this country?
- How do practices and expectations within health care settings reflect
  ethnocentrism regarding behaviours such as these?
- How might ethnocentrism or stereotyping affect interaction with others,
  especially within a nursing setting?

Cultural Values and Beliefs

Because culture is one of the key organizing concepts of nursing, nurses need to be
actively learning about:

> the health beliefs and values of clients. [This kind of active learning]
> include[s exploring] how these influence their response to health care
> and beliefs about self-care in health and illness, the role of health care
> providers and hospitalization, birth practices, death and dying, family
> involvement, spirituality, customs, rituals, food and alternative or
> traditional therapies. This encourages respectful and open exploration
> of client attitudes, beliefs, perceptions and goals. (CNA, 2000)*

Cultural values and beliefs guide our thinking, being, and doing in patterned ways.
Beliefs about health and practices related to health and healing are some of the patterns
influenced by culture that are significant in providing health care. Such beliefs and
practices manifest in both direct and subtle ways, and sensitivity to them can affect
patient outcomes and satisfaction with care. It is helpful to recognize a distinction
between **disease**, which is demonstrated through pathophysiological or biomedical
signs and diagnostic features, and **illness**, which is a personal or subjective experience
of suffering and is contrasted with health. The way we experience illness, and express
that experience to others, often flows from how our culture teaches us to be sick in a
social context (Emson, 1987; Jennings, 1986). Transcultural issues are often present in
nursing situations, but may not be identified as such. Instead, patients may be labelled
as stoic, unco-operative, noncompliant, strange, or "crazy" because of choices they
make, and their health and care may be compromised. Leininger (1991) has delineated
principles of transcultural care, human rights, and ethical considerations that offer
guidance for nurses in dealing with transcultural issues; these are listed in Figure 17–1.
Although she offers these principles as a guide particularly for transcultural nurses,
they apply as well to other nurses. In light of these principles, many nursing practices
derived from the Western biomedical model may benefit from re-evaluation.

---

* "Cultural Diversity: Changes and Challenges", *Nursing Now: Issues and Trends in Canadian Nursing*
Number 7 © 2000 Canadian Nurses Association. Reprinted with permission. Further reproduction prohibited.

FIGURE 17–1 **TRANSCULTURAL CARE PRINCIPLES, HUMAN RIGHTS, AND ETHICAL CONSIDERATIONS**

1. Human beings of any culture in the world have a right to have their cultural care values known, respected and appropriately used in nursing and other health care services.

2. Human cultures have diverse and universal modes of caring and healing practices that need to be recognized and used by professional nurses to function effectively and therapeutically with people of different cultures.

3. Care is the essence of nursing and a basic human need for growth, healing, well-being, recovery, and survival.

4. Cultural care is a critical component influencing human health, well-being, and recovery from illnesses or disabilities.

5. Every culture has at least two major types of health care systems, namely, the *folk (generic, lay or indigenous) care system* and the *professional care system* which influences their health outcomes, and the transcultural nurse is challenged to use this knowledge to guide nursing care decisions and actions.

6. All professional nurses are challenged to respect common human needs and humanistic aspects of people care worldwide, and also the divergent care expressions, meaning, and practices.

7. Transcultural nurses are expected to respect Western and non-Western cultures which often have different values, beliefs, and norms to assess and understand human beings.

8. Transcultural nursing principles and practices are the arching framework for all nursing care practices which differ from nursing practices that rely on traditional medical symptoms, diseases and treatment regimes.

9. Since transcultural nursing focuses upon *comparative cultural* care values, beliefs and practices of cultures, the nurse is expected to work with individuals, families, groups, cultures, subcultures and institutions that reflect cultural care variabilities.

10. Nurses with transcultural knowledge are expected to respond appropriately to *culture care differences* and *similarities* in order to ease or ameliorate a human condition or lifeway, and to help clients face death.

11. Ethical and moral differences and similarities exist among human cultures which necessitates that nurses recognize, respect, and respond appropriately to such variabilities.

12. It is essential that transcultural nurses be open-minded and willing to learn from cultural informants about their human values, beliefs, needs and practices in order to make appropriate nursing care plans, judgments and actions.

13. The ability of the nurse to listen, use silence and envision the client's or family's human condition or cultural circumstance with its positive or less positive features is important in transcultural nursing.

(Continued)

14. Transcultural nursing often requires that nurses communicate with clients in their native language to know, learn and understand individuals, families and groups of different cultures.

15. Transcultural nurses are challenged to identify what constitutes ethical or moral principles and norms of cultures and not assume that all cultures are alike.

16. Transcultural nurses are expected to guide other nurses who have not been prepared in transcultural nursing in order to prevent marked ethnocentrism, cultural imposition practices, and inappropriate ethical and moral judgments about clients.

17. Transcultural nursing reflects that an individual or group of a designated culture are active participants and decision-makers in culture care practices in order to develop and maintain creative and effective professional care practices.

18. Clients of diverse or similar cultures have a right to have their caring life styles and expressions known and used in transcultural nursing in order to promote client health or well-being.

19. Transcultural nursing takes into account the world view, environmental context, ethnohistory, social structure features (including the religious, kinship, philosophic, economic, political, technological and cultural values), language, expressions, gender and age difference of people.

20. Transcultural nursing is concerned with the assessment of caregiver and carereceiver [sic] expressions, beliefs and lifeways that often go beyond nurse-client dyadic relationship to that of care relationships with families, groups, institutions and communities in order to facilitate congruent care practices and to avoid unfavorable culture care conflicts, stress and negligent care practices.

21. Since ethical, moral and legal systems of human values [sic] and rights exist in all cultures, it is the task and responsibility of transcultural nurses to discover these dimensions with key and general informants and in diverse cultural contexts.

22. Human care rights tend to be covert and embedded in social structure, cultural values and world view of clients, and so the transcultural nurse is challenged to discover these dimensions mainly through qualitative research methods.

23. Transcultural nurses recognize that cultures are complex, dynamic and change over time and in varying ways.

24. Transcultural nurses recognize that many cultures and subcultures in the world have not been studied and yet nurses are expected to care for all peoples, including minorities.

25. Transcultural nursing is a major breakthrough for new nursing knowledge and practices that do not follow the traditional nursing or medical disease, symptom and illness models.

Transcultural Care Principles, Human Rights and Ethical Considerations, Leininger, M. (1991) *Journal of Transcultural Nursing*, 3, 21–23. Reprinted by Permission of SAGE Publications.

Incorporating cultural assessment into care with patients is an important part of a comprehensive nursing assessment. This assessment facilitates better understanding of sometimes overlooked factors that influence health behaviours and decisions. Cultural assessment helps nurses to appropriately identify and understand the meaning of behaviours that might otherwise be judged negatively or be confusing to the nurse (Breton, 2000; Engebretson & Headley, 2000; Giger & Davidhizar, 1995). We must recognize that each person is culturally unique, and that not all persons in a particular cultural group believe or respond the same way. Cultural assessment includes exploration of six cultural phenomena that are evident in all cultural groups: communication, space, social organization, time, environmental control, and biological variation (Engebretson & Headley, 2000; Giger & Davidhizar, 1999). Such exploration enables nurses to identify areas where modifications in care can be incorporated so that care is more culturally congruent. Although the process may also reveal divergent beliefs that are difficult to accommodate within the current health care system, acknowledging differences may help the patient and family to feel more comfortable within the system. For example, when assessing eating patterns and food preferences, the nurse might discover that the patient commonly eats only two meals a day, consisting of burritos in the morning and rice and beans in the evening. Typical hospital food and a three-meals-a-day pattern might not be appetizing for this patient. The patient's nutrition may suffer, and she may perceive that she is not being fed. By arranging for the patient to have culturally similar foods at similar times, the nurse provides more culturally congruent care.

Because Canadian nurses are expected to learn about cultural diversity, knowledge, skills, and attitudes about culture are included in the *1999 CNA Blueprint* for the Registered Nurse Examination. These competencies are: demonstrating consideration for client diversity; providing culturally sensitive care (e.g., openness, sensitivity, recognizing culturally based practices and values); and incorporating cultural practices into health promotion activities.

In order to be able to begin to provide culturally relevant and competent care, the CNA (2000) articulates four nursing responsibilities: to perform cultural assessments, use cultural knowledge, understand communication, and form partnerships. As noted below, from a 2000 article in *Canadian Nurse*, these four responsibilities, alongside strategies to improve responsiveness and awareness at a personal and professional level, are key to developing cultural competence.

Cultural assessment challenges nurses to examine their own attitudes and values about health, illness, and health care. When nurses understand the differences between their own values and beliefs and those of their clients, they can appreciate the strength of both. The plan of care can then become mutually respectful and effective.

Cultural knowledge includes learning about the health beliefs and values of clients. It includes how these influence their response to health care, and beliefs about self-care in health and illness, the role of health care providers and hospitalization, birth practices, death and dying, family involvement, spirituality, customs, rituals, food, and alternative or traditional therapies. This encourages respectful and open exploration of client attitudes, beliefs, perceptions, and goals.

Verbal and nonverbal communication between client and provider can be a barrier to accessibility of services. The use of facial expressions, body language, and norms related to eye contact are examples of nonverbal communication differences that need to be understood. Listening, respecting, and being open are essential. Specialized health care interpreters can be more effective than volunteer translators in interpreting both the words and the meaning of health information in a culturally accurate context.

Partnership among clients, providers, and funding agencies is essential to developing a system that incorporates culturally diverse practices into health care services while optimizing health outcomes for the client. Partners can establish health care needs and mutual goals for individuals and communities, and facilitate client choice (Canadian Nurses Association, 2000).*

 CASE PRESENTATION

Cultural Differences

Angie is a home care nurse in Manitoba. She has been working with the family of a newborn child with complex needs. The family have lived in Canada all their lives and are practising Muslims. The child is now at home, with significant supports for the complex technology and therapy that the child requires on a daily basis. The parents, both well-educated professionals, have learned quickly how to provide the complexity of care that their child requires.

Today Angie is called on an emergent basis by her manager to attend to the family. This morning the child died at home. When Angie arrives, the emergency services are already there and they have called the medical examiner, as is the practice with deaths of unknown causes. The family are distraught and Angie tries to comfort them.

The paramedics inform the family that an autopsy will have to be performed and that the medical examiner will come to collect the child's body for this purpose. The family agree. The child's mother asks the paramedic when the autopsy might be performed. He replies that he is unsure, but likely within 72 hours.

Both parents turn to Angie for help. They tell her that their religious traditions require burial rituals to be performed, if at all possible, within 24 hours of death at their mosque. The paramedic, overhearing, says gently to the family that this is almost impossible, with the volume of cases to which the medical examiner must attend. He goes on to say that this is not unusual, and it is "always" the case that people have to wait this long.

---

* "Cultural Diversity: Changes and Challenges" *Nursing Now: Issues and Trends in Canadian Nursing* © 2000 Canadian Nurses Association. Reprinted with permission. Further reproduction prohibited.

? THINK ABOUT IT

How Can Nurses Develop Cultural Competence?

- In what way is there a demonstrable lack of cultural competence?
- How can Angie help to make the care, from all, at this point, to be more culturally sensitive?
- In this case, what strategies do you see as an important step in helping to avoid this situation recurring?
- For now, if you were Angie, what would you do to advocate for your clients?

Culture and the Health Care System

Concepts of health and healing, of right and wrong, of what is proper and what is not, are rooted in culture. Cultures have different explanatory models regarding health and illness that reflect their beliefs about the causes, symptoms, and treatments of illness, and response to dying and death. Our explanatory model helps us to recognize, respond to, interpret, cope with, and make sense of illness and other life experiences (Engebretson & Headley, 2000).

Transcultural issues arise when nurses, patients, and families hold differing views of what is important or necessary regarding health, recovery, illness, or the dying process. The contemporary health care system is not user-friendly when it comes to incorporating diversity. By virtue of its history, the system reflects predominantly middle-class, European American, Judeo-Christian, paternalistic values and perspectives (Kavanagh, 1993). This system includes the attitude that the health care provider knows what is "best for the patient," as viewed from the health provider's perspective.

The health provider's perspective generally derives from a combination of two cultural orientations. The primary cultural orientation is the biomedical model, and the secondary cultural orientation is the provider's personal cultural background. If the patient's perspective is different from this model and is not considered, dilemmas may emerge. Consider, for example, a situation in which the physician, who is schooled in the Western biomedical model, views death as "the enemy" to be overcome at all costs. The patient, who comes from an Aboriginal culture, views death as a part of life that one prepares for by being in harmony with one's surroundings. Medical or surgical interventions that may prolong the patient's life for a few weeks, which would be very important in the physician's worldview, may be very low on the list of considerations for this patient.

We must be aware that the health care system is a different culture from that of most of the patients served by the system. The language, values, norms, behaviours, rituals, and environment are generally unfamiliar to those who seek its services. Even people who belong to the same dominant culture in society as their health care providers are often strangers when they enter the institutions of the system. For those who do not belong to the dominant culture, negotiating the system can be a formidable task. Lack of understanding of language, procedures, expectations, and other elements of the culture can lead to miscommunication, unclear decisions, and a sense of powerlessness or lack of control. Ethical dilemmas may arise due to misunderstandings. Consider the case of a mentally alert ninety-year-old woman who, after her doctor of thirty-five years retired, sought care from a new young physician. After a few visits she stopped going to see him, even though she was having serious health problems, because, in her perception, he did not do anything for her. Essentially, he did not talk with her nor spend the kind of time with her that her former physician had, and instead gave her medicines that she felt made her sick and that she did not need.

In turn, the physician may have also felt that he was providing thorough and holistic care. He may have decided that the priority of care was not to have long discussions, but to carefully and thoroughly treat the elderly woman's medical problems. In examining common problems such as these, we often discover that while the problem appears to be an issue of diverse or conflicting values and practices, usually it is simply a matter of miscommunication, lack of effective communication, or a lack of the time to understand the priorities of the other.

When we speak of values such as autonomy, beneficence, justice, or the right to self-determination, we must ask from whose perspective these values are understood—that of the nurse or that of the patient. This same question is appropriate regarding definitions of health. For example, many cultures place a higher emphasis on loyalty to the group than on the self-reliance and autonomy valued within the broader North American Culture (Andrews, 1999; Davis, 1999; Ludwick & Silva, 2000). Health care decisions in these cultures are often made by a group such as the family, community, or society, rather than by the individual.

As Ellis and Early (2006) note, Aboriginal persons define themselves as part of a collective and a community. Their identity is rooted within a community and a deep sense of the shared is part of their culture and everyday decision making processes. This paradigm can be contrasted to that of what we consider to be mainstream North American culture, in which great worth is placed on the individual; therefore, individual decision making in matters related to health care is valued, and even cherished, above all. For Aboriginal persons, health is maintained by a connection to not only the environment, but also the community around oneself (University of Victoria, 2008). These ideas are not new as fundamental parts of Aboriginal culture. But for some nurses, these ideas and values may not be in "alignment" with the traditional North American biomedical model, which is part of much of our health care system.

Cultural assessment provides insight into the congruence, or lack thereof, between patients' and nurses' values and understandings of health. Consider, for example, a situation in which the nurse believes that health includes being able to be a productive member of society and that health problems provide opportunities for one to grow and become more self-actualized. The patient, on the other hand, believes that his work-related injury is an act of *fate* and focuses on being free of pain and able to "get around." If the differing perceptions of health are not recognized and addressed, efforts to have the patient participate in rehabilitation and job retraining or to utilize nonpharmacological measures for pain control may meet with much resistance and, justifiably, patient dissatisfaction.

Legal Considerations Related to Transcultural Issues

Cultural misunderstandings can provide fertile ground for litigation. Communication—verbal, nonverbal, and written—is always of the utmost importance. When a patient's first language is different from that of the nurse, we must determine the extent of the patient's understanding of the nurse's language. When the patient uses another language (including sign language), having an interpreter fluent in the patient's language is essential. If the interpreter is a member of the patient's family, the translation may be filtered through the perspective of the family member. Consider, for example, an elderly Cambodian man who is in the hospital and not doing well. His grandson serves as interpreter. The grandson was born in this country and is embarrassed by his grandfather's "old" ways. When the man says that he needs a particular traditional herbal tea each afternoon in order to get well (which is available in a local ethnic store), the grandson translates this generically as "tea." Even though the nurse responds by making sure that the patient has tea each afternoon, the patient's needs are not met.

The language in which we explain procedures and consent forms presents other issues. Be sure that the patient or family member is able to read the language in which the form is written, and that all the terms used are understood. If the form needs to be interpreted for the patient, it is essential that the interpreter understands the procedure and that an appropriate person is available to clarify any areas of uncertainty. Many hospitals and health care agencies have translators available. Additionally, many health care practitioners and staff speak languages other than English, and can assist. People may indicate that they understand when they do not, in order to avoid offending the nurse or being considered ignorant. One way of dealing with this is having patients describe in their own words what they have been told. Most importantly, adequate time must be set aside to explain procedures and consent processes to those who may require additional time or the services of a translator.

SUMMARY

Issues of gender and culture have profound effects upon nursing practice and health care. Nursing has been faced with gender issues since the early days of the profession and these issues pervade our practice roles and views. Nursing's role and status has been coloured by societal expectations of women and the feminization of nursing care. Considerations of gender can have an influence on salaries and job status, communication and interactions with other health care professionals and patients, perceptions of abilities, and stereotypical expectations of how nurses should look and act. Men in the profession also face challenges in dealing with societal stereotypes in a female-dominated profession. Awareness of the kinds of unique issues encountered by nurses of all genders helps nurses to recognize inequities and to develop strategies for effective, equitable change. In addition to paying attention to issues of gender, nurses must be attentive to cultural aspects of care. The diversity of cultures and spiritual expressions within our society requires that nurses be able to identify concerns and issues in these areas and address them competently and confidently. Familiarity with the values, beliefs, and practices of various cultures is a useful adjunct to careful cultural assessments with patients. Self-awareness regarding our own cultural values, beliefs, and expressions is necessary in order to address these areas with patients. Such awareness enables us to act from our own cultural perspectives, while taking care not to impose these views on others. Part of providing holistic nursing care means being attuned to issues of culture and gender that can have an impact on nurses who are working within diverse professional groups, and on those to whom we provide care. In reflecting upon the care we provide in light of the issues identified in this chapter, care planning can become much more relevant to the individual patient's cultural and gender-based expressions and experiences.

CHAPTER HIGHLIGHTS

- Controversy exists regarding how the title of the person caring for the sick relates to the gender of the person providing care. Both women and men in nursing must deal with social stereotyping regarding expected roles and behaviours.

- Societal expectations of women and paternalistic ideology throughout history have led to discrimination in nursing, though gender discrimination may exist for both women and men in different nursing settings.

- Issues of comparable worth relative to gender are of concern in nursing, particularly in areas of salary and positions of prestige and responsibility.

- Nurses need to be alert to sexual harassment and employ strategies to combat it.

- Gender-based differences in styles and patterns of communication can affect all areas of nursing practice, requiring attentiveness to effective communication with patients and colleagues in order to foster better patient outcomes.

- Sexism, occurring in both subtle and overt ways, continues to be an issue in nursing, and harassment and discrimination based on sexual orientation may be underrecognized.

- Since culture influences beliefs and behaviours regarding health and healing, cultural assessment is integral to a comprehensive nursing assessment.

- Providing effective nursing care within the diversity of our multicultural society requires cultural competence on the part of nurses. Cultural competence can help prevent dilemmas from arising when there are differences in cultural perspective between patient and nurse.

DISCUSSION QUESTIONS AND ACTIVITIES

1. One frequently cited political action strategy is to build coalitions with "powerful persons of like mind" (Hamilton, 1996). If nurses in your community are to become empowered, with whom would they build coalitions?

2. Read an article on how nursing students learn to care. Do you think that men learn about, or express, caring differently than women? How does this relate to your experiences as a student nurse? How does this relate to Begany's (1994) images of nurturer or handmaiden?

3. What stereotypes of nurses are present in your community or national media? What types of "get well" cards are in your local card shop? What do you think it will take to change these and other stereotypes about nurses?

4. What is the gender makeup of your local nursing administration? How many women are in positions of authority or power within your health care setting?

5. Observe gender-based communication patterns between nurses and physicians. Consider your own style of communication with same-gender and other-gender friends and colleagues. What patterns do you identify? How might these patterns affect your professional interactions? Are there areas that need to be modified in order to promote more effective communication?

6. Explore various Web sites to find the guidelines regarding sexual harassment that are offered by the Canadian Nurses Association and other professional organizations.

7. Consider how your cultural values affect personal choices regarding health and healing. Discuss this with other students, noting similarities and differences.

8. What aspects of the dominant culture or cultures within the health care system are difficult for you as a nurse? Identify personal conflicts and the beliefs and values underlying them.

9. Recall a time when you or someone you know experienced a conflict with persons within the health care system. What values, beliefs, or understandings contributed to this conflict?

10. Discuss patient health care choices or behaviours based upon cultural beliefs or gender differences that might present a dilemma for you. Consider how you would approach the situation in a professional manner and describe the ethical stance that would guide your decisions.

11. Reflect upon how the social construction of gender and culture may have an impact on access to and treatment within the health care system, issues of social justice, and marginalization.

REFERENCES

Aboriginal Nurses Association of Canada (2009). *Cultural Competence and Cultural Safety in Nursing Education.* Aboriginal Nurses Association of Canada: Ottawa.

Achterberg, J. (1990). *Woman as healer.* Boston, MA: Shambhala.

Anderson, F., J. Maloney, D. Oliver, D. Brown & M. Hardy (1996). Nurse-physician communication: Perceptions of nurses at an army medical center. *Military Medicine, 161,* 411–415.

Andrews, M. M. (1999). Cultural diversity in the health care workforce. In M. M. Andrews & J. S. Broyle, *Transcultural concepts in nursing care* (3rd ed., pp. 471–506).

Anonymous. (2007). New Canada-wide group promotes men in nursing. *The Canadian Nurse, 103*(8), p. 7.

Begany, T. (1994). Your image is brighter than ever. *RN, 57,* 28–35.

Benokraitis, N. V., & J. R. Feagin (1995). *Modern sexism: Blatant, subtle, and covert discrimination* (2nd ed.). Englewood Cliffs, NJ: Prentice-Hall.

Bernardi, A. (1996, Winter). Untitled. [Letter to the editor]. Interaction, *Newsletter of the American Assembly for Men in Nursing,* p. 3.

Breton, J. H. (2000). Treating beyond color: Health issues for minority women. *Advance for Nurse Practitioners,* (November), 65–68, 101.

Campbell-Heider, N., & C. Hart (1993). Updating the nurse's bedside manner. *Image, 25,* 133–139.

Canadian Labour Congress. (2005). *Pay equity.* Retrieved June 15, 2012, from http://www.canadianlabour.ca/issues/pay-equity

Canadian Nurses Association. (2000). Cultural diversity: Changes and challenges. *The Canadian Nurse. 96:2.*

Canadian Nurses Association. (2011). *2009 Workplace profile of registered nurses in Canada.* Ottawa: Author.

Chinn, P. L. (1991). *Anthology on caring.* New York: National League of Nursing Press.

Corser, W. D. (1998). A conceptual model of collaborative nurse-physician interactions: The management of traditional influences and personal tendencies. *Scholarly Inquiry for Nursing Practice, 12*(4), 343–346.

Davis, A. J. (1999). Global influence of American nursing: Some ethical issues. *Nursing Ethics: An International Journal for Health Care Professionals, 6*(2), 118–125.

Department of Justice Canada. (2001). *Canadian Human Rights Act* (R.S., 1985, c. H-6). Government of Canada: Ottawa. Retrieved August 15, 2008, from http://laws.justice.gc.ca/en/showdoc/cs/H-6///en?page=1.

Department of Justice, Government of Canada. (1982). *Charter of Rights and Freedoms. Schedule B. Constitution Act, 1982.* Retrieved August 17, 2008, from http://laws.justice.gc.ca/en/const/annex_e.html#I.

Ekstrom, D. N. (1999). Gender and perceived caring in nurse-patient dyads. *Journal of Advanced Nursing, 29*(6), 1393–1401.

Ellis, J., & C. Hartley (2003). *Nursing in today's world* (8th ed.). Philadelphia, PA: Lippincott.

Ellis, J. B., & M. A. Early (2006). Reciprocity and constructions of informed consent: Researching with indigenous populations. *International Journal of Qualitative Methods, 5*(4), Article 1. Retrieved July 11, 2008, from http://www.ejournals.library.ualberta.ca/index.php/IJQM/article/view/4356/3803.

Emson, H. E. (1987). Health, disease and illness: Matters for definition. *Canadian Medical Association Journal, 136*(8), 811–813.

Engebretson, J. C., & J. A. Headley (2000). Cultural diversity and care. In B. M. Dossey, L. Keegan & C. E. Guzzetta, *Holistic nursing: A handbook for practice* (3rd ed., pp. 283–310). Gaithersburg, MD: Aspen.

Feist-Price, S. (1994). Cross-gender mentoring relationships: Critical issues. *Journal of Rehabilitation, 60*, 13–17.

Giger, J. N., & R. E. Davidhizar (1995). *Transcultural nursing: Assessment and intervention* (2nd ed.). St. Louis, MO: Mosby.

Giger, J. N., & R. E. Davidhizar (1999). *Transcultural nursing: Assessment and intervention* (5th ed.). St. Louis, MO: Mosby.

Gilloran, A. (1995). Gender differences in care delivery and supervisory relationship: The case of psychogeriatric nursing. *Journal of Advanced Nursing, 21*, 652–658.

Grigsby, K., & M. Megel (1995). Caring experiences of nurse educators. *Journal of Nursing Education, 34*, 411–418.

Hamilton, P. (1996). *Realities of contemporary nursing*. Menlo Park, CA: Addison-Wesley.

International Council of Nurses. (2006). *The ICN code of Ethics for nursing*, Geneva, Switzerland: Imprimerie Fornara.

International Council of Nurses. (2007). *Position statement on ethical nurse recruitment*. Geneva: ICN. Retrieved January 19, 2009, from http://www.icn.ch/psrecruit01.htm.

Jennings, D. (1986). The confusion between disease and illness in clinical medicine. *Canadian Medical Association Journal, 135*(8), 865–870.

Kane, D., & B. Thomas (2000). Nursing and the "F" word. *Nursing Forum, 35*(2), 17–24.

Kavanagh, K. (1996). Social and cultural dimensions of health and health care. In J. Creasia & B. Parker, eds., *Conceptual foundations of nursing practice* (pp. 285–308). St. Louis, MO: Mosby.

Kavanagh, K. H. (1993). Transcultural nursing: Facing the challenges of advocacy and diversity/universality. *Journal of Transcultural Nursing, 5*, 4–13.

Leininger, M. (1991). Transcultural care principles, human rights, and ethical considerations. *Journal of Transcultural Nursing, 3*, 21–22.

Leininger, M. (2002). Culture care theory: A major contribution to advance transcultural nursing knowledge and practice. *Journal of Transcultural Nursing, 13*(3), 189–192.

Lewenson, S. B. (1996). *Taking charge: Nursing suffrage & feminism in America, 1873–1920*. New York: National League of Nursing Press.

Ludwick, R. & M. C. Silva (August 14, 2000). Nursing around the world: Cultural values and ethical conflicts. *Online journal of issues in nursing*. Retrieved January 8, 2001, from http://www .nursingworld.org/ojin/ethicol/ethics_4.html.

Madison, J., & V. Minichiello (2000). Recognizing and labeling sex-based and sexual harassment in the health care workplace. *Journal of Nursing Scholarship, 32*(4), 405–410.

Maier-Lorentz, M. M. (2008). Transcultural nursing: Its importance in nursing practice. *Journal of Cultural Diversity, 15*(1), 37–44.

Marinaki v. Human Resources Development Canada (2000), TD 3/00 (C.H.R.T.).

Meadus, R. J., & J. Creina Twomey (2007). Men in nursing: Making the right choice. *The Canadian Nurse, 103*(2), 13–6.

Nightingale, F. (1859/1992). *Notes on nursing: What it is, and what it is not*. London: Harrison & Sons.

Ontario Human Rights Commission. (2008). *Sexual harassment. Your rights and responsibilities*. Retrieved January 2, 2009, from http://www.ohrc.on.ca/en/issues/sexual_harassment.

Peter, E., & R. Gallop (1994). The ethic of care: A comparison of nursing and medical students. *Image, 26,* 47–51.

Porter, S. (1992). Women in a women's job: The gendered experience of nurses. *Sociology of Health and Illness, 14*(4), 510–526.

Propst, M. (1996). Registered nurses' practice and perspective toward sexuality in women's health. *Southern Nursing Research Society Abstracts,* 83.

Racher, F. E. & R. C. Annis (2007). Respecting culture and honoring diversity in community practice. *Research and Theory for Nursing Practice, 21*(4), 255–270.

Reskin, B., & I. Padavic (1994). *Women and men at work*. Thousand Oaks, CA: Pine Forge Press.

Shortell, S., J. Zimmerman, D. Rousseau, R. Gillies, D. Wagner, E. Draper, W. Knaus & J. Duffy (1994). The performance of intensive care units: Does good management make a difference? *Medical Care, 32,* 508–525.

Squires, T. (1995). Men in nursing. *RN, 58,* 26–28.

Statistics Canada. (2005). *Population by religion, by provinces and territories*. Retrieved January 19, 2009, from http://www.statcan.gc.ca/tables-tableaux/sum-som/l01/cst01/demo30a-eng.htm.

Statistics Canada. (2006). *2006 Census*. Retrieved August 26, 2012, from http://www12.statcan.gc.ca/census-recensement/2006/dp-pd/92-596/index.cfm?Lang=eng.

Stein, L. (1967). The nurse-doctor game. *Archives of General Psychiatry, 16,* 699–703.

Stein, L., D. Watts & T. Howell (1990). The doctor-nurse game revisited. *New England Journal of Medicine, 322,* 546–549.

Stevens, P. (1995). Structural and interpersonal impact of heterosexual assumptions on lesbian health care clients. *Nursing Research, 44,* 25–30.

Sullivan, E. J. (2000). Men in nursing: The importance of gender diversity. *Journal of Professional Nursing, 16*(5), 253–254.

Tannen, D. (1990). *You just don't understand: Women and men in conversation*. New York: Ballantine.

Tosh-Kennedy, T. (2007). Increasing the numbers. *The Canadian Nurse, 103*(2), 17.

Twenge, J. (2006). *Generation Me: Why today's young Americans are more confident, assertive, entitled—and more miserable than ever before.* New York: Free Press.

The United Nations Committee on the Elimination of Discrimination against Women (CEDAW). (1979). *Convention on the Elimination of all Forms of Discrimination against women*: New York: United Nations.

University of Victoria. (2008). *Cultural safety: Peoples' experiences of colonization in relation to health care.* Modules 1, 2 and 3.

U.S. Department of Health and Human Services Health Resources and Services Administration (HRSA) (2010). *The Registered Nurse Population: Findings from the 2008 National Sample Survey of Registered Nurses.* Rockville, MD: HRSA.

Valentine, P. E. B. (1995). Management of conflict: Do nurses/women handle it differently? *Journal of Advanced Nursing, 22*, 142–149.

Valentine, P. E. B. (2010). A gender perspective on conflict management strategies of nurses. *Journal of Nursing Scholarship, 33*(1), 69–74.

van Ooijen, E., & A. Charnock (1995). How men and women view the world: A sexual perspective. *Nursing Times, 91*, 38–39.

Vere-Jones, E. (2008). Why are there so few men in nursing? *Nursing Times, 104*(9), 18.

Waters, C. (1996). Professional development in nursing—A culturally diverse postdoctoral experience. *Image, 28*, 47–50.

Williams, C. (1995). Hidden advantages for men in nursing. *Nursing Administration Quarterly, 19*, 63–70.

Zurlinden, J. (1997). *Lesbian and gay nurses.* Albany, NY: Delmar.

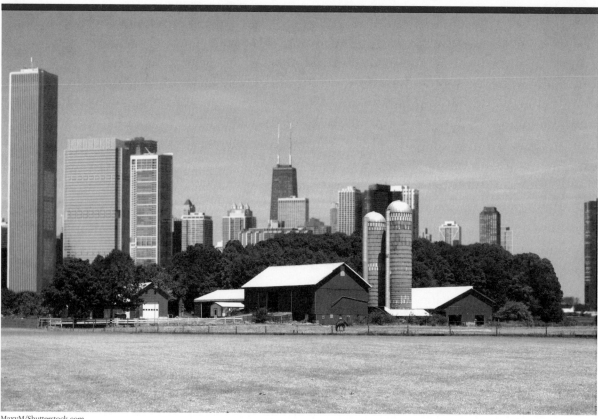

MaxyM/Shutterstock.com

CHAPTER **18**
RURAL AND ABORIGINAL NURSING IN CANADA

OBJECTIVES

1. To discuss the different health problems and challenges facing urban and rural Canada.
2. To define rural and remote nursing.
3. To articulate the unique professional role of the rural nurse.
4. To highlight the professional and practice challenges of rural nursing.
5. To discuss Aboriginal health in Canada.
6. To identify unique health problems and challenges related to Aboriginal health.
7. To articulate the role of the nurse in Aboriginal health care and promotion.

INTRODUCTION

For many, the idea of a life working and living in a rural area is idyllic. The notion of an escape from the hectic pace, crowding, and anonymity of city living is, for many, a positive prospect. With an estimated 20 percent of Canadians living in rural areas (Human Resources and Skills Development Canada, 2006), alongside an increasing demand and need for health services in rural areas, rural health is an area that will require more attention from nurses, professional bodies, and policy makers at all levels of government. As more active recruitment of nurses into rural areas continues in urban nursing schools, the topic will be one that educators must also address.

RURAL NURSING

For many new graduates contemplating employment opportunities, the idea of living in a rural town or in the countryside, and providing nursing care to a small popu-lation, with a more independent practice and closer, more personal relationships with patients, is very appealing. With increased communications technology and the Internet, along with social networking, being in a rural setting no longer means being socially or professionally as isolated, as many nurses have been in the past. However, from what we know about rural nursing, it can present its own unique challenges. Often working with limited resources, having an ever-expanding scope of practice and very few opportunities for privacy in a small rural town, may, for many, offset the advantages of living and working closer to nature and being removed from the concrete jungle. For some nurses, the move to rural nursing may be a return to an area where they grew up or otherwise have a connection. Or, some nurses might make the decision to practice rural nursing because of a positive rural clinical expe-rience in their undergraduate education (Lea and Cruikshank, 2005), although, for many nurses being educated in large urban centres, the opportunity to experience a more rural clinical setting is rare. One thing is very clear from what we know about rural nursing, and that is that rural nursing is a specialty unto itself, with diverse roles and scope of practice, professional challenges and professional rewards that are quite different from those of a nurse working in a large downtown hospital in a busy city like Vancouver, Ottawa, or Montreal.

Canada's Rural Environments

If you ask people what "rural" means, most people tend to try to define "rural" by what it is *not*, that is, it is "non-urban." When we think about rural areas, we typically think about areas with less population density that are relatively distant from urban centres. Rural areas tend to be defined by having a more widely scattered population, and their "rural-ness" exists in gradations or iterations. For example, rural areas closer to cities will experience more influence from the cities, as compared to rural areas farther away from urban centres, or large cities. (Public Health Agency of Canada [PHAC], 2006) Because many rural areas close to cities exist as "bedroom communities" or "bedroom suburbs" within what is known as a "commuter belt," many who live in these areas commute to the city to work and return home to a more rural area each night. Thus, these kinds of rural areas will have certain kinds of infrastructures, such as highways and roads, along with easier access to cities by public transportation, that support commuting lifestyles. They will also experience what we call "urban sprawl" as cities tend to grow outwards, both geographically and in influence, and extend into the surrounding rural areas.

Our definition of rural affects the number of people we identify as living in a rural area. In Canada, anywhere between 20 and 30 percent of Canadians are defined as living in a rural environment (PHAC, 2006). From a demographic perspective, when compared to urban areas, a higher proportion of the rural population consists of dependent persons, with a higher population of children and youth (up to 19 years of age) and seniors (age 65 and older). Migration patterns play a role in this distribution, as youth in rural areas move to cities to find a wider variety of opportunities, and older people may leave the cities to retire in more rural settings (PHAC, 2006).

In general, evidence suggests that, on average, families tend to have lower incomes in rural areas compared with those in urban areas. Average levels of education are lower in many rural populations (PHAC, 2006). There has been a trend noted over the last fifteen years of more new immigrants and visible minorities in cities and more urbanized areas (PHAC, 2006). Urban areas also tend to be more ethnically diverse, although this trend may be changing.

From a population health perspective, it is important to examine the many contextual and interrelated factors that can contribute to people's health and well-being in order to guide policy-makers. A population health approach typically has a strong **social justice** aspect, in that one of its goals is to reduce inequities between groups and populations. Through the kinds of data that a population health approach uncovers, such an approach also aims to make recommendations about ways to reduce inequities between populations in terms of health outcomes or access to health care (Federal/Provincial/Territorial Advisory Committee on Population Health [FPT-ACPH], 1996). This approach considers much more than the health status of individuals within a population. It also considers the complex interaction of contextual factors that can contribute, directly or indirectly, to the health of individuals, communities, and populations. Factors that can be considered include the physical environment, weather, the economy, dominant discourses, cultures, the political system, the health care system, use of and access to health care, and other factors related to the social determinants of health (PHAC, 2006).

A population approach can be helpful when looking at rural health, because what is being examined is the health of a population with very different kinds of health-related and lifestyle factors than populations living in urban environments. One drawback is that a population approach may not fully enable us to appreciate the differences *between* one rural population and another. If we consider Canada's various rural populations, there are significant differences between the lives of people living in rural areas within an hour's drive to Toronto or Ottawa, say, and people living in much more remote rural areas such as northern Alberta or many parts of Newfoundland and Labrador (PHAC, 2006). But as a start, and as a way to appreciate both the similarities and differences in health and wellness between those in rural areas and those in urban areas, a population health approach makes sense.

Rural Health

While urban and rural populations in Canada share many of the same kinds of health problems, there are also some unique health issues, concerns, and problems found in rural communities. The Public Health Agency of Canada conducted a pan-Canadian study examining the health and health-related issues in rural areas in 2006, and the report resulting from that study presents a broad and inclusive picture of rural health across the country (PHAC, 2006). The report presents some clear findings of significant differences in health and illness between those living in urban areas and those living in rural areas. Those in rural areas have been found to have a higher incidence of smoking and obesity, alongside lower rates "healthy heart" practices, such as healthy diets, increased physical activity, and smoking cessation activities. While there is a higher rate of mortality due to respiratory disease in rural areas, women in some rural areas closer to cities report much less respiratory disease, e.g. asthma, than comparable women in urban environments.

Deaths due to circulatory disease, suicide, and injuries are more common in rural areas than in urban areas, but these kinds of problems vary with the "degree of ruralness." In other words, those who live in rural areas that are farther from urban centres are reported to be at a higher risk for such kinds of problems (PHAC, 2006). Deaths from motor vehicle accidents are more common for those living in rural areas, likely because people must drive longer distances for day-to-day activities in rural areas. While descriptive studies, such as the one by the Public Health Agency of Canada (2006), do not prove causation, it is clear that living in a rural area implies different kinds of health concerns and problems than living in an urban area.

In addition to looking at patterns of health status, it is important to consider issues related to health *care* in rural areas. People in rural areas may have less access to emergency care, specialized care, and intensive care. It is easy to see that if a woman suffered a massive heart attack on a downtown street in Toronto or Calgary, she would be in an emergency room in minutes, and have access to critical cardiac care or surgery, if required, within a matter of hours. In fact, a woman who has a heart attack in downtown Toronto may well be able to *choose* which urban acute-care cardiac centre she wishes to be taken to. A similar woman suffering a similar heart attack in a remote or rural area may well have an increased chance of dying, as the closest hospital may be many hours away and there may be a lack of specialized services available at the closest centre. Many patients who arrive with critical illnesses at remote or very rural hospitals require transport to more specialized hospitals in bigger centres in order to access specialized or critical care or to undergo surgery. With some diseases or acute illnesses, a wait to access specialized care may contribute to increased complications or risk of death. Access to timely health care, and to the right health care, continues to be a challenge in rural areas across Canada (MacLeod, Kulig, Stewart & Pitblado, 2004). Of course, that doesn't mean access to timely and appropriate care in *urban* areas is without challenges. Challenges related to accessing care in urban environments do exist, but they are significantly different in nature than those experienced by rural dwellers.

THE CHALLENGES OF RURAL NURSING

Rural nurses are "as diverse as the settings they work in" (MacLeod *et al.*, 2004, p. 27). The uniqueness of rural and remote nursing is emphasized in the literature, and we know already that rural nursing differs from nursing in urban centres for reasons that are directly related to geographical isolation, limited access to health care resources, a more varied and broader scope of practice, and different types of social connections and networks in rural areas (Zibrik, MacLeod & Zimmer, 2010).

The challenges of having a more autonomous and isolated practice, with a scope of practice that evolves out of need, rather than in an organized or planned way, is why many nurses in rural or remote settings have characterized themselves as a "jack of all trades, master of none" (Hegney, McCarthy, Rogers-Clark & Gorman, 2002, p. 179).

There is still relatively little literature on what rural nursing is, and the challenges rural nurses face that are distinct from those in urban centres have yet to be fully explored and described. However, a number of nursing scholars have begun to describe what it means to be a nurse in a rural or remote setting in Canada. Groups like the Canadian Association for Rural and Remote Nursing (CARRN) (see Figure 18-1), an associate group of the Canadian Nurses Association (CNA), and the Rural

FIGURE 18–1 **OBJECTIVES OF THE CANADIAN ASSOCIATION FOR RURAL AND REMOTE NURSING**

> ### The objectives of the Canadian Association for Rural and Remote Nursing include:
>
> - To promote the development and dissemination of standards of practice
> - To facilitate communication and networking
> - To present the views of the CARRN to government, educational, professional and other appropriate bodies
> - To explicate the evolving roles and functions of rural and remote nurses
> - To identify and promote educational opportunities
> - To promote the conduct and dissemination of research
> - To collaborate with the key stakeholders on the development of sound health policy for those living in rural and remote Canada
>
> "Rural and Remote Nursing Practice Parameters" © 2008, Canadian Association for Rural and Remote Nursing/Canadian Nurses Association. Reprinted with permission. Further reproduction prohibited.

Nursing Organization (RNO) in the U.S., have helped to highlight the unique role of the rural nurse and to advocate for increased attention to, and resources for, nurses who practice in rural settings.

Professionalism in Rural Nursing

Maintaining professionalism in a rural setting may be quite different from doing so in an urban acute-care hospital. Having overlapping professional and personal roles and interacting with community members in both these roles, on a consistent basis, may make it difficult to maintain clear professional boundaries.

Professionalism is one aspect of nursing that contributes to nurses' satisfaction with their work, across a variety of settings. What does it mean to be professional for rural nurses, and how is this different from their counterparts in urban environments?

Professionalism is a collective notion that refers to the aims, the conduct, and the attributes that distinguish a group of persons who are professionals from non-professionals. The Registered Nurses Association of Ontario (RNAO) has published a *Best Practice Guideline* outlining what it means to be a professional nurse. In this document, eight attributes of nursing professional practice are identified, as follows: Knowledge, spirit of inquiry, accountability, autonomy, advocacy, innovation and visionary, collegiality and collaboration, ethics and values (RNAO, 2007). These attributes pertain to nurses across a variety of practice settings and contexts. However, in reality, many of them may be actualized differently, according to where a nurse practices. For example, autonomy in nursing practice may look quite different in a busy urban urgent care clinic where teamwork and interdisciplinary approaches are the norm, than in a small remote town where two nurses make up the entire staff most days in the local health clinic. Having an autonomous practice in a remote or rural setting may not be a privilege of a profession, but rather an inevitability related to the reality of practice. As another example, consider the RNAO's mention of innovation. Innovation for a rural nurse may be enacted simply because of a lack of supplies or resources. In such a situation, a rural nurse may be very capable of adapting inadequate or out-of-date equipment very well in order to meet the needs of his or her patients, or may be creative in advocating for newer, more up-to-date equipment. A rural nurse may have no choice but to be an innovator who can problem-solve independently. When faced with little to no IV fluids, or while waiting for a shipment, an innovative rural nurse with significant experience might mix up normal saline by hand, on a stove, by boiling a mixture of salt and water, and letting it cool (Community Care Access Centre, 2012).

The literature suggests that nurses in rural and remote settings share many concerns in terms of being able to practice as effectively as nurses in more urban environments. However, nurses in rural areas have different concerns when it comes to being able to engage in professional practice, ranging from dealing with inadequate equipment to having access to continuing education and opportunities for teamwork, coping with a broad and difficult-to-define scope of practice, and fostering a sense of community and overlapping professional and personal roles (Henderson Betkus and MacLeod,

2004; Kulig *et al.*, 2009; Penz, Stewart, D'Arcy and Morgan, 2008; Zibric, MacLeod and Zimmer, 2010).

Boundaries, Obligations, and Confidentiality

Nurses working in many rural areas are faced with the reality of being very visible in the communities where they work. They are embedded within communities where people know each other, and are often aware of each others' habits and lifestyles. Higher visibility within a smaller community can be a challenge for a rural nurse, who may find his or her work-life and leisure time overlapping, as the interactions are with many of the same people. The waitress at a local restaurant may be a patient, as might the cashier at a local grocery store. Anonymity is difficult, and may well be impossible, for a nurse in a rural setting. As one nurse in a study noted, "there is no place to hide" (Zibric, MacLeod and Zimmer, 2010, p. 26). It is almost impossible, for many rural nurses, to clearly separate their work and personal life, as highlighted in Mark's case, later in this chapter.

Being embedded or enmeshed within a community can present both challenges and rewards. For many, working in a busy urban clinic where patients rarely return or are seen once or twice without the ability to follow up can, over time, be frustrating or feel less rewarding. Having long-standing relationships with patients and being able to see those patients through a variety of health challenges and life events, on the other hand, can be very rewarding. It also gives a nurse the opportunity to provide more holistic nursing care, including health teaching and health promotional activities, and to follow up with patients regarding the effectiveness of these kinds of interventions. Additionally, some nurses quite like the experience of being approached in public places by patients asking advice or asking quick questions about their health or illness. While such interactions do imply a considerable overlap between work and personal life for the nurse, and imply that there is no real time off from being a nurse, some nurses value these expressions of trust and rapport with their patients, who are also their neighbours and members of the same community. Some nurses have said that it makes them feel more professional, more respected, and an integrated community member to be approached by patients and the public in this way (Kulig *et al.*, 2009; Zibric, MacLeod & Zimmer, 2010). This, in turn, contributes to a stronger sense of accountability to community members and patients and is an important and unique aspect of rural nursing (Shellian, 2002). For many nurses, this is the most satisfying part of their work life, and this sustainable connection with their community alongside a strong sense of accountability is highly valued.

This closeness to the community can present challenges, however, and an important one is related to confidentiality (Henderson Betkus & MacLeod, 2004; Rosenthal, 2000; Zibric, MacLeod & Zimmer, 2010). Rural nurses in one study reported that they were often approached by community members asking, out of concern, about their ill relatives, friends, or neighbours (Zibric, MacLeod & Zimmer, 2010). While a clear expectation of nurses is that confidentiality of patients must be protected, this obligation may be more difficult to manage in a small community setting. Not providing information may be seen as implying that one is unfriendly, standoffish, or detached. Worse, a nurse who appropriately safeguards information in such a situation may be seen as someone who is unable to understand the local community and its norms. While it may be a local norm that community members talk about others over coffee or at a local store, this cannot be something that a rural nurse takes part in, as nurses everywhere are trusted by their patients to keep their secrets and preserve confidentiality (Shellian, 2002). This does not change in a rural setting, although meeting this requirement may prove challenging in practice. The rural nurse must find a clear way to set these kinds of boundaries and to explain the professional commitment to confidentiality. This is, one suspects, more easily said than done, and the challenge of maintaining confidentiality in rural nursing is one that is arises frequently in the literature.

CASE PRESENTATION

Mark grew up in a rural area of northern Alberta and moved to Calgary to get his Bachelor's Degree in Nursing. After graduation, he worked in a busy critical care environment in one of the city's hospitals and gained valuable experience working in a fast-paced and demanding unit. Mark's father recently died and his mother, now living alone in the house where Mark grew up, has told Mark how much she misses him. Mark also misses his mother and the quaint, small prairie town where he grew up, with its sense of community and laid-back lifestyle. His partner, Jamal, grew up on a farm in Manitoba and works from home as a freelance writer. Mark and Jamal make the decision to move from Calgary back to the small town where Mark grew up and where everyone knows him. Mark is warmly welcomed back to the community and the small hospital where he, and most people in the town, were born. Mark is happy that he made the move, but finds it challenging to be faced, on almost a daily basis, with questions about patients' health from members of those patients' families. When he and Jamal are in the hardware store in town, the owner, whose daughter is in hospital, asks Mark, "How is Alyssa today? I know she had some tests and I thought she would know the results today. I've been busy working all weekend, so I haven't been by to see her for a few days." Mark knows that Alyssa and her father have had a tense and difficult relationship over the years. He also knows that Alyssa has had very bad news yesterday from the physician regarding her prognosis, and that she doesn't want her parents to know. However, Alyssa's parents often babysat Mark when his parents had to be away, and he feels close to them, as you would to an uncle and aunt, so he feels torn. He understands Alyssa's father's request and that he does care, but he also knows he must respect Alyssa's confidentiality and her specific request for non-disclosure. When he tells her father that he can't give any information to him and why, her father responds by saying, "Marky, it's me asking. Not some stranger. You can tell me, can't you? I mean, we're like family!"

In this case, we see a real life example of how the closeness of a community can contribute to professional challenges for a rural nurse who has strong roots in the area and is trusted and known by so many people in a small town or a close-knit community. When Mark is at the hardware store, he is not working as a nurse and he knows how to differentiate between these roles, yet for the rest of the community, these two roles are not differentiated and Mark is seen, at all times, as both the nurse and the boy who grew up with, and remains close to, so many in the small town. Mark is understandably conflicted, torn between carrying out his professional obligations to protect Alyssa's confidentiality and managing his personal obligations to be caring to those he is closest to. Mark's professional role is seen, by others, as perhaps less important than the role he has as a community member in a place where most people are connected, in a very personal way, to others. It may be more difficult—but no less important—in a case like Mark's, to maintain professionalism through keeping information confidential. As Mark is well aware, our professional obligations cannot be compromised in order to keep others happy. Alyssa, like any other patient, has trusted Mark to keep her information confidential and, as a Registered Nurse, he owes his patients that obligation. Many of us might say that it seems straightforward that Mark should maintain confidentiality, but in the moment, it seems that it would be a challenge for Mark to find the right kinds of words and explanation to present to Alyssa's father and to try to set the kinds of professional and personal boundaries that are most challenging in a setting like this. One tactic might simply be for Mark to encourage Alyssa's father to go visit her and facilitate a family discussion, thus maintaining Alyssa's control over her own information while acknowledging her father's caring interest.

Working with Constraints

In all areas of health care, limited resources pose challenges. From complex care to family practice, lack of sufficient funding, lack of proper equipment, and lack of adequate human resources all have a noticeable impact upon the ability to provide high-quality nursing care. But in a rural or remote setting, not having the right equipment may be a serious problem for an isolated nurse who is managing a specialized problem, one that requires particular equipment, or more up-to-date equipment than is at hand. In terms of human resources, while many urban hospitals may have nursing resource pools or a significant casual pool, along with agency nurses to draw from in cases of short-staffing, the available "resource pool" for a rural hospital may consist of the small handful of nurses who are already on duty. In times of staff shortages or very bad weather, having nursing staff present in a rural hospital may be a very different challenge than in the city, where nurses may be travelling a much shorter distance to work and there may be a number of options for relief nurses to fill staffing quotas. Health human resource issues in rural settings also mean that often, the nurse will have to take on roles of other health care professionals. Without timely access to a physiotherapist, occupational therapist, or speech pathologist, an innovative nurse might need to quickly learn key kinds of exercises and therapy to help facilitate the recovery of a stroke patient. More than simply providing ancillary services, nurses must take on these roles in many areas where hospitals or small communities do not have allied health professionals on staff on a daily basis (Rosenthal, 2000).

Many rural nurses note that they work not only without access to proper equipment but also without access to supportive resources, such as specialized or continuing education. Most opportunities for continuing education require that nurses leave the rural areas where they work. This may be impractical, as it involves nurses leaving not only their workplace, but also their families and homes, to get a speciality certificate, or to obtain a Master's or an advanced degree. For nurses living in cities with universities or colleges, accessing continuing education may still be challenging, but it does not typically involve leaving their families or homes for long periods. It may be difficult for a small rural hospital to send nurses to universities or colleges located elsewhere, as there may be a lack of relief staff in place, and it can be costly. Some rural employers may be unwilling or unable to provide funding for travel, living, and tuition costs, and this may place continuing education simply out of reach for many nurses in rural settings.

The trend towards more modular and on-line courses being offered in nursing education may help nurses in rural and remote areas to access continuing and graduate education. These kinds of innovative educational models are ideal for nurses who can access courses from home or travel for more intensive programs requiring less time spent away from home and work.

Having resources and equipment that are adequate, readily available, and up-to-date, on one hand, and access to educational opportunities, on the other, have been found to be two significant predictors of job satisfaction for nurses working alone in rural and remote areas (Andrews *et al.*, 2005). This is echoed in other Canadian studies as a significant factor related to rural and remote job satisfaction, but it is not discussed in detail in the literature (Penz, Stewart, D'Arcy & Morgan, 2008), perhaps because much of the decision-making regarding equipment acquisition and resource allocation still typically lies outside the direct control of front line nurses.

Scope of Practice

Often, the scope of practice of nurses in rural settings is determined by necessity, rather than strictly defined, as might be the case for a nurse working on a specialty unit of a large urban hospital (Rosenthal, 2000). Scope of practice, for rural and remote nurses, is very different and much less rigidly defined. It is typically extended beyond what we might expect of a nurse in a more structured urban setting who works as part of a large multi-disciplinary team on a daily basis. While nurses in some large hospitals may not put IVs in (as an IV team does this), may not routinely draw blood (as a venipuncture team does this), or may not administer respiratory treatments (as respiratory therapists do this), a rural nurse or a nurse in a remote setting may not have anyone else to depend upon. They may not have a team made up of allied health professionals, but rather just a small team of other nurses and/or a physician. Without the daily presence of other kinds of allied health professionals, many nurses end up carrying out what would be the jobs of the respiratory therapist, the speech pathologist, or the physiotherapist, simply out of necessity to provide high quality holistic nursing care. Thus, scope of practice may be driven by the needs of the patient population presenting to the rural nurse.

How, then, do rural nurses learn the wide variety of skills that they might need at any moment? One way is by cross-training, which involves nurses teaching nurses about other kinds of practice areas and then learning further on the job by experience (Rosenthal, 2000). As Rosenthal puts it, rural nurses often learn through "trial by fire" (p. 24B), as they are faced with critical situations and may be the only person available, or the best-qualified nurse on the team of nurses in a small rural hospital, and they essentially learn through actually performing a clinical skill. The rural nurse's broad scope of practice is emphasized throughout the literature, and it is often pointed out that rural nurses learn through "the Boy Scout school of nursing" (Zibrik, MacLeod & Zimmer, 2010), in which the emphasis is on *being prepared*. Excellent assessment skills and the ability to remain calm in a critical or urgent situation, while having knowledge of one's own skills and competencies (and the limits of these), are some key skills of a competent rural nurse, consistently faced with unpredictable and diverse patient-care challenges.

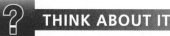

THINK ABOUT IT

- In light of what you now know about the professional and practice challenges faced by rural and remote nurses, what might be important attributes for rural nurses?

- What would you think are the greatest challenges in transitioning from an urban nursing role to rural nursing?

- Can you ever see yourself in a rural or remote nursing role? Why or why not?

Rural nurses have, as noted, very different kinds of professional challenges than their urban counterparts. However, despite the unique professional challenges of being a nurse in a rural or remote setting, there are many unique opportunities and rewards. Rural nurses have strong ties to and respect from their community, a practice that is dynamic, diverse and patient-centred, a greater level of autonomy in many cases, and a broader scope of practice developed through becoming proficient in roles that often fall to other professionals in an urban allied health network.

ABORIGINAL HEALTH IN CANADA

We know that, in any discussion of population health, the social determinants of health are an important starting point in assessing the health of a group or community.

In examining the impact of the social determinants of health on communities, groups, and even individuals, we can begin to highlight inequities and vulnerabilities that may leave people more likely to have an additional burden of health-related problems. When we look at the social determinants of health of Aboriginal groups and peoples of Canada, we see that there are distinct historical, socioeconomic, and political legacies that have had an impact upon the social factors that have directly affected the health and well-being of communities and the individual men, women, and children living in those communities (Reading & Wein, 2009; Wilkinson & Marmot, 1998).

By "Aboriginal" persons, we are referring to individuals who self-identify as being a part of at least one Aboriginal group, which may include First Nations (North American Indian), Métis, or Inuit (Eskimo), those who are members of an Indian Band or First Nation, or those who identify as a Treaty Indian or Registered Indian (as defined by the *Indian Act* of Canada) (Statistics Canada, 2007). In discussing the social determinants of health and Aboriginal persons, care must be taken to acknowledge and understand the complexity of the historical processes that have led to what we find today in terms of patterns of Aboriginal health. The effects of colonization and the forcing of colonial systems and institutions into the lives of Aboriginal people only a few generations ago has had a notable impact across all groups of Aboriginal people. In some cases, there are marked differences between various Aboriginal groups in terms of health outcomes and status. For example, First Nations people have been most affected by government policies and initiatives, including especially the *Indian Act* of 1876. The *Act* outlines what is required in order to claim Indian status, and it gives the federal government the right to decide who is and is not classified as a person with Indian status, and what lands will or will not be designated as Indian lands. Additionally, the *Act* identifies that health care to First Nations people will be provided by the federal government directly. This differs from the usual provision of health care, which is under provincial jurisdiction with federal guidance.

Issues of self-identity, self-determination and lack of inclusion in decision-making processes have affected many Aboriginal persons and communities. Through colonization and subsequent sociocultural and political processes, many of these communities and individuals have suffered from discrimination, racism, social isolation, and inadequate access to the basic necessities of life and health care (Reading & Wien, 2009).

Four important areas to highlight in our discussion of the health and well-being of Aboriginal persons include: the physical environment (including housing), poverty, education, and health behaviours. While many Aboriginal persons report their health as being good, identifiable chronic health problems such as cardiovascular disease, diabetes, and respiratory disease are widespread in many Aboriginal communities (MacMillan *et al.*, 2003; Reading & Wien, 2009). The information for the following discussions of the factors that have an impact upon the health of Aboriginal persons and communities includes extensive data from the National Collaborating Centre for Aboriginal Health report prepared by Reading and Wein (2009).

Factors Affecting the Health of Aboriginal Persons

The physical environment has a significant effect on the health of any person. Safe and affordable housing, healthy sanitary conditions, and access to clean water are all things we consider basic necessities of life in Canada. However, many Aboriginal people experience a severe lack of adequate, safe, and affordable housing, poor sanitary conditions, and little or no access to clean running water. Lack of affordable, well-built, and safe housing has resulted in many problems related to overcrowding and poor ventilation, including respiratory problems in Aboriginal children and adults and a rise in the incidence of communicable diseases such as tuberculosis on reserves, where housing is often a serious problem. Overcrowding due to substandard housing can further contribute to more efficient spreading of common viral and infectious diseases, and is linked to mental health problems, such as depression, along with family tensions and estrangement.

Food insecurity is another problem in many Aboriginal communities, especially those that are more remote. When we state that a household enjoys "food security," we mean that the members of that household can access a sufficient quantity and variety of foods so that they are not in fear of hunger or extreme starvation. In cases of food insecurity, which can occur in degrees, there are typically problems with food distribution or production, such as a lack of transportation to provide food to remote locations or a changing climate that no longer supports the growth and sustainability of particular crops or livestock. Across the world, many people suffer from food insecurity, undernourishment, and starvation. Extreme hunger is typically linked to extreme poverty, but other factors, such as climate, socio-political forces, civil war, and population growth can also play roles in extreme food insecurity. In Canada's Aboriginal communities, food security is typically related to poverty, politics, and transportation. The cost of transporting typical market foods (the kind we would find in a grocery store in a large city) to some Aboriginal communities is high, resulting in food being more expensive once on the shelves, or never getting to such communities at all, due to cost constraints. Lack of access to nutrient-dense and healthy foods (which tend to be more expensive to provide and buy) is felt to be linked to poor health outcomes in Aboriginal communities, including increased rates of obesity, diabetes, and cardiovascular disease. Traditional foods and foods acquired through contemporary hunting may also be out of reach, in terms of costs, for many Aboriginal families and communities.

Lack of access to clean and safe water is another concern for Aboriginal communities, many of which do not have access to running water that is safe to drink. Tap water in many homes is not safe for drinking and water must be brought in, and paid for, by families and individuals. Unsafe water is a serious issue that can contribute to many health-related problems, due to exposure to toxins, heavy metals, and other contaminants. The term "water security" is also now being used to describe populations or communities' sustainable access to clean, safe running water.

Many Aboriginal communities face very high rates of poverty. Poverty is linked to a variety of negative outcomes in terms of health and well-being and is one of the most important social determinants of health, as it has implications for so many other social determinants. High rates of poverty in communities can be linked to social exclusion, lower social cohesion or "sense of community," increased crime, and mental health problems, including anxiety, low self-esteem, depression, and hopelessness. Hopelessness and depression can in turn contribute to problems such as alcoholism and drug addiction. High rates of poverty in Aboriginal communities mean that these serious *sequelae*, which are related to cyclic poverty, are common problems. Poverty and social exclusion are related to high levels of unemployment and low levels of education. In many Aboriginal communities, there is inadequate education and children must leave their homes on the reserve to get schooling past grade eight. Many youth drop out of high school without completing their education. Without a high school diploma, job prospects are few and the cycle of poverty continues.

Access to health care for on-reserve Aboriginal populations is a continuing problem. The inadequacy of small local clinics, often poorly staffed with long wait times for service, contributes to this problem. Many Aboriginal persons also have difficulty in obtaining traditional or culturally-competent care. Additionally, many reserves and Aboriginal communities do not have a dedicated health facility or clinic at all, and hence are without access to the services of a nurse or physician. Emergency services are few, and in the case of more remote areas or reserves, may indeed be non-existent. The costs involved in travelling in order to access basic health care (the true cost of which may include paying for child care, overnight accommodation, and more) is burdensome to families already suffering from poverty, and this is an additional, significant barrier to accessing health care. Add to this the costs of possibly paying for services such as dental care, physiotherapy, or eye care, and it is easy to see how many Aboriginal persons affected by poverty carry serious health-related burdens.

CASE PRESENTATION

Attawapiskat First Nation is an isolated community located in northern Ontario at the mouth of the Attawapiskat River, at James Bay. Serious problems in health, housing, and security have persisted for the approximately 1800 residents since a large diesel oil spill in 1979. Since 2008, a state of emergency has been declared three times for grave problems including potential flooding, massive sewage backup destroying what was already limited housing for 90 people, and most recently, for very low temperatures in the context of severely inadequate housing, as many residents have been forced to live in tents and temporary shelters (CBC News Canada, 2011). Furthermore, since the elementary school was closed in 2000 after health problems related to the diesel spill were uncovered, there has been no new school built for community children, in spite of three separate government promises to do so. The government response has been lacking in the provision of

(Continued)

any kind of practical or sustainable solutions; temporary assistance has come from the Red Cross. The media have tried to highlight the truly alarming conditions that the residents of Attawapiskat are living in (Arsenault, 2011). Without adequate shelter, clean living conditions, adequate schooling, running water, or working phone lines, the Attawapiskat community continues to be a community at serious risk for a myriad of problems.

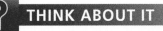

THINK ABOUT IT

- The crisis in Attawapiskat is not the first crisis in housing and living conditions for those Aboriginal and First Nations people living in remote areas or on reserves. These problems have caught the attention of the global media and the United Nations, but the problems persist, despite outcries for change and social justice (United Nations, 2007).

- What kinds of factors or legacy issues have had an effect on the governmental response or lack thereof?

- In this community, everyone is at serious risk. When you take a closer look at the problems, which community members are at the most risk, and why?

- If you were a nurse practicing in the community or healing centre in Attawapiskat, what are some interventions or actions you could take, to advocate for the community?

Aboriginal Nursing

In referring to **Aboriginal nursing**, many people are referring to nurses who work in Aboriginal communities, while others are instead referring to Aboriginal persons who work as Registered Nurses. Most of the time, the term "Aboriginal nursing" refers to anyone involved in providing nursing care in Aboriginal communities, while the term **Aboriginal nurse** refers to a person who self-identifies as an Aboriginal person and who is also a nurse. As of 2008, there are only about 3250 self-identified Aboriginal nurses in Canada (Gregory, Pijl-Zieber, Barsky & Daniels, 2008). Groups like the Aboriginal Nurses Association of Canada, an affiliate group of the Canadian Nurses Association, have raised the profile of Aboriginal nurses and have helped introduce important ideas such as cultural safety and culturally-competent care in the context of Aboriginal nursing. Research centres such as The National Collaborating Centre for Aboriginal Health at the University of Northern British Columbia also carry out extensive health-related research that helps to inform policy-makers and decision-makers who set policies that have an impact on how nursing care can be provided to these communities. As you can see from their key objectives in the text box below, one important goal is to work directly to improve the well-being and health of Aboriginal communities, as well as working with health professionals who serve these communities.

FIGURE 18–2 **KEY OBJECTIVES OF THE ABORIGINAL NURSING ASSOCIATION OF CANADA**

The Association's key objectives were updated in 2010 to be more reflective of the current changing health, social, and political environment.

a. To work with communities, health professionals and government institutions on Aboriginal Health Nursing issues and practices within the Canadian Health system that address particular interest and concern in Aboriginal communities with a view to benefiting Aboriginal peoples of Canada by improving their health and well-being, physically, mentally, socially and spiritually.

b. To engage and conduct research on Aboriginal Health Nursing and access to health care as related to Aboriginal Peoples.

c. To consult with government, non-profit and private organizations in developing programs for applied and scientific research designed to improve health and well-being in Aboriginal Peoples.

d. To develop and encourage the teaching of courses in the educational system on Canadian Aboriginal health, Indigenous knowledge, cultural safety in nursing and the health care system and/or other educational resources and supports.

e. To promote awareness in both Canadian and International Aboriginal and non-Aboriginal communities of the health needs of Canadian Aboriginal people.

f. To facilitate and foster increased participation of Aboriginal Peoples involvement in decision-making in the field of health care.

g. To strengthen partnerships and develop resources supporting the recruitment and retention of more people of Aboriginal ancestry into nursing and other health sciences professions.

h. To disseminate such information to all levels of community.

Reprinted with permission from the Aboriginal Nurses Association of Canada. www.anac.on.ca

---

On First Nations reserves, health and nursing care is funded by the federal government, and nurses who provide care in these settings are typically employed by Health Canada.

A 2006 report on Aboriginal nursing attempted to describe the nature of Aboriginal nursing in rural and remote communities through detailed surveys of rural and remote nurses, including those who self-identified as First Nations, Métis, or Inuit (Stewart *et al.*, 2006). Many who responded to the survey reported being the first point of contact for health care in their communities, and a significant proportion reported working in a nursing station or outpost setting, living far away from a major centre and without a physician living in their community. One important fact that the results of this survey identify is that some Aboriginal nurses feel that their education did not prepare them for the realities of their jobs and that they would like further education in order to provide effective nursing care. This need for further education is identified by other scholars, along with a need for increased attention and resources to support recruitment and retention of Aboriginal nurses (Gregory, Pijl-Zieber, Barsky & Daniels, 2008).

The themes found in surveys of Aboriginal nurses reflect, to some degree, the themes identified in research involving rural nurses in general, which we have discussed already in this chapter. However, Aboriginal nursing brings added complexity: many Aboriginal nursing graduates state that providing culturally sensitive, competent, community-driven care is something that is not emphasized, or included, in curricula in most nursing schools, and as a result, such graduates feel unprepared for this challenge. One theme identified in this study that is significantly different from surveys of non-Aboriginal rural nurses is their reported experience of abuse while working as an Aboriginal nurse, which was significantly higher (37%) than reported by their non-Aboriginal counterparts (30%). Types of abuse reported included physical abuse and assault, sexual harassment, and assault and verbal abuse or threats. Another interesting finding is that many Aboriginal nurses said that they practiced with a lack of physician services and allied health services, and that the only reasonable year-long access to such communities is by plane. The same number of non-Aboriginal and Aboriginal nurses in the survey identified that they were, in fact, the sole providers of health care for their community, and a high percentage of the total respondents pointed to the importance of technology—including Internet access and Telehealth—to being able to provide care (Stewart *et al.*, 2006). Overall, many respondents reported that they enjoyed their work and that the focus on community and community health was something that provided satisfaction and meaning in their nursing practice, a theme that we see echoed in other discussions of rural and remote nursing.

While there are notable differences between non-Aboriginal and Aboriginal nursing, and between those in less rural and more remote locations, we see a number of common concerns and rewards related to nursing in communities outside of large cities, across Canada. While we pointed out at the outset of this chapter that it is difficult to generalize about rural areas or rural nurses, we can say that there are identifiable challenges and rewards that are unique to nurses providing care across a variety of rural and Aboriginal settings.

Recommendations for the Future of Rural and Aboriginal Nursing

One of the most important goals of talking about and conducting research on rural and remote nursing is to develop an understanding of just what rural and remote nursing looks like, in order to better ground policy recommendations in the actual practice of rural nurses. Those in positions of power who are policy-makers or administrators must be able to appreciate that while nurses across Canada practice according to provincial standards, the nature of nursing work varies significantly among settings, and a key example of this is the way nursing work varies between urban settings and rural environments. Further documenting the quantitative data and qualitative experience of rural and remote nurses will help to provide a more complete picture of what it means to be a rural nurse and help to better inform evidence-based decisions that will have an effect on rural nursing care (Penz, Stewart, D'Arcy & Morgan, 2008). Recruitment and retention strategies for big-city hospitals must necessarily be quite different from strategies for outpost nursing positions, and ways of best supporting nurses who are located in urban centres will be very different from effective supporting of nurses in remote areas served only by plane. Community involvement and support are clearly important predictors of satisfaction and success in rural nursing (Penz, Stewart, D'Arcy & Morgan, 2008). The challenges and barriers that rural nurses face, and the rewards that they seek, make theirs a unique specialty that will be in increasing demand. As that demand exacerbates the existing shortage of nurses who are able and willing to work in rural and remote areas, we will need to pay closer attention to including discussion and teaching of rural and Aboriginal health in nursing school curricula, increasing supports for Aboriginal nursing students, and facilitating access to opportunities for nursing students to experience clinical placements in rural settings (Zibrik, MacLeod & Zimmer, 2010).

With an aging nursing workforce, we may in addition see a different kind of shortage of nurses across sectors, including in rural nursing. To increase job satisfaction and retention of nurses already working in rural and remote areas, providing opportunities for additional relevant training, certification, and continuing education that is accessible, innovative, and tailored to nurses in these kinds of settings will be an important consideration for universities and colleges across Canada (Henderson Betkus & MacLeod, 2004).

SUMMARY

All of the factors shaping health care, and the health of Canadians, affect more than just those living in big cities. Rural populations, while being affected by the same kinds of trends that affect us all, are unique populations, and are affected in significant and different ways by their geography than are urban dwellers. Nurses providing care and working with Aboriginal populations must be attentive to the unique cultural, social, and historical contexts and legacies that have had an impact on the well-being of Aboriginal persons. Sensitivity to the unique needs and priorities of these populations is an absolute requirement of nurses who choose to practice in these communities. The nurse in a rural, remote, or Aboriginal community is an important provider of health care and advocate for an ever-evolving nation of diverse communities and populations.

CHAPTER HIGHLIGHTS

- Rural health is an area that will require more attention from not only nurses and professional nursing bodies, but also from policy makers at all levels of government.

- In Canada, anywhere between 20 and 30 percent of Canadians are defined as living in a rural environment.

- Deaths due to circulatory disease, suicides, injuries, and motor vehicle accidents are more common in rural areas than in urban areas.

- Those living in rural areas may have less access to emergency care, specialized care, and intensive care.

- Access to timely health care, and to the right health care, continues to be a challenge in rural areas across Canada.

- There is still relatively little literature on what rural nursing is, and the challenges rural nurses face that are distinct from those in urban centres have yet to be fully explored and described.

- Rural nursing differs from nursing in urban centres for reasons that are directly related to geographical and professional isolation, increased autonomy, limited access to health care resources, a more varied and broader scope of practice, and different types of social connections and networks.

- Often, the scope of practice of nurses in rural settings is determined by necessity, rather than strictly defined, as might be the case for a nurse working on a specialty unit of a large urban hospital.

- Being able to innovate and adapt is a key attribute of an effective rural nurse.

- With improved communications technology, including the Internet and social networking, being in a rural setting no longer means being or professionally as isolated as many nurses have been in the past.

- For many nurses in rural and Aboriginal settings, the strong sense of community and their sustainable connection to the community is the most satisfying part of their work life.

- Nurses working in many rural areas are faced with the reality of being very visible, and embedded in the communities in which they work.

- All nurses must protect the confidentiality of patients, and this obligation may be more difficult to negotiate in a small community setting.

- Many rural nurses note that they work without access to proper, up-to-date equipment and supportive resources, such as adequate staffing and specialized or continuing education.

- Having resources and equipment that are adequate, readily available, and up-to-date, as well as access to educational opportunities. are two significant predictors of job satisfaction for nurses working alone in rural and remote areas.

- There are distinct historical, socioeconomic, and political legacies that have had an impact upon the social determinants of health and the well-being of Aboriginal communities and the individual men, women, and children living in them.

- Issues of self-identity, self-determination, and lack of inclusion in decision-making processes have affected many Aboriginal persons.

- Safe and affordable housing, clean sanitation conditions, and access to clean water are all things we consider to be basic necessities of life in Canada.

- Many Aboriginal people experience a severe lack of adequate, safe, and affordable housing, as well as experiencing poor sanitation conditions and little or no access to clean running water.

- In Aboriginal communities, food security is typically related to poverty, politics, and transportation.

- Many Aboriginal communities are affected by issues related to overcrowding, such as an increase in communicable diseases like tuberculosis and viral illnesses, mental health issues, and family tensions.

- High rates of poverty in Aboriginal communities are linked to social exclusion, lower social cohesion or "sense of community," increased crime, and mental health problems, including anxiety, low self-esteem, depression, and hopelessness.

- Access to health care for on-reserve Aboriginal populations is a continuing problem.

- Many Aboriginal nurses are the first point of contact for health care in their community, and a significant number report working in a nursing station or outpost setting, living far from a major centre and without a physician living in their community.

- The added complexity of providing culturally-sensitive and competent, community-driven care is something that many Aboriginal nursing graduates state is not emphasized or included in curricula in nursing schools, and they report feeling unprepared for this challenge.

- Surveyed nurses in rural and Aboriginal communities report that they enjoy their work and that the focus on community and community health is something that provides satisfaction and meaning in their nursing practice.

- Further documenting the quantitative data and qualitative experience of rural and remote nurses will help to provide a more complete picture of what it means to be a rural nurse and help to better inform evidence-based decisions that have an effect on rural nursing care.

- There should be greater emphasis on the discussion and teaching of rural and Aboriginal health in nursing school curricula, on providing supports for Aboriginal nursing students, and facilitating access to opportunities for nursing students to experience clinical placements in rural settings.

DISCUSSION QUESTIONS AND ACTIVITIES

1. Describe the unique health concerns in rural settings compared to urban environments.

2. List and describe what you consider to be key attributes for an effective rural nurse.

3. What are some strategies you might think about that rural nurses could use to handle issues related to confidentiality?

4. Imagine you were designing a recruitment campaign to attract nurses to rural and remote settings. What are some highlights and rewards of rural nursing you would emphasize?

5. What are some strategies you can identify for increasing awareness of, and providing resources for, nurses in rural and Aboriginal communities?

6. Think about your career vision. Does nursing in a rural or Aboriginal setting play a part in your career vision? Why or why not?

7. What do you see might be the effect of ever-increasing urbanization on the well-being and lifestyles of those living in rural areas? How do you foresee increased urbanization affecting the health of those living in rural areas?

8. Think about your own nursing program. Have you learned about rural health or rural nursing? Do you have opportunities to access clinical placements in rural settings? If not, how will you aim to learn more about this nursing specialty?

REFERENCES

Aboriginal Nurses Association of Canada (2010). *A.N.A.C. Objectives*. Ottawa: Aboriginal Nurses Association of Canada. Retrieved on August 21, 2012 from: http://www.anac.on.ca/

Andrews, M. E., M. J. Stewart, J. R. Pitblado, D. G. Morgan, D. Forbes & C. D'Arcy (2005). Registered nurses working alone in rural and remote Canada. *Canadian Journal of Nursing Research, 37*(1), 14–33.

Arsenault, A. (2011). *Reporter's Notebook (CBC Canada)*. Retrieved on May 29, 2012 from http://www.youtube.com/watch?v=adKggXHA1uM

Canadian Association for Rural and Remote Nursing (CARRN) (2009). *Rural and remote practice parameters: A Discussion Document*. Retrieved from http://www.carrn.com/files/NursingPracticeParametersJanuary08.pdf on January 11, 2012.

CBC News Canada (2011). *Attawapiskat crisis sparks political blame game*. Retrieved on May 29, 2012 from http://www.cbc.ca/news/canada/sudbury/story/2011/12/01/attawapiskat-thursday.html

Community Care Access Centres (2012). *How to make normal saline*. Retrieved May 28, 2012 from http://www.ccac-ont.ca/Upload/mh/General/Preparing_Normal_Saline.pdf

Federal/Provincial/Territorial Advisory Committee on Population Health (FPT-ACPH). (1996). *First report on the Health of Canadians (1996)*. Committee on Population Health, Ottawa, ON.

Gregory, D., E. M. Pijl-Zieber, J. Barsky & M. Daniels (2008). Aboriginal nursing education in Canada: An update. *The Canadian Nurse*, 104(4), 24–28.

Hegney, D., A. McCarthy, C. Rogers-Clark & D. Gorman (2002). Why nurses are attracted to rural and remote practice. *Australian Journal of Public Health, 10*(3), 178–186.

Henderson Betkus, M., & L. MacLeod (2004). Retaining public health nurses in rural British Columbia. *Canadian Journal of Public Health, 95*(1), 54–58.

Human Resources and Skills Development Canada (2006). *Canadians in Context - Geographic Distribution.* Retrieved from http://www4.hrsdc.gc.ca/.3ndic.1t.4r@-eng.jsp?iid=34 on January 15, 2012.

Kulig, J. C., N. Stewart, K. Penz, D. Forbes, D. Morgan & P. Emerson (2009). Work setting, community attachment, and satisfaction among rural and remote nurses. *Public Health Nursing, 26*(5), 430–439.

Lea, K., & M. Cruikshank (2005). Factors that influence the recruitment and retention of graduate nurses in rural health care facilities. *Collegian, 12*(2), 22–27.

MacLeod, M., J. Kulig, N. Stewart & R. Pitblado (2004). *Nursing practice in rural and remote Canada. Final report to Canadian Health Services Research Foundation.* Retrieved from http://ruralnursing.unbc.ca/ on January 20, 2012.

MacLeod, M. L., J. C. Kulig, N. J. Stewart, J. R. Pitblado & M. Knock (2004). The nature of nursing practice in rural and remote Canada: This three-year ongoing study is already revealing that nursing in rural and remote Canada is complex and deserves formal recognition, as well as financial and educational support. *The Canadian Nurse, 6*, 27–31.

MacMillan, H. L., C. A. Walsh, E. Jamieson, M. Y.-Y. Wong, E. J. Faries, J. McCue, A. B. MacMillan, D. R. Offord & The Technical Advisory Committee of the Chiefs of Ontario (2003). The health of Ontario First Nations people: Results from the Ontario First Nations Regional Health Survey. *Canadian Journal of Public Health, 94*(3), 168–172.

Penz, K., N. J. Stewart, C. D'Arcy & D. Morgan (2008). Predictors of job satisfaction for rural acute care Registered Nurses in Canada. *Western Journal of Nursing Research, 30*(7), 785–800.

Public Health Agency of Canada. (2006). *How Healthy Are Rural Canadians? An Assessment of Their Health Status and Health Determinants.* Canadian Institutes of Health Research. ISBN 13: 978-1-55392-881-2 (PDF). Retrieved from: http://www.phac-aspc.gc.ca/publicat/rural06/pdf/rural_canadians_2006_report_e.pdf on December 28, 2011.

Reading, C. L. R., & F. Wien (2009). *Health Inequalities and Social Determinants of Aboriginal Peoples' Health.* National Collaborating Centre for Aboriginal Health. Prince George, British Columbia. Retrieved from: http://www.nccah-ccnsa.ca/docs/social%20determinates/NCCAH-Loppie-Wien_Report.pdf on January 20, 2012.

Registered Nurses' Association of Ontario (2007). *Professionalism in Nursing.* Registered Nurses' Association of Ontario. Toronto, Canada. Retrieved from http://www.rnao.org/Storage/28/2303_BPG_Professionalism.pdf on January 20, 2012.

Rosenthal, K. (2000). Rural nursing: Is it the right choice for you? *American Journal of Nursing, 100*(4), 24A–24B.

Shellian, B. (2002). Primer on rural nursing. *Alberta RN, 58*(2), 5.

Statistics Canada (2007). *How Statistics Canada Identifies Aboriginal Peoples.* Retrieved from http://www.statcan.gc.ca/pub/12-592-x/12-592-x2007001-eng.htm#a2 on January 21, 2012.

Stewart, N. J., J. C. Kulig, K. Penz, M. E. Andrews, S. Houshmand, D. G. Morgan, M. L. P. MacLeod, J. R. Pitblado & C. D'Arcy (2006). *Aboriginal nurses in rural and remote Canada: Results from a national survey*. Saskatoon, Saskatchewan: University of Saskatchewan, College of Nursing. R06-2006.

United Nations (2007). *United Nations expert on adequate housing calls for immediate attention to tackle national housing crisis in Canada*. Retrieved May 29, 2012 from http://www.unhchr.ch/huricane/huricane.nsf/0/90995D69CE8153C3C1257387004F40B5?opendocument

Wilkinson, R., & M. Marmot (1998). *Social determinants of health: the solid facts*. Geneva: World Health Organization.

Zibrik, K. J., M. L. P. MacLeod & L. V. Zimmer (2010). Professionalism in rural acute-care nursing. *Canadian Journal of Nursing Research, 42*(1), 20–36.

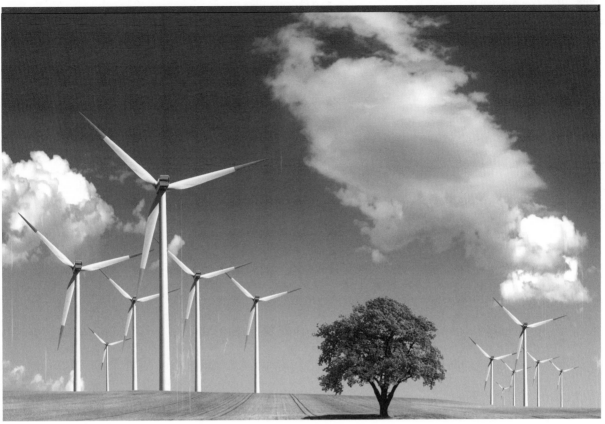

WDG Photo/Shutterstock.com

CHAPTER **19**
EMPOWERMENT FOR NURSES

Based on an earlier version of this chapter by Barbara C. Banonis

OBJECTIVES

After completing this chapter, the reader should be able to:

1. Describe the concepts of power and empowerment.
2. Discuss personal empowerment and its importance within nursing.
3. Discuss the relationship among professional empowerment, principled behaviour, and nursing practice.
4. Describe the role of diversity in empowerment.
5. Discuss the notion of whistleblowing.

6. Discuss the meaning of patient empowerment and describe the role of nursing in the empowerment of patients.

7. Describe the attitudes of nurses, and the knowledge and skills of nurses that help to enable empowerment.

8. Describe factors that enhance or block patient empowerment.

INTRODUCTION

In this chapter, we will discuss the importance of empowering nurses and patients. To deal with the complex issues facing nursing today, nurses are required to exercise integrity, accountability, and courage. Nurses have the responsibility, authority, and power to make principled choices. Additionally, the empowerment of patients is an important element of nursing care that derives from an appreciation that patients have the ability to discern their own needs and make decisions about their own lives and health. Being an enabler of empowerment requires nurses to relinquish power and embrace the patient as an equal partner. Nurses can facilitate empowerment by working directly with patients and through addressing social, political, and environmental factors that affect the empowerment of individuals and communities. In the midst of an ever-changing and challenging health care environment, in which issues of power and control continue to affect patient care, it is imperative that nurses be both empowered and competent enablers of patient empowerment. In this chapter, we will discuss empowerment in a variety of nursing contexts: personal empowerment, professional empowerment, and the empowerment of both nursing students and of patients.

Nurses have the power to make a difference by acting in principled ways in all areas of their lives and practice. However, as has been evident throughout the discussions in this book, many factors mitigate against nurses claiming this power. Gordon and Buresh (2000) note that nursing, as a profession, although the largest group of health care professionals, is still markedly invisible and silent. In health care forums across the country, the voice of nursing is largely unheard. A larger and related concern is the lack of public knowledge about just what it is that nurses do in their work. While the public continues to hold nursing in high esteem, deeming nurses as some of the most trusted professionals, members of the public actually have little knowledge about the kind of work that nurses do. Furthermore, as a profession, we have only begun to understand how to publicize our work and attend to our image as a profession. Nurses need to develop skills in communication, empowerment, and acting collectively in order to function fully in their legitimate roles within health care and optimize their professional capabilities and roles. Nurses must be aware of values, beliefs, and other factors affecting personal decision making, and expand their knowledge of ethical principles, legal considerations, and issues facing nursing. Understanding **power** and **empowerment** can help in developing strategies for action in this regard.

The word *"power"* is often understood in terms of strength, force, or control, but the primary dictionary definition of the term, derived from its Latin root "potere," is "the ability to do or act, capability of doing or accomplishing something" (*The Random House Dictionary of the English Language*, 1987). To have power, then, means having the ability to do or act; and to *"empower"* is to facilitate the ability of another person to do or to act.

Empowerment is more difficult to define. Since the term is overused in a number of contexts, it is understandably difficult to agree upon one simple definition (Bradbury-Jones, Sambrook & Irvine, 2007). Rodwell suggests that **empowerment** is a "helping process whereby groups of individuals are enabled to change a situation, given skills, resources, opportunities and authority to do so. It is a partnership which respects and values self and others—aiming to develop positive beliefs in self and the future" (1996, p. 309). Similarly, Ellis-Stoll and Popkess-Vawter (1998) describe empowerment as a participative process, or partnership between a nurse and patient, that is designed to assist in changing unhealthy behaviours. This partnership is viewed by some as a social process of recognizing, promoting, and enhancing patients' abilities to meet their own needs, solve their own problems, and mobilize the necessary resources in order to feel in control of their own lives (Connelly, Keele, Kleinbeck, Schneider & Cobb, 1993; Fulton, 1997). Kuokkanen and Leino-Kilpi note that empowerment may also be seen as a "process of personal growth and development" (2000, p. 273). Bolton & Brookings (1998) describe empowerment as the capacity of disenfranchised people to understand and become active participants in the matters that affect their lives, suggesting that a personal attitude that change is possible is important for empowerment to occur. Gurka (1995) reflects that empowerment is a philosophy or world view flowing from belief in each person's inherent worth, and a process of self-discovery that involves creating a vision, taking risks, making choices, and behaving in authentic ways. Empowerment requires respect for an individual's personal beliefs and goals, as well as trust in the person's ability to make decisions, take action, and be accountable for the actions. Although the sharing of knowledge through education is important for empowerment, the literature clearly indicates that emotional and social support is essential as well.

In-depth analyses of the construct suggests that empowerment is both a process and an outcome, taking different forms with different people and contexts (Ellis-Stoll & Popkess-Vawter, 1998; Gibson, 1991; Hawks, 1992; Rodwell, 1996; Ryles, 1999). It is also worthwhile to note that empowerment is often referred to as a "construct" rather than a "concept," as it is a possibility, and not something that one can observe directly (Herbert, Gagnon, Rennick and O'Loughlin, 2009). Because of this, empowerment needs to be defined by the people concerned. Empowerment is a transactional process involving or occurring within a relationship with others. This relationship includes mutually beneficial interactions aimed at strengthening rather than weakening; power sharing through mutual sharing of knowledge, resources, and opportunities; and respect for self and others. Empowerment is nurtured by collaborative efforts that focus on solutions rather than problems, and on strengths, rights, and abilities rather than deficits. Empowerment derives from a feminine perspective of *power with* or *power to*, which implies sharing responsibility, knowledge, and resources; collaboration for goal achievement; incorporating diversity; valuing the contributions of each person; and valuing the process. In contrast is the traditionally masculine view of *power over* that incorporates a sense of paternalistic control, struggle for and protection of limited resources, separation of leaders and followers, expediency, and results even at the expense of persons (Chinn, 1995).

Empowerment can seem like a rather abstract term, and you may be wondering what being empowered looks and feels like. Certainly, two people in the same circumstances can have different experiences of empowerment. Nurse scholars use a variety of descriptive terms when discussing people who are empowered. These include *positive self-concept, personal satisfaction, self-efficacy, sense of mastery regarding self and the environment, sense of control, sense of connectedness, self-development, feeling of hope, the ability to make changes, self-determination, action orientation, authority, autonomy, capability of social intercourse, caring, choosing, self-confidence, courage, decision-making ability, emancipatory power, endurance, expertise, freedom, influence, instrumental exercise of power, participation, resilience, rights, self-control, solidarity, strength, sturdiness, taking a position, assertiveness, coercion, enabling,* and *freedom to make choices* (Bolton & Brookings, 1998; Byrne, 1999; Chavasse, 1992; Connelly *et al.*, 1993; Ellis-Stoll & Popkess-Vawter, 1998; Fulton, 1997; Hartrick & Schreiber, 1998; Hawks, 1992; Jones, O'Toole, Hoa, Chau, & Muc, 2000; Klakovich, 1995; Kuokkanen & Leino-Kilpi, 2000; Laschinger, Wong, McMahon, & Kaufmann, 1999; Rodwell, 1996; Ryles, 1999; Wallerstein & Bernstein, 1988). Although not all of these attributes are necessarily part of every experience of empowerment, they provide markers that help us identify the process and presence of empowerment.

Empowerment implies choice on the part of those being empowered. Individuals and groups must ultimately motivate and empower themselves. This process requires self-awareness, positive self-esteem, commitment to self and others, and the desire and ability to make decisions. Responsibility and accountability for our actions and having the authority to act are implicit in the ability to choose. The concept of empowering patients has emerged as nursing has directed its ethical focus to advocacy for patients. Adherence to principles discussed throughout this book, particularly respect for persons, autonomy, justice, and beneficence, makes it incumbent upon nurses to involve patients in making decisions about their own health and care. Some patients have both the desire and the skills to take charge of their lives; some have the desire but need assistance or support; while others have limitations in both ability and desire. Negotiating within a system that has traditionally placed decision-making authority and power primarily within the hands of physicians requires skill, support, and a strong sense of personal empowerment.

Through the empowerment process, we can enable others to develop awareness of areas that need change, foster a desire to take action, and share resources, skills, and opportunities that support the change. Rodwell (1996) notes that it is self-awareness and resources, rather than the services provided to persons, that lead to self-empowerment. Enhanced self-esteem, personal satisfaction, sense of connectedness, the ability to set and reach goals, a sense of control over life and change processes, and a sense of hope and direction are outcomes of empowerment.

ASK YOURSELF

What Makes You Feel Empowered?

- Consider a situation in which you felt empowered. Describe factors contributing to your sense of empowerment.

- Recall a time when you felt disempowered. What contributed to this sense? How might you have felt more empowered in that situation?

- Nursing students often feel disempowered by virtue of their position relative to instructors, faculty members, and the Registered Nurses they work with. Reflect on your own experience as a student nurse. What made you feel disempowered? What helped you to feel better supported and empowered?

- Patients often describe feelings of disempowerment as a result of feeling that health care practitioners are acting in a paternalistic or overly protective manner, or as a result of feeling uninformed or left out of decision-making processes. Reflect on the way you interact with patients. Do you approach patients in a way that includes them in decisions, keeps them informed, and allows them the freedom to articulate and explore what they consider to be their best interests?

- Reflect on a patient care situation in which a patient required extra time and information from you in order to help make a decision regarding their care and you were rushed, impatient, and unable to take the time to spend with the patient. How do you think the patient felt?

- Look at your own working conditions. Do you have input into the environment and milieu of the unit or agency where you work? Are you able to provide feedback about decisions that will affect patient care or your own satisfaction with your practice? Are you allowed some degree of autonomy in how you choose to approach day-to-day situations, as well as more significant issues?

PERSONAL EMPOWERMENT

The power or nursing to make a difference in care with patients derives from many factors. In order to serve as credible models of empowerment for others, we must demonstrate congruence between values and behaviours in our own lives. Personal integrity implies an ability to be honest with and care for ourselves, as well as to respond to the needs of others. Often nurses, and especially women, have learned to value caring for others before or instead of caring for self. A true value for human life must include value for our own life as well. We must attend to ourselves and treat ourselves with the same respect and dignity we afford others. Personal empowerment begins with actions that support the meeting of our own needs and self-actualization. It is from our personal stores of creativity, empowerment, and health that we are able to inspire, teach, and assist others in achieving their potential.

In principle, many nurses would agree with the concept of care for self; however, actions often conflict with this acknowledged belief. Nurses often agree to work additional hours even when they are exhausted; consume large amounts of caffeine and sugar to boost waning energy; go home to care for children, spouse, and friends; and collapse into bed only to get up and do it all again the next day because they feel limited power to do otherwise. What causes a person to behave in a way that conflicts with their stated values? Often the person has learned conflicting messages. A belief in caring for ourselves may conflict with a learned belief that caring for others is more admirable or important than caring for ourselves. Many people find that they have feelings of guilt if they are not putting others ahead of themselves. We emphasize the idea of a fiduciary duty for health care professionals who are caring for patients. This duty, when considered in the context of health care, encompasses the notion of putting others' needs ahead of our own. Many nurses—women and men—are socialized to put the needs of others before their own needs. While it is admirable to care for others ahead of oneself, doing so disproportionately or while neglecting oneself is neither constructive nor healthy, and will ultimately result in an inability to provide competent or thoughtful care to others.

Some people feel very little control over any area of their lives. Others may feel empowered to make decisions in some situations but not in others—for example, a person may actively make decisions in the home environment while feeling like a pawn of the system at work. The sense of power that nurses have in their personal lives may affect their perception of empowerment in the professional arena and *vice versa*. Burnout, job dissatisfaction, and limited professional commitment all affect the quality of patient care, and all are often associated with feelings of powerlessness (Moss, 1995). Attributes of empowerment noted in the previous section reflect important considerations for self-empowerment on both the personal and professional level.

In order to be able to facilitate empowerment in others, we must first develop our own personal empowerment. This means valuing ourselves and "listening inwardly to your own senses as well as listening intently and actively to others, consciously taking in and forming strength" (Chinn, 1995, p. 3). Self-awareness is necessary, since self-perception has a direct link to quality of patient care (Moss, 1995). Such awareness requires attentiveness to factors that influence our thoughts, feelings, actions, and reactions in the present circumstance, and reflective consideration of such influences on past experiences, as well as an ability to critically look toward the future.

Self-awareness of this kind involves recognizing old or repetitive thought patterns and changing those that no longer support a creative, actualizing life. Extreme self-criticism, being overly judgmental of oneself or others, and engaging in consistent negative thinking can be particularly confining or limiting, in terms of self-actualization. Old thinking can be updated with new knowledge. Questioning the origin of particular thoughts can reveal ideas that were true at one time but are no longer true. For example, a child who was always told that she did not know enough to make a decision, and that mother knew best, may become an adult who still consults her mother before making decisions. Seeking alternative views of situations, and learning logical or critical thinking skills, are other ways to restructure thought patterns.

Feelings are transient signals that alert us to what is positive or objectionable in a situation. Owning our feelings means acknowledging and exploring the reasons that we might be reacting in a particular way, rather than blaming other persons or situations for our feelings. People may experience different feelings in similar situations. For example, a grave diagnosis may elicit a variety of feelings in different persons. Some people's reactions might include fear, panic, trepidation, or extreme anxiety. Other people may experience feelings of despair or disbelief. Some may describe feelings of resignation, powerlessness, or anger. Still others may even demonstrate feelings of hope, relief, or feeling a sense of direction in their life. Feelings and reactions are as diverse as the persons who have them. While events may be the triggers of certain feelings, it is important to note that feelings are elicited *within the person* and not *within the event*.

It is important to try to articulate and take ownership of personal values and, in doing so, claim our ability to make choices. When experiencing a lack of control in life, we should identify both internal and external barriers to having control, consider the degree of control we wish to have, and explore what we need to do and are willing to risk in order to exercise some degree of control. Consciously acting based upon a clear evaluation of the current situation, rather than acting automatically, is one way to own our behaviour. Taking ownership of behaviour requires being able to see options and being realistic about those options. Believing there are no viable options can result in feeling powerless, trapped, or victimized. Even when we do not believe we can change a current unacceptable situation immediately, we can make a plan for change and set that plan into motion one step at a time. A *victim* waits and hopes something or someone else will change; makes excuses for not taking action (time, cost, fatigue, and the like); blames people, places, or things for the situation; and is trapped and unaware of options. An *empowered person* decides to be accountable for personal responses, makes plans, considers options, develops strategies for change, and acts on plans by doing what is necessary to succeed. Even in a situation where it may be impossible to exercise control or have access to realistic options, empowered persons are able to reflect on what they have learned from the situation or event and prospectively consider how such a situation might be approached differently in the future.

Personal empowerment "is growth of personal strength, power, and ability to enact one's own will and love for self in the context of love and respect for others . . . [and] is only possible when individuals express respect and reverence for all other forms of life and ground the energy of the Self as one with the earth" (Chinn, 1995, p. 3). A commitment to personal growth and self-care, developing a positive sense of self, and an awareness of strengths and abilities as well as limitations, and then drawing on our supports and sources of connectedness will foster this process. It is essential that we trust ourselves and our knowledge and abilities and are courageous in taking risks. Empathy with others, appreciation of diversity, tolerance, flexibility, and willingness to compromise empower a person. Empowerment requires being true to ourselves and our values while respecting the diverse choices of others.

PROFESSIONAL EMPOWERMENT

Professional empowerment is built upon the foundational elements of personal accountability and the support of nursing colleagues. In order to deal in a principled way with issues and dilemmas arising within health care settings, nurses must feel personally and professionally empowered to act on sometimes difficult choices. Many factors affect nursing actions in the professional arena, including personal attitudes and self-concept; the structural and functional interrelatedness of health care systems; political, economic, and social forces; and interactions with patients and colleagues. Barriers to empowerment exist within the community of nursing, and are also imposed from external sources. Curtin points out that "many nurses are unwilling to assume responsibility for decision making and that nursing has failed to develop an adequate support system for nurses" (1982, p. 10). Sadly, thirty years later, Curtin's observations are still quite accurate.

Empowerment requires nurses to become knowledgeable about and address systemic issues as well as interpersonal issues. Such issues include recognizing the need for changing the power base within the current health care system, moving from a paternalistic, hierarchical model of control toward one that values collaboration, and the power of the collective. Nurses must become involved in shared decision making and in the formation of institutional policies as part of this process (Chandler, 1991; Moss, 1995).

It is thought that empowerment and feelings of being empowered are influenced as much by the structures and environments one works in as the personal and professional attributes of individual nurses. Qualities of an empowered nurse can include being honest, maintaining autonomy and expertise in practice, being future-oriented and goal-driven, and being socially skilled and able to promote a positive working environment (Babendo-Mould, Iwasiw, Andrusyszyn, Laschinger & Weston, 2012; Kuokkanen & Leino-Kilpi, 2001).

The effect of nurses' empowerment in the health care environment can have personal, institutional, and patient care implications. In terms of nursing management and health systems, some authors view empowerment as a method for delegating authority and sharing power and a strategy for improving the productivity of nurses. Laschinger and colleagues (1999) report that empowered nurses are more likely to initiate and sustain independent behaviours to accomplish task objectives in the face of difficulty, thereby increasing work effectiveness. One study suggests a link between staff nurses' perceptions of their work effectiveness and workplace empowerment (Laschinger and Wong, 1999). The authors identify three factors that have a positive impact on empowerment: access to the structures of information, support, and resources. Moss (1995) relates empowerment to increased efficiency, job satisfaction, and better patient care. In contrast, Moss notes that feelings of powerlessness are associated with job dissatisfaction and low levels of professional commitment, which are barriers to quality patient care. This author links nurses' perceptions of themselves to quality of patient care, reflecting that nurses who are burned out and dissatisfied are more inclined to give only the most routine care. Klakovich (1995) proposes that only an empowered work force can be effective in an environment of patient-focused care and shared governance. Inherent in this perspective is a sense that each person is free to make choices, and that those who are empowered, both internally and by the system, feel more in control of their lives, and are able to act in appropriate, meaningful ways and do what they truly want to do.

A related concept is the notion of emancipation actions in nursing, described by Kendall (1992). Some feel that this is an extension of the concept of empowerment. Derived from work by Habermas (1971) and others, the notion of emancipatory nursing refers to not merely helping those who might be oppressed, marginalized, or disenfranchised to cope with the difficulties or challenges in their lives, but actually fighting back against the socially constructed barriers that oppress them. Acting in an advocacy role by simply facilitating coping with difficulties is not enough, according to Kendall. Instead, this new type of empowered caring involves "living, teaching, encouraging and activating emancipatory behaviors, rather than relying heavily on the concepts of coping and adaptation" (Kendall, 1992, p. 2).

Nevertheless, nurses can and do feel disempowered in their work settings, and instead of feeling empowered or enacting emancipatory nursing actions, they may choose the *victim* stance, which relinquishes power to the system, or they may challenge the system. Dealing with the system requires skills in conflict management, negotiation, and effective communication. Challenging the system can take many forms. Being a change agent begins with the nurse's personal presence and attitude as an individual.

As a cohesive group and as individuals, nurses can address social and economic constraints on nursing and health care through their involvement in professional organizations and through becoming politically active. Participation on institution boards or committees that focus on patient care and professional practice concerns is another way to challenge the system, as is speaking out about unsafe or questionable practices. Speaking out is sometimes referred to as **whistleblowing**. However, speaking out or challenging the status quo is not always the same as whistle-blowing. The term "whistleblowing" comes from the image of someone blowing a shrill whistle, loud enough to jolt others away from the "false harmony" (Ray, 2006, p. 438) of the *status quo*, to pay attention to perceived inequities, incompetence, abuse, or danger, usually within or from outside an organization or hierarchy.

Whistleblowing should always be a last resort when looking at ways to deal with unsafe, unethical, illegal, or challenging practices in the workplace—only used when all other legitimate ways of approaching a problem have failed. Whistleblowing is not without risks, as well as significant physical and emotional side effects for those who choose this method to speak out. In one nursing study, stress-induced effects were noted both in nurses who chose to blow the whistle and in those who did not choose to do so when dealing with a difficult situation (McDonald, 2002). It is not surprising that simply being involved in a situation that one identifies as potentially dangerous or unethical can induce feelings similar to any stressful situation; however, these things and others must be taken into account before deciding to "blow the whistle."

The Canadian Nurses Association notes that whistleblowing should be considered only after all other ways of addressing a problem have been tried. They continue, stating that there might be a moral right on behalf of nurses to disclose cases of public harm and, in some cases, even a moral obligation to do so. The association also notes that having a right to speak up does not imply that one ought to then engage in whistleblowing (Baker, 1988). Three things must be explored before deciding to blow the whistle. First, there must be serious harm or potential harm to the public involved. Second, one must have reported the problem, issue, or events appropriately through the hierarchy of the organization. Finally, and most importantly, perhaps, the whistleblower must be convinced or have evidence that the act of speaking out in this manner will likely result in positive or desired change (Baker, 1988).

Empowerment incorporates divergent and conflicting solutions to problems based on choosing to support others rather than choosing divisiveness (Chinn, 1995; Gibson, 1991). It implies embracing diversity and moving from fear of that which is different to appreciation of the strength derived from, and unity contained in, diversity. Nurses need to recognize that systems exert control, in part, by fostering divisiveness among workers in order to deter unity of opposition to system policies. When nurses unite with and support colleagues who challenge harmful or potentially harmful practices, they are personally and professionally empowered.

Challenging unjust, unprofessional, or unethical practices is not an easy decision, and may entail risk for nurses. Feeling empowered to take a stand requires personal integrity and support from others. Before whistleblowing, consider the following:

- Determine if you are ready, both personally and professionally, to take action through personal reflection and consultation with others.
- Consult a lawyer or your professional association for legal advice.
- Use a journal to document instances that give you concern and that compromise care, creating a paper trail that includes dates, times, and outcomes of unsafe or inappropriate care. Make a copy of all documentation and keep all electronic communication.
- Remember when communicating by e-mail to never make any statements you would not want attributed to you on the front page of a newspaper.
- Speak only the truth, state only the facts, and follow the institution's chain of command to the letter before contacting an outside agency.
- Build leadership skills and unity among your colleagues.
- Most of all, contribute to developing a strong sense of ethical integrity in your nursing community. Pay attention to issues of inequity or threats to others' integrity, find places to initiate discussions about ethical and practical challenges, and create safe places to voice concerns.

Nurses need to be willing to struggle with difficult questions and arrive at decisions that flow from their own internal values and perspectives, rather than looking for the *right* answer to come from an external source. Empowerment implies accountability for our own choices and actions. Jameton (1984) points out that people pretend they are forced to do things when they are not. He gives the example of a nurse who instructs a patient to take a medication because the physician ordered it, noting that both patient and nurse pretend that they must act because of the physician's order, although each could make another choice. Reflecting that nurses who choose to work in systems such as hospitals are accountable for their actions despite the existence of systemic problems affecting health care, Jameton writes,

> If one fails to resist exploitation, incompetence, and corrupt practices, one becomes responsible for them. If one resists them, one enters into conflict with conventional conceptions of behavior for employees and thereby risks reprisals. One has to choose between complicity and self-sacrifice, or enter the uncomfortable middle ground of irony. Ethics does not give a clear answer as to which one must choose. Instead, one is free to move in the direction of the kind of world one personally desires to create. (1984, p. 289)

We must decide whether we prefer a world in which we are empowered in the professional arena, or one in which we are controlled by others. The choices we make influence the outcome.

Empowerment for Evolving Professional Nurses

Nursing students often struggle with the notion of empowerment as they move through their education towards graduation and fully independent practice. Nursing still has a reputation for "eat[ing] their young" (Daiski, 2004, p. 46), and reports persist of nursing students feeling disempowered through a variety of experiences: being excluded, silenced, treated insensitively, bullied, or being made to feel inadequate, incapable, or powerless. These findings tell us that there is still much to explore and change about the way nursing students are educated and supported (Bradbury-Jones, Sambrook & Irvine, 2007; Daiski, 2004). While nursing students may feel empowered in discussions in the classroom, their clinical practice experiences while in school and as new graduates may lead them to feel disempowered, discouraged, and not supported (McKenna, Smith, Poole & Coverdale, 2003). Research about the self-esteem of nursing students is limited, but what there is demonstrates links between empowerment, self-esteem, and autonomy in reaching goals; much needs to be still explored (Bradbury-Jones, Sambrook & Irvine, 2007; Mailloux, 2006; McKenna, Smith, Poole & Coverdale, 2003). With significant documented problems in the recruitment and retention of new graduate nurses, we know that not enough is being done to create safe, supportive and empowering work environments and that many new nurses feel this in a strong enough way to leave the professional altogether within two years of graduating (Lavoie-Tremblay, O'Brien-Pallas, Gélinas, Desforges & Marchionni, 2008). The authors go on to note that many new nurses, feeling devalued and without support, describe an imbalance between the perceived rewards of the work and the efforts put forth, as individuals. It is clear that further supporting nursing students today in the creation of safe and empowering environments will have a significant impact upon the profession tomorrow—our future clinical teachers and managers in nursing are, in fact, the students of today.

NURSES AND PATIENT EMPOWERMENT

Although empowerment is something that comes from within a person, nurses can serve as enablers of the process. Enabling the empowerment process requires a paradigm shift away from the paternalistic attitude of knowing what is best for the patient. Instead, we recognize and accept that patients are essentially responsible for their own health and have the ability to discern what they need, make decisions, and direct their own destinies. In order to make appropriate decisions, however, people may need information and support.

Gibson describes empowerment in the health care arena as "a social process of recognizing, promoting and enhancing people's abilities to meet their own needs, solve their own problems and mobilize the necessary resources in order to feel in control of their own lives . . . a process of helping people to assert control over the factors which affect their health" (1991, p. 339). In light of this description and nursing's focus on patient advocacy, nurses are called to be enablers of the empowerment process with patients, families, and communities. Certain attitudes, knowledge, and skills are basic to fulfilling this role.

Attitudes of Nurses That Enable Empowerment

A view of the nurse as an advocate, facilitator, and resource rather than merely one who provides services for patients is basic to enabling the empowerment of patients (Ellis-Stoll & Popkess-Vawter, 1998; Fulton, 1997; Gibson, 1991). Nurses must learn to surrender their need for control, developing instead attitudes of collaboration and mutual participation in decision making. This requires self-reflection on the part of the nurse, through which the nurse confronts personal values and the subtle, and not-so-subtle, benefits of being in a position of power. It is essential that nurses make a commitment to being with patients as they struggle with their questions and issues and seek meaning in the process. Relinquishing control also means that nurses need to accept decisions made by patients and families, even when they are different from what the nurse might do or suggest. Respect for persons, which includes valuing others and mutual trust, is key (Gibson, 1991; Rodwell, 1996; Ellis-Stoll & Popkess-Vawter, 1998; Ryles, 1999).

Nursing Knowledge and Skills Necessary for Enabling Empowerment

Information presented throughout this book provides a foundation for facilitating the empowerment process. Paying attention to ethical principles and to the processes of decision making fosters empowerment. Being aware of how values develop and how they affect choices enables nurses to be think more clearly about their own perspectives, so as to foster integrity and avoid imposing personal values on others. Knowledge of social, cultural, political, economic, and other forces affecting a person's options and health choices is essential.

Empowerment is an interactive process. As in many other areas of nursing, effective communication is necessary for facilitating empowerment. The ability to listen with our whole being and to trust intuitive as well as intellectual understanding is important. Reflective listening allows us to help people to recognize their own strengths, abilities, and personal power. Active listening also helps people to develop an awareness of the root causes of problems and to determine their readiness to take action for change.

If it is determined that the patient does not want to be empowered, nursing interventions need to be provided in a way that acknowledges their own strengths, rather than in a way that patients may experience as controlling (Gibson, 1991). This means approaching patients with an attitude of trust in their ability to know what they need, and to incorporate behaviours such as offering patients choices about aspects of their care over which they can have some control. For example, a patient who is hospitalized for intravenous antibiotic therapy for a serious cardiac infection may feel that she has little choice over whether or not to actually have the antibiotic, but can have some degree of choice over where her intravenous line is inserted, and the timing of the medication administration.

Having the opportunities and resources needed for understanding and changing our world is part of the empowerment process. Nurses must have knowledge of factors affecting a patient's health and health care decisions in order to help provide or share the necessary resources. Such knowledge includes awareness of the patient's and family's values and decision-making style; cultural context; social, political, and economic influences on our options; and health care system constraints.

We also recognize that individual responsibility for health is necessarily tempered by social and economic factors. Gibson (1991) suggests that nurses need to focus health promotion efforts on the macro social level, attending to conditions that control, influence, and produce health or illness in people. Efforts as individuals, within professional organizations, and within communities, aimed at providing access to health care for all, provide a broad base of support for empowerment.

Nurses must approach patients as equal partners. Skilful collaboration and negotiation, which incorporate power sharing and mutually beneficial interactions, enable empowerment. Relinquishing professional power returns power to the patient.

ENHANCING PATIENT CAPACITY FOR DECISION MAKING

The ability to make decisions regarding our own lives and destinies requires a basic level of cognitive functioning and sense of control over life processes and change processes. Empowerment originates in self-esteem; it is developed through a sense of connectedness, responsibility, and opportunities for choice; and is supported through perceived meaning and hope in life (Rodwell, 1996).

Helping patients through the process of self-discovery facilitates empowerment by enabling them to decide what they want to do based on an appreciation of who they are. Empowerment, according to Purtilo and Meier (1993), arises out of a person's ability to reflect upon and understand oneself. This may require facilitating a patient's self-awareness on many levels, such as identifying personal values, sources of these values, where and to whom they feel connected, and where and how they experience control in life. Following the decision-making process discussed in Chapter 6 can facilitate empowerment with patients.

Determining whether a person functions primarily from a sense of internal or external locus of control can be useful. **Locus of control** refers to beliefs about the ability to control events in our life. People who believe that they are able to influence or control the things that happen to them are considered to have an **internal locus of control**. On the other hand, people who feel that forces outside themselves direct or rule their lives—whether generalized forces such as fate or other persons who are perceived to be more powerful—are considered to have an **external locus of control**. Persons who are internally motivated are more likely to perceive themselves as having the power to make choices and control their own lives, and to be motivated to make necessary changes. Those who are externally motivated tend to be more fatalistic, expecting their lives to be controlled by powerful others, and less likely to enact personal power (Dawson, 1994; Miller, 1993).

ASK YOURSELF

How Does Locus of Control Affect Empowerment?

- Reflect on how you have thought through significant decisions in your life. Do you consider that you are more internally or externally motivated? Give specific examples to support your self-assessment.

- In working with patients, what would you consider indications of an internal and external locus of control?

- How would your approach to facilitating empowerment be different with persons who exhibit an internal locus of control compared to those with an external locus of control?

Fostering Patient Empowerment

We can facilitate empowerment in others by being role models of self-empowerment. As noted previously, a belief that patients have the right and ability to make choices regarding their health, and other areas of their lives, is basic to empowerment. Patients need to be given opportunities for choice regarding small as well as major decisions. This means that there needs to be participatory decision making, involving collaboration and negotiation, in what we might consider the "less important" decisions regarding things in all areas of health care. For example, involving patients in making decisions about when they will bathe, what foods to include in their diet, or when to take their medications is as important to empowerment as their participation in decision making regarding life-support measures. Because of social, environmental, and other factors, some people have had limited opportunities for making choices and may need education, practice, and encouragement in this area. Offering options and developing strategies to enhance the patient's ability to set and reach goals are important parts of the nursing role. Connelly *et al.* (1993) suggest that choosing implies having both the freedom and the courage to choose from different options. Support is an important part of the encouraging process.

Support can take many forms. We provide support by determining what patients identify as empowering to them and encouraging these choices, behaviours, or attitudes. Caring relationships, in which experiences are shared and patients are accepted for who they are, offer support. Having at least one other person who supports a choice made or a stance that a person takes enhances the likelihood that the person will follow through on the decision.

Having knowledge and having the necessary resources available are prerequisites for considering options and making choices. In order to enable empowerment, we may have to provide resources or help patients discover how to access resources. In some instances, this may mean becoming politically and socially active regarding health care issues affecting vulnerable populations. We need to develop strategies that enhance patients' abilities to acquire the knowledge they need. This may mean working with

THINK ABOUT IT

Outcomes of Patient Empowerment

Upholding the view that patients know what they need opens up the probability that some patients will make decisions that are not consistent with what the nurse or other health team members think is best. Such decisions may have a relatively minor impact on a patient's or family's health and well-being, or may be judged to have potentially serious outcomes for the patient or family.

- What factors need to be considered when dealing with decisions involving differing values between patients and nurses?
- Give examples of situations in which patient empowerment might potentiate an ethical dilemma for you. Reflect on how you would approach such a situation.
- If you feel a patient is making an unwise decision, how would you respond? How should you respond?
- Discuss your view regarding any limits or constraints on patient empowerment.

patients and communities to identify both health concerns and socioculturally relevant approaches to dealing with these concerns. We foster empowerment by promoting processes that encourage the mutually respectful exchange of ideas, and analysis of concerns and potential solutions. Success in achieving goals must be defined from the perspective of the patient or community.

BARRIERS TO EMPOWERMENT

Empowerment involves a willingness to take risks, to move beyond what is known, and perhaps comfortable, to the unknown. It often requires a change in self-perception, developing a different vision of who we are. This can stimulate anxiety and fear. Nurses need to recognize such barriers and appreciate that not everyone wants to take the risks and assume the responsibility that empowerment demands. Patients who may be used to the more traditional patriarchal model of the health care professional–patient relationship may have difficulty with or be uncomfortable when given the opportunity to have the "power" to make decisions about their own care, preferring to relinquish such decision-making power to physicians or other health care professionals, like nurses. This also arises from a belief that medical or nursing knowledge is of greater value than patients' own knowledge of self. Ideally, specific physiological, biomedical, and nursing knowledge, as well as the particular context and situation of a patient, are all important considerations in providing quality care. Paternalistic attitudes within the health care system have fostered reliance on health care providers to determine what patients need for health. Other barriers include patients' lack of knowledge of resources or strategies that promote empowerment, dependency, apathy, mistrust, and being labelled by staff (Connelly *et al.*, 1993). Social, cultural, economic, or political factors can present barriers, such as limitation of resources, control of knowledge about options, locking people into traditional roles and expectations, social labelling that stereotypes and devalues certain people or behaviours, and restriction of access to resources. Patients may also feel hesitant to take part in decision making for fear of making poor decisions or decisions that their medical provider might feel are irresponsible or inappropriate. Often, patients feel that they are being blamed for their decisions, especially decisions regarding lifestyle habits (e.g., smoking, alcohol use, risky sexual practices, a poor diet). Furthermore, they may feel that the notion of being empowered is, to some degree, an empty and overused concept, as it is invoked so frequently and in such divergent contexts, such as direct-to-consumer advertisements for drugs (only in the United States but frequently viewed on American television channels by Canadians), advocacy groups, policy makers, and politicians, who all quote the best interests of patients and the goal of empowerment, until it loses any real meaning (Tomes, 2007). Lack of empowerment of professionals, and their inability to relinquish power to patients, hinder patient empowerment as well. Honouring patient decisions may be very threatening to nurses who do not appreciate that patients know what they need.

One important barrier to the empowerment of patients is a fundamental lack of or inability to practise patient-centred care. In their discussion on patient-centredness,

Mead and Bower (2000) talk about the kinds of factors that affect the ability of physicians, specifically, to engage in patient-centred care. While patient-centred care is different from empowerment, it is certainly a prerequisite at least. This phenomenon, while contextualized in the physician–patient relationship, is also highly relevant to relationships patients have with other health care professionals. The authors identify five categories of factors that influence patient-centred care. These are patient factors, physician (or health care professional) factors, consultation-level influences, professional context influences, and shapers. Patient factors include things like attitudes and expectations, level of knowledge, age, and gender. Health care professional factors include attitudes, values, level of knowledge and expertise, age, gender, and knowledge of patient. Consultation-level influences are things like how frequent interruptions are during a patient-professional interaction, physical barriers, time limitations, communication barriers, and the presence of third parties. Professional context influences include professional norms, performance incentives, accreditation, and policies. Finally, shapers include formal and informal learning of patients via the media, personal experiences of both the health care professional and the patient, and socioeconomic background (Mead and Bower, 2000). This is interesting, because, before we can, as nurses, begin to think about empowering patients, we must first reflect on whether or not we are facilitating patient-centred care and ensuring that we examine these kinds of influences on our ability to put our patients and their interests first. Only after we do that can we claim to be in a position, both reflectively and practically, to empower others.

SUMMARY

Empowerment is a complex and multifaceted concept. Awareness of attitudes about nursing's role in health care and factors that shape these attitudes enables nurses to identify more effectively what supports or diminishes both personal and professional empowerment. Attentiveness to personal empowerment, which includes integrity, accountability, and courage, is fundamental to addressing empowerment issues within the context of professional practice for all nurses, from novices to experienced practitioners and nurse educators. Patient empowerment is an important element of nursing care that derives from an appreciation that patients have the ability to discern their own needs and make decisions about their own lives and health. Becoming an enabler of empowerment requires that nurses learn to relinquish power and embrace the patient as a partner. Self-awareness, respect for others, and effective communication skills serve as foundations for the process. Nurses can facilitate empowerment by working directly with patients and through addressing social, political, and environmental factors affecting empowerment of individuals and communities. In the midst of an ever-changing and challenging health care environment in which issues of power and control continue to affect patient care, nurses must be competent enablers of patient empowerment. Empowerment for nurses requires remembering *who* we are, recognizing that *knowing* must be the same as *doing*, and following our own vision of nursing.

CHAPTER HIGHLIGHTS

- Empowerment, which is both process and outcome, derives from a feminine perspective of *power to* or *power with*, reflecting a supportive partnership based on mutual love and respect that enables people to change situations given the necessary resources, knowledge, skills, and opportunities. Empowerment comes from within a person and involves choice; we cannot empower another.

- The ability to deal with health care issues and dilemmas in a principled way derives from personal and professional empowerment and requires attentiveness to intrapersonal, interpersonal, and systems issues.

- Personal empowerment requires self-awareness and is characterized by maintaining personal integrity in the midst of a loving response to the choices of others. Self-concept and sense of power in a nurse's personal life affects nursing care and a nurse's ability to enable empowerment in others.

- Recognizing unity in diversity and incorporating divergent views and solutions empowers nurses and others.

- Defining nursing according to nursing's own vision is an act of empowerment that implies accountability for our own choices and actions, with awareness that each choice helps create the kind of world and environment within which nurses must practise.

- Patient empowerment, which is both a process and an outcome, relates to ethical principles and flows from nursing's focus on patient advocacy.

- Although nurses cannot empower patients, they can be enablers of empowerment, a process that requires recognition and acceptance that patients have the ability to discern what they need, to make decisions, and to direct their own destinies.

- Empowerment is interactive and requires knowledge of personal values and needs for control, mutual trust, and respect, effective communication and reflective listening skills, and the willingness to accept patient decisions regardless of whether the nurse thinks they are best or not.

- Empowerment requires us to first reflect on whether or not we are truly practising "patient-centred" care.

- Fostering patient empowerment requires knowledge of social, political, cultural, economic, and environmental factors affecting a person's options and health choices and may involve addressing health promotion efforts on the macro social level.

- Empowerment is fostered through self-discovery, enhanced self-esteem, a sense of connectedness, support, opportunities for choice, and having needed resources, knowledge, and skills.

- Empowerment strategies that mesh with a person's or community's sociocultural context are more effective.

DISCUSSION QUESTIONS AND ACTIVITIES

1. Where or when in your life do you feel most or least personally empowered? Think about the factors affecting your feelings of empowerment or disempowerment in these situations or contexts.

2. Review Chapters 5 and 6 and reflect on how your values and current phase of development affect your sense of personal empowerment.

3. Describe a situation in which you took responsibility for your own feelings or actions.

4. Describe a time when you found yourself blaming others or assuming a victim stance.

5. Discuss with classmates factors prompting each stance and how you felt in each situation.

6. What aspects of empowerment do you think are most important in nursing practice settings? Support your perspective.

7. Describe a personal experience as a patient within the health care system in which you felt that you were empowered. What or who contributed to the empowerment process for you?

8. In your clinical setting, observe nurses that you work with, and describe attitudes and behaviours that either foster or block empowerment with patients.

9. Discuss factors within the health care system that work to inhibit patient empowerment.

10. What would indicate to you that a patient might not want to be empowered? How would you approach and work with this patient?

REFERENCES

Babendo-Mould, Y., C. L. Iwasiw, M. Andrusyszyn, H. K. S. Laschinger & W. Weston (2012). Effects of clinical practice environments of clinical teacher and nursing student outcomes. *Journal of Nursing Education, 51*(4), 217–225.

Baker, J. (1988). Confidentiality and when to blow the whistle. As cited in *Ethics in Practice. Canadian Nurses Association*. November 1999. C.N.A.: Ottawa.

Bolton, B., & J. Brookings (1998). Development of a measure of intrapersonal empowerment. *Rehabilitation Psychology, 43*(2), 131–142.

Bradbury-Jones, C., S. Sambrook & F. Irvine (2007). The meaning of empowerment for nursing students: a critical incident study. *Journal of Advanced Nursing, 59*(4), 342–351.

Byrne, C. (1999). Facilitating empowerment groups: Dismantling professional boundaries. *Issues in Mental Health Nursing, 19*, 55–71.

Chandler, G. E. (1991). Creating an environment to empower nurses. *Nursing Management, 22*, 20–23.

Chavasse, J. M. (1992). New dimensions of empowerment in nursing—and challenges. *Journal of Advanced nursing, 17,* 1–2.

Chinn, P. (1995). *Peace and power: Building communities for the future.* New York: National League of Nursing Press.

Connelly, L. M., B. S. Keele, V. M. Kleinbeck, J. K. Schneider & A. K. Cobb (1993). A place to be yourself: Empowerment from the client's perspective. *IMAGE: Journal of Nursing Scholarship, 25*(4), 297–303.

Curtin, L. (1982). Autonomy, accountability and nursing practice. *Topics in Clinical Nursing, 4,* 7–14.

Daiski, I. (2004). Changing nurses' disempowering relationship patterns. *Journal of Advanced Nursing, 48*(1), 43–50.

Dawson, M. S. (1994). Using locus of control to empower student nurses to be professional. *Nursing Forum, 29,* 10–15.

Ellis-Stoll, C. C., & S. Popkess-Vawter (1998). A concept analysis on the process of empowerment. *Advances in Nursing Science, 21*(2), 62–68.

Fulton, Y. (1997). Nurses' views on empowerment: A critical social theory perspective. *Journal of Advanced Nursing, 26,* 529–536.

Gibson, C. H. (1991). A concept analysis of empowerment. *Journal of Advanced Nursing, 16,* 354–361.

Gordon, S., & B. Buresh (2000). *From silence to voice: What nurses know and must communicate to the public.* Canadian Nurses Association: Ottawa.

Gurka, A. M. (1995). Transformational leadership: Qualities and strategies for the CNS. *Clinical Nurse Specialist, 9,* 169–174.

Habermas, J. (1971). *Knowledge and Human Interests.* Boston: Beacon Press.

Hartrick, G., & R. Schreiber (1998). Imaging ourselves: Nurses' metaphors of practice. *Journal of Holistic Nursing, 16*(4), 420–434.

Hawks, J. H. (1992). Empowerment in nursing education: Concept analysis and application to philosophy, learning and instruction. *Journal of Advanced Nursing, 17,* 609–618.

Herbert, R. J., A. J. Gagnon, J. E. Rennick & J. L. O'Loughlin (2009). A systematic review of questionnaires measuring health-related empowerment. *Research and Theory for Nursing Practice: An International Journal, 23*(2), 107–132.

Jameton, A. (1984). *Nursing practice: The ethical issues.* Englewood Cliffs, NJ: Prentice-Hall.

Jones, P. S., M. T. O'Toole, N. Hoa, T. T. Chau & P. D. Muc (2000). Empowerment of nursing as a socially significant profession in Vietnam. *Journal of Nursing Scholarship, 32*(3), 317–321.

Kendall, J. (1992). Fighting back: Emancipatory nursing actions. *Advances in Nursing Science, 15*(2), 1–15.

Klakovich, M. (1995). Development and psychometric evaluation of the reciprocal empowerment scale. *Journal of Nursing Management, 3*(2), 127–143.

Kuokkanen, L., & H. Leino-Kilpi (2000). Power and empowerment in nursing: Three theoretical approaches. *Journal of Advanced Nursing, 31*(1), 235–241.

Kuokkanen, L. & H. Leino-Kilpi (2001). The qualities of an empowered nursing and the factors involved. *Journal of Nursing Management, 9,* 273–280.

Laschinger, H. K., & C. Wong (1999). Staff nurse empowerment and collective accountability: Effect on perceived productivity and self-rated work effectiveness. *Nursing Economics, 17*(6), 308–316.

Laschinger, H. K., C. Wong, L. McMahon & C. Kaufmann (1999). Leader behavior impact on staff nurse empowerment, job tension, and work effectiveness. *JONA, 29*(5), 28–39.

Lavoie-Tremblay, M., L. O'Brien-Pallas, C. Gélinas, N. Desforges & C. Marchionni (2008). Addressing the turnover issue among new nurses from a generational standpoint. *Journal of Nursing Management, 16,* 724–733.

Mailloux, C. G. (2006). The extent to which students' perceptions of faculties' teaching strategies, students' context, and perceptions of learner empowerment predict perceptions of autonomy in BSN students. *Nursing Education Today, 26,* 578–585.

McDonald, S. (2002). Physical and emotional effects of whistle blowing. *Journal of Psychosocial Nursing & Mental Health Services, 40*(1), 14–27. Retrieved September 6, 2008, from ProQuest Nursing & Allied Health Source database. (Document ID: 103437026).

McKenna, B., N. Smith, S. Poole, & J. Coverdale (2003). Horizontal violence: experiences of Registered Nurses in the first year of practice. *Journal of Advanced Nursing, 42*(1), 90–96.

Mead, N., & P. Bower (2000). Patient-centredness: A conceptual framework and review of the empirical literature. *Social Science and Medicine, 51,* 1087–1110.

Miller, C. M. (1993). Trajectory and empowerment theory applied to care of patients with multiple sclerosis. *Journal of Neuroscience Nursing, 25,* 343–348.

Moss, M. T. (1995). Foundations of nursing empowerment. *Nursing Economics, 13,* 112–114.

Purtilo, R. B., & R. H. Meier (1993). Team challenges: Regulatory constraints and patient empowerment. *American Journal of Physical Medicine & Rehabilitation, 72,* 327–330.

Random House dictionary of the English language, second edition unabridged. (1987). New York: Random House.

Ray, S. (2006). Whistle-blowing and organizational ethics. *Nursing ethics, 13*(4), 438–445.

Rodwell, C. M. (1996). An analysis of the concept of empowerment. *Journal of Advanced Nursing, 23,* 305–313.

Ryles, S. M. (1999). A concept analysis of empowerment: Its relationship to mental health nursing. *Journal of Advanced Nursing, 29*(3), 600–607.

Tomes, N. (2007). Patient empowerment and the dilemmas of late-modern medicalisation. *Lancet, 369,* 698–700.

Wallerstein, N., & E. Bernstein (1988). Empowerment education: Freire's ideas adapted to health education. *Health Education Quarterly, 15*(4), 379–394.

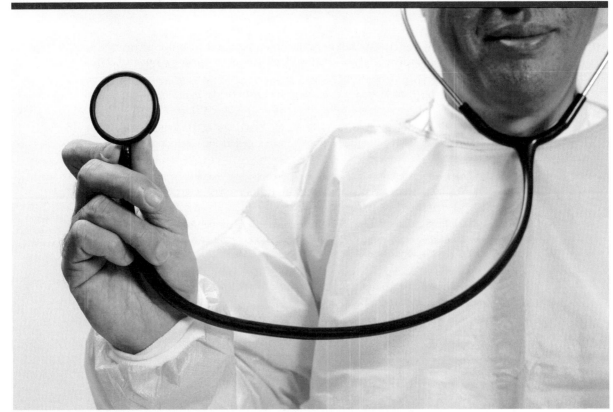

Apple's Eyes Studio/Shutterstock.com

APPENDIX **A**

THE CANADIAN NURSES ASSOCIATION CODE OF ETHICS FOR REGISTERED NURSES

PREAMBLE

The Canadian Nurses Association's *Code of Ethics for Registered Nurses*[1] is a statement of the ethical[2] **values**[3] of **nurses** and of nurses' commitments to persons with health-care needs and **persons receiving care**. It is intended for nurses in all contexts and

---

[1] In this document, the terms *registered nurse* and *nurse* include nurses who are registered or licensed in extended roles, such as nurse practitioners.

[2] In this document, the terms *moral* and *ethical* are used interchangeably based upon consultation with nurse ethicists and philosophers. We acknowledge that not everyone concurs in this usage.

[3] Words or phrases in bold print are found in the glossary. They are shown in bold only on first appearance.

domains of nursing practice[4] and at all levels of decision-making. It is developed by nurses for nurses and can assist nurses in practising ethically and working through ethical challenges that arise in their practice with individuals, **families**, communities and public health systems.

The societal context in which nurses work is constantly changing and can be a significant influence on their practice. The quality of the work environment in which nurses practise is also fundamental to their ability to practise ethically. The code of ethics is revised periodically (see Appendix A [All Appendices refer to those in the *Code of Ethics*. They are not included here.]) to ensure that it is attuned to the needs of nurses by reflecting changes in social values and conditions that affect the public, nurses and other **health-care providers**, and the health-care system (see Appendix B, for a list of societal changes envisioned to affect nursing practice in the coming decade). Periodic revisions also promote lively dialogue and create greater awareness of and engagement with ethical issues among nurses in Canada.

PURPOSE OF THE CODE

The *Code of Ethics for Registered Nurses* serves as a foundation for nurses' ethical practice. The specific values and ethical responsibilities expected of registered nurses in Canada are set out in part I. Endeavours that nurses may undertake to address social **inequities** as part of ethical practice are outlined in part II.

The code provides guidance for ethical relationships, responsibilities, behaviours and decision-making, and it is to be used in conjunction with the professional standards, laws and regulations that guide practice.

It serves as a means of self-evaluation and self-reflection for ethical nursing practice and provides a basis for feedback and peer review. The code also serves as an ethical basis from which nurses can **advocate** for **quality work environments** that support the delivery of safe, **compassionate**, competent and ethical care.

Nurses recognize the privilege of being part of a self-regulating profession and have a responsibility to merit this privilege. The code informs other health-care professionals as well as members of the public about the ethical commitments of nurses and the responsibilities nurses accept as being part of a self-regulating profession.

FOUNDATION OF THE CODE

Ethical nursing practice involves core ethical responsibilities that nurses are expected to uphold. Nurses are accountable for these ethical responsibilities in their professional relationships with individuals, families, groups, populations, communities and colleagues.

---

[4]In this document, *nursing practice* refers to all areas of nursing practice, including direct care (which includes community and public health), education, administration, research and policy development.

As well, nursing **ethics** is concerned with how broad societal issues affect **health** and **well-being**. This means that nurses endeavour to maintain awareness of aspects of **social justice** that affect health and well-being and to advocate for change. Although these endeavours are not part of nurses' core ethical responsibilities, they are part of ethical practice and serve as a helpful motivational and educational tool for all nurses.

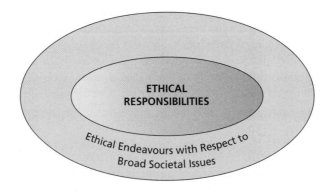

http://www.cna-nurses.ca/cna/documents/pdf/publications/ CodeofEthics2002_e.pdf. Reprinted with permission from the Canadian Nurses Association.

The code is organized in two parts:

PART I:

Part I, "Nursing Values and Ethical Responsibilities," describes the core responsibilities central to ethical nursing practice. These ethical responsibilities are articulated through seven primary values and accompanying responsibility statements, which are grounded in nurses' professional relationships with individuals, families, groups, populations and communities as well as with students, colleagues and other health-care professionals. The seven primary values are:

1. Providing safe, compassionate, competent and ethical care
2. Promoting health and well-being
3. Promoting and respecting informed decision-making
4. Preserving dignity
5. Maintaining privacy and confidentiality
6. Promoting justice
7. Being accountable

PART II:

Ethical nursing practice involves endeavouring to address broad aspects of social justice that are associated with health and well-being. Part II, "Ethical Endeavours," describes endeavours that nurses can undertake to address social inequities.

USING THE CODE IN NURSING PRACTICE

Values are related and overlapping. It is important to work toward keeping in mind all of the values in the code at all times for all persons in order to uphold the dignity of all. In health-care practice, values may be in conflict. Such value conflicts need to be considered carefully in relation to the practice situation. When such conflicts occur, or when nurses need to think through an ethical situation, many find it helpful to use an ethics model for guidance in ethical reflection, questioning and decision-making (see Appendix C).

Nursing practice involves both legal and ethical dimensions. Still, the law and ethics remain distinct. Ideally, a system of law would be completely compatible with the values in this code. However, there may be situations in which nurses need to **collaborate** with others to change a law or policy that is incompatible with ethical practice. When this occurs, the code can guide and support nurses in advocating for changes to law, policy or practice. The code can be a powerful political instrument for nurses when they are concerned about being able to practise ethically.

Nurses are responsible for the ethics of their practice. Given the complexity of ethical situations, the code can only outline nurses' ethical responsibilities and guide nurses in their reflection and decision-making. It cannot ensure ethical practice. For ethical practice, other elements are necessary, such as a commitment to do good; sensitivity and receptiveness to ethical matters; and a willingness to enter into relationships with persons receiving care and with groups, populations and communities that have health-care needs and problems. Practice environments have a significant influence on nurses' ability to be successful in upholding the ethics of their practice. In addition, nurses' self-reflection and dialogue with other nurses and health-care providers are essential components of ethical nursing practice. The importance of the work environment and of reflective practice is highlighted below.

QUALITY WORK ENVIRONMENTS

Nurses as individuals and as members of groups advocate for practice settings that maximize the quality of health outcomes for persons receiving care, the health and well-being of nurses, organizational performance and societal outcomes (Registered Nurses' Association of Ontario [RNAO], 2006 [All references refer to those in the *Code of Ethics*. They are not included here.]). Such practice environments have the organizational structures and resources necessary to ensure safety, support and respect for all persons in the work setting. Other health-care providers, organizations and policy-makers at regional, provincial/territorial, national and international levels strongly influence ethical practice.

NURSES' SELF-REFLECTION AND DIALOGUE

Quality work environments are crucial to ethical practice, but they are not enough. Nurses need to recognize that they are **moral agents** in providing care. This means that they have a responsibility to conduct themselves ethically in what they do and how they interact with persons receiving care. Nurses in all facets of the profession need to reflect on their practice, on the quality of their interactions with others and on the resources they need to maintain their own well-being. In particular, there is a pressing need for nurses to work with others (i.e., other nurses, other health-care professionals and the public) to create the **moral communities** that enable the provision of safe, compassionate, competent and ethical care.

Nursing ethics encompasses the breadth of issues involved in health-care ethics, but its primary focus is the ethics of the everyday. How nurses attend to ethics in carrying out their daily interactions, including how they approach their practice and reflect on their ethical commitment to the people they serve, is the substance of **everyday ethics**.

In their practice, nurses experience situations involving ethics. The values and responsibility statements in the code are intended to assist nurses in working through these experiences within the context of their unique practice situations.

TYPES OF ETHICAL EXPERIENCES AND SITUATIONS

When nurses can name the type of ethical concern they are experiencing, they are better able to discuss it with colleagues and supervisors, take steps to address it at an early stage, and receive support and guidance in dealing with it. Identifying an ethical concern can often be a defining moment that allows positive outcomes to emerge from difficult experiences. There are a number of terms that can assist nurses in identifying and reflecting on their ethical experiences and discussing them with others:[5]

Ethical problems involve situations where there are conflicts between one or more values and uncertainty about the correct course of action. Ethical problems involve questions about what is right or good to do at individual, interpersonal, organizational and even societal levels.

Ethical (or moral) uncertainty occurs when a nurse feels indecision or a lack of clarity, or is unable to even know what the moral problem is, while at the same time feeling uneasy or uncomfortable.

Ethical dilemmas or questions arise when there are equally compelling reasons for and against two or more possible courses of action, and where choosing one course of action means that something else is relinquished or let go. True dilemmas are infrequent in health care. More often, there are complex ethical problems with multiple courses of actions from which to choose.

---

[5]These situations are derived from CNA, 2004b; Fenton, 1988; Jameton, 1984; and Webster & Baylis, 2000.

Ethical (or moral) distress arises in situations where nurses know or believe they know the right thing to do, but for various reasons (including fear or circumstances beyond their control) do not or cannot take the right action or prevent a particular harm. When values and commitments are compromised in this way, nurses' identity and **integrity** as moral agents are affected and they feel moral distress.

Ethical (or moral) residue is what nurses experience when they seriously compromise themselves or allow themselves to be compromised. The moral residue that nurses carry forward from these kinds of situations can help them reflect on what they would do differently in similar situations in the future.

Ethical (or moral) disengagement can occur if nurses begin to see the disregard of their ethical commitments as normal. A nurse may then become apathetic or disengage to the point of being unkind, non-compassionate or even cruel to other health-care workers and to persons receiving care.

Ethical violations involve actions or failures to act that breach fundamental duties to the persons receiving care or to colleagues and other health-care providers.

Ethical (or moral) courage is exercised when a nurse stands firm on a point of moral principle or a particular decision about something in the face of overwhelming fear or threat to himself or herself.

PART I: NURSING VALUES AND ETHICAL RESPONSIBILITIES

Nurses in all domains of practice bear the ethical responsibilities identified under each of the seven primary nursing values.[6] These responsibilities apply to nurses' interactions with individuals, families, groups, populations, communities and society as well as with students, colleagues and other health-care professionals. The responsibilities are intended to help nurses apply the code. They also serve to articulate nursing values to employers, other health-care professionals and the public. Nurses help their colleagues implement the code, and they ensure that student nurses are acquainted with the code.

A. Providing Safe, Compassionate, Competent and Ethical Care

Nurses provide safe, compassionate, competent and ethical care.

Ethical responsibilities:

   1. Nurses have a responsibility to conduct themselves according to the ethical responsibilities outlined in this document and in practice standards in what they do and how they interact with persons receiving care as well as with families, communities, groups, populations and other members of the health-care team.

---

[6]The value and responsibility statements in the code are numbered and lettered for ease of use, not to indicate prioritization. The values are related and overlapping.

2. Nurses engage in compassionate care through their speech and body language and through their efforts to understand and care about others' health-care needs.

3. Nurses build trustworthy relationships as the foundation of meaningful communication, recognizing that building these relationships involves a conscious effort. Such relationships are critical to understanding people's needs and concerns.

4. Nurses question and intervene to address unsafe, non-compassionate, unethical or incompetent practice or conditions that interfere with their ability to provide safe, compassionate, competent and ethical care to those to whom they are providing care, and they support those who do the same. See Appendix D.

5. Nurses admit mistakes[7] and take all necessary actions to prevent or minimize harm arising from an adverse event. They work with others to reduce the potential for future risks and preventable harms. See Appendix D.

6. When resources are not available to provide ideal care, nurses collaborate with others to adjust priorities and minimize harm. Nurses keep persons receiving care, families and employers informed about potential and actual changes to delivery of care. They inform employers about potential threats to safety.

7. Nurses planning to take job action or practising in environments where job action occurs take steps to safeguard the health and safety of people during the course of the job action. See Appendix D.

8. During a natural or human-made disaster, including a communicable disease outbreak, nurses have a duty to provide care using appropriate safety precautions. See Appendix D.

9. Nurses support, use and engage in research and other activities that promote safe, competent, compassionate and ethical care, and they use guidelines for ethical research[8] that are in keeping with nursing values.

10. Nurses work to prevent and minimize all forms of violence by anticipating and assessing the risk of violent situations and by collaborating with others to establish preventive measures. When violence cannot be anticipated or prevented, nurses take action to minimize risk to protect others and themselves.

---

[7]Provincial and territorial legislation and nursing practice standards may include further direction regarding requirements for disclosure and reporting.

[8]See *Ethical* Research *Guidelines for Registered Nurses* (CNA, 2002) and the *Tri-Council Policy Statement: Ethical Conduct for Research Involving Humans* (Canadian Institutes of Health Research, Natural Sciences and Engineering Research Council of Canada, & Social Sciences and Humanities Research Council, 1998).

B. Promoting Health and Well-Being

Nurses work with people to enable them to attain their highest possible level of health and well-being.

Ethical responsibilities:

1. Nurses provide care directed first and foremost toward the health and well-being of the person, family or community in their care.

2. When a community health intervention interferes with the individual rights of persons receiving care, nurses use and advocate for the use of the least restrictive measures possible for those in their care.

3. Nurses collaborate with other health-care providers and other interested parties to maximize health benefits to persons receiving care and those with health-care needs, recognizing and respecting the knowledge, skills and perspectives of all.

C. Promoting and Respecting Informed Decision-Making

Nurses recognize, respect and promote a person's right to be informed and make decisions.

Ethical responsibilities:

1. Nurses, to the extent possible, provide persons in their care with the information they need to make informed decisions related to their health and well-being. They also work to ensure that health information is given to individuals, families, groups, populations and communities in their care in an open, accurate and transparent manner.

2. Nurses respect the wishes of capable persons to decline to receive information about their health condition.

3. Nurses recognize that capable persons may place a different weight on individualism and may choose to defer to family or community values in decision-making.

4. Nurses ensure that nursing care is provided with the person's informed consent. Nurses recognize and support a capable person's right to refuse or withdraw consent for care or treatment at anytime.

5. Nurses are sensitive to the inherent power differentials between care providers and those receiving care. They do not misuse that power to influence decision-making.

6. Nurses advocate for persons in their care if they believe that the health of those persons is being compromised by factors beyond their control, including the decision-making of others.

7. When family members disagree with the decisions made by a person with health-care needs, nurses assist families in gaining an understanding of the person's decisions.

8. Nurses respect the informed decision-making of capable persons, including choice of lifestyles or treatment not conducive to good health.

9. When illness or other factors reduce a person's capacity for making choices, nurses assist or support that person's participation in making choices appropriate to their capability.

10. If a person receiving care is clearly incapable of consent, the nurse respects the law on capacity assessment and substitute decision-making in his or her jurisdiction (Canadian Nurses Protective Society [CNPS], 2004).

11. Nurses, along with other health-care professionals and with substitute decision-makers, consider and respect the best interests of the person receiving care and any previously known wishes or advance directives that apply in the situation (CNPS, 2004).

D. Preserving Dignity

Nurses recognize and respect the intrinsic worth of each person.

Ethical responsibilities:

1. Nurses, in their professional capacity, relate to all persons with respect.

2. Nurses support the person, family, group, population or community receiving care in maintaining their dignity and integrity.

3. In health-care decision-making, in treatment and in care, nurses work with persons receiving care, including families, groups, populations and communities, to take into account their unique values, customs and spiritual beliefs, as well as their social and economic circumstances.

4. Nurses intervene, and report when necessary,[9] when others fail to respect the dignity of a person receiving care, recognizing that to be silent and passive is to condone the behaviour. See Appendix D.

5. Nurses respect the physical privacy of persons by providing care in a discreet manner and by minimizing intrusions.

6. When providing care, nurses utilize practice standards, best practice guidelines and policies concerning restraint usage.

7. Nurses maintain appropriate professional boundaries and ensure their relationships are always for the benefit of the persons they serve. They recognize the potential vulnerability of persons and do not exploit their trust and

---

[9]See footnote 7.

dependency in a way that might compromise the therapeutic relationship. They do not abuse their relationship for personal or financial gain, and do not enter into personal relationships (romantic, sexual or other) with persons in their care.

8. In all practice settings, nurses work to relieve pain and suffering, including appropriate and effective symptom and pain management, to allow persons to live with dignity.

9. When a person receiving care is terminally ill or dying, nurses foster comfort, alleviate suffering, advocate for adequate relief of discomfort and pain and support a dignified and peaceful death. This includes support for the family during and following the death, and care of the person's body after death.

10. Nurses treat each other, colleagues, students and other health-care workers in a respectful manner, recognizing the power differentials among those in formal leadership positions, staff and students. They work with others to resolve differences in a constructive way. See Appendix D.

E. Maintaining Privacy and Confidentiality

Nurses recognize the importance of privacy and confidentiality and safeguard personal, family and community information obtained in the context of a professional relationship.

Ethical responsibilities:

1. Nurses respect the right of people to have control over the collection, use, access and disclosure of their personal information.

2. When nurses are conversing with persons receiving care, they take reasonable measures to prevent confidential information in the conversation from being overheard.

3. Nurses collect, use and disclose health information on a need-to-know basis with the highest degree of anonymity possible in the circumstances and in accordance with privacy laws.

4. When nurses are required to disclose information for a particular purpose, they disclose only the amount of information necessary for that purpose and inform only those necessary. They attempt to do so in ways that minimize any potential harm to the individual, family or community.

5. When nurses engage in any form of communication, including verbal or electronic, involving a discussion of clinical cases, they ensure that their discussion of persons receiving care is respectful and does not identify those persons unless appropriate.

6. Nurses advocate for persons in their care to receive access to their own health-care records through a timely and affordable process when such access is requested.

7. Nurses respect policies that protect and preserve people's privacy, including security safeguards in information technology.

8. Nurses do not abuse their access to information by accessing health-care records, including their own, a family member's or any other person's, for purposes inconsistent with their professional obligations.

9. Nurses do not use photo or other technology to intrude into the privacy of a person receiving care.

10. Nurses intervene if others inappropriately access or disclose personal or health information of persons receiving care.

F. Promoting Justice

Nurses uphold principles of justice by safeguarding human rights, equity and fairness and by promoting the public good.

Ethical responsibilities:

1. When providing care, nurses do not discriminate on the basis of a person's race, ethnicity, culture, political and spiritual beliefs, social or marital status, gender, sexual orientation, age, health status, place of origin, lifestyle, mental or physical ability or socio-economic status or any other attribute.

2. Nurses refrain from judging, labelling, demeaning, stigmatizing and humiliating behaviours toward persons receiving care, other health-care professionals and each other.

3. Nurses do not engage in any form of lying, punishment or torture or any form of unusual treatment or action that is inhumane or degrading. They refuse to be complicit in such behaviours. They intervene, and they report such behaviours.

4. Nurses make fair decisions about the allocation of resources under their control based on the needs of persons, groups or communities to whom they are providing care. They advocate for fair treatment and for fair distribution of resources for those in their care.

5. Nurses support a climate of trust that sponsors openness, encourages questioning the status quo and supports those who speak out to address concerns in good faith (e.g., whistle-blowing).

G. Being Accountable

Nurses are accountable for their actions and answerable for their practice.

Ethical responsibilities:

1. Nurses, as members of a self-regulating profession, practise according to the values and responsibilities in the *Code of Ethics for Registered Nurses* and in keeping with the professional standards, laws and regulations supporting ethical practice.

2. Nurses are honest and practise with integrity in all of their professional interactions.

3. Nurses practise within the limits of their competence. When aspects of care are beyond their level of competence, they seek additional information or knowledge, seek help from their supervisor or a competent practitioner and/ or request a different work assignment. In the meantime, nurses remain with the person receiving care until another nurse is available.

4. Nurses maintain their fitness to practise. If they are aware that they do not have the necessary physical, mental or emotional capacity to practise safely and competently, they withdraw from the provision of care after consulting with their employer or, if they are self-employed, arranging that someone else attend to their clients' health-care needs. Nurses then take the necessary steps to regain their fitness to practise.

5. Nurses are attentive to signs that a colleague is unable, for whatever reason, to perform his or her duties. In such a case, nurses will take the necessary steps to protect the safety of persons receiving care. See Appendix D.

6. Nurses clearly and accurately represent themselves with respect to their name, title and role.

7. If nursing care is requested that is in conflict with the nurse's moral beliefs and values but in keeping with professional practice, the nurse provides safe, compassionate, competent and ethical care until alternative care arrangements are in place to meet the person's needs or desires. If nurses can anticipate a conflict with their conscience, they have an obligation to notify their employers or, if the nurse is self-employed, persons receiving care in advance so that alternative arrangements can be made. See Appendix D.

8. Nurses identify and address conflicts of interest. They disclose actual or potential conflicts of interest that arise in their professional roles and relationships and resolve them in the interest of persons receiving care.

9. Nurses share their knowledge and provide feedback, mentorship and guidance for the professional development of nursing students,novice nurses and other health-care team members. See Appendix D.

PART II: ETHICAL ENDEAVOURS

There are broad aspects of social justice that are associated with health and well-being and that ethical nursing practice addresses. These aspects relate to the need for change in systems and societal structures in order to create greater **equity** for all. Nurses should endeavour as much as possible, individually and collectively, to advocate for and work toward eliminating social inequities by:

   i. Utilizing the principles of primary health care for the benefit of the public and persons receiving care.

    ii. Recognizing and working to address organizational, social, economic and political factors that influence health and well-being within the context of nurses' role in the delivery of care.

    iii. In collaboration with other health-care team members and professional organizations, advocating for changes to unethical health and social policies, legislation and regulations.

    iv. Advocating for a full continuum of accessible health-care services to be provided at the right time and in the right place. This continuum includes health promotion, disease prevention and diagnostic, restorative, rehabilitative and palliative care services in hospitals, nursing homes, home care and the community.

    v. Recognizing the significance of social determinants of health and advocating for policies and programs that address these determinants.

    vi. Supporting environmental preservation and restoration and advocating for initiatives that reduce environmentally harmful practices in order to promote health and well-being.

    vii. Working with individuals, families, groups, populations and communities to expand the range of health-care choices available, recognizing that some people have limited choices because of social, economic, geographic or other factors that lead to inequities.

    viii. Understanding that some groups in society are systemically disadvantaged, which leads to diminished health and well-being. Nurses work to improve the quality of lives of people who are part of disadvantaged and/or vulnerable groups and communities, and they take action to overcome barriers to health care.

    ix. Advocating for health-care systems that ensure accessibility, universality and comprehensiveness of necessary health-care services.

    x. Maintaining awareness of major health concerns such as poverty, inadequate shelter, food insecurity and violence. Nurses work individually and with others for social justice and to advocate for laws, policies and procedures designed to bring about equity.

    xi. Maintaining awareness of broader global health concerns such as violations of human rights, war, world hunger, gender inequities and environmental pollution. Nurses work individually and with others to bring about social change.

    xii. Advocating for the discussion of ethical issues among health-care team members, persons in their care, families and students. Nurses encourage ethical reflection, and they work to develop their own and others' heightened awareness of ethics in practice. See Appendix C.

    xiii. Working collaboratively to develop a moral community. As part of the moral community, all nurses acknowledge their responsibility to contribute to positive, healthy work environments.

GLOSSARY

The glossary is intended to provide nurses with a common language for their reflections and discussions about nursing ethics. It may also be instructive, since nurses who read the glossary terms are more likely to investigate these concepts further, especially if they are unfamiliar. The glossary does not necessarily provide formal definitions of terms, but rather it presents information in a manner and language that is meant to be helpful and accessible. Some terms in the glossary are not included in the main body of the code but are in the appendices, others may not appear exactly as noted in the text, and others may not be included in the text but may be useful to nurses in their ethical reflection and practice.

Advance Directives A person's written wishes about how and what decisions should be made if they become incapable of making decisions for themselves. In decisions about life-sustaining treatment, advance directives are meant to assist with decisions about withholding or withdrawing treatment. Also called living wills or personal directives.

Adverse Events Unexpected, undesirable incidents resulting in injury or death that are directly associated with the process of providing health care or health services to a person receiving care (Hebert, Hoffman & Davies, 2003).

Advocate Actively supporting a right and good cause; supporting others in speaking for themselves or speaking on behalf of those who cannot speak for themselves.

Boundaries A boundary in the nurse-person relationship is the point at which the relationship changes from professional and therapeutic to unprofessional and personal (College and Association of Registered Nurses of Alberta [CARNA], 2005a [All references refer to those in the *Code of Ethics*. They are not provided here]).

Capable Being able to understand and appreciate the consequences of various options and make informed decisions about one's own care and treatment.

Collaborate Building consensus and working together on common goals, processes and outcomes (RNAO, 2006).

Compassionate The ability to convey in speech and body language the hope and intent to relieve the suffering of another. Compassion must coexist with competence. "Compassion is a relational process that involves noticing another person's pain, experiencing an emotional reaction to his or her pain, and acting in some way to help ease or alleviate the pain" (Dutton, Lilius & Kanov, 2007).

Competency The integrated knowledge, skills, judgment and attributes required of a registered nurse to practise safely and ethically in a designated role and setting. (Attributes include, but are not limited to, attitudes, values and beliefs.)

Confidentiality The ethical obligation to keep someone's personal and private information secret or private (Fry & Johnstone, 2002).

Conflict of Interest Occurs when a nurse's personal or private interests interfere with the interests of a person receiving care or with the nurse's own professional responsibilities (College of Registered Nurses of British Columbia [CRNBC], 2006c).

Consent   *See Informed consent.*

Conscientious Objection   A situation in which a nurse requests permission from his or her employer to refrain from providing care because a practice or procedure conflicts with the nurse's moral or religious beliefs (CRNBC, 2007).

Cultures   The processes that happen between individuals and groups within organizations and society, and that confer meaning and significance; the health-care system has its own culture(s) (Varcoe & Rodney, 2002).

Determinants of Health   These include income and social status, social support, education and literacy, employment and working conditions, physical and social environments, biology, genetic endowment, personal health practices and coping skills, healthy child development, health services, gender and culture (Public Health Agency of Canada, 2003).

Diversity   The variation between people in terms of a range of factors such as ethnicity, national origin, race, gender, ability, age, physical characteristics, religion, values, beliefs, sexual orientation, socio-economic class or life experiences (RNAO, 2007a).

Duty to Provide Care   Nurses have a professional duty and a legal obligation to provide persons receiving care with safe, competent, compassionate and ethical care. There may be some circumstances in which it is acceptable for a nurse to withdraw from care provisions or to refuse to provide care (CRNBC, 2007; College of Registered Nurses of Nova Scotia [CRNNS], 2006a). See Appendix D.

Equitable   Determining fairness on the basis of people's needs.

Equity   In health care, the fulfillment of each individual's needs as well as the individual's opportunity to reach full potential as a human being (Canadian Nurses Association [CNA], 2006).

Ethics   The moral practices, beliefs and standards of individuals and/or groups (Fry & Johnstone, 2002).

Everyday Ethics   How nurses pay attention to ethics in carrying out their common daily interactions, including how they approach their practice and reflect on their ethical commitments to persons receiving care and those with health-care needs.

Fairness   Equalizing people's opportunities to participate in and enjoy life, given their circumstances (Caplan, Light & Daniels, 1999), and society's equitable distribution of resources (in health care this means an expectation of equitable treatment).

Family/Families   In matters of caregiving, family is recognized to be those people identified by the person receiving care or in need of care as providing familial support, whether or not there is a biologic relationship. However, in matters of legal decision-making it must be noted that provincial legislation is not uniform across Canada and may include an obligation to recognize family members in priority according to their biologic relationship (CNA, 1994).

Fitness to Practise   All the qualities and capabilities of an individual relevant to his or her capacity to practise as a registered nurse, including, but not limited to, freedom from any cognitive, physical, psychological or emotional condition and dependence on alcohol or drugs that impairs his or her ability to practise nursing (CRNBC, 2006a; CRNNS, 2006b).

Global Health   The optimal well-being of all humans from the individual and the collective perspective. Health is considered a fundamental right and should be equally accessible by all (CNA, 2003).

Health   A state of complete physical, mental (spiritual) and social well-being, not merely the absence of disease (CNA, 2007; World Health Organization [WHO], 2006).

Health-Care Providers   All those who are involved in providing care; they may include professionals, personal care attendants, home support workers and others (CNA, 1994).

Health-Care Team   A number of health-care providers from different disciplines (often including both regulated professionals and unregulated workers) working together to provide care for and with individuals, families, groups, populations or communities.

Health Promotion   A continuing process of enabling people to increase their control over and improve their health and well-being.

Human Rights   The rights of people as expressed in the *Canadian Charter of Rights and Freedoms* (1982) and the *United Nations Universal Declaration of Human Rights* (1948), and as recorded in the CNA position statement *Registered Nurses and Human Rights* (CNA, 2004a).

Incapable/Incapacity   Failing to understand the nature of the treatment decisions to be made, as well as the consequences of consenting to treatment or declining treatment.

Inequity   An instance of unjust or unfair treatment of each individual's needs; health inequity means a lack of equitable access and opportunity for all people to meet their health needs and potential (CNA, 2006).

Informed Consent   The process of giving permission or making choices about care. It is based on both a legal doctrine and an ethical principle of respect for an individual's right to sufficient information to make decisions about care, treatment and involvement in research. In the code, the term *informed decision-making* is primarily used to emphasize the choice involved.

Integrity   (1) For persons receiving care, integrity refers to wholeness,and protecting integrity can mean helping them to become whole and complete again; (2) for health-care providers, showing integrity means consistently following accepted moral norms. Implicit in integrity is soundness, trustworthiness and consistency of convictions, actions and emotions (Burkhart & Nathaniel, 2002).

Interdisciplinary   The integration of concepts across different disciplines. An interdisciplinary team is a team of people with training in different fields: such teams are common in complex environments such as health care (RNAO, 2007b) and may also be referred to as interprofessional teams.

Intersectoral   All sectors of society (government, community and health).

Justice   Includes respecting the rights of others, distributing resources fairly,and preserving and promoting the common good (the good of the community).

Moral Agent/Agency The capacity or power of a nurse to direct his or her motives and actions to some ethical end; essentially, doing what is good and right.

Moral Climate In health care, the implicit and explicit values that drive health-care delivery and shape the workplaces in which care is delivered (Rodney, Hartrick Doane, Storch & Varcoe, 2006).

Moral Community A workplace where values are made clear and are shared, where these values direct ethical action and where individuals feel safe to be heard (adapted from Rodney & Street, 2004). Coherence between publicly professed values and the lived reality is necessary for there to be a genuine moral community (Webster & Baylis, 2000).

Nurse(s) In this code, refers to registered nurses, including nurses in extended roles such as nurse practitioners.

Person/Persons Receiving Care An individual, family, group, community or population that accesses the services of the registered nurse; may also be referred to as client(s) or patient(s).

Primary Health Care "Primary health care is essential health care based on practical, scientifically sound and socially acceptable methods and technology made universally accessible to individuals and families in the community through their full participation and at a cost that the community and country can afford to maintain at every stage of their development in the spirit of self-reliance and self-determination. It forms an integral part both of the country's health system, of which it is the central function and main focus, and of the overall social and economic development of the community. It is the first level of contact of individuals, the family and community with the national health system bringing health care as close a spossible to where people live and work, and constitutes the first element of acontinuing health care process" (WHO, 1978).

Privacy (1) Physical privacy is the right or interest in controlling or limiting the access of others to oneself; (2) informational privacy is the right of individuals to determine how, when, with whom and for what purposes any of their personal information will be shared.

Public Good The good of society or the community, often called the common good.

Quality Practice Environments Practice environments that have the organizational and human support allocations necessary for safe, competent and ethical nursing care (CNA, 2001).

Social Determinants Of Health Factors in the social environment, external to the health-care system, that exert a major and potentially modifiable influence on the health of populations (Evans, 1994). See also *Determinants of health*.

Social Justice The fair distribution of society's benefits and responsibilities and their consequences. It focuses on the relative position of one social group in relation to others in society as well as on the root causes of disparities and what can be done to eliminate them (CNA, 2006).

Substitute Decision-Maker An individual designated by operation of a provincial or territorial statute or in an advance directive of a person in care to make decisions about health care and treatment on the person's behalf (CNA, 1994).

Unregulated Care Provider Paid providers who are neither licensed nor registered by a regulatory body (CRNBC, 2006b).

Values Standards or qualities that are esteemed, desired, considered important or have worth or merit (Fry & Johnstone, 2002).

Violence Includes any abuse of power, manipulation or control of one person over another that could result in mental, emotional, social or physical harm.

Vulnerable Groups Groups disadvantaged by attitudes and systems in society that create inequities.

Well-Being A person's state of being well, content and able to make the most of his or her abilities.

Whistle-Blowing Speaking out about unsafe or questionable practices affecting people receiving care or working conditions. This should be resorted to only after a person has unsuccessfully used all appropriate organizational channels to right a wrong and has a sound moral justification for taking this action (Burkhardt & Nathaniel, 2002).

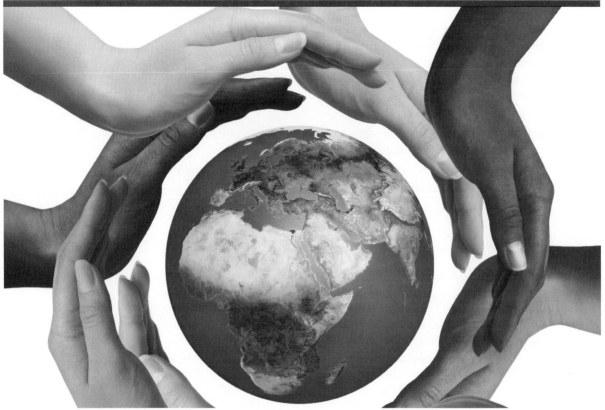

APPENDIX B

THE ICN CODE OF ETHICS FOR NURSES

An international code of ethics for nurses was first adopted by the International Council of Nurses (ICN) in 1953. It has been revised and reaffirmed at various times since, most recently with this review and revision completed in 2005.

PREAMBLE

Nurses have four fundamental responsibilities: to promote health, to prevent illness, to restore health and to alleviate suffering. The need for nursing is universal.

Inherent in nursing is respect for human rights, including cultural rights, the right to life and choice, to dignity and to be treated with respect. Nursing care is respectful of and unrestricted by considerations of age, colour, creed, culture, disability or illness, gender, sexual orientation, nationality, politics, race or social status.

Nurses render health services to the individual, the family and the community and co-ordinate their services with those of related groups.

THE ICN CODE

The *ICN Code of Ethics for Nurses* has four principal elements that outline the standards of ethical conduct.

ELEMENTS OF THE CODE

1. Nurses and People

The nurse's primary professional responsibility is to people requiring nursing care.

In providing care, the nurse promotes an environment in which the human rights, values, customs and spiritual beliefs of the individual, family and community are respected.

The nurse ensures that the individual receives sufficient information on which to base consent for care and related treatment.

The nurse holds in confidence personal information and uses judgement in sharing this information.

The nurse shares with society the responsibility for initiating and supporting action to meet the health and social needs of the public, in particular those of vulnerable populations.

The nurse also shares responsibility to sustain and protect the natural environment from depletion, pollution, degradation and destruction.

2. Nurses and Practice

The nurse carries personal responsibility and accountability for nursing practice, and for maintaining competence by continual learning.

The nurse maintains a standard of personal health such that the ability to provide care is not compromised.

The nurse uses judgement regarding individual competence when accepting and delegating responsibility.

The nurse at all times maintains standards of personal conduct which reflect well on the profession and enhance public confidence.

The nurse, in providing care, ensures that use of technology and scientific advances are compatible with the safety, dignity and rights of people.

3. Nurses and the Profession

The nurse assumes the major role in determining and implementing acceptable standards of clinical nursing practice, management, research and education.

The nurse is active in developing a core of research-based professional knowledge.

The nurse, acting through the professional organisation, participates in creating and maintaining safe, equitable social and economic working conditions in nursing.

4. Nurses and Co-Workers

The nurse sustains a co-operative relationship with co-workers in nursing and other fields.

The nurse takes appropriate action to safeguard individuals, families and communities when their health is endangered by a co-worker or any other person.

Suggestions for Use of the ICN Code of Ethics for Nurses

The *ICN Code of Ethics for Nurses* is a guide for action based on social values and needs. It will have meaning only as a living document if applied to the realities of nursing and health care in a changing society.

To achieve its purpose the *Code* must be understood, internalised and used by nurses in all aspects of their work. It must be available to students and nurses throughout their study and work lives.

Applying the Elements of the *ICN Code of Ethics for Nurses*

The four elements of the *ICN Code of Ethics for Nurses*: nurses and people, nurses and practice, nurses and the profession, and nurses and co-workers, give a framework for the standards of conduct. The following chart will assist nurses to translate the standards into action. Nurses and nursing students can therefore:

- Study the standards under each element of the *Code*.
- Reflect on what each standard means to you. Think about how you can apply ethics in your nursing domain: practice, education, research or management.
- Discuss the *Code* with co-workers and others.
- Use a specific example from experience to identify ethical dilemmas and standards of conduct as outlined in the *Code*. Identify how you would resolve the dilemmas.
- Work in groups to clarify ethical decision making and reach a consensus on standards of ethical conduct.
- Collaborate with your national nurses' association, co-workers, and others in the continuous application of ethical standards in nursing practice, education, management and research.

Element of the Code # 1: NURSES AND PEOPLE		
Practitioners and Managers	**Educators and Researchers**	**National Nurses' Associations**
Provide care that respects human rights and is sensitive to the values, customs and beliefs of all people.	In curriculum include references to human rights, equity, justice, solidarity as the basis for access to care.	Develop position statements and guidelines that support human rights and ethical standards.
Provide continuing education in ethical issues.	Provide teaching and learning opportunities for ethical issues and decision making.	Lobby for involvement of nurses in ethics review committees.
Provide sufficient information to permit informed consent and the right to choose or refuse treatment.	Provide teaching/ learning opportunities related to informed consent.	Provide guidelines, position statements and continuing education related to informed consent.
Use recording and information management systems that ensure confidentiality.	Introduce into curriculum concepts of privacy and confidentiality.	Incorporate issues of confidentiality and privacy into a national code of ethics for nurses.
Develop and monitor environmental safety in the workplace.	Sensitise students to the importance of social action in current concerns.	Advocate for safe and healthy environment.

Element of the Code # 2: NURSES AND PRACTICE		
Practitioners and Managers	**Educators and Researchers**	**National Nurses' Associations**
Establish standards of care and a work setting that promotes safety and quality care.	Provide teaching/ learning opportunities that foster life long learning and competence for practice.	Provide access to continuing education, through journals, conferences, distance education, etc.

| Establish systems for professional appraisal, continuing education and systematic renewal of licensure to practice. | Conduct and disseminate research that shows links between continual learning and competence to practice. | Lobby to ensure continuing education opportunities and quality care standards. |
| Monitor and promote the personal health of nursing staff in relation to their competence for practice. | Promote the importance of personal health and illustrate its relation to other values. | Promote healthy lifestyles for nursing professionals. Lobby for healthy work places and services for nurses. |

Element of the Code # 3: NURSES AND PROFESSION		
Practitioners and Managers	**Educators and Researchers**	**National Nurses' Associations**
Set standards for nursing practice, research, education and management.	Provide teaching/learning opportunities in setting standards for nursing practice, research, education and management.	Collaborate with others to set standards for nursing education, practice, research and management.
Foster workplace support of the conduct, dissemination and utilisation of research related to nursing and health.	Conduct, disseminate and utilise research to advance the nursing profession.	Develop position statements, guidelines and standards related to nursing research.
Promote participation in national nurses' associations so as to create favourable socio-economic conditions for nurses.	Sensitise learners to the importance of professional nursing associations.	Lobby for fair social and economic working conditions in nursing. Develop position statements and guidelines in workplace issues.

Element of the Code # 4: NURSES AND CO-WORKERS		
Practitioners and Managers	**Educators and Researchers**	**National Nurses Associations**
Create awareness of specific and overlapping functions and the potential for inter-disciplinary tensions.	Develop understanding of the roles of other workers.	Stimulate co-operation with other related disciplines.
Develop workplace systems that support common professional ethical values and behaviour.	Communicate nursing ethics to other professions.	Develop awareness of ethical issues of other professions.
Develop mechanisms to safeguard the individual, family or community when their care is endangered by health care personnel.	Instil in learners the need to safeguard the individual, family or community when care is endangered by health care personnel.	Provide guidelines, position statements and discussion fora related to safeguarding people when their care is endangered by health care personnel.

DISSEMINATION OF THE ICN CODE OF ETHICS FOR NURSES

To be effective the *ICN Code of Ethics for Nurses* must be familiar to nurses. We encourage you to help with its dissemination to schools of nursing, practising nurses, the nursing press and other mass media. The Code should also be disseminated to other health professions, the general public, consumer and policy-making groups, human rights organisations and employers of nurses.

GLOSSARY OF TERMS USED IN THE *ICN CODE OF ETHICS FOR NURSES*

Co-operative relationship	A professional relationship based on collegial and reciprocal actions, and behaviour that aim to achieve certain goals.
Co-worker	Other nurses and other health and non-health related workers and professionals.
Family	A social unit composed of members connected through blood, kinship, emotional or legal relationships.
Nurse shares with society	A nurse, as a health professional and a citizen, initiates and supports appropriate action to meet the health and social needs of the public.
Personal health	Mental, physical, social and spiritual wellbeing of the nurse.
Personal information	Information obtained during professional contact that is private to an individual or family, and which, when disclosed, may violate the right to privacy, cause inconvenience, embarrassment, or harm to the individual or family.
Related groups	Other nurses, health care workers or other professionals providing service to an individual, family or community and working toward desired goals.

GLOSSARY

Aboriginal nurse A person who self-identifies as an Aboriginal person and who is also a nurse. (p. 458)

Aboriginal nursing Most often refers to anyone involved in providing nursing care in Aboriginal communities. (p. 458)

Accountability The state of being answerable to someone for something one has done. (p. 194)

Active voluntary euthanasia An act in which the physician both provides the means of death for a patient, such as a lethal dose of medication, and administers it. (p. 294)

Activism A passionate approach to everyday activities that is committed to seeking a more just social order through critical analysis, provocation, transformation, and rebalancing of power. (p. 360)

Act utilitarianism A basic type of utilitarianism that suggests people choose actions that will, in a specific situation, result in more overall good. (p. 31)

Administrative law The branch of law that consists mainly of the legal powers granted to administrative agencies by the legislature, and the rules those agencies make to carry out their powers. (p. 151)

Advance directives Instructions that indicate which health care interventions to initiate or withhold, or that designate someone who will act as a surrogate in making such decisions, in the event that a person loses decision-making capacity. (p. 256)

Allocative policies Policies designed to provide net benefits to some distinct group or class of individuals or organizations, at the expense of others, in order to ensure that public objectives are met. (p. 349)

Alternative therapies Therapies that are used in place of conventional treatments. (p. 290)

Anonymity In a study, the situation in which even the researcher cannot link information with a particular participant. (p. 314)

Appeals to conscience Personal and subjective beliefs, founded on a prior judgment of rightness or wrongness, that are motivated by personal sanction rather than external authority. (p. 211)

Assault The unjustifiable attempt or threat to touch a person without consent that results in fear of immediately harmful or threatening contact. (p. 160)

Assisted suicide A situation in which patients receive the means of death from someone, such as a physician, but activate the process themselves. (p. 294)

Authenticity The quality of being genuine and consistent over time. (p. 91)

Authority The state of having legitimate power and sovereignty. (p. 199)

Autonomy An ethical principle that literally means self-governing. It denotes having the freedom to make independent choices. (p. 49)

Axiology   The branch of philosophy that studies the nature and types of values, which may include the study of aesthetics as well as the study of ethics. (p. 87)

Battery   The unlawful touching of another, or the carrying out of threatened physical harm, including any wilful, angry, and violent or negligent touching of another's person, clothes, or anything attached to his or her person or held by him or her. (p. 160)

Beneficence   The ethical principle that requires one to act in ways that benefit another. In research, this implies the protection from harm and discomfort, including a balance between the benefits and risks of a study. (p. 59)

Caring   This involves "emotional commitment to, and deep willingness to act on behalf of, persons with whom one has a significant relationship." (Beauchamp & Childress, 2008, p. 36). (p. 39)

Cartesian philosophy   A widespread belief during the Renaissance related to Descartes' proposal that the universe is a physical thing, and all therein is analogous to machines that can be analyzed and understood, and that the mind and body are separate entities. (p. 12)

Case law   Principles of law arising out of judicial opinions and decisions. *See* common law. (p. 151)

Categorical Imperative   The Kantian maxim stating that no action can be judged as right which cannot reasonably become a law by which every person should always abide. (p. 34)

Character ethics   Theories of ethics, sometimes called virtue ethics, related to the concept of innate moral virtue. (p. 37)

Charter of Rights and Freedoms   A comprehensive list of the rights, freedoms, and privileges applicable to all Canadian citizens. (p. 150)

Cheating   Dishonesty and deception regarding examinations, projects, or papers. (p. 304)

Civil law   (also called private law) The law that determines a person's legal rights and obligations in many kinds of activities involving other people. (p. 153)

Code of nursing ethics   Explicit declaration of the primary goals and values of the profession that indicate the profession's acceptance of the responsibility and trust with which it has been invested by society. (p. 195)

Coercion   Actual or implied threat of harm or penalty for not participating in a research project, or offering excessive rewards for participation in the project. (p. 311)

Common law   A system of law, also known as case law, based largely on previous court decisions. In this system, decisions are based upon earlier court rulings in similar cases, or precedents. Over time, these precedents take on the force of law. This is the basis of the legal system in Canada, except in the province of Quebec, where the legal system is based on French civil law. (p. 151)

Communitarian theories   Theories of justice that place the community, rather than the individual, the state, the nation, or any other entity, at the centre of the value system; that emphasize the value of the public good; and that conceive of values as being rooted in communal practices. (p. 379)

Compassion A focal virtue combining an attitude of active regard for another's welfare with an imaginative awareness and emotional response of deep sympathy, tenderness, and discomfort at the other person's misfortune or suffering. (p. 39)

Competence A person's ability to make meaningful life decisions. A declaration of incompetence involves legal action with a ruling by a judge that the person is unable to make such life decisions. (p. 281)

Complementary therapies Therapies that are used alongside conventional therapies. (p. 290)

Concern for welfare A fundamental ethical principle in the conduct of research referring to the obligation of the researcher to protect research participants from potential risk of harm and ensure that research has potential for benefit. (p. 311)

Confidentiality The ethical principle that requires nondisclosure of private or secret information with which one is entrusted. In research, confidentiality refers to the researcher's assurance to participants in studies that information provided will not be made public or available to anyone other than those involved in the research process without the participant's consent. (p. 69)

Conscientiousness A person acts in a conscientious way, according to Beauchamp and Childress (2008), if he or she consistently, with explicitly good intentions, tries to do what is right, after putting an effort into determining what constitutes the "right" choice of action. (p. 40)

Consent A complex legal and ethical notion, arising from autonomy and dignity, which states that persons have the right to decide what can and cannot be done to them. In law, it is often referred to as the right to be free from interference. In health care, it is an absolute necessity to obtain consent from patients or participants in research prior to carrying out any interventions or actions. (p. 161)

Consequentialism A theory of ethics, sometimes called utilitarianism. In this theory, the moral worth of an action or choice is evaluated based on the consequences or outcomes as opposed to the intentions or duties of the moral agent. (p. 30)

Constitutional law A formal set of rules and principles that describe the powers of government and the rights of the people. (p. 150)

Contract An agreement between two or more people that can be enforced by law. (p. 153)

Contract law A type of law that deals with the rights and obligations of people who make contracts. (p. 155)

Controlled act An act that can only be carried out by a qualified member of a designated profession. (p. 198)

Covert values Expectations that are not in writing that are often identified only through participation in, or controversies within, an organization or institution. (p. 97)

Criminal Code of Canada It is the formal articulation of all offenses and procedures. (p. 153)

Criminal law A type of law that deals with crimes, or actions considered harmful to society. (p. 153)

Cultural awareness Knowledge about values, beliefs, and behaviours in cultures other than one's own. (p. 426)

Cultural competence Skill in dealing with transcultural issues, which is demonstrated through cultural awareness and cultural sensitivity. (p. 426)

Cultural safety This "involves the recognition that we are all bearers of culture and we need to be aware of and challenge unequal power relations at the individual, family, community, and societal level" (University of Victoria, 2008, p. 1) (p. 429)

Cultural sensitivity The ability to incorporate a patient's cultural perspective into nursing assessments, and to modify nursing care in order to be as congruent as possible with the patient's cultural perspective. (p. 426)

Culture is a complex phenomenon that can be defined as the worldview, lifestyle, shared knowledge, symbols, and rules for guiding behaviour and creating shared meaning within a group of persons. (p. 426)

Decision-making capacity The ability of a person to understand all information about a health condition, to communicate understanding and choices, and to reason and deliberate; and the possession of personal values and goals that guide the decision. (p. 279)

Declaration of Helsinki Principles issued by the World Medical Assembly to guide clinical research in 1964; revised in 1975, 1983, 1989, 1996, 2000, and most recently in 2008. (p. 308)

Defamation Harm that occurs to a person's reputation and good name, diminishes others' value or esteem, or arouses negative feelings toward the person, by the communication of false, malicious, unprivileged, or harmful words. (p. 161)

Deontology Related to the term "duty," deontology is a group of ethical theories based upon the rationalist view that the rightness or wrongness of an act depends upon the nature of the act, rather than the consequences that occur as a result of it. Also called formalism. (p. 34)

Discernment A focal virtue of sensitive insight, acute judgment, and understanding that eventuates in decisive action. (p. 39)

Distributive justice Application of the ethical principle of justice that relates to fair, equitable, and appropriate distribution in society, determined by justified norms that structure the terms of social co-operation. Its scope includes policies that allot diverse benefits and burdens such as property, resources, taxation, privileges, and opportunities. (p. 76)

Diversity The experience within nursing of differences among colleagues and patients in areas such as gender, age, socioeconomic position, sexual orientation, health status, ethnicity, race, and culture. (p. 426)

Do not resuscitate (DNR) orders Written directives placed in a patient's medical chart indicating that cardiopulmonary resuscitation is to be avoided. (p. 251)

Durable power of attorney Allows a competent person to designate another as a surrogate or proxy to act on her or his behalf in making health care decisions in the event that he or she loses the capacity to make decisions. (p. 279)

Duty to care A legal principle referring to the obligation imposed on someone to act, or refrain from acting, so as not to cause harm to another person. (p. 157)

Egalitarian theories   Theories of justice that promote ideals of equal distribution of social benefits and burdens, and recognize the social obligation to eliminate or reduce barriers that prevent fair equality of opportunity. (p. 378)

Empirical   Knowledge gained through the processes of observation and experience. (p. 8)

Empowerment   A construct or process of helping and partnership, enacted within a context of mutual respect, through which individuals and groups are enabled to grow and develop, and are provided with the skills, resources, opportunities, and autonomy to do so. (p. 468)

Ethical dilemma   Occurs when there are conflicting moral claims. *See also* Moral dilemma. (p. 123)

Ethical principles   Basic and obvious moral truths that guide deliberation and action. Major ethical principles include autonomy, beneficence, non-maleficence, veracity, confidentiality, justice, and fidelity. (p. 49)

Ethical space   An environment in which ethical deliberation, reflection, debate, and discussion over values and beliefs is encouraged and supported. (p. 42)

Ethical treatment of data   Includes integrity of research protocols and honesty in reporting findings. (p. 319)

Ethic of care   An approach to ethical decision making that is grounded in relationships and mutual responsibility. (p. 111)

Ethic of justice   An approach to ethical decision making that is based on objective rules and principles, in which choices are made from a stance of separateness. (p. 111)

Ethics   The study of social morality, and philosophical reflection on its norms and practices. (p. 26)

Ethnocentrism   Judging the behaviours of someone from another culture by the standards of one's own culture. (p. 428)

Euthanasia   Causing the painless death of a person in order to end or prevent suffering. (p. 245)

Expertise   The characteristic of having a high level of specialized skill and knowledge. (p. 189)

Explicit consent   Either verbal or written consent, specifically articulating the patient's agreement to a particular treatment or procedure. (p. 165)

External locus of control   The belief that one's life is directed or ruled by forces outside oneself, whether these be generalized forces, such as fate, or other persons who are perceived as being more powerful. (p. 480)

External standards of nursing practice   Guides for nursing care that are developed by non-nurses, legislatures, or institutions. (p. 196)

False imprisonment   The unlawful, unjustifiable detention of a person within fixed boundaries, or an act intended to result in such confinement. (p. 161)

Fidelity   An ethical principle related to the concept of faithfulness and the practice of keeping one's promises. (p. 75)

Fiduciary   Someone who has an ethical duty to act in the best interests of another; this involves an ethical obligation to act in a way that protects others and furthers their best interests. (p. 307)

Fiduciary duty   A duty in which the nurse sets aside his or her own agenda, needs, or feelings, in order to place the patient in a position of priority. (p. 307)

Focal virtues   Virtues considered to be core values, and more pivotal than others in characterizing a virtuous person, including compassion, discernment, trustworthiness, integrity, and conscientiousness. (p. 39)

Formalism   A term often used to refer to deontology. (p. 34)

Fraud   A deliberate deception for the purpose of securing an unfair or unlawful gain. (p. 159)

Full disclosure   Indicates that a research participant must be fully informed of the nature of a study, anticipated risks and benefits, time commitment, expectations of the participant and the researcher, and the right to refuse to participate. (p. 311)

Globalization   A set of processes or goals aiming to integrate economic, social, political, and trade systems across political boundaries. (p. 100)

Grassroots lobbying   Lobbying efforts that involve mobilizing a committed constituency to influence the opinions of policy makers. (p. 360)

Guardian *ad litem*   A court-appointed guardian for a particular action or proceeding; such a guardian may not oversee all of the person's affairs. (p. 257)

Health policies   Authoritative decisions focusing on health that are made in the legislative, executive, or judicial branches of government and are intended to direct or influence the actions, behaviours, or decisions of others; their lifestyles and personal behaviours; and improvements in the availability, accessibility, and quality of their health care services. (p. 348)

Hedonism   The pursuit of pleasure as the highest achievable ***good***. (p. 31)

Implied consent   Consent that is inferred from a person's actions, presence, or informed co-operation. (p. 165)

Informed consent   A process by which patients are informed of the possible outcomes, alternatives, and risks of treatments, and are required to give their consent freely. This implies legal protection of a patient's right to personal autonomy by providing the opportunity to choose a course of action, including the right to refuse medical recommendations and to choose from available therapeutic alternatives. *In research*, this refers to consent to participate in a research study, after the research purpose, expected commitment, risks and benefits, any invasion of privacy, and ways that anonymity and confidentiality will be addressed, have all been explained. (p. 55)

Integrity   Refers to adherence to moral norms that is sustained over time. Implicit in integrity is trustworthiness and consistency in convictions, actions, and emotions. (p. 40)

Intentional infliction of emotional distress   Also known as "intentional infliction of mental distress" or the "tort of outrage," this is a relatively new tort claim in Canada, allowing for a claim to be made against someone who acts in a heinous, reckless, or extreme way, resulting in emotional distress for another. (p. 162)

Intentional torts   Wilful or intentional acts that violate another person's rights or property. (p. 159)

Internal locus of control The belief that one is able to influence or control things that happen in one's own life. (p. 480)

Internal standards of nursing practice Standards of nursing practice that are developed within the profession of nursing. (p. 195)

Invasion of privacy Includes intrusion on the patient's physical and mental solitude or seclusion, public disclosure of private facts, publicity that places the patient in a false light in the public eye, or appropriation for the defendant's benefit or advantage of the patient's name or likeness. (p. 160)

Involuntary euthanasia Euthanasia practised without consent. In this case, the person is, for some reason, incapable or unable to consent to euthanasia. The decision should be based on clear ideas about the authentic wishes of the individual, if he/she could consent. (p. 294)

Judicial decisions Authoritative court decisions that direct or influence the actions, behaviours, or decisions of others. (p. 349)

Justice An ethical principle that relates to fair, equitable, and appropriate treatment in light of what is due or owed to persons, recognizing that giving to some will deny receipt to others who might otherwise have received these things. *In research*, justice implies the rights of fair treatment and privacy, including anonymity and confidentiality. (p. 76)

Kantianism A deontological theory of ethics based upon the writings of the philosopher Immanuel Kant. (p. 34)

Law The system of enforceable principles and processes that governs the behaviour of people in respect to relationships with others and with the government. (p. 147)

Libel Printed defamation by written words and images that injure a person's reputation or cause others to avoid, ridicule, or view the person with contempt. (p. 162)

Libertarian theories Theories of distributive justice that propose that the just society protects the rights of property and liberty of each person, allowing citizens to improve their circumstances by their own effort. (p. 379)

Living wills Legal documents, developed voluntarily by persons, giving directions to health care providers related to withholding or withdrawing life support if certain conditions exist. (p. 279)

Lobbying The art of persuasion — attempting to convince a legislator, a government official, the head of an agency, or an official to comply with a request — whether it is convincing them to support a position on an issue or to follow a particular course of action. (p. 359)

Locus of control Beliefs about the ability to control events in one's life. (p. 480)

Loyalty Showing sympathy, care, and reciprocity to those with whom we appropriately identify; working closely with others toward shared goals; keeping promises; making mutual concerns a priority; sacrificing personal interests to the relationship; and giving attention to these over a substantial period of time. (p. 222)

Material rules Rules by which distributive justice decisions regarding entitlement are made. (p. 373)

Medical futility Situations in which medical interventions are judged to have no medical benefit, or in which the chance for success is low. (p. 245)

Misrepresentation of personal performance This includes submitting work that has been taken from another and representing it as your own, allowing someone else to write an exam using your name, or not being forthright with academic records or documents. (p. 305)

Moral autonomy The process of moving away from simply adopting the values and beliefs of others who influence us, to a state of taking responsibility for our values and beliefs, embracing them as our own and demonstrating them through our actions. (p. 88)

Moral courage When one takes action for strong moral reasons, and those actions carry the risk of adverse consequences or potential negative outcomes for oneself. *See also* Steadfastness. (p. 127)

Moral development A product of the sociocultural environment in which one lives and develops that reflects the intellectual and emotional process through which one learns and incorporates values regarding right and wrong. (p. 107)

Moral dilemma A situation in which a conflict between two or more moral imperatives exists. *See also* Ethical dilemma. (p. 124)

Moral disengagement When a person feels that his or her views, contributions, and ethical concerns are not valued by the institution or agency, that person can, over time, become disengaged or far less invested in his or her nursing role and practice. (p. 127)

Moral distress The reaction to a situation in which there are moral problems that seem to have clear solutions, yet one is unable to follow one's moral beliefs because of external or institutional restraints. This may manifest itself in anger, frustration, dissatisfaction, and poor performance in the work setting. (p. 97)

Moral integrity A focal virtue that relates to soundness, reliability, wholeness, an integration of character, and fidelity in adherence to moral norms sustained over time. (p. 40)

Moral outrage A state that occurs when someone else in the health care setting performs an act the nurse believes to be immoral. In cases of moral outrage, the nurse does not participate in the act and therefore does not feel responsible for wrong, but feels powerlessness to prevent it. (p. 126)

Moral philosophy The philosophical discussion of what is considered to be good or bad, right or wrong. (p. 26)

Moral reasoning Refers to the thoughtful examination and evaluation of right and wrong, good and bad. *See also* Moral thought. (p. 5)

Moral residue When nurses find that they are being asked to compromise their values time and time again, this can lead to moral residue, which may include feelings of guilt, inadequacy, and powerlessness. (p. 127)

Moral thought Individuals' cognitive examination of right and wrong, good and bad. (p. 88)

Moral uncertainty A state that occurs when one senses that there is a moral problem, but is not sure of the morally correct action; when one is unsure what moral principles or values apply; or when one is unable to define the moral problem. (p. 122)

Moral values   Preferences or dispositions that reflect right or wrong, should or should not, in human behaviour. (p. 88)

Naturalism   A view of moral judgment that regards ethics as depending on human nature and psychology. (p. 27)

Negligence   Omitting to do something that a reasonable person, guided by those ordinary considerations that ordinarily regulate human affairs, would do, or doing something that a reasonable and prudent person would not do. (p. 156)

Noncompliance   Denoting an unwillingness on the part of the patient to participate in health care activities that have been recommended by health care providers. (p. 58)

Non-maleficence   An ethical principle related to beneficence that requires one to act in such a manner as to avoid causing harm to another, including deliberate harm, risk of harm, and harm that occurs during the performance of beneficial acts. (p. 62)

Nuremberg Code   A set of principles for the ethical conduct of research. (p. 308)

Nursing process   A model commonly used for decision making in nursing. (p. 128)

Obligation   Being required to do something by virtue of a moral rule, a duty, or some other binding demand, such as a particular role or relationship. (p. 212)

Overt values   Values of individuals, groups, institutions, and organized systems that are explicitly communicated through philosophy and policy statements. (p. 96)

Palliative care   A comprehensive, interdisciplinary, and total care approach, focusing primarily on the comfort and support of patients and families who face illness that is chronic or not responsive to curative treatment. (p. 241)

Parentalism   A more modern, gender-neutral alternative to the term **paternalism,** which applies to professionals who restrict others' autonomy, usually to protect that person from perceived or anticipated harm or with a goal of acting in that person's best interests. (p. 56)

Paternalism   A gender-biased term that literally means acting in a "fatherly" manner, the traditional view of which implies well-intentioned actions of benevolent decision making, leadership, protection, and discipline, which, in the health care arena, manifest in the making of decisions on behalf of patients without their full consent or knowledge. (p. 56)

Philosophy   The intense and critical examination of beliefs and assumptions. (p. 25)

PIPEDA   The *Personal Information Protection and Electronic Documents Act* is a federal law that deals with the privacy of personal information for all Canadians. (p. 175)

Plagiarism   Taking another's ideas or work and presenting them as one's own. (p. 305)

Policies   Plans of action that guide actions—of governments, institutions, corporations, communities, etc. Policies often reflect the values and beliefs of the majority, or of those directly responsible for creating the policy. (p. 347)

Policy formulation   A phase of the policy-making process that includes such actions as agenda setting and the subsequent development of legislation. (p. 350)

Policy implementation   A phase of the policy-making process that follows the enactment of legislation and includes taking the actions and making the additional decisions necessary to implement legislation, such as rule making and policy operation. (p. 350)

Policy modification   A phase of the policy-making process that exists to improve or perfect legislation previously enacted. (p. 350)

Politics   Refers to anything that involves groups of persons making decisions or influencing how decisions are made or resources are allocated. The term implies both action and thought. (p. 347)

Power   The ability to do or act; the capability of doing or accomplishing something. (p. 468)

Practical dilemma   A situation in which moral claims compete with non-moral claims. (p. 124)

Privacy   The condition of not having personal information about oneself known by others. (p. 69)

Private law   The law that determines a person's legal rights and obligations in many kinds of activities involving other people. *See* Civil law. (p. 153)

Profession   A complex, organized occupation preceded by a long training program geared toward the acquisition of exclusive knowledge necessary to provide a service that is essential or desired by society, leading to a monopoly that provides autonomy, public recognition, prestige, power, and authority for the practitioner. (p. 185)

Professionalism   A collective notion that refers to the aims, the conduct, and the attributes that distinguish a group of persons who are professionals from non-professionals. (p. 449)

Public law   Law that defines a person's rights and obligations in relation to government, and describes the various divisions of government and their powers. (p. 154)

Quality of life   A subjective appraisal of well-being and the factors that make life worth living and contribute to a positive experience of living. (p. 238)

Rationalism   A view of moral judgment that regards truth as necessary, universal, and superior to the information received from the senses; having an origin in the nature of the universe, or in the nature of a higher being. (p. 27)

Regulatory policies   Policies that are designed to influence the actions, behaviours, and decisions of others through directive techniques. (p. 349)

Respect for persons   An attitude by which one considers others to be worthy of high regard. (p. 49)

Right to fair treatment   In research, assures equitable treatment of participants in the research selection process, during the study, and after the completion of the study. (p. 313)

Right to privacy   The right to be left alone or to be free from unwanted publicity. In research, this is the right of research participants to determine when, where, and what kind of information is shared, with an assurance that information and observations will be treated with respect and kept in strict confidence. (p. 160)

Rules or regulations   Policies that are established to guide the implementation of laws and programs. (p. 349)

Rule utilitarianism   A type of utilitarianism that suggests people choose rules that, when followed consistently, will maximize the overall good. (p. 31)

Sanctity of life The belief that all human life should be valued, no matter what and at all costs. (p. 237)

Scope of practice A description of the procedures, actions, and responsibilities of a health care professional. Also refers to clearly defined parameters or boundaries of duties and commitments. (p. 198)

Self-awareness Conscious awareness of one's thoughts, feelings, physical and emotional responses, and insights in various situations. (p. 92)

Sexism The assumption that members of one sex are superior to those of the other. (p. 424)

Slander Defamation that occurs when one speaks unprivileged or false words about another. (p. 162)

Social justice The aim to and processes by which, as a society, we can achieve a more equitable distribution of resources, burdens, and benefits. Social justice is based upon principles of equality and solidarity, with attention to human rights and the inherent dignity of all persons. (p. 446)

Spectrum of urgency A spectrum depicting the degree of urgency in health care decision making, ranging from minor and non-urgent to severe and very urgent. (p. 227)

Standards of nursing practice Written documents outlining minimum expectations for nursing care. (p. 195)

Statutes or laws Legislation that has been enacted by legislative bodies and approved by the executive branch of government. (p. 349)

Statutory (legislative) law Formal laws written and enacted by federal or provincial/territorial legislatures. (p. 151)

Steadfastness The quality of remaining loyal or true despite, or in the face of, adversity. *See also* Moral courage. (p. 127)

Stereotyping Expecting all persons from a particular group to behave, think, or respond in a certain way, based on preconceived ideas. (p. 428)

Submission of false information It may include actions such as submitting a false statement (e.g., a medical certificate) to avoid completing an assignment or writing an exam, submitting false academic records, or altering official academic documents. (p. 305)

Sympathy Sharing, in imagination, of others' feelings. (p. 28)

Theory A proposed explanation for a class of phenomena. (p. 109)

Tort A wrong or injury that a person suffers because of someone else's action, either intentional or unintentional. The action may cause bodily harm; damage a person's property, business, or reputation; or make unauthorized use of a person's property. (p. 153)

Trustworthiness A focal virtue that results in recognition by others of one's consistency and predictability in following moral norms. (p. 40)

Undue Influence A situation in which one makes another person feel obligated to make a particular decision constrained in his or her choices. This term is frequently used to describe feelings of obligation based on already-standing relationships in the recruitment of potential participants for research studies. (p. 311)

Unintentional torts Torts that occur when an act or omission causes unintended injury or harm to another person. (p. 156)

Unity An attribute of a profession, as a united whole, to articulate and embrace shared values, principles, and virtues. (p. 200)

Utilitarianism A moral theory which holds that an action is judged as good or bad in relation to the consequence, outcome, or end result derived from it, as opposed to the intentions or duties of the moral agent. Also called consequentialism. (p. 30)

Utilitarian theories Theories of distributive justice that distribute resources based on the premise of the greatest good for the greatest number of people. These theories place social good before individual rights. (p. 379)

Utility The property of usefulness in any object, whereby it tends to produce benefit, advantage, pleasure, good, or happiness, or prevent mischief, pain, evil, or unhappiness. (p. 30)

Values Ideals, beliefs, customs, modes of conduct, qualities, or goals that are highly prized or preferred by individuals, groups, or society. (p. 87)

Values clarification Refers to the process of becoming more conscious of and naming what one values or considers worthy. (p. 91)

Values conflict Internal or interpersonal conflict that occurs in circumstances where personal values are at odds with those of patients, colleagues, or the institution. (p. 95)

Veracity A moral value also known as telling the truth. (p. 64)

Victim blaming Holding the people burdened by social conditions accountable for their own situations and responsible for needed solutions. (p. 405)

Virtue ethics Theories of ethics, usually attributed to Aristotle, which represent the idea that an individual's actions are based upon innate moral virtue. Also called character ethics. (p. 37)

Whistleblowing Speaking out about unsafe or questionable practices affecting patient care or working conditions. This should be resorted to only after a person has unsuccessfully used all appropriate organizational channels to right a wrong, and has a sound moral justification for taking this action. (p. 475)

References

Beauchamp, T., & J. Childress (2008). Principles of biomedical ethics (6th ed.). New York: Oxford University Press.

University of Victoria. (2008). Cultural safety: Peoples' experiences of colonization in relation to health care. Modules 1, 2 and 3.

INDEX

Aboriginal health, 454–461
  Aboriginal nursing, 458–460
  factors affecting, 456–458
  future of nursing, 460–461
  sense of community, 436
Aboriginal nurse, defined, 458
Aboriginal Nurses Association of Canada, 458, 459
Abortion, 291–293
Absolute homelessness, 395
Abuse
  intimate-partner violence, 397–400
  reporting of, 75, 76, 298
Academic honesty, 304–307, 319–320
Accessibility principle, Canada Health Act, 79
Access to health care, 337–338
Accountability, 194–199
  codes of nursing ethics, 195
  mechanisms of, 194–199
  nursing theory and practice derived from research, 199
  in practice, 178
  scope of practice, 198
  standards of nursing practice, 195–197
A.C. et al. v. Director of Child and Family Services (2008), 169
Achterberg, J., 11, 12, 416
Active euthanasia, 294
Active voluntary euthanasia, 294
Activism, 360
Act Respecting the Protection of Confidential Disciplinary Proceedings of Health Professions (Nova Scotia), 196
Acts, 153
Act utilitarianism, 31–32

Administrative law, 151
Advance care planning, 281–285
Advance directives, 171, 256–257, 278–285
Advanced practice nursing, 226–227
Adverse events, 158
Advocacy, 230–231
Africa, 309
AIDS. *See* HIV/AIDS
AJN (*American Journal of Nursing*), 187
Allocative policies, 349
Alma-Ata Declaration, 334
Alternative medicine, 290–291
Altruism, 186, 219
American Journal of Nursing (AJN), 187
American Nurses Association (ANA), 194, 195
Anonymity, 314
Appeals to conscience, 211
Appearance of nurses, 423–424
Aquinas, Thomas, 9
Aristotle, 37–38
Artificial sources of nutrition, 254–255
Assault, 160
Assisted Human Reproduction Act, 350
Assisted suicide, 294
Attawapiskat First Nation, 457–458
Attorney for personal care. *See* Substitute decision-maker (SDM)
Authenticity, 91
Authority
  professional, 199–200
  unethical research concerning, 310
Auton, Connor, 375
Auton (Guardian ad litem of) v. British Columbia (Attorney General), 375

Autonomy, 49–59
  barriers to, 55
  elements of, 50–52
  informed consent and, 55–56
  moral, 89
  noncompliance and, 53–54, 58–59
  paternalism/parentalism, 56–58,
      270–273
  professional, 189–193
  in rural nursing, 449
  social issues and, 404–405
  threats to, 51–52
  values formation and, 88
  violations of patient, 53–55
Awareness of beliefs and values, 21
Axiology, 87

Battery, 160–161
Beauchamp, T., 39–41, 66
Beauchamp, T. L., 355
Beletz, E., 188, 189, 202
Beliefs
  awareness of, 21
  and culture, 430–435
  spirituality and religion, 6–7
  See also Values
Beneficence, 59–62, 236–237, 270–271,
      404
Bentham, Jeremy, 30–31
Best Practice Guideline, 449
Bigotry, 425
Biomedical model, 435
Bixler, Genevieve, 187
Bixler, Roy, 187
Blaming, victim, 405–406
Bok, S., 68
Boundaries, in rural nursing, 450–452
Bower, P., 483
Brain death, 259
Britain, nursing in, 12
British North America Act, 150, 326, 331
Buber, Martin, 25
Buddha, 25
*Building on Values: The Future of Health
    Care in Canada*, 334
Bulgin, Sanchia, 163

Bullying, 223, 225
Business records, 173

California, 416
California Supreme Court, 74
Callahan, S., 131
CAM (complementary and alternative
    medicine), 290–291
Canada
  health care delivery, 77–78, 331–335
  history of nursing in, 12–16
  homelessness in, 394–395
  legislative process, 151–154
  poverty in, 392–394
  racism in, 402–403
  regulatory policies, 349
  See also Health care delivery
Canada Act, 150
Canada Health Act, 78–79, 330, 333, 372,
      374
Canada Health and Social Transfer
    payment system (CHST), 333
Canadian Adverse Events Study, 158
Canadian Association for Rural and
    Remote Nursing (CARRN), 448
Canadian Environment Protection Act,
    350
Canadian Hospice Palliative Care
    Association, 244
Canadian Human Rights Commission,
    224–225
Canadian Institute of Child Health, 392
Canadian Mental Health Association, 329
Canadian National Association of Trained
    Nurses (CNATN), 14
Canadian Nurses Association (CNA)
  accountability, 194
  advance directives, 256
  Code of Ethics, 73–74, 96, 200–201,
      214, 229
  cultural values and beliefs, 430
  future goals for nursing, 15
  lobbying, 359
  medical futility, 245
  nurses role in policy formulation, 357
  origin of, 14

scope of practice, 198
value of nursing history, 3–4
See also Code of Ethics for Registered Nurses
Canadian Policy Research Network (CPRN), 356
Canadian Red Cross Society, 15, 330
Canadian Society for Superintendents of Training Schools for Nurses, 14
Capacity to consent, 167–168
Cardiac death, 259
Cardiopulmonary resuscitation (CPR), 251–252
Care
  duty to, 157
  ethic of, 111, 115–117
  human focus of, 261–262
  technology and, 261–262
Caring
  curing versus, 12
  ethic of, 111–113
  gender and, 418–420
  virtue of, 39
CARRN (Canadian Association for Rural and Remote Nursing), 448
Cartesian philosophy, 12
Case law, 151
Case Presentations
  Aboriginal health, 457–458
  academic honesty, 306–307
  advance directives, 283–285
  allocation of resources, 385–386
  beneficence, 60–61, 63–64
  confidentiality, 70, 72–73, 296–298, 451
  conflicting duties, 28
  conflict of values, 95–96, 99, 292–293
  consent, 167–168, 171–172, 276–277
  cultural differences, 434–435
  distributive justice, 376–377
  DNR orders, 252–253
  economic factors in nursing care, 217
  elder care, 400–401
  end-of-life technology, 257–258
  ethical dilemmas, 22–24
  ethical theory, 43–45
  ethics of justice/care, 117

intimate-partner violence, 399–400
lifestyle choices, 288–289
loyalty conflicts, 220
medical futility, 246–247, 248–250
noncompliance versus autonomy, 53–54
nurse–institution relationship, 217, 220
nurse-physician relationship, 227–228
patient autonomy, 271–272
practical dilemmas, 215–216, 220
privatization of health care, 382–383
research ethics, 314–315, 316–317, 319–320
rights and duties, 36–37
socioeconomic influences, 393–394, 396–397
standards of nursing practice, 196–197
utilitarianism, 33–34
values development, 114–115
Categorical imperative, 34–35
Catholic Church, 8–10, 12, 415–416
Center for Practical Bioethics, 385
Chang, C. F., 384
Chaoulli v. Quebec, 382–383
Character ethics, 37–41
Charter of Rights and Freedoms, 150–151, 176–177, 332, 374, 402, 421–422
Cheating, 304
Child abuse, reporting of, 75
Children, consent capacity of, 168–170
Children's Aid Societies, 329
Children's Hospital of Winnipeg, 202–203
Childress, J., 39–41, 66, 355
Chinn, P., 472, 473
Choices, life-and-health, 285–286
  CAM, 290–291
  confidentiality, 296–298
  controversial choices, 291–296
  recommended treatment and, 286–298
Christianity, 8–10, 12
CHST (Canada Health and Social Transfer payment system), 333
Civil law, 153, 155
Civil Marriage Act, 415–416

Cleanliness, 13

CNA. *See* Canadian Nurses Association

CNATN (Canadian National Association of Trained Nurses), 14

Code of Ethics, (CNA), 73–74, 96, 200–201, 214, 229

Code of Ethics for Nurses (ICN), 61, 69, 192, 212–214, 357

Code of Ethics for Registered Nurses, (CNA)
  accountability, 194
  advance directives, 282
  autonomy, 192
  confidentiality, 69
  decision-making processes, 59
  lifestyle choices, 286
  nursing practice, 358
  preventing/removing harm, 61–62
  professional relationships, 209
  scope of practice, 214

Codes of ethics, personal, 27

Coercion, 311, 315

Cognitive development, 109–110

Colleagues, relationships with, 201–202, 221–225

Collective culture, 201

College of Nurses of Ontario, 128–129

College of Registered Nurses of British Columbia, 191

College of Registered Nurses of Nova Scotia, 191

Common law, 151–152

Communicable disease outbreak, ethical considerations for, 62

Communication
  about advance directives, 283
  decision making at end of life, 255–256
  doctor–nurse game, 422–423
  gender and, 422–424
  nurse–patient, 423–424
  transcultural, 437
  truth-telling, 64–69

Communitarian theories of justice, 379–380

Compassion, 39

Competence
  cultural, 426, 428–429
  establishing, 281
  expertise, 189
  and gender, 425

Complementary and alternative medicine (CAM), 290–291

Comprehensiveness principle, *Canada Health Act*, 78

Computerized documentation, 174–175

Concealed homelessness, 395

Confidentiality, 69–75, 160–164, 175–178, 314, 450–452

Confucius, 25

Conscience, appeals to, 211

Conscientiousness, 40

Consent, 164–172
  adults with diminished capacity, 170–172
  capacity to, 167–168
  children's capacity to, 168–170
  defined, 161
  explicit, 165
  implied, 165
  informed, 166
  organ donation and, 259–260
  treatment- and provider-specific, 166–167
  voluntary, 165–166

Consent to Treatment and Health Care Directives Act (Prince Edward Island), 164

Consequentialism, 30

Constitution Act, 150

Constitutional law, 150–151

Contract law, 155–156

Contracts, 153, 155

Control, locus of, 480

Controlled acts, 198

Controlled Drugs and Substances Act, 154, 350

Core professional values, 201

Costs. *See* Economics

Covert values, 97

CPR (cardiopulmonary resuscitation), 251–252

CPRN (Canadian Policy Research Network), 356
Crimean War, 13
Criminal Code of Canada, 153, 154, 294
Criminal law, 153, 154
Critical social theory, 4
Cross-gender mentoring relationships, 420
Cultural assessment, 433, 437
Cultural awareness, 426
Cultural competence, 426, 428–429
Cultural Competence and Cultural Safety in Nursing Education, 429
Cultural safety, 429–430
Cultural sensitivity, 426
Culture
    assessment of, 433, 437
    autonomy and, 50
    defined, 426
    health care delivery, 435–437
    understanding, 428
    values and beliefs, 100, 107, 430–435
Curtin, Leah, 226, 230, 255, 474

Daniels, N., 372
Data, ethical treatment of, 319–320
Death
    assisted suicide, 294
    attitudes toward, 239–241
    euthanasia, 245, 294
    organ transplants and, 259–260
    See also End-of-life care
deBlois, J., 370
Deception, 67
Decision making
    capacity to consent, 167–172
    enhancing patient capacity for, 479–482
    evaluating outcomes of action, 140
    nursing and, 25
    participants in, 133–135, 139
    processes, 132–138
    scientific process and, 130
    thought processes and, 54
    See also Choices, life-and-health; Ethical decision making; Problem solving

Declaration of Alma-Ata, 334
Declaration of Helsinki, 308–309, 312
Defamation, 161–162
Degazon, C., 201
Deontology, 34–37
Department of Health and Human Services, U.S., 309
Descartes, René, 11–12
DeVries, C. M., 359–360
Dilemmas
    ethical, 21–24, 123–124
    moral, 122, 123–124
    practical, 124, 215–216, 220
    See also Problem solving
Dilley, K. B., 230
Direct lobbying, 361
Discernment, 39
Discipline, professional, 200, 230
Discrimination, 225, 402, 416–422, 425–426
Disease
    versus illness, 430
    outbreaks of, 62
Distribution of resources, 378
Distributive justice, 371–380
    defined, 371
    distribution of resources, 378
    entitlement and, 373–377
    fairness in, 377–378
    principle of, 76–78
    theories of, 378–380
Diversity
    appreciating, 21
    defined, 426
    understanding, 428–429
DNR orders, 251–254
Dock, Lavinia Lloyd, 14
Doctor–nurse game, 422–423
Documentation, 173–178
    accountability in practice, 178
    privacy and confidentiality, 175–178
    technology and, 174–175
Doig, C. J., 259
Donabedian, A., 199
Donation after brain death (DBD), 259–260

Donation after cardiac death (DCD), 259–260
"Do no harm" principle, 62–64, 236–237, 403–404
Douglas, Tommy, 330, 332
Dress, 423–424
Drummond Report, 335
Dueck, Tyrell, 169–170
Durable powers of attorney, 279
Durant, W., 38
Duties
  conflicting, 28
  rights and, 36–37
Duty to care, 157
Duty to warn, 74, 298
Dying, attitudes toward, 239–241. *See also* Death

"Eating your young," 223, 229, 477
Economics, 367–389
  distributive justice and, 371–380
  medical futility and, 250
  overview, 367–371
  recent trends, 380–386
  standards of nursing practice affected by, 216–218
Education, 189, 453
Egalitarian theories of justice, 378–379
Elder abuse, 76
Elder population, 400–401
Election to public office, 363–364
Electronic records, 174–175
Ellin, Joseph, 67
Emancipatory nursing, 475
Embodiment, 42
Emotional distress, 162
Emotions, owning, 473
Empathy, 5
Empiricism, 8–9
Empowerment, 467–487
  barriers to, 482–483
  characteristics of, 478–479
  decision making, 4
  locus of control and, 480
  overview, 467–471
  patient, 478–482

patient-centred care and, 482–483
  personal, 471–474
  professional, 474–478
End-of-life care, 234–268
  advance directives, 278–279
  decision making, 255–260
  DNR orders, 251–254
  medical futility, 245–255
  nursing practice and technology, 260–262
  overview, 235
  palliative care, 241–245
  quality of life, 237–245
  technology in, 235–237
Entitlement, 373–377
Entrepreneurial health care model, 370
Established Programs Financing Act, 332
Ethical decision making, 121–143
  acting on, 136, 140
  application of process, 138–140
  claim identification, 132–133, 138–139
  data gathering, 132–133, 138–139
  emotions and, 130–131
  evaluating outcomes of action, 137–138, 140
  guide for, 137–138
  identification of options, 135–136, 139–140
  key participant identification, 133–135, 139
  moral perspective, 133–135, 139
  nursing and, 128–129
  outcome determination, 135, 139
  overview, 121–122
  problems, 122–128
  process of, 132–138
  scientific process and, 130
  See also Problem solving
Ethical dilemmas, 21–24, 123–124
Ethical principles, 48–84
  applied to social issues, 403–405
  autonomy, 49–59
  beneficence, 59–62
  confidentiality, 69–75
  fidelity, 75–76
  justice, 76–78

non-maleficence, 62–64
overview, 48–49
respect for persons, 49
veracity, 64–69
Ethical space, 42
Ethical theory, 20–47
deontology, 34–37
feminist/relational ethics, 41–45
naturalism, 27–28
overview, 20–25
philosophy and, 25–28
rationalism, 28
utilitarianism, 30–34
virtue ethics, 37–41
Ethical treatment of data, 319–320
Ethic of caring, 111–113, 115–116
Ethic of justice, 111, 115–116
Ethics
defined, 26
dilemmas, 21–24, 123–124
law and, 147–149
nursing and, 24–25
in policy making, 355
problems, 122–128
research, 307–319
theories of, 28–37
See also specific codes of ethics by name;
terms beginning with Ethical
Ethnocentrism, 428, 429–430
Europe, history of nursing in, 8–12
Euthanasia, 245, 294
Expertise, 189
Explicit consent, 165
External locus of control, 480

Face-to-face lobbying, 360
Fair distribution, 377–378
Fair treatment, right to, 313
False imprisonment, 161
False information, submission of, 305, 320
Family conferences on end-of-life care,
242–243
Farquhar, M., 238
Federal responsibilities in health care
delivery, 326–335
Feminist ethics, 41–45

Feminization of nursing, 7, 416
Fenwick, Ethel, 14
Ferguson v. Hamilton (1983), 174
Fidelity, 75–76
Fiduciary duty, 307–308
Fiduciary relationship, 212
FIPPA (*Freedom of Information and Pro-
tection of Privacy Act* of Ontario),
72, 176
First Ministers' Health Accord, 334
Flaherty, M. J., 226
Flexner, Abraham, 186
Focal virtues, 39–41
Food and Drugs Act, 350
Food insecurity, in Aboriginal
communities, 456
Foot, Phillipa, 38–39
Foreseeability, 74, 158
Formalism, 34–36
Four humours, 10
Fowler, J. W., 107
Fowler, M., 188
France, nursing in, 12
Fraud, 159–160
*Freedom of Information and Protection of
Privacy Act* (Alberta), 72
*Freedom of Information and Protection
of Privacy Act* (FIPPA) (Ontario),
72, 176
Full disclosure, 311
Futility, medical. *See* Medical futility

Gay men, 416, 425–426
Gender, 414–426
communication and, 422–424
discrimination, 417–420
doctor–nurse game, 422–423
historical perspective, 415–417
intimate-partner violence, 397–400
mentoring and, 420
nurse-physician relationships, 226
nursing and, 6–7, 416
overview, 414–415
paternalism, 56–58
and autonomy, 270–273
sexism, 424–425

sexual harassment, 420–422
sexual orientation, 425–426
societal expectations, 416–417
See also Men; Women
Gibson, C. H., 478
Gibson, J., 130
Gilligan, Carol, 111–113
Global health care delivery, 338–340
Globalization, 100
Golden mean, 38
Golden Rule, 5, 79
Good, 31, 60
Governor General of Canada, 152
Grassroots lobbying, 360
Grey Nuns, 14
Guardian *ad litem*, 257
Gunshot wounds, mandatory reporting
    of, 72

Hagerdorn, S., 360
Harassment
    sexual, 420–422
    workplace, 224–225
Harm
    non-maleficence, 62–64, 236–237,
        403–404
    prevention/removal of, 61–62
    types of, 312
Harm principle, 73
Hartman Value Profile, 98
*Health Care [Consent] and Care Facility
    [Admission] Act of British Columbia*,
    164
Health Care Consent Act (Ontario), 164,
    165
Health care decision-making groups,
    participation in, 25
Health care delivery, 324–344
    access to, 337–338
    Canadian history of, 331–335
    challenges in, 335–338
    federal and provincial responsibilities
        in, 326–335
    global concerns, 338–340
    history of, 328–335
    medically necessary services, 338

overview, 324–326
political issues in, 353–354
privatization of, 382–383
right versus privilege of, 340, 373–374
teamwork, 229
U.S., 79, 370–371, 384–385
Health Care Directives Act (Manitoba),
    164
Health for All by the Year 2000, WHO,
    15
Health Information Act (Alberta), 72, 176
Health Information Protection Act
    (Saskatchewan), 176
Health issues in rural areas, 447–448
*The Health of Canadians: The Federal
    Role*, 334
Health policy, 346–366
    ethics in policy making, 355
    lobbying, 359–364
    nursing as political force, 352–354
    overview, 346–347
    politics and, 347–348, 356–357,
        363–364
    process, 350–352
    research and, 355–356
Health Professions Act (Alberta), 198, 349
Health Professions Act (British Columbia),
    196
Health promotion, role of values in, 101
Hébert, Marie Rollet, 12
Hedonism, 31
Helping, motivation for, 5–6
Henderson, Virginia, 56–57
Heterosexism, 425
Hidden homelessness, 395
Hippocratic Oath, 69
HIV/AIDS
    allocation decisions based on lifestyle
        choices, 287
    confidentiality concerning, 72
    drug trials in Africa, 309
    testing for, 167, 294–296
Holmes, B., 160
Homelessness, 394–397
Homophobia, 425
Homosexuality, 425–426

Honesty, 38, 194
Honesty, academic, 304–307
Hooker, Worthington, 32
Horizontal violence, 223
Hospital Construction Grants Program, 330
Hospital Insurance and Diagnostic Services Act, 332
Hospitals, 12–13, 329–330
Hôtel-Dieu de Montréal, 12–13
House of Commons, 152
Housing, Aboriginal, 456
Human focus of care, 261–262
Humphreys, Laud, 310–311

ICES (Institute for Clinical Evaluative Sciences), 356
ICN (International Council of Nurses), 14
Illness, versus disease, 430
Immigrants, 338, 402, 426–427
Implied consent, 165
Imprisonment, false, 161
Independent skilled health care, 16
Indian Act, 455
Indictable offences, 155
Indirect lobbying, 361
Infant mortality, 244–245, 339
Informed consent, 273–278
    autonomy and, 55–56
    elements of, 274–277
    information and, 274–275
    legal aspects of, 166
    nursing role and responsibilities, 277–278
    research ethics and, 315–317
    voluntariness, 276–277
Innovation, in rural nursing, 449
Institute for Clinical Evaluative Sciences (ICES), 356
Institutions
    nurses' relationships with, 216–221
    policies, 348
    values, 96–99
Instruction directive, 282
Integrity, 40, 91, 304

Intentional infliction of emotional distress, 162
Intentional torts, 159
Internal locus of control, 480
Internal standards of nursing practice, 195
International Convention on the Elimination of All Forms of Racial Discrimination, 402
International Council of Nurses (ICN), 14
Intimate-partner violence, 397–400
Invasion of privacy, 160
Involuntary euthanasia, 294

Jameton, A., 3, 188–189, 192, 219, 222, 477
Jecker, N. S., 239
Jennings, C., 360
Job selection, influence of values on, 97–99
The Joint Statement on Preventing and Resolving Conflicts Involving Health Care Providers and Persons Receiving Care, 246, 248
The Joint Statement on Resuscitative Interventions, 251
Journaling, 93–94
Judicial decisions, 349
Justice
    autonomy and, 273
    as ethical principle, 76–78
    ethic of, 111, 115–117, 371
    research ethics, 313–315
    social issues and, 403
    See also Distributive justice

Kant, Immanuel, 34–36
Kantianism, 34–36
Kavanagh, K., 424, 425
Kendall, J., 475
King, Martin Luther, Jr., 149
Kirby, M. J. L., 374
Kirby Report, 383
Knowledge, patient's, 55
Knowledge, philosophy of, 26
Kohlberg, Lawrence, 110–111

Kolesar v. Jeffries, 174
Kolkmeier, L. G., 93

Labour Code, 225
Lalonde, Marc, 332
Lalonde Report, 332
Language
    and informed consent, 276–277
    transcultural communication, 437
    used in lobbying, 363
    victim blaming, 405–406
    of violence, 406–407
Law, 146–182
    accountability and, 178
    administrative, 151
    branches of, 154–156
    case, 151
    civil, 153, 155
    common, 151–152
    consent and, 164–172
    constitutional, 150–151
    contract, 155–156
    criminal, 153, 154
    defined, 147
    documentation and, 173–178
    end-of-life technology, 256–258
    ethics and, 147–149
    legislative, 151
    legislative process in Canada, 151–154
    negligence, 156–160
    overview, 146–147
    privacy/confidentiality and, 71–72, 74,
        160–164
    private, 153, 155
    public, 154–155
    regarding workplace violence/harass-
        ment, 225
    sources of, 150–151
    statutory, 151, 152
    tort, 153, 156
Laws, 349
Lazar, N., 171
Legislative law, 151
Letter writing, lobbying through, 361–362
Libel, 162
Libertarian theories of justice, 79, 379

Licensure, 75
Life-sustaining technologies. *See*
        End-of-life care
Listening skills, 479
Literature, nursing versus medical
    on paternalism, 57
    on veracity, 66–67
Living donors, 260
Living wills, 256, 279, 281–282
Lo, B., 295
Lobbying, 359–364
    direct, 361
    face-to-face, 360
    grassroots, 360
    indirect, 361
    language used in, 363
    political campaigns, 363–364
Lockwood, M., 69
Locus of control, 480
Loyalty
    to colleagues, 202, 222
    conflicts in, 220
    defined, 222
    to institutions, 218, 220–221
    nurse–patient relationship, 76
Lying, 66–67
Lyon, B., 192–193

Madison, J., 421
Maier-Lorentz, M. M., 428
Malpractice, 163
Managed-care system, 384–385
Mance, Jeanne, 12–13
Mandatory reporting, 72, 298
Markus, A., 69
Material rules, 373
Mature minors, 168
McDonald, M., 136
Mead, N., 483
Media, lobbying through, 362
Medical Care Act, 330
Medical futility, 245–255
    artificial sources of nutrition, 254–255
    DNR orders, 251–254
    economics and, 250, 369
Medically necessary services, 338

Medicare program, 332, 349
Medications
 coverage of, 349
 errors, 159
Men
 gender stereotyping, 7
 increasing number of male nurses, 418
 intimate-partner violence against, 398
Men in Nursing Interest Group (MINIG),
  420
Mental distress, intentional infliction of,
  162
Mental illnesses, treatment of in Middle
  Ages, 9
Mentoring relationships, cross-gender,
  420
Mentors, moral, 231
Middle Ages, 8–11
Milgram, Stanley, 310
Mill, John Stuart, 31, 73
Mind-body distinction, 11–12
Minichiello, V., 421
MINIG (Men in Nursing Interest Group),
  420
Misconduct, professional, 222
Misrepresentation of personal
  performance, 305
Moore, Lawrence, 74
Moral autonomy, 89
Moral courage, 127–128
Moral development
 Gilligan's theory, 111–113
 Kohlberg's theory, 110–111
 See also Values development
Moral dilemmas, 122, 123–124
Moral disengagement, 127
Moral distress, 97, 122, 124–126
Moral integrity, 40, 91, 210, 230–231
Morality
 defined, 26
 dilemmas, 122, 123–124
 disengagement, 127
 distress, 97, 122, 124–126
 and nursing, 3
 outrage, 126
 problems, 122–128

uncertainty, 122–123
 See also Ethics; *terms beginning with*
  Moral
Moral mentors, 231
Moral outrage, 126
Moral philosophy, 26
Moral reasoning, 5–6
Moral residue, 127
Moral response, 113–115, 134
Moral thought, 88
Moral uncertainty, 122–123
Moral values, 88
Motivation for helping, 5–6
*Municipal Freedom of Information and
  Protection of Privacy Act* (Ontario),
  176
Munson, R., 57
Murphy v. LaMarsh, 161
Mutual respect, 42

*The National Collaborating Centre for
  Aboriginal Health*, 458
National health systems model, 77–78,
  369
Naturalism, 27–28
Negligence, 156–160, 163
*A New Perspective on the Health of Cana-
  dians*, 332
NHBD (non-heart-beating organ
  donations), 259
Nietzsche, Friedrich, 79
Nightingale, Florence, 7, 13–14
Nightingale Pledge, 40–41, 69
Noncompliance, 52, 53–54, 58–59
Non-heart-beating organ donations
  (NHBD), 259
Non-maleficence, 62–64, 236–237,
  403–404
Norris, P., 370
Notes, nursing, 173–174
Nuremberg Code, 308, 309
Nurse–patient relationship
 communication, 423–424
 empowerment through, 478–482
 guiding families through end-of-life
  care decisions, 242–243

loyalty, 76
obligations in, 212–213
trust, 24, 66
Nurses' relationships
importance of trust, 66
with institutions, 216–221
loyalty in, 76
with nurses, 201–202, 221–225
with physicians, 226–228
Nursing
advance care planning, 281–285
ancient times, 8
Canadian history, 12–16
decision making, 128–129
DNR orders, 251–254
gender and, 6–7, 416
influence of social need, 5–6
informed consent and, 277–278
and lobbying, 359–364
men in, 7, 418
Middle Ages, 8–11
morality and, 3
motivation for, 5–6
overview, 2–4
politics and, 352–354, 356–357
Renaissance and Reformation, 11–13
and research, 317–318
social need, 5–6
societal expectations, 416–417
spirituality and religion, 6–7
technology and, 260–262
See also Rural nursing
Nursing considerations, 115–117
Nursing education, 189, 453
Nursing notes, 173–174
Nursing orders, in Middle Ages, 9–10
Nursing process, 128–129
Nursing professional associations, 357
Nursing students. *See* Students, nursing
Nutrition, artificial sources of, 254–255

Obligations, 212–213, 450–452
Occupational Health and Safety (OHS) Regulation Act (Alberta), 349
Occupational Health and Safety Act (Ontario), 349

Office for Human Research Protection, 309
Omery, A., 87
Ontario College of Nurses, 191
Ontario Human Rights Commission, 421
Oppressed group behaviours, 224
Organizational values, conflict between personal and, 98
Organ procurement and transplantation, 259–260
O'Rourke, K., 370
Outrage, moral, 126
Overt values, 96

Palliative care, 241–245, 256, 261
Pandemics, 62
Parent, W. A., 69
Parentalism, 56–58
Parliament, 152
Paternalism, 56–58, 270–273
Patient-centred care, 482–483
Patients
advance directives, 171, 256–257, 278–285
autonomy of, 51–52, 270–273
beliefs about death and dying, 240
choices concerning life and health, 286–298
communication with, 423–424
consent of, 164–172
decision-making capacity, 279–281
empowerment, 478–482
informed consent, 273–278
knowledge possessed by, 55
lifestyle choices, 285–289
obligations to, 212–213
overview, 269–270
paternalism, 270–273
quality of life, 239
requests for confidentiality, 296–298
treatment of in Middle Ages, 9
values, 99–102
See also Choices, life-and-health
Pay gap, 417–418
Pender, N. J., 101
Personal code of ethics, 27
Personal empowerment, 471–474

Personal harassment, 224–225
Personal Health Information Protection Act (Ontario), 72, 176
Personal Information Protection Act (PIPA) (Alberta), 72, 176
Personal Information Protection and Electronic Documents Act (PIPEDA), 71, 175–176
Personal performance, misrepresentation of, 305
Personal visits, lobbying through, 362–363
Persons, respect for, 49, 311–312
Pfoutz, S. K., 384
Philosophy, 25–28
Philosophy of knowledge, 26
Philosophy of practice, 26
Physicians
    doctor–nurse game, 422–423
    lying to patients, 68
    nurses' relationships with, 226–228
Piaget, Jean, 109–110
PIPA (*Personal Information Protection Act* of Alberta), 72, 176
PIPEDA (*Personal Information Protection and Electronic Documents Act*), 71, 175–176
Plagiarism, 305
Plans of care, ability to follow, 58–59
Poddar, Prosenjit, 74
Policies
    defined, 347
    types of, 348
    See also Health policy
Policy formulation, 350, 351–352, 355
Policy implementation, 350, 352
Policy-making bodies, participation in, 25
Policy modification, 350, 352, 355
Policy Research Initiative (PRI), 356
Political-party activity, 363
Politics
    defined, 347
    issues in health care, 353–354
    lobbying in, 359–364
    nursing and, 352–354, 356–357
    political campaigns, 363–364

Portability principle, Canada Health Act, 78–79
Position Statement on Ethical Nurse Recruitment, 425–426
Poverty, 337, 392–394, 456–457
Powelson, Harvey, 74
Power
    defined, 469
    power over, 470
    power to, 469–470
    power with, 469–470
    See also Empowerment
Practical dilemmas, 124, 215–216
Practice, philosophy of, 26
Practice Standard for Ethics, 128–129
Premiums on health care, 373
Prescription drug coverage, 58–59, 349
President's Commission for the study of Ethical Problems in Medicine and Biomedical and Behavioral Research (U.S.), 375
PRI (Policy Research Initiative), 356
Price, S. A., 384
Primary health care, 336
Primary Health Care Transition Fund, 334
Privacy, 69–71, 160–164, 175–178, 313–314
Privacy Act, 71, 175
Privacy Commissioner of Canada, 72
Private law, 153, 155
Private-sector expenditures on health care, 333
Privatization of health care, 382–383
Privilege, health care as, 340, 373–374
Problem solving, 210–216
    clarification of obligations, 212–213
    considering alternatives, 214
    determining nature of problem, 213–214
    developing respectful solutions, 214–216
    personal values and, 211–212
Professional empowerment, 474–478
Professionalism in rural nursing, 449–450
Professional issues, 183–207
    accountability, 194–199
    authority, 199–200
    autonomy, 189–193

discipline, 200, 230
expertise, 189
overview, 183–184
profession defined, 185
status of profession, 184–189
unity, 200–203
Professional nursing associations, 14, 201
Professional relationships, 208–233
moral integrity and, 210, 230–231
nurse–institution, 216–221
nurse–nurse, 221–225
nurse–physician, 226–228
overview, 208–209
problem solving, 210–216
teamwork, 229–230
workplace harassment, 224–225
Proposition 8 (California), 416
Provider-specific consent, 166–167
Providing nursing care at the end of life,
282
Provincial responsibilities in health care
delivery, 326–335
Proxy decision makers, 171, 279
Proxy directive, 282
Public administration principle, Canada
Health Act, 78
Public Health Agency of Canada, 391
Public health nursing, 15, 329–330
Public insurance health care model, 370
Public law, 154–155
Public office, election to, 363–364
Public policies, 348

Quality of life, 237–245
defined, 236, 238
issues of life, death, and dying,
239–241
palliative care, 241–245
treating patients, 239
Quarantine Act, 350
Quinlan, Karen, 257
Quinn, C. A., 57

Racism, 402–403
Rand, Ayn, 25–26, 219
Raphael, D., 393

Raphael, D. D., 28, 35
Rationalism, 28
Rawls, John, 379
Ray, S., 475
Reed, P. G., 188–189
Reformation, and nursing, 11–13
Registered Nurses Act (Newfoundland),
198
Registered Nurses Act (Saskatchewan), 198
Registered Nurses Association of Ontario
(RNAO), 449
Registration, 75
Regulated Health Professions Act in On-
tario (RHPA), 196, 198, 349
*Regulated Health Professions Statutes
Amendment Act* (Manitoba), 349
Regulations, 153, 191, 349
Regulatory policies, 349–350
Relational ethics, 41–45
Relative homelessness, 395
Religion, 6–7
Renaissance, 11–13
Reporting misconduct, 222
Research
health policy, 355–356
nursing theory/practice and, 199
Research ethics, 307–319
characteristics of, 317–319
concern for welfare, 312
informed consent, 315–317
justice, 313–315
respect for persons, 311–312
violations of, 310–311
vulnerable populations, 317
Respect for persons, 49, 311–312
RHPA (*Regulated Health Professions Act*
in Ontario), 196, 198, 349
Rights
fair treatment, 313
health care services, 340, 373–374
privacy, 160, 313–314
RNAO (Registered Nurses Association of
Ontario), 449
Rodwell, C. M., 469
Roman Catholic Church. *See* Catholic
Church

Romanow Report, 336, 383–384
Royal Assent, 152
Rules, 349
Rule utilitarianism, 31
Rural nursing, 444–461
   Aboriginal nursing, 454–461
   accessibility to health services, 337
   boundaries, obligations, and confidentiality, 450–452
   challenges of, 448–454
   overview, 444–445
   professionalism in, 449–450
   rural environments in Canada, 445–447
   rural health, 447–448
   scope of practice, 453–454
   working with constraints, 452–453
Rushton, C. H., 245
R. v. Dyment (1988), 177

Salaries, 417–418
Same-sex marriage, 415–416
Sanctity of life, 237
SARS (Severe Acute Respiratory Syndrome), 62, 351
Saskatchewan Hospitalization Act, 332
Saskatchewan Medical Care Insurance Act, 332
Schiavo, Terri, 257–258
Scholarship, 303–323
   academic honesty, 304–307
   ethical treatment of data, 319–320
   overview, 303–304
   research issues and ethics, 307–319
   on social issues, 407
Science
   effect on medical perspectives, 239
   and ethical decision making, 130
   during Renaissance, 11–12
Scofield, G. R., 253
Scope of practice, 198, 453–454
SDM (substitute decision-maker), 171, 279, 280, 281
Second World War, 308
Secular nursing orders, in Middle Ages, 9–10
Selanders, L. C., 4

Self-awareness
   and empowerment, 470, 472
   enhancing, 92–94
   values clarification and, 90–94
Self-regulation, 191–192
Self-sacrifice, 219
Senate, 152
Seroka, A. M., 88
Severe Acute Respiratory Syndrome (SARS), 62, 351
Sexism, 424–425
Sexual activity, unethical research concerning, 310–311
Sexual harassment, 420–422
Sexual orientation, 425–426
Shaw, H., 201
Sherwin, W., 270–271
Shore, Lisa, 163
Silencing behaviours, 224
Slander, 162
Smith, M. D., 57
Smoke-Free Environment Act (Newfoundland), 153
Smoke-free Ontario Act (Ontario), 153
Smoking laws, 153
Snively, Mary Agnes, 14
Social issues, 390–413
   elder population, 400–401
   ethical principles applied to, 403–405
   homelessness, 394–397
   intimate-partner violence, 397–400
   overview, 390–391
   poverty, 392–394
   racism, 402–403
   scholarship on, 407
   vulnerable populations, 405–407
Social justice, 446
Social need, influence of, 5–6
Social policies, 348
Social programs, 329
Social Union Framework Agreement, 333
Societal expectations, gender-related, 416–417
Socrates, 25
Spectrum of urgency, 227
Spirituality and religion, 6–7

Starson v. Swayze, 167–168

Statutes, 349

Statutory law, 151, 152

Steadfastness, 127

Stereotyping, 428

Stevens, P. E., 4

Students, nursing
  bullying of, 223
  empowerment, 477–478
  mentorship of, 229

Submission of false information, 305, 320

Substitute decision-maker (SDM), 171, 279, 280, 281

Substitute Decisions Act (Ontario), 164

Summary offences, 155

Superstition, in medicine during Middle Ages, 10

Supreme Court of Canada, 152, 420

Sympathy, 28

Syphilis, unethical research concerning, 310

Tarasoff, Tatiana, 74

TCPS 2 (*Tri Council Policy Statement on the Ethical Conduct of Research*), 309

Teamwork, 229–230

Tearooming, 310–311

Technology
  beneficence, 236–237
  benefits and challenges of, 235–236
  current issues in use of, 237
  documentation, 174–175
  end-of-life care, 235–237
  non-maleficence, 236–237
  nursing practice, 260–262

Teenage rebellion, 89

Theory, defined, 109

Thomas, J., 113–115, 134

Thought processes of patients, 54

Tissue procurement and transplantation, 259–260

Tobacco Act, 153

Tobacco Act (Quebec), 153

Tobacco Control Act (Saskatchewan), 153

Tort law, 156

Tort of outrage, 162

Torts
  defined, 153
  intentional, 159
  unintentional, 156

Transcultural issues, 426–437
  care principles, 431–432
  cultural safety, 429–430
  cultural understanding, 428
  diversity, 428–429
  health care system, 435–437
  legal considerations, 437
  values and beliefs, 430–435
  values development, 107–108

Treatment
  consent, 166–167
  patient choice concerning, 286–298

Tri Council Policy Statement (TCPS 2), 309

The Tri Council Policy Statement: Ethical Conduct for Research Involving Humans, 316

Trust and trustworthiness, 40, 64–69, 194

Truth-telling, 64–69, 87

Tube feeding, 254–255

Tunajek, S., 223

Tuskegee Syphilis Study, 310

Undue influence, 311

Uniforms, 423–424

Unintentional torts, 156

United Nations Convention on the Elimination of All Forms of Discrimination Against Women, 417

United States
  Department of Health and Human Services, 309
  health care delivery, 79, 370–371, 384–385
  health care fraud, 159–160
  right to health care, 375

Unity, professional, 200–203

Universal Declaration of Human Rights, 374

Universal health care, 77–78

Universality principle, Canada Health
Act, 78
University nursing degree programs, 330
University-trained physicians, in Middle
Ages, 10
Urgency, spectrum of, 227
Utilitarianism, 30–34
act, 31–32
justice and, 379
rule, 31, 32–34
Utility, 30

Values
acquisition of, 88–90
of children, and capacity to consent,
168
conflict of, 95–96, 97–99
core professional, 201
covert, 97
culture and, 430–435
defined, 87–88
institutional, 96–99
moral, 88
overt, 96
patient choices and nurses', 53–54
patients', 99–102
problem solving and, 211–212
in professional situations, 94–102
self-awareness, 21, 90–94
Values clarification, 86–105
acquisition of values and, 88–90
conflict and, 95–96
defined, 91
institutional values and, 96–99
moral values, 88
overview, 86–87
patients and, 99–102
professional situations and, 94–102
self-awareness and, 90–94
values defined, 87–88
Values development, 106–120
gender and, 111–113
Gilligan's study of, 111–113
Kohlberg's theory, 110–111
nursing considerations, 115–117
overview, 106–107

Piaget's theory, 109–110
theoretical perspectives on, 109–115
Thomas's theory, 113–115
transcultural considerations in, 107–108
Vanderbilt, M. W., 359–360
Veatch, R., 60
Veracity, 64–69
Victim blaming, 405–406
Victorian Order of Nurses, 330
Violence
intimate-partner, 397–400
language and, 406–407
Virtue ethics, 37–41
Voluntary consent, 165–166
Vulnerability principle, 74–75
Vulnerable populations, 71, 317, 405–407

Wages, gender and, 417–418
Waiting lists, 339–340
Waluchow, W., 134
Warn, duty to, 74, 298
Water insecurity, in Aboriginal communities, 456
Welfare, concern for, 312
Welfare programs, 329
Whistleblowing, 126, 475–476
WHO (World Health Organization), 15,
242, 334, 391
Williams, Christine, 418, 419
Williams, J. R., 274
Witch hunts, in Middle Ages, 10–11
Women
as healers in historical perspective, 7,
8, 9–11, 12–15
intimate-partner violence against,
397–400
moral development of, 111–113
pay gap, 417–418
role in nursing profession, 6–7
sexual harassment, 420–422
societal expectations concerning,
416–417
view of during Middle Ages, 9
See also Gender
Work ethic, 79
Working conditions, 218–219

Working Through Ethical Situations in Nursing Practice, 128–129
Workplace harassment, 224–225, 420–422
Workplace incivility, 222–224
World Health Organization (WHO), 15, 242, 334, 391

World Wars, nursing during, 14
Written consent forms, 315

Youth Criminal Justice Act, 154

Zurlinden, J., 425